TRADITIONAL CHINESE MEDICINE

TRADITIONAL CHINESE MEDICINE

Edited by

Chun-Su Yuan MD PhD

Cyrus Tang Professor
Director, Tang Center for Herbal Medicine Research
University of Chicago Pritzker School of Medicine
Illinois, USA

Eric J. Bieber MD

Chair, Obstetrics and Gynecology
Chief Medical Officer, Geisinger Wyoming Valley and Geisinger South Wilkes-Barre
Senior Vice President, Geisinger Health Systems
Wilkes-Barre/Danville, Pennsylvania, USA

Brent A. Bauer MD

Director
Complementary and Integrative Medicine Program
Professor of Medicine at Mayo Medical School
Mayo Clinic, Rochester, Minnesota, USA

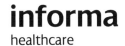

Originally published as part of:

Chun-Su Yuan, Eric J Bieber, and Brent A Bauer, *Textbook of Complementary and Alternative Medicine,*

Second Edition. Informa Healthcare, 2006.
This edition published in 2011 by Informa Healthcare, Telephone House, 69-77 Paul Street, London EC2A 4LQ, UK.
Simultaneously published in the USA by Informa Healthcare, 52 Vanderbilt Avenue, 7th floor, New York, NY 10017, USA.

A CIP record for this book is available from the British Library.

ISBN-13: 978-1-8418-4842-6

Orders may be sent to: Informa Healthcare, Sheepen Place, Colchester, Essex CO3 3LP, UK
Telephone: +44 (0)20 7017 5540
Email: CSDhealthcarebooks@informa.com
Website: http://informahealthcarebooks.com/

For corporate sales please contact: CorporateBooksIHC@informa.com
For foreign rights please contact: RightsIHC@informa.com
For reprint permissions please contact: PermissionsIHC@informa.com

Typeset by MPS Limited, a Macmillan Company

Printed and bound by CPI Group (UK) Ltd, Croydon, CR0 4YY

Transferred to Digital Print 2011

Contents

Contributors

Michael K. Ang-Lee MD
Department of Anesthesia
Western Washington Medical Group
Everett, WA
USA

Anoja S. Attele DDS MD
Department of Pathology
University of Illinois at Chicago
Chicago, IL
USA

Han H. Aung MD
Tang Center for Herbal Medicine Research
University of Chicago
Chicago, IL
USA

Daniel Basila
Tang Center for Herbal Medicine Research
University of Chicago
Chicago, IL
USA

Brent A. Bauer MD
Complementary and Integrative Medicine Program
Mayo Clinic
Rochester, MN
USA

Todd T. Brown MD
Division of Endocrinology and Metabolism
Johns Hopkins University School of Medicine
Baltimore, MD
USA

Wei-Tien Chang MD
Department of Emergency Medicine
National Taiwan University Hospital
National Taiwan University College of Medicine
Taiwan

Lucy Dey MD
Diabetes/Endocrine Section
Chicago Medical School at Rosalind Franklin
  University
VA Medical Center
North Chicago, IL
USA

Adrian S. Dobs MD MHS
Division of Endocrinology and Metabolism
Johns Hopkins University School of Medicine
Baltimore, MD
USA

Deborah J. Engen BS CMT
Occupational Therapy
Mayo Clinic
Rochester, MN
USA

Monica E. Jones LAc MAcOM
Holistic Health Professionals
Neptune, NJ
USA

Mark C. Lee MD
General Internal Medicine
Mayo Clinic
Rochester, MN
USA

Chunyi Lin MA IQM
Spring Forest Healing Center
St. Louis Park, MN
USA

Nisha J. Manek MD
Rheumatology
Mayo Clinic
Rochester, MN
USA

David D. McFadden MD MPH
General Internal Medicine
Mayo Clinic
Rochester, MN
USA

Sangeeta R. Mehendale MD PhD
Department of Anesthesia and Critical Care
  and Tang Center for Herbal Medicine Research
University of Chicago
Chicago, IL
USA

Jonathan Moss MD PhD
Department of Anesthesia and Critical Care
  and Institutional Review Board
University of Chicago
Chicago, IL
USA

Victoria Rand MD
California Pacific Medical Center
San Francisco, CA
USA

Wallace Sampson MD
Stanford University School of Medicine
  and The Scientific Review of Alternative Medicine
Los Altos, CA
USA

Zuo-Hui Shao MD
Section of Emergency Medicine
Department of Medicine
University of Chicago
Chicago, IL
USA

Yukihiro Shoyama PhD
Laboratory of Medicinal Resourses Regulation
Faculty of Pharmaceutical Sciences
Kyushu University
Fukuoka
Japan

Mi-Yeon Song OMD PhD
Department of Oriental Rehabilitation Medicine
College of Oriental Medicine
Kyung Hee University
Dongdaemun-gu
Seoul
Korea

Feng Sun PhD MD
Department of Medicine
University of Alberta
Edmonton, Alberta
Canada

Shusheng Tai PhD
Department of Medicine
University of Alberta
Edmonton, Alberta
Canada

Terry L. Vanden Hoek MD
Section of Emergency Medicine
Department of Medicine
  and the Emergency Resuscitation Center
University of Chicago
Chicago, IL
USA

Chong-Zhi Wang PhD
Tang Center for Herbal Medicine Research
University of Chicago Pritzker School of Medicine
Chicago, IL
USA

Yong Gao Wang MD MBA LAc
Department of Physiology
Loyola University of Chicago
Maywood, IL
USA

Sheila M. Wicks MD MBA
Tang Center for Herbal Medicine Research
University of Chicago
Chicago, IL
USA

Ji An Wu PhD
Department of Pharmaceuticals and New Technology
Pharmaceutical Products Division
Abbott Laboratories
Abbott Park, IL
USA

Jing-Tian Xie MD
Tang Center for Herbal Medicine Research
University of Chicago
Chicago, IL
USA

Bob Xu CMD MS
American Chinese Medical Association
  and Center for Holistic and Herbal Therapy
Plainfield, IL
USA

Wen Xuan MD
Chicago First Chinese Acupuncture and Medical
  Center
Chicago, IL
USA

Stevenson Xutian PhD
Department of Medicine
University of Alberta
Edmonton, Alberta
Canada

Fay A. Yao BS
Division of Endocrinology and Metabolism
Johns Hopkins University School of Medicine
Baltimore, MD
USA

Chun-Su Yuan MD PhD
Department of Anesthesia and Critical Care
  and Tang Center for Herbal Medicine Research
University of Chicago Pritzker School of Medicine
Chicago, IL
USA

Definitions and regulatory status

M. C. Lee

HISTORICAL BACKGROUND

The federal regulation of food, drugs, and supplements was fairly limited until the last century. One of the first laws passed by Congress was the Pure Food and Drugs Act of 1906 in the effort to broadly prohibit the mislabeling or adulteration of food. Although it represented a step in the regulation of consumables, it did not provide any specific provisions for dietary supplements or in the regulation of the safety or effectiveness of drugs. It served to establish minimal standards for quality, purity, and strength[1].

Due to the limitations of the Pure Food and Drugs Act of 1906, Congress put forth the Federal Food, Drug, and Cosmetic Act (FDCA) in 1938. Public outcry regarding the deaths associated with elixir of sulfanilamide poisoning spawned this legislation focused on drug safety and established food standards of identity. The FDCA also established, for the first time, a category of foods 'for special dietary use'[2]. The Food and Drug Administration (FDA) subsequently spread regulations regarding labeling requirements for dietary supplements and foods and established quantitative minimum daily requirements. However, much of the burden of safety monitoring was placed on the FDA.

In 1958, Congress amended the FDCA to shift the responsibility of proving the safety of food and drug ingredients from the FDA to manufacturers. This new amendment essentially provided the FDA with premarket approval of 'food additives'. Food additives were defined as 'any substance, the intended use of which results, or may reasonably be expected to result, directly or indirectly, in its becoming a component or otherwise affecting the characteristics of food'[3]. The FDA also applied this broad definition to the regulation of dietary supplements, to protest from the public and dietary supplement manufacturers. Through the initiation of the recommended daily allowance, the FDA placed restrictions on the potency and combinations of vitamins and minerals in dietary supplements, further polarizing the public.

This public outrage spawned the Proxmire Amendment of 1976 that prohibited the FDA from:

(1) Establishing maximum limits on the potency of any synthetic or natural vitamin or mineral;

(2) Classifying any natural or synthetic vitamin or mineral (or combination thereof) as a drug solely because it exceeds the level of potency which (the FDA) determines is nutritionally rational or useful; and

(3) Limiting the combination or number of any synthetic or natural vitamin, mineral, or other ingredient of food.

In the years following the Proxmire Amendment the FDA relaxed its efforts to impugn manufacturers, making way for a growth in the industry. By the 1980s, many supplement manufacturers began to make health claims that were not substantiated or sanctioned by the FDA, leading to the Nutrition Labeling and Education Act (NLEA) of 1990.

The NLEA was enacted by Congress in 1990 to provide mandatory nutrition labeling for most food products intended for human consumption. It also gave the FDA broad authority to regulate health claims made by manufacturers and it opened the door for the FDA to regulate what is now known as dietary supplements since they were perceived to be a subset of food meant for human consumption. As a result of this legislation, a grassroots campaign from supplement consumers and manufacturers swelled to test the FDA's regulatory authority.

DIETARY SUPPLEMENT HEALTH AND EDUCATION ACT OF 1994

In response to the pressure and lobbying exerted by the dietary supplement industry, Congress passed legislation to amend the FDCA. President Clinton signed into law the Dietary Supplement Health and Education Act (DSHEA) on 25 October 1994. The DSHEA created the dietary supplement category that is distinct from food and drugs, and allowed the industry to promote their products without the requirement of providing proof of efficacy, safety, or quality control.

Definitions

The DSHEA defined a dietary supplement as:

(1)   A product (other than tobacco) intended to supplement the diet that bears or contains one or more of the following ingredients:

   (a)   A vitamin;
   (b)   A mineral;
   (c)   An herb or other botanical;
   (d)   An amino acid;
   (e)   A dietary substance for use by man to supplement the diet by increasing the total dietary intake; or
   (f)   A concentrate, metabolite, constituent, extract, or combination of any ingredient described in clause (a), (b), (c), (d), or (e);

(2)   A product intended for ingestion in a pill, capsule, tablet, or liquid form;

(3)   Not used as a conventional food or as the sole item of a meal or diet; and

(4)   Labeled as a dietary supplement.

Safety implications

Through creating and defining the class of agents known as dietary supplements, the DSHEA, in effect, removed the FDA's responsibility to oversee and regulate the dietary supplement industry. Whereas drug manufacturers are required to perform tests to determine safety and efficacy prior to introduction to the market, dietary supplement manufacturers are not held to this standard. Supplement manufacturers are not required to perform safety, efficacy, or purity tests on their products prior to human consumption. As a result, shortly following the passing of the DSHEA in 1994, the supplement market became flooded with a myriad of untested products. Although the majority of supplements are believed to be safe, many have subsequently been found to be harmful. The DSHEA put the burden of responsibility for ensuring safety of the supplement industry on the FDA. This is accomplished through an arduous process of reporting and documenting multiple adverse events from dietary supplements before the FDA can take action to restrict their use.

After the FDA received hundreds of adverse event reports on the use of ephedra (ma huang) in 1997, it sought to restrict dosages while promoting strong warning labels. The supplement industry again mounted a grassroots campaign to counter the FDA's efforts – ultimately succeeding in thwarting the FDA's proposals. It took an additional 5 years of FDA investigation until ephedra was banned in 2004. Although at the present time ephedra-containing products are difficult to acquire, manufacturers have since replaced such products with 'ephedra-free' versions containing similar stimulants such as bitter orange (*Citrus aurantium*) and caffeine.

Since 1994, there have been reports of adverse events caused by many other dietary supplements, resulting in FDA restrictions and safety warnings in products. Aristolochia (aristolochic acid) is a Chinese herbal supplement that is a known carcinogen and that has been associated with renal failure. Chaparral, germander, comfrey, and kava are herbs associated with hepatic failure and death that share a wealth of adverse reports resulting in FDA consumer warnings. Yohimbe and bitter orange are herbal stimulants that have been associated with cardiac related complications similar to ephedra. Other adverse events have been associated with unintended product contamination, such as the substitution of foxglove (*Digitalis lanata*) for the herbal ingredient plantain, or with heavy metal preservation with lead and arsenic in Asian preparations. There likely remain many potentially dangerous dietary supplements; however, under the current DSHEA legislation, identification and action lags behind patient safety.

Consumer use and market implications

Dietary supplement sales have become one of the fastest growing segments in the sales industry. With the advent of DSHEA, the food supplement industry grew from an estimated 246 million dollars in 1994[4], to 1.3–1.7 billion dollars in 2001[5], to 4.2 billion dollars in 2003[6]. Although other factors exist to account for the rapid increase in the use of dietary supplements in the United

States over the past decade, such as the Internet and easy access to dietary supplements, the DSHEA's effect on the food supplement industry mirrored the exponential growth in popularity and use by consumers. In the year 2000, the FDA estimated that 158 million Americans used dietary supplements including vitamins[7]. This is in stark contrast to a 1997 survey that demonstrated that alternative medical therapies, primarily herbals, were used by 83 million people in the United States[8]. According to a 1997 survey[4], the top ten herbal supplements sold in the USA were:

(1) Ginkgo;

(2) Ginseng;

(3) Garlic;

(4) Echinacea/goldenseal;

(5) St John's wort;

(6) Saw palmetto;

(7) Grapeseed extract;

(8) Evening primrose oil;

(9) Cranberry;

(10) Valerian.

Purity

The DSHEA authorized the FDA to establish 'good manufacturing practices' regarding the preparation, packaging, and storage of dietary supplements. Although intended to provide guidelines to ensure purity and safety of dietary supplements, the DSHEA empowered supplement manufacturers to police themselves, resulting in varying and unmonitored compliance. In 1995, *Consumer Reports* analyzed ten readily available ginseng products comparing the quantified levels of ginsenocides[9]. Although the manufacturers' packaging suggested standardized herb amounts, the studied ginseng brands displayed wide variations in purity. Several preparations even lacked significant amounts of ginsenocides. Fortunately, subsequent *Consumer Reports* analyses, in December 2000, of common dietary supplements (St John's Wort, SAM-e, and kava suggest improved standardization. However, consumer awareness still needs to be heightened as most dietary supplements in the United States are not standardized to an active ingredient, as is the case in Europe.

Health claims

The DSHEA limits manufacturers' ability to claim that their product prevents or treats a disease or disorder (disease claim). However, supplement manufacturers are allowed to express how their product may affect the body in the form of structure–function claims without FDA authorization. These claims are statements that describe the effect a dietary supplement may have on the structure or function of the human body. However, prior to the FDA publication on Structure/Function Claims Small Entity Compliance Guide in January 2000[10], the distinction between a structure–function and a disease claim was at times unclear. Despite the FDA's clarification, the distinction is still sometimes blurred (Table 1.1).

All structure–function claims are required by law to be accompanied by the disclaimer 'This statement has not been evaluated by the Food and Drug Administration. This product is not intended to diagnose, treat, cure, or prevent any disease'. However, the manufacturer is responsible for ensuring the accuracy and truthfulness of structure–function claims. Any disease claim must be approved by the FDA prior to marketing the product. Ultimately, it is the Federal Trade Commission (FTC) who regulates advertising for dietary supplements sold to consumers.

Table 1.1 Contrasting examples of structure–function and disease claims

Structure–function claim	*Disease claim*
Provides relief of occasional constipation	provides relief of chronic constipation
Promotes prostate health	relieves symptoms of benign prostatic hyperplasia (BPH)
Promotes digestion	relief of persistent heartburn
Suppresses appetite to aid weight loss	suppresses appetite to treat obesity
Helps maintain normal cholesterol levels	lowers cholesterol

CONCLUSION

The limited regulatory environment for dietary supplements sold in the USA creates unique challenges for patients and consumers. It also creates a special opportunity for physicians to educate and inform. By highlighting the limited government supervision and the relative lack of quality controls, physicians can bring awareness to their patients. Already, patients and consumers are showing signs of increasing sophistication, as evidenced by the growth in third party, quality verification programs. As quality products become more readily distinguishable, patients and consumers will have at least one problem addressed in their quest to successfully incorporate dietary supplements into their health management.

References

1. Kaczka KA. From herbal Prozac to Mark McGuire's tonic: how the Dietary Supplement Health and Education Act changed the regulatory landscape for health products. J Contemp Health Law Policy 2000; 17: 463–99
2. Federal Food, Drug, and Cosmetic Act 21 USC §343(j), 1995
3. Food Additives Amendments of USC § 301(s), 1958
4. The Complete German Commission E Monographs – Therapeutic Guide to Herbal Medicines. Portland, OR: American Botanical Council, 1999
5. HerbalGram. 2003; 60: 48–53
6. HerbalGram. 2005; 66: 63
7. Goldman P. Herbal medicines today and the roots of modern pharmacology. Ann Intern Med 2001; 135: 594–600
8. Eisenberg DM, Davis RB, Ettner SL, et al. Trends in alternative medicine use in the United States, 1990–1997: results of a follow-up national survey. J Am Med Assoc 1998; 280: 1569–75
9. Herbal roulette. Consumer Reports 1995; Nov: 689–705
10. FDA. Structure/Function Claims Small Entity Compliance Guide, 21 CFR Part 101. Rockville, MD: Food and Drug Administration, 2000

Commonly used herbal medicines 2

M. K. Ang-Lee and D. Basila

ALOE

Common names: aloe, aloe vera, Barbados aloe, Cape aloe, Curaçao aloe, Zanzibar aloe, kumari (Sanskrit name), lu hui (Chinese name).

Background

Aloe, a member of the lily (Liliaceae) family (Figure 2.1), has been used medicinally for thousands of years. Of the several hundred species, *Aloe vera* is the most extensively used topically. Other species such as *Aloe barbadensis* (Curaçao aloe) and *Aloe capensis* (Cape aloe) are more frequently used internally.

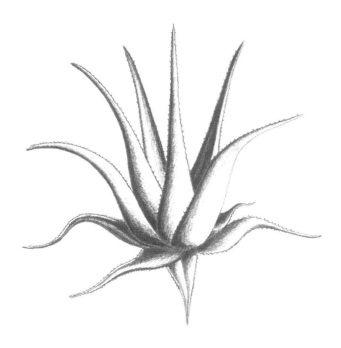

Figure 2.1 *Aloe vera*

Uses

Aloe gel, a clear jelly-like substance obtained from the inner parenchymal tissue of the leaf, is used for topical wound healing. It has been investigated for use in wounds caused by incisions[1], burns[2], radiation[3], dermabrasion[4], frostbite[5], pressure[6], and psoriasis[7,8]. The healing effect of aloe has been shown in animal models[9–11]. In humans, however, clinical trials have reported inconsistent results. An aloe extract in hydrophilic cream improved healing of psoriatic skin lesions[7], while an aloe vera gel was found no better than placebo in treating psoriasis[8]. Aloe gel accelerated wound healing in patients who underwent full-face dermabrasion[4]. In patients with aphthous stomatitis, aloe did not deter the development of oral mucosal ulcers[12], but acemannan, an isolated aloe gel polysaccharide, accelerated healing of ulcers and reduced pain[13]. *Aloe vera* gel did not prevent skin injury from radiation therapy[3]. In patients with wounds healing by secondary intention, aloe may have been detrimental to wound healing[1]. These inconsistent results may be explained by differences in preparations, treatment regimens, patient populations, and study methodologies.

In addition to topical administration, aloe is also taken orally. The latex of the plant, a yellow juice extracted from the superficial pericyclic cells, contains anthraquinones. Anthraquinones, particularly aloe-emodin, induce the active secretion of water and electrolytes into the lumen of the bowel. Laxative effects follow approximately 9 h after ingestion. Oral aloe has been advocated to heal gastrointestinal ulcers[14], treat AIDS[15], treat inflammatory bowel disease[16], lower blood sugar in patients with diabetes[17], treat and prevent cancer[18], and lower blood lipid levels[19]. A recent phase II trial showed oral aloe vera to be ineffective in improving quality-of-life in head and neck neoplasm patients receiving radiation[20]. Although preliminary data suggest that aloe is potentially effective in some of the above conditions, more evidence is necessary before clinicians should recommend oral aloe.

Phytochemistry and pharmacology

Aloe extract contains many compounds, not all of which have been characterized. Identified compounds include polysaccharides, lectins, anthranoids, salicylates, cholesterol, triglycerides, magnesium lactate, and carboxypeptidase. Of these compounds, the polysaccharides and lectins are the most important. Acemannan, a proprietary aloe polysaccharide, has been used in several clinical trials.

Many mechanisms have been proposed to explain the wound-healing effects of aloe. The simplest of these is that aloe acts as a moisturizing agent. However, many aloe constituents are pharmacologically active, and some have anti-inflammatory effects[21]. For example, magnesium lactate inhibits the production of histamine by blocking the enzyme histidine decarboxylase. Aloe also contains natural salicylates, and other substances may inhibit the production of inflammatory mediators such as bradykinin and thromboxane. Furthermore, aloe may have antibacterial[2] and antiviral activity[22]. The gel polysaccharides, particularly acemannan, have immunostimulatory effects *in vitro*[23]. Some constituents of aloe may have antimutagenic effects[24]. Aloe may alter vascular tone, improving blood supply to wounded tissue.

Safety

The topical use of aloe is generally safe, although cases of allergic dermatitis and minor burning sensations have been reported[25–27]. The internal use of aloe is contraindicated in cases of intestinal obstruction, inflammatory bowel disease, appendicitis, and abdominal pain of unknown origin[28]. Long-term internal use can lead to electrolyte loss and dehydration and increase the risk (relative risk of 3.0) of colorectal cancer[29].

Internal use during pregnancy or while breastfeeding is not recommended.

Preparations and dosage

Aloe is an ingredient in a wide variety of cosmetic and health-care products. The benefits of commercially available products are unknown, because many only contain minimal amounts of aloe[30]. However, some aloe gel products are available that contain more than 95% pure aloe gel. For topical use, recommendations are to apply liberally as needed. When used internally, the typical dosage is 20–30 mg of anthraquinones/day[31].

ECHINACEA

Common names: purple coneflower, red sunflower, black sampson.

Background

There are nine species of *Echinacea*, a member of the daisy family (Figure 2.2). Three species, *Echinacea angustifolia*, *Echinacea purpurea*, and *Echinacea pallida*, are used for medicinal purposes. The most commonly studied is *Echinacea purpurea*, used for the prophylaxis and treatment of viral, bacterial, and fungal infections, particularly those of upper respiratory origin. Compelling evidence supporting its use in upper respiratory infections is lacking[32,33]. Echinacea is also used as an immunostimulant after chemo- and radiation therapy, an adjunct in cancer treatment, and a topical promoter of wound healing.

Phytochemistry and pharmacology

Echinacea contains alkylamides, alkaloids, caffeic acid esters, polysaccharides, flavonoids, polyacetylenes, and essential oils. Pharmacologic activity cannot be attributed to a single compound, although the lipophilic fraction, which contains the alkylamides (primarily the dodeca-2,4,8,10-tetraenoic acid isobutylamides), polyacetylenes, and essential oil, appears to be more active than the hydrophilic fraction.

Echinacea has a number of immunomodulatory effects. *In vitro*, it activated immune cells, increased cytokine production, and inhibited hyaluronidase[34]. *In vivo*, it activated natural killer cells in humans[35], and increased production of immunoglobulins (Ig)G and M in rats[36]. In 2005, a large-scale, randomized, double-blind study of echinacea's effectiveness in decreasing the length and severity of rhinovirus infection was conducted. The study found echinacea to have no significant effect regardless of whether administration was prior to infection, after infection, or both[37].

Safety

Echinacea appears to have a low potential for toxicity and mutagenicity[38]. In a preliminary investigation it was not harmful during pregnancy[39], nevertheless the lack of

Although the pyrrolizidine alkaloids in echinacea lack the 1,2-unsaturated necrine ring system associated with hepatotoxicity in other pyrrolizidine alkaloid-containing plants such as comfrey, concerns of potential hepatotoxicity have also been raised[46].

The pharmacokinetics of echinacea have not been studied.

Preparations and dosage

Several preparations are available. The fresh aerial parts of the plant can be pressed to yield a juice that is stabilized with alcohol. The usual dosage is 6–9 ml of expressed plant juice or its equivalent as an extract per day. Preparations can also be made from plant root, and the usual dosage is 0.9 g of cut root several times daily.

EPHEDRA

Commmon names: ma huang, epitonin.

Background

Ephedra is an herbal medication obtained from the woody stems of *Ephedra sinica* (Figure 2.3), a shrub native to the semiarid and desert areas of Asia, Europe, and Africa. *Ephedra sinica* is the most commonly used species for medicinal purposes, but other species have also been described. This herbal medication has a long history in traditional Chinese medicine, in which it is known as ma huang, where it has been used to treat respiratory ailments for thousands of years[47].

Uses

Ephedra was traditionally given to induce perspiration and to treat respiratory conditions including asthma, bronchitis, allergic rhinitis, and upper respiratory tract infections. Today, it is still used to treat respiratory disorders. The German Commission E has approved ephedra for diseases of the respiratory tract with mild bronchospasm in adults and children over the age of six[38]. The World Health Organization has determined its effectiveness in treating nasal congestion and asthma[48]. The known pharmacologic effects of ephedrine, the major active alkaloid in ephedra, suggest that ephedra is an effective bronchodilator.

Ephedra has gained popularity as an aid to weight loss; in 1998, 2% of obese Americans and 1% of the

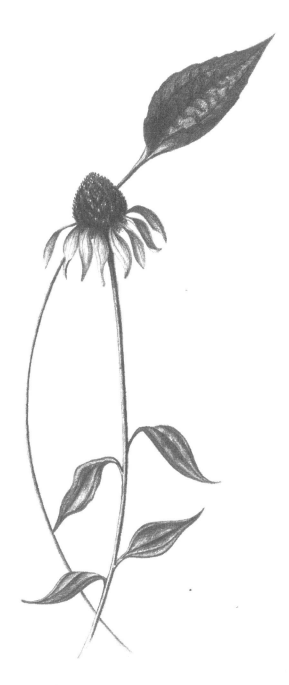

Figure 2.2 *Echinacea purpurea*

substantive data indicates use during pregnancy should remain cautious[40–42]. Echinacea has been associated with allergic reactions, including one reported case of anaphylaxis, and therefore should be used with caution in patients with asthma, atopy, or allergic rhinitis[43,44]. Its immunomodulatory effects may diminish the effectiveness of immunosuppression in patients such as organ transplant recipients. Moreover, immunosuppression is possible if echinacea is taken long-term (> 8 weeks)[45].

general population took over-the-counter weight-loss products containing ephedra[49–51]. These figures could increase in subsequent years, particularly in light of a Food and Drug Administration (FDA) proposal in 2001 to withdraw approval of phenylpropanolamine, another popular over-the-counter drug for weight loss[52]. Ephedrine is often combined with caffeine to promote weight loss by increasing thermogenesis and reducing appetite[51,53,54]. In a randomized controlled trial, an ephedra/caffeine preparation produced significant weight loss in obese subjects[55]. However, in that study, 23% of the actively treated subjects withdrew because of side-effects.

Ephedra has also gained popularity as an ergogenic (physical performance enhancing) aid. Individual ephedrine alkaloids did not affect physical performance[56], but the combination of ephedrine and caffeine improved physical performance as determined by exercise time to exhaustion[50,57]. This combination of ephedrine and caffeine may be unsafe, because it also causes greater tachycardia than either placebo or ephedrine alone. Moreover, ephedrine is a banned substance in amateur sporting events and is likely to disqualify athletes in drug-tested events[56].

'Herbal ecstasy' preparations that are advertised as safe alternatives to illegal street drugs contain ephedra[58,59]. The labels of such preparations claim or imply that they produce euphoria and increase awareness, energy, and sexual sensation.

Phytochemistry and pharmacology

Unlike those in many herbs, the pharmacologically active constituents in ephedra are well characterized. They consist of ephedrine and ephedrine-related alkaloids, primarily pseudoephedrine, norephedrine, methylephedrine, and norpseudoephedrine. Commercial preparations may be standardized to ephedra alkaloid content, but content can vary considerably among manufacturers[60].

Ephedrine, the primary alkaloid in ephedra, is a noncatecholamine sympathomimetic agent that exhibits α_1, β_1, and β_2 activity by acting directly at adrenergic receptors and by indirectly releasing endogenous norepinephrine (noradrenaline). Ephedrine has caused dose-dependent increases in blood pressure and heart rate[61]. However, ephedra inconsistently increased heart rate and blood pressure in healthy, normotensive volunteers after a single dose[62].

The pharmacokinetics of ephedrine have been studied in humans. It has an elimination half-life of

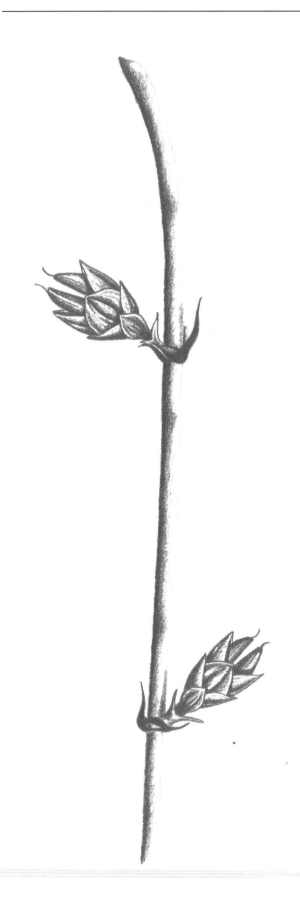

Figure 2.3   *Ephedra sinica*

4.85–6.47 h and is excreted unchanged in urine[63]. The pharmacokinetics of ephedrine do not depend on whether it is taken alone or in unprocessed ephedra[62].

Safety

The use of ephedra has raised serious safety concerns. Its sympathomimetic effects have been associated with adverse events in the central nervous and cardiovascular systems including hypertension, arrhythmias, stroke, seizures, and death[64]. Most of these adverse events have occurred in healthy young or middle-aged adults who used ephedra for weight loss and for increasing energy[65,66]. In at least one case, ephedra has also been associated with eosinophilic myocarditis[67]. As a result, ephedra should be avoided by those with hypertension, cardiovascular disease, cerebrovascular disease, seizure disorders, thyrotoxicosis or pheochromocytoma. It should not be taken with caffeine or other stimulants. It should also be avoided by pregnant or nursing women and by those taking monoamine oxidase (MAO) inhibitors and cardiac glycosides.

The long-term abuse of dietary supplements containing ephedrine has been reported to cause radiolucent kidney stones that, by some estimates, account for 0.064% of all cases of nephrolithiasis[68].

A major concern is lack of consistency of extract composition with variation in the herb source and inadequate chemical analysis of herbal extracts[69]. Poorly defined constituent ingredients and inconsistent herbal composition caused by agricultural practices in various geographic locations add to potential toxicity[70,71]. Ephedra extract contains multiple alkaloids and possibly other undefined ingredients that could explain health risks associated with ephedra[70]. In one study, 11 of 20 ephedra-containing dietary supplements tested either failed to list the ephedrine content on the label or varied in excess of 20% from the actual content and the claim on the label[72]. In 2004, the US FDA banned all dietary supplements containing ephedra alkaloids[73].

Preparations and dosage

In case of use outside of North America, ephedra should be used with caution, especially when in combination with caffeine and/or exercise[74,75]. It should not be taken for prolonged periods of time, during pregnancy, or while breastfeeding[76]. Use should be extremely restricted in the young and the elderly[77]. Daily doses of ephedra alkaloids should be limited to 24 mg/day.

GARLIC

Common names: stink weed, ajo, da suan (Chinese name), rashona (Sanskrit name), clove garlic.

Background

Garlic is the common name for *Allium sativum*, a member of the lily family (Figure 2.4). It is predominantly consumed for its aromatic qualities in food but has a history of medicinal use dating back to Egyptian times.

Uses

Garlic has been studied for its potential to modify the risk of atherosclerosis by reducing blood pressure, thrombus formation, and serum lipid and cholesterol levels. It may even promote the regression of atherosclerotic plaque[78]. Garlic has also been promoted for treatment and prevention of cancer and infectious diseases.

Evidence of the therapeutic efficacy of garlic in lowering serum cholesterol is compelling, although the effect appears to be modest[79]. A meta-analysis determined that the consumption of one-half to one clove of garlic per day decreased total serum cholesterol levels by an average of 9%[80]. In a German multi-center randomized controlled trial, standardized garlic powder tablets reduced serum cholesterol levels by 12% and triglyceride

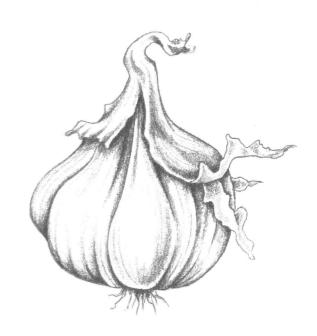

Figure 2.4 Garlic *(Allium sativum)*

levels by 17% in patients with hyperlipidemia[81]. However, not all studies have found that garlic reduced serum cholesterol[82–84]. It did not have a significant effect on children with familial hyperlipidemia[85]. Differences may be explained by variations in treatment regimens, patient populations, study methodology, and publication bias.

Little is known about the mechanism of the cholesterol-lowering effect of garlic. In isolated rat hepatocytes, garlic inhibited acetate uptake and interfered with cholesterol biosynthesis[86]. This mechanism has yet to be demonstrated in humans[83]. Garlic may also decrease the susceptibility of lipoproteins to oxidation[87]. The cholesterol-lowering effect of garlic may be mediated by a reduction in food intake[88].

Although garlic lowers blood pressure in animals, there is insufficient evidence to support the antihypertensive effect of garlic[89,90]. Garlic may be useful in cases of mild hypertension but should not replace lifestyle modification and drug therapy. In nulliparous parturients, garlic therapy during the third trimester reduced the incidence of hypertension but not the incidence of pre-eclampsia[91].

Phytochemistry and pharmacology

Garlic contains organosulfur compounds, adenosine, trace minerals, and amino acids. The pharmacologic effects are attributed to the sulfur-containing compounds, particularly allicin and its transformation products. When garlic is cut or crushed, alliin, the first compound found in nature to display optical isomerism at a sulfur as well as a carbon atom, is exposed to the enzyme alliinase and converted to allicin.

Garlic's constituents and their transformation products inhibit platelet aggregation dose-dependently. This activity is predominantly attributed to allicin[92], ajoene (4,5,9-trithiadodeca-1,6,11-triene-9-oxide)[89], and methyl allyl trisulfide[93,94]. The inhibition of platelet aggregation by ajoene appears to be irreversible[95] and may potentiate the effect of other compounds such as prostacyclin, forskolin, indomethacin, and dipyridamole[96]. The mechanism behind these effects is unclear, although some investigators have implicated the cyclo-oxygenase pathway[89]. Others have found a direct interaction with the platelet fibrinogen receptor[97]. Still other possibilities surround the exogenous adenosine in garlic[98] and inhibition of endogenous adenosine deamination and cyclic AMP phosphodiesterase[89]. The extent of garlic's antiplatelet activity *in vivo* is uncertain. In volunteers, inhibition of platelet aggregation to 5-hydroxytryptamine was transient but potent[86]. Another study showed no

such activity[99]. Garlic may also act as an anticoagulant by promoting fibrinolysis, which has been demonstrated in volunteers[100].

Little is known about the mechanism by which garlic may lower blood pressure. This effect may be mediated by nitric oxide[101,102], or by an as yet unknown mechanism[103]. Allicin decreased pulmonary vascular resistance in isolated rat lungs independently of nitric oxide, ATP-sensitive potassium channels, activation of cyclo-oxygenase, and changes in bronchomotor tone.

The pharmacokinetics of garlic's constituents are poorly understood. Allicin is not found in the blood after garlic consumption[104]. It is unstable and converts readily into mono-, di-, tri- and polysulfides, sulfur oxide, and other compounds such as ajoene[105]. These organosulfur compounds readily react with cysteine in the intestinal tract or circulation[106]. The sulfur-containing compounds found in the body after consumption of garlic are not known. Pharmacokinetic studies in animals have provided little insight[107,108].

Safety

The anticoagulant effect of garlic has raised concerns about bleeding in garlic users. One elderly patient developed a spontaneous epidural hematoma that was attributed to frequent garlic ingestion[109]. Although unreliable, bleeding times were significantly elevated when the patient was hospitalized and returned to normal 3 days after the discontinuation of garlic.

Preparations and dosage

The usual dosage is 4 g (approximately two cloves) of fresh bulb or its equivalent as an extract or tincture per day[110]. Much larger doses (up to 28 cloves/day) have been advocated, and the development of concentrated garlic preparations has made these doses achievable[111]. Commercial garlic preparations may be standardized to a fixed alliin and allicin content.

GINKGO

Common names: maidenhair, yin-hsing (Chinese name), silver apricot, duck foot tree, fossil tree.

Background

Ginkgo is derived from the leaf of *Ginkgo biloba* (Figure 2.5), also known as the maidenhair or fossil tree. It is the

although results are mixed, preliminary evidence is generally promising[115–123].

The use of ginkgo has also been advocated and scrutinized for the treatment of peripheral vascular disease[124], age-related macular degeneration[125,126], vertigo[127–129], tinnitus[130], sexual dysfunction[131–133], and altitude sickness[134]. Studies have led to generally mixed results for treatment of the above disorders with ginkgo. A consensus is forming that ginkgo is ineffective in treating tinnitus[135–139].

Phytochemistry and pharmacology

Ginkgo contains a number of active compounds. Those believed to be responsible for its pharmacologic effects are the terpenoids and flavonoids. The terpenoids include the sesquiterpene bilobalide and ginkgolides A, B, C, and J. The flavonoids are ginkgo-flavone glycosides that include kaempferol, quercetin, and isorhamnetin derivatives.

Ginkgo appears to alter vasoregulation[140], to act as an antioxidant[141], to modulate neurotransmitter and receptor activity[142,143], and to inhibit platelet-activating factor (PAF)[144]. The antioxidant and free radical scavenging effects have been attributed to the flavonoids, because they inhibit the expression of inducible nitric oxide synthase[145,146]. Ginkgolide B was a potent inhibitor of PAF in laboratory animals and humans[147]. PAF is an ether-linked phospholipid that mediates a diverse number of processes including stimulation of the inflammatory response, induction of platelet aggregation, and modulation of neuronal function[148]. Inhibition of PAF protects against hypoxia-induced neuronal injury[149,150]. Ginkgo may also have a non-PAF-mediated inhibitory effect on platelet aggregation in stressed laboratory animals, a finding that, if confirmed in humans, may be significant[151]. Ginkgo inhibited MAO in laboratory animals[152,153], but not in humans[154].

Bilobalide and ginkgolides A and B are highly bioavailable when administered orally. Glucuronidation appears to be part of the metabolism of the flavonoids[155]. Elimination half-lives of ginkgolides A and B and bilobalide after oral administration are 4.5, 10.6, and 3.2 h, respectively[156].

Safety

Although serious adverse effects have not been reported in clinical trials in relatively small numbers of patients, the anticoagulant effects of ginkgo have been associated with bleeding complications[157,158]. There are four

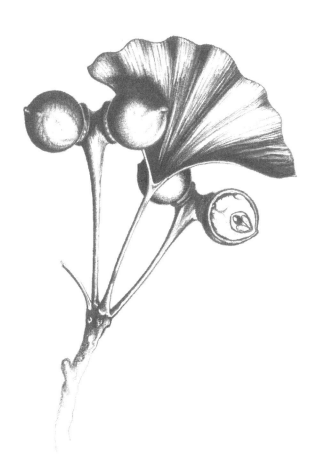

Figure 2.5   *Ginkgo biloba*

oldest living species of tree in existence today; fossils of the Ginkgo tree date as far back as 200 million years. An individual tree can live as long as 1000 years. In traditional Chinese medicine, *Ginkgo biloba* was used to make medicinal teas.

Uses

Ginkgo is primarily used to treat cognitive impairment, particularly Alzheimer's disease. A multi-center, randomized, placebo-controlled, double-blind trial showed that ginkgo extract (EGb 761) stabilized or improved cognitive function in patients with Alzheimer's disease and multi-infarct dementia[112]. In a meta-analysis of studies investigating the use of ginkgo for dementia or cognitive impairment, researchers concluded that ginkgo had a small but significant effect on objective measures of cognitive function in patients with Alzheimer's disease[113,114]. Whether ginkgo can improve cognitive function in healthy people is under active investigation;

reported cases of spontaneous intracranial bleeding[159–162], one case of spontaneous hyphema[163], and one case of post-operative bleeding[164] associated with ginkgo use. Interactions between ginkgo and prescription medications have been indicated, with particular concern for negative interactions in elderly subjects[165–169].

Hypersensitivity to ginkgo preparations is possible. Use during pregnancy or by nursing mothers is not recommended.

Preparations and dosage

Ginkgo is usually prepared as a dried leaf extract. The two ginkgo extracts used in clinical trials, EGb 761 and LI 1370, undergo extensive processing and are standardized to ginkgo-flavone glycoside and terpenoid content. The recommended dosage of ginkgo extract is 120–240 mg/day in two or three divided doses.

GINSENG

Common names: Panax, redberry, tartar root, five fingers, American ginseng, Chinese ginseng, Korean ginseng, Asian ginseng.

Background

Ginseng is an herbal medication derived from the root of the *Panax* genus of plants (Figure 2.6). It has been used for several thousands of years in Asia and its purported medicinal properties have reached mythic proportions. The use of ginseng in America dates back to the eighteenth century. Daniel Boone traded ginseng, and in his diary, George Washington mentioned gathering the herb.

Among the species used for pharmacologic effects, Asian ginseng (*Panax ginseng*), American ginseng (*Panax quinquefolius*), and Japanese ginseng (*Panax japonicus*) are commonly described. Other 'varieties' such as Siberian ginseng (*Eleintherococcus senticosus*) and Brazilian ginseng (*Pfaffia paniculata*) are unique plants with different pharmacologic effects that may nevertheless be included in commercially available ginseng preparations.

Uses

Brekham, an early pioneer in the study of ginseng, labeled it an 'adaptogen' because it appeared to protect the body against stress and restore homeostasis[170].

Ginseng has been advocated for virtually every purpose including general health[171], fatigue[172,173], immune function[174], cancer[175–178], cardiovascular disease[179,180], diabetes mellitus[181], cognitive function[182], viral infections[183], sexual function[184,185], and athletic performance[186,187]. Although ginseng has therapeutic potential and measurable pharmacologic activity, compelling evidence is lacking to support its use for any specific indication[188]. The German Commission E has approved ginseng as therapy for fatigue and decreased concentration and work capacity[189].

Phytochemistry and pharmacology

Constituents found in most ginseng species include ginsenosides, polysaccharides, peptides, polyacetylenic alcohols and fatty acids. Most pharmacologic actions are

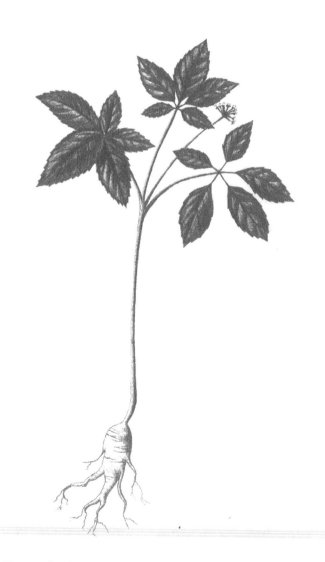

Figure 2.6   Ginseng

attributed to the ginsenosides that belong to a group of compounds known as steroidal saponins, steroid molecules with attached sugar residues. More than 20 ginsenosides have been isolated.

The pharmacologic profile of ginseng is broad and incompletely understood because of the many heterogeneous and sometimes opposing effects of different ginsenosides[190]. The underlying mechanism of action of the ginsenosides appears to be similar to that for steroid hormones. Actions on virtually every organ system have been described.

One of the most promising therapeutic uses of ginseng surrounds the regulation of carbohydrate metabolism and blood glucose. In patients with type 2 diabetes mellitus, ginseng lowered post-prandial blood glucose compared to placebo when taken 40 min before or at the same time as a glucose challenge[181]. In healthy subjects without diabetes mellitus, ginseng lowered post-prandial blood glucose compared to placebo only if taken 40 min before a glucose challenge.

Data from animal studies suggest that ginseng may have beneficial effects in the central nervous system. Ginsenosides prevented scopolamine-induced memory deficits in laboratory animals by increasing central cholinergic activity[191,192]. The compounds may also protect neurons from ischemic damage[193] and facilitate learning and memory by enhancing nerve growth[194]. The effect of ginseng on pain pathways needs further investigation. Ginsenosides had non-opioid-mediated analgesic properties in laboratory animals[195,196], but attenuated the analgesic effects of opiates[197,198]. Ginsenosides appear to modulate neurotransmission through γ-aminobutyric acid (GABA)[199,200] and by inhibiting neurotransmitter reuptake[201].

The results of investigations of the cardiovascular effects of ginseng are often contradictory, depending on the compounds tested and the organ system in which they are tested[202]. Stimulation of endogenous nitric oxide release has been implicated in the cardiovascular and antioxidant effects of ginsenosides. In humans, normal doses of ginseng did not appear to affect blood pressure and heart rate, although extremely high doses were associated with hypertension[203]. Ginseng may protect against myocardial reperfusion injury. In a preliminary study, cardioplegia solution containing ginseng extract improved post-bypass myocardial function in patients having mitral valve surgery[204].

Ginsenosides have anticarcinogenic and immunomodulatory effects. Several individual ginsenosides suppressed tumor cell growth, induced cell differentiation, regulated programmed cell death, and inhibited

metastasis[190]. Results of a cohort study showed that ginseng consumers had a lower risk for several different types of cancer compared to those who did not consume ginseng, suggesting that ginseng may have non-organspecific anticarcinogenic effects[205]. Ginsenosides also enhanced humoral and cell-mediated immune responses in laboratory animals[206–208], and potentiated the response to vaccination in humans[209].

The pharmacokinetics of ginsenosides Rg1, Re, and Rb2 have been investigated in rabbits[210]. The elimination half-lives of these three ginsenosides ranged from 0.8 h for ginsenoside Re to 7.4 h for ginsenoside Rb2. The degree of protein binding may explain the wide variation in half-lives between different ginsenosides.

Safety

Early descriptions of a 'ginseng abuse syndrome'[203] characterized by hypertension and central nervous system excitation have since been challenged, although a number of case reports have cautioned against the indiscriminate use of ginseng. The estrogen-like effects of ginseng have been associated with postmenopausal vaginal bleeding and mastalgia[211–214]. An interaction between ginseng and the MAO inhibitor phenelzine resulted in headache, tremors, and mania[215]. There is a case report of angiogram-confirmed, self-limited cerebral arteritis associated with ginseng overdose[216]. Ginseng was also associated with a significant decrease in warfarin anticoagulation in one case[217]. It is not known whether ginseng can cause the same side-effects as those described from longterm steroid use.

Another potential safety issue surrounding the use of ginseng concerns its effects on coagulation pathways. Ginsenosides inhibit platelet aggregation *in vitro*[218,219], and prolong both thrombin time and activated partial thromboplastin time in rats[220]. These findings await confirmation in humans.

Use during pregnancy or while breastfeeding is not recommended.

Preparations and dosage

Ginseng root is either dried to yield 'white ginseng' or steamed and then dried to yield 'red ginseng'. Commercial ginseng extract preparations standardized to ginsenoside content are available. The recommended daily dose is 100–200 mg of ginseng extract once daily. Dosages of ginseng extract up to 600 mg three times daily have been advocated[221].

KAVA

Common names: intoxicating pepper, kawa, kava kava, ava pepper.

Background

Kava is an herbal medication derived from the dried root of the pepper plant *Piper methysticum* (Figure 2.7). Kava has a long history of use as a ceremonial intoxicant in the South Pacific islands. It was relatively unknown to the rest of the world until missionaries introduced it into Australian aboriginal society in the 1980s[222,223]. The missionaries intended kava to substitute for alcohol which was abused by the aboriginal population. Unfortunately, kava misuse became an additional public health problem, and it was eventually outlawed in many aboriginal communities. Australian physicians provided many of the earliest descriptions of the medical effects of kava[224,225].

Uses

Kava has gained popularity as an over-the-counter anxiolytic and sedative. It is purported to be a safe alternative to benzodiazepines. Kava and alcohol do not appear to have synergistic effects on cognitive and psychomotor impairment[226]. Several randomized controlled trials have compared kava to placebo for the treatment of anxiety (diagnosed by DSM-III-R criteria)[227–231], situational anxiety[232], and anxiety associated with menopause[233–235]. A meta-analysis of clinical trials suggested that kava has therapeutic potential in the treatment of the symptoms of anxiety[236–239]. Kava has been advocated for the treatment of insomnia, but its effect on sleep in humans has not been well characterized[240].

Phytochemistry and pharmacology

Kava contains many pharmacologically active constituents that act synergistically to produce effects greater than those achieved with any single compound[241–243]. The kavalactones, also known as kavapyrones or α-pyrones, are responsible for most of the pharmacologic effects[244–249]. The six major kavalactones that have been identified are kawain, dihydrokawain, methysticin, dihydromethysticin, yangomin, and desmethoxyyangonin[250].

Kava produces dose-dependent effects on the central nervous system. The antiepileptic and neuroprotective properties of kavalactones have been demonstrated in animal models[247,248,251]. Kavalactones produced centrally mediated skeletal muscle relaxation *in vivo* and smooth muscle relaxation *in vitro*[248]. Unlike other central nervous system depressants, kava does not depress cognitive function or electroencephalographic event-related potentials[239,252,253]. However, the ability of kavalactones to increase barbiturate sleep time significantly has been demonstrated in animals[242,254]. Kavalactones also have significant local anesthetic properties. Kawain is equipotent to cocaine in producing topical anesthesia[248].

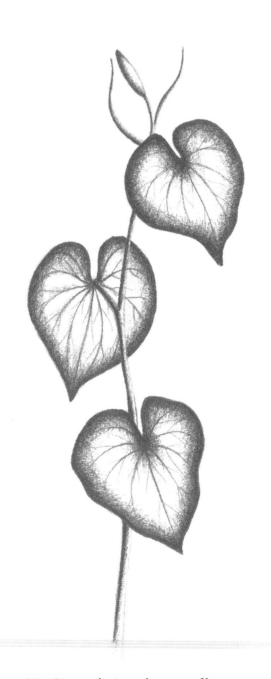

Figure 2.7   *Piper methysticum,* the source of kava

The mechanism of action of kava has not been fully elucidated, but multiple effector sites are involved. The anxiolytic and sedative effects of kava suggest that it potentiates GABA inhibitory neurotransmission. The first investigation addressing this effect found no evidence of binding in the mouse brain frontal cortex or cerebellum[255]. A later investigation showed that kavalactones mediate their effect through $GABA_A$ in the limbic structures of the brain[241]. In that study, the kavalactones and pentobarbital also produced a synergistic effect on [^{3}H]muscimol binding to GABA. Kavalactones inhibit voltage-dependent sodium and calcium channels *in vitro*, possibly explaining the antiepileptic and local anesthetic effects[256–259]. Kava may exert its effects through neurotransmitters such as dopamine and serotonin, but evidence of this is less compelling[260,261].

Peak plasma levels occur 1.8 h after an oral dose, and the elimination half-life of kavalactones is 9 h[262]. In rats, unchanged kavalactones and their metabolites undergo renal and fecal elimination[243].

Safety

In Germany, kava has been linked to 24 cases of liver toxicity culminating in one death and three liver transplants. Kava extracts were banned in the European Union and Canada in 2003[263]. Kava may potentiate the sedative effects of prescription medications[264]. With frequent use, kava produces 'kava dermopathy', characterized by reversible scaly cutaneous eruptions[265]. Kava may have abuse potential, but whether long-term use results in addiction, tolerance, and acute withdrawal after abstinence has not been satisfactorily investigated.

Kava is one of the top-selling herbs in the USA[266]. In spite of safety concerns of recent reports of liver toxicity related to use of kava products in humans[267,268], the FDA has not taken any action against kava products.

Use during pregnancy or while breastfeeding is not recommended.

Preparations and dosage

The recommended dose is 150–300 mg of kava extract divided into two doses or 50–240 mg of kavalactones per day[269].

MILK THISTLE

Common names: Marian thistle, St Mary's thistle, wild artichoke.

Background

Milk thistle is the common name for *Silybum marianum* (Figure 2.8), a member of the daisy family native to the Mediterranean. The therapeutic uses of milk thistle have been recognized for at least 2000 years. It was first used for liver and gallbladder disorders just as it is today. Silymarin, the biologically active flavonoid complex, is extracted from the seed of the plant.

Uses

Milk thistle has been advocated for the prophylaxis and treatment of liver disorders including cirrhosis[270,271] and alcoholic, viral, and toxic hepatitis[272–275]. Although inconclusive, available evidence suggests that milk thistle is potentially useful in some clinical situations. In a randomized controlled trial, it was reported that silymarin significantly improved survival in patients with cirrhosis (4-year survival of 58% in the treatment group and 39% in the placebo group)[276]. The subgroup analysis in this

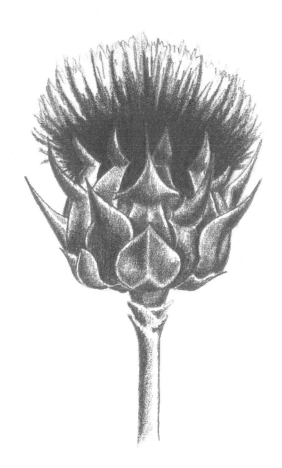

Figure 2.8 *Silybum marianum*, the milk thistle

study indicted that silymarin was effective in patients with alcoholic cirrhosis and in patients whose liver disease was initially rated as Child's Class A. Several clinical trials have demonstrated that silymarin significantly lowers serum liver enzyme and bilirubin levels in patients with cirrhosis and hepatitis[277–279]. In other controlled trials, however, silymarin did not improve survival or retard progression of disease in patients with alcoholic cirrhosis[280–283]. Milk thistle is effective in decreasing mortality caused by the ingestion of *Amanita phalloides*, the highly hepatotoxic deathcap mushroom[284].

Phytochemistry and pharmacology

The active compounds in milk thistle are the flavonolignane isomers, silybin, silidianin, and silichristine. Of these, silybin is the most prevalent and biologically active. Multiple mechanisms explain the hepatoprotective effects of milk thistle. Silymarin acts as an antioxidant, scavenging free radicals and inhibiting free radical production and lipid peroxidation[285–290]. Silymarin may protect against hepatotoxins by altering cell membrane permeability and receptor antagonism[291]. Data from *in vitro* studies suggest that silymarin may facilitate hepatocyte regeneration by effecting DNA expression[292]. In a rat model, silymarin conjugant with vitamin C supplements protected liver tissue from lead toxicity[293].

Only 20–50% of silymarin is absorbed from the gastrointestinal tract. Peak plasma concentrations occur 2–4 h after an oral dose, and the elimination half-life is approximately 6 h[294].

Safety

Milk thistle is generally safe[295,296]. The most frequently reported adverse effects are nausea and vomiting, urticaria, pruritis, and dyspepsia. Allergic reactions may stem from the development of IgE and IgG antibodies[297]. No drug interactions with milk thistle have been reported.

Use during pregnancy or while breastfeeding is not recommended.

Preparations and dosage

Commerical extracts of milk thistle are typically standardized to a silymarin content of 70–80%. Tea preparations are not recommended because silymarin is poorly water soluble. The recommended dosage is 100–200 mg of silymarin twice daily.

SAW PALMETTO

Common names: dwarf palmetto, pan palm, sabal.

Background

Saw palmetto is the common name for *Serenoa repens* (Figure 2.9), a dwarf palm tree native to Florida and other parts of the southeastern USA. The urologic effects of the saw palmetto berry were recognized by native Americans who used it as a source of food. Saw palmetto preparations today consist of refined extracts of the dried ripe berry.

Uses

Saw palmetto extract is used to treat symptoms associated with benign prostatic hypertrophy (BPH), a condition found in approximately 40% of men in their fifties and 90% of men in their eighties[298,299]. It is often used as first-line treatment for BPH in Europe[300], and in Germany herbal medications account for more than 90% of all drugs prescribed for the treatment of BPH.

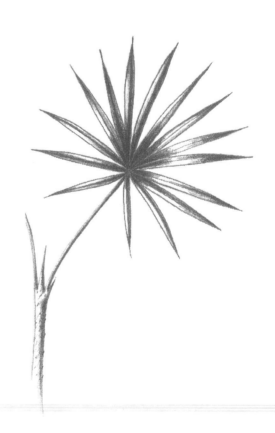

Figure 2.9 *Serenoa repens*, the saw palmetto

In a meta-analysis of 18 randomized controlled trials that compared saw palmetto extract to placebo or standard medical therapies, saw palmetto extract improved urinary symptoms and flow measures significantly compared to placebo[301,302]. These improvements were comparable to those achieved with finasteride. Saw palmetto extract is less expensive and associated with a significantly lower incidence of impotence compared to finasteride[302]. Others have reached similar conclusions, but caution that most trials were significantly limited by methodologic flaws, small patient numbers, and brief treatment intervals[303].

It is not known whether saw palmetto extract can prevent long-term complications of BPH such as acute urinary retention or the need for surgery. Saw palmetto extract does not affect levels of serum prostate-specific antigen[304].

Saw palmetto has been used to treat various other urologic conditions and respiratory conditions such as chronic bronchitis, laryngitis, and nasal inflammation.

Phytochemistry and pharmacology

The major constituents of saw palmetto are fatty acids and their glycerides (triacylglycerides and monoacylglycerides), carbohydrates, steroids, flavonoids, resin, pigment, tannin, and volatile oil[305]. The pharmacologic activity of saw palmetto has not been attributed to a single compound.

The mechanism of action of saw palmetto is not known, but multiple mechanisms have been proposed. Data from *in vitro* studies support the widely held belief that saw palmetto extract, like finasteride, inhibits 5α-reductase[303,306]. However, results of *in vivo* studies of inhibition of 5α-reductase by saw palmetto have been inconsistent[303]. Other hypotheses are that saw palmetto exerts its effects by inhibition of dihydrotestosterone binding to the androgen receptors in the prostate[307], inhibition of estrogen receptors[308], blocking of prolactin receptor signal transduction[309], interference with fibroblast proliferation[310], induction of apoptosis[311], inhibition of α_1 adrenergic receptors[312], and attenuation of the inflammatory response[313,314].

The pharmacokinetics of the constituents of saw palmetto have not been studied.

Safety

Adverse effects attributed to saw palmetto are mild and usually gastrointestinal in nature[307]. The long-term safety of saw palmetto extract has not been studied.

However, it has a long history of safe use in Europe. Saw palmetto should be discontinued before undergoing surgery, because it may be associated with excessive intraoperative bleeding[315].

Use during pregnancy or while breastfeeding is not recommended.

Preparations and dosage

Liposterolic extracts are used in virtually all investigational studies. Commercial preparations may be standardized to fatty acid and sterol content. The recommended daily dose is 1–2 g saw palmetto berry or 320 mg of lipid soluble extract[305].

ST JOHN'S WORT

Common names: amber, goatweed, klamath weed, hardhay.

Background

St John's wort is the common name for *Hypericum perforatum* (Figure 2.10), a flowering plant that can be found in Europe, Asia, Africa, Australia, and the Americas. It is so named because its yellow flower was traditionally gathered for the feast of St John the Baptist. The herbal medication comes from the aerial parts of the plant harvested shortly before or during flowering.

Uses

St John's wort has been used since the Middle Ages for neuralgia, depression, and various 'nervous' conditions. Today, St John's wort is primarily used as an antidepressant. It has the largest market share of antidepressants in Europe with $6 billion in sales in 1988. The popularity of St John's wort is reflected in the large number of clinical trials, meta-analyses, and reviews of its effectiveness as an antidepressant, which have concluded that it is more effective than placebo in the treatment of mild to moderate depression and has a low incidence of side-effects[316–325]. In the treatment of major depression, however, St John's wort is not effective[326–328]. Moreover, it is unclear whether St John's wort is as effective as conventional antidepressants. Some reviews concluded that St John's wort and the older tricyclic antidepressants were equally effective[317–319,329]. Others concluded that St John's wort was less effective than tricyclic antidepressants[322]. Still others believe that there is insufficient

acylphloroglucinols (hyperforin and adhyperforin), flavonol glycosides, biflavones, proanthocyanidins, and phenylpropanes (chlorogenic acid and caffeic acid). Among these constituents, hypericin and hyperfornin have received the most scientific interest. Hypericin was originally considered the active component in St John's wort, and commercial preparations are standardized to hypericin content. Recent evidence suggests that hyperforin and its analogs play a larger role in the pharmacologic effects[337–338]. Because hyperforin is an unstable compound and is susceptible to oxidative degradation, its concentration in St John's wort may vary considerably[339].

St John's wort inhibits reuptake of serotonin, norepinephrine, and dopamine[337,340–342]. This property appears to be different from that found in conventional antidepressants. St John's wort also had antinociceptive effects in mice similar to those seen with tricyclic antidepressants[343].

Initially, MAO inhibition was considered a possible mechanism of action. Later studies have shown, however, that the inhibition of MAO by St John's wort is clinically non-significant[337,344–346]. Adverse events that would be expected with MAO inhibition have not been reported with St John's wort.

The pharmacokinetics of hypericum extract have been studied. After oral administration in human volunteers, the median half-life for absorption was 0.6 h, the median half-life for distribution was 6.0 h, and the median half-life for elimination was 43.1 h[347]. In another study, peak plasma levels of hypericum extract were obtained 3–3.5 h after oral dosing, and the elimination half-life was 9 h. Plasma concentration time curves fit a two-compartment model[348]. Hypericin and pseudohypericin are most likely to be conjugated and excreted in the bile[347].

Safety

When St John's wort is taken by healthy patients, it is generally well tolerated. Adverse effects include photosensitivity, rash, nausea, fatigue, and restlessness[322,349,350]. Serotonin syndrome was reported in patients taking St John's wort alone[349,351], or in combination with conventional antidepressants[352]. In patients who may have subclinical or undiagnosed bipolar disorder, induction of mania was also reported[353–356].

Patients taking prescription medications should be cautious taking St John's wort, since significant herb–drug interactions can occur[357]. It induces cytochrome P450 enzymes and increases the metabolism of

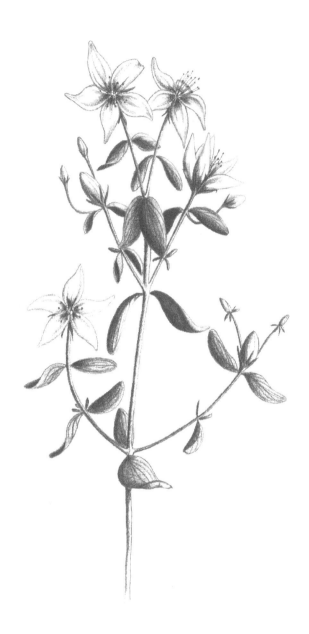

Figure 2.10 *Hypericum perforatum*, St John's wort

evidence to compare St John's wort to conventional antidepressants and have called for more studies comparing St John's wort to the newer serotonin reuptake inhibiting antidepressants[323,330]. The methodology of many studies has been criticized with the implication that firm conclusions about the efficacy of St John's wort are premature[318,328,331–336].

Phytochemistry and pharmacology

The constituents of St John's wort are the naphthodianthrones (hypericin and pseuodohypericin),

protease inhibitors, oral contraceptives, cyclosporin, warfarin, digoxin, and many other concomitantly administered drugs. The metabolic activity of the cytochrome P450 3A4 isoenzyme is most affected, and its metabolic activity is approximately doubled[358–360]. This isoform is the most abundant hepatic enzyme, responsible for the oxidative metabolism of over 50% of all conventional medications subject to cytochrome P450 oxidative metabolism. Interactions with substrates of the 3A4 isoform including indinavir[361], ethinylestradiol[362], and cyclosporin[363–366] have been documented. In one series of 45 organ transplant patients, St John's wort was associated with an average decrease of 49% in blood cyclosporin levels[367]. Another group reported two cases of acute heart transplant rejection associated with this particular pharmacokinetic interaction[368]. In addition to the 3A4 isoform, the cytochrome P450 2C9 isoform may also be induced. The anticoagulant effect of warfarin, a substrate of the 2C9 isoform, was reduced in seven reported cases. A study of renal transplant patients showed St John's wort significantly decreased the efficacy of administered immunosuppressants, thereby increasing patient susceptibility to organ rejection[369].

St John's wort also affects digoxin pharmacokinetics, possibly by altering a P-glycoprotein transporter[370]. In volunteers, co-administration of St John's wort led to a 26% reduction in the C_{max} and a 33% reduction of the C_{trough} of digoxin.

Use during pregnancy or by nursing mothers is not recommended.

Preparations and dosage

St John's wort extracts are commercially available, and many are standardized to hypericin content. The recommended daily dose of St John's wort is 2–4 g of St John's wort or 0.2–1 mg of hypericin[371].

VALERIAN

Common names: all-heal, garden heliotrope, vandal root, capon's tail, amantilla, setwall.

Background

Valerian is the common name given to the herbal medication derived from the root of the *Valeriana* genus of plants, pink-flowered perennials (Figure 2.11) native to the temperate areas of the Americas, Europe, and Asia. The different species of valerian used in various parts of the world – *Valeriana officinalis* in northern Europe, *Valeriana angstifolia* in China and Japan, *Valeriana wallichii* in India – are all used for essentially the same purpose. *Valeriana officinalis* is the species most commonly available and studied.

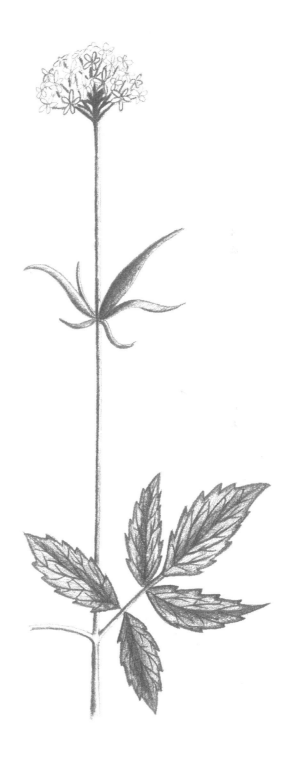

Figure 2.11 *Valeriana officinalis*, the source of valerian

Uses

Valerian is used as a sedative to treat insomnia and anxiety[372,373]. Virtually all herbal sleep-aid preparations contain valerian. During World War I, 'shell-shocked' soldiers were treated with valerian. Valerian also promotes smooth muscle relaxation and may be used to treat gastro-intestinal hyperactivity.

Phytochemistry and pharmacology

Valerian contains multiple chemical constituents that act synergistically. These include volatile oils (sesquiterpenes and monoterpenes), valepotriates, alkaloids, and lignans[374–377]. The sesquiterpenes are considered the primary source of the pharmacologic effects[378]. At least 17 sesquiterpenes have been characterized[379]. Some commercial preparations are standardized to the content of valerenic acid, a sesquiterpene that is not known to exist elsewhere in nature. The valepotriates have also been characterized and consist of a furanopyranoid monoterpene skeleton found in glycosylated forms known as iridoids. At least 37 valepotriates have been isolated. They act as prodrugs that are metabolized into compounds more active than the parent compound[380]. The pharmacologic action of the other constituents of valerian is unclear. Seven alkaloids have been isolated but not well studied. GABA and various amino acids have been isolated from the aqueous portion of valerian, but their bioavailability remains in question[378].

Valerian produced dose-dependent sedation and hypnosis in preclinical studies[381–383]. The sesquiterpenes and, to a lesser extent, the valepotriates, increased barbiturate sleep time in animals. Valerian extract 11.2 g/kg was equivalent to diazepam 3 mg/kg in doubling hexobarbital sleep time in mice[272]. Valerian had weak anticonvulsant properties in mice[384]. In isolated guinea-pig ileum, relaxation of smooth muscle by valerian was peripherally mediated[385].

In humans, valerian produced dose-dependent electroencephalogram changes consistent with sedation[386,387]. The pharmacodynamic studies of valerian in humans have focused on the sleep setting. Modest improvements in subjective ratings of sleep were reported, but objective measurements were inconsistent[388–391]. Subjective and objective measurements of sleep improved after multiple but not single-dose treatment[392].

The biologic activity of valerian is consistent with the modulation of GABA inhibitory neurotransmission. Constituents of valerian extract have effects at the GABA$_A$ receptor[393,394]. Valerian extract influenced presynaptic components of GABA-ergic neurons, although the mechanism of action was unclear. It also influenced GABA synaptosomal release[395,396], inhibited GABA reuptake[394], and inhibited GABA breakdown[397].

The subjective effects of valerian are short-lived with no demonstrable psychomotor effects the morning after treatment[398]. Multiple doses per day are needed for treatment of anxiety, and the peak effect occurs 1–2 h after oral administration.

Safety

Short-term use of valerian is safe[399,400]. Because of its GABA receptor activity, the long-term use of valerian may be associated with a benzodiazepine-like withdrawal syndrome. In fact, valerian attenuated benzodiazepine withdrawal in rats[401]. In one patient, the long-term use of valerian was associated with a life-threatening benzodiazepine-like withdrawal syndrome after surgery[397].

Use during pregnancy or while breastfeeding is not recommended.

Preparations and dosage

Commercial valerian preparations consist of the dried extract of the root and may be standardized to a minimum level of valerenic acid or other selected constituents. As a sleep aid, the recommended dosage of valerian extract is 400–900 mg taken 30 min before bedtime. For anxiety, the recommended dosage of valerian extract is 220 mg of extract three times daily. The daily dosage of valerian extract should not exceed 1800 mg, and it is not meant for long-term use[400].

References

1. Schmidt JM, Greenspoon JS. Aloe vera dermal wound gel is associated with a delay in wound healing. Obstet Gynecol 1991; 78: 115–17

2. Rodriguez-Bigas M, Cruz NI, Suarez A. Comparative evaluation of aloe vera in the management of burn wounds in guinea pigs. Plast Reconstr Surg 1988; 81: 386–9

3. Williams MS, Burk M, Loprinzi CL, et al. Phase III double-blind evaluation of an aloe vera gel as a prophylactic agent for radiation-induced skin toxicity. Int J Radiat Oncol Biol Phys 1996; 36: 345–9

4. Fulton JE Jr. The stimulation of postdermabrasion wound healing with stabilized aloe vera gel–polyethylene oxide dressing. J Dermatol Surg Oncol 1990; 16: 460–7

5. McCauley RL, Heggers JP, Robson MC. Frostbite: methods to minimize tissue loss. Postgrad Med 1990; 88: 73–7

6. Thomas DR, Goode PS, LaMaster K, Tennyson T. Acemannan hydrogel dressing versus saline dressing for pressure ulcers. A randomized, controlled trial. Adv Wound Care 1998; 11: 273–6

7. Syed TA, Ahmad SA, Holt AH, et al. Management of psoriasis with Aloe vera extract in a hydrophilic cream: a placebo-controlled, double-blind study. Trop Med Int Health 1996; 1: 505–9

8. Paulsen E, Korsholm L, Brandrup F. A double-blind, placebo-controlled study of a commercial aloe vera gel in the treatment of slight to moderate psoriasis vulgaris. J Eur Acad Dermatol Venereol 2005; 19: 326–31

9. Chithra P, Sajithlal GB, Chandrakasan G. Influence of aloe vera on the healing of dermal wounds in diabetic rats. J Ethnopharmacol 1998; 59: 195–201

10. Somboonwong J, Thanamittramanee S, Jariyapongskul A, Patumraj S. Therapeutic effects of aloe vera on cutaneous microcirculation and wound healing in second degree burn model in rats. J Med Assoc Thai 2000; 83: 417–25

11. Reynolds T, Dweck AC. Aloe vera leaf gel: a review update. J Ethnopharmacol 1999; 68: 3–37

12. Garnick JJ, Singh B, Winkley G. Effectiveness of a medicament containing silicon dioxide, aloe, and allantoin on aphthous stomatitis. Oral Surg Oral Med Oral Pathol Oral Radiol Endod 1998; 86: 550–6

13. Plemons JN, Rees TD, Binnie WH, et al. Evaluation of acemannan in the treatment of recurrent aphthous stomatitis. Wounds 1994; 6: 40–5

14. Blitz J, Smith JW, Gerard JR. Aloe vera gel in peptic ulcer therapy: preliminary report. J Am Osteopath Assoc 1963; 62: 731–5

15. Montaner JS, Gill J, Singer J, et al. Double-blind placebo-controlled pilot trial of acemannan in advanced human immunodeficiency virus disease. J Acquir Immune Defic Syndr Hum Retrovirol 1996; 12: 153–7

16. Angmead L, Feakins RM, Goldthorpe S, et al. Randomized, double-blind, placebo-controlled trial of oral aloe vera gel for active ulcerative colitis. Aliment Pharmacol Ther 2004; 19: 739–47

17. Ghannam N, Kingston M, Al Meshaal IA, et al. The antidiabetic activity of aloes: preliminary clinical and experimental observations. Horm Res 1986; 24: 288–94

18. Sakai R. Epidemiologic survey on lung cancer with respect to cigarette smoking and plant diet. Jpn J Cancer Res 1989; 80: 513–20

19. Vogler BK, Ernst E. Aloe vera: a systematic review of its clinical effectiveness. Br J Gen Pract 1999; 49: 823–8

20. Su CK, Mehta V, Ravikumar L, et al. Phase II double-blind randomized study comparing oral aloe vera versus placebo to prevent radiation-related mucositis in patients with head-and-neck neoplasms. Int J Radiat Oncol Biol Phys 2004; 60: 171–7

21. Vazquez B, Avila G, Segura D, Escalante B. Anti-inflammatory activity of extracts from Aloe vera gel. J Ethnopharmacol 1996; 55: 69–75

22. Andersen DO, Weber ND, Wood SG, et al. In vitro virucidal activity of selected anthraquinones and anthraquinone derivatives. Antiviral Res 1991; 16: 185–96

23. Stuart RW, Lefkowitz DL, Lincoln JA, et al. Upregulation of phagocytosis and candidicidal activity of macrophages exposed to the immunostimulant acemannan. Int J Immunopharmacol 1997; 19: 75–82

24. Lee KH, Kim JH, Lim DS, Kim CH. Anti-leukaemic and anti-mutagenic effects of di(2-ethylhexyl)phthalate isolated from Aloe vera Linne. J Pharm Pharmacol 2000; 52: 593–8

25. Morrow DM, Rapaport MS, Strick RA. Hypersensitivity to aloe. Arch Dermatol 1980; 116: 1064–5

26. Shoji A. Contact dermatitis to Aloe arborescens. Contact Dermatitis 1982; 8: 164–7

27. Hunter D, Frumkin A. Adverse reactions to vitamin E and Aloe vera preparations after dermabrasion and chemical peel. Cutis 1991; 47: 193–6

28. Anon. Aloe. In Gruenwald J, Brendler T, Jaenicke C, eds. PDR for Herbal Medicines, 2nd edn. Montvale, NJ: Medical Economics Company, 2000: 16–20

29. Siegers CP, von Hertzberg-Lottin E, Otte M, Schneider B. Anthranoid laxative abuse – a risk for colorectal cancer? Gut 1993; 34: 1099–101

30. Pribitkin ED, Boger G. Herbal therapy: what every facial plastic surgeon must know. Arch Facial Plast Surg 2001; 3: 127–32

31. Anon. Aloe. In Blumenthal M, Busse WR, Goldberg A, et al., eds. The Complete German Commission E Monographs: Therapeutic Guide to Herbal Medicines, 1st edn. Boston, MA: Integrative Medical Communications, 1998

32. Melchart D, Linde K, Fischer P, Kaesmayr J. Echinacea for preventing and treating the common cold. Cochrane Database Syst Rev 2000; 2: CD000530

33. Caruso TJ, Gwaltney JM Jr. Treatment of the common cold with echinacea: a structured review. Clin Infect Dis 2005; 40: 807–10

34. Pepping J. Echinacea. Am J Health-Syst Pharm 1999; 56: 121–2

35. Gan XH, Zhang L, Heber D, Bonavida B. Mechanism of activation of human peripheral blood NK cells at the single cell level by Echinacea water soluble extracts: recruitment of lymphocyte-target conjugates and killer cells and activation of programming for lysis. Int Immunopharmacol 2003; 3: 811–24

36. Rehman J, Dillow JM, Carter SM, et al. Increased production of antigen-specific immunoglobulins G and M following in

vivo treatment with the medicinal plants Echinacea angustifolia and Hydrastis canadensis. Immunol Lett 1999; 68: 391–5

37. Turner RB, Bauer R, Woelkart K, et al. An evaluation of Echinacea angustifolia in experimental rhinovirus infections. N Engl J Med 2005; 353: 341–8

38. Mengs U, Clare CB, Poiley JA. Toxicity of Echinacea purpurea. Acute, subacute and genotoxicity studies. Arzneimittelforschung 1991; 41: 1076–81

39. Gallo M, Sarkar M, Au W, et al. Pregnancy outcome following gestational exposure to echinacea: a prospective controlled study. Arch Intern Med 2000; 160: 3141–3

40. Huntley AL, Thompson Coon J, Ernst E. The safety of herbal medicinal products derived from Echinacea species: a systematic review. Drug Safety 2005; 28: 387–400

41. Gallo M, Koren G. Can herbal products be used safely during pregnancy? Focus on echinacea. Can Fam Physician 2001; 47: 1727–8

42. Tsui B, Dennehy CE, Tsourounis C. A survey of dietary supplement use during pregnancy at an academic medical center. Am J Obstet Gynecol 2001; 185: 433–7

43. Mullins RJ, Heddle R. Adverse reactions associated with echinacea: the Australian experience. Ann Allergy Asthma Immunol 2002; 88: 42–51

44. Mullins RJ. Echinacea-associated anaphylaxis. Med J Aust 1998; 168: 170–1

45. Boullata JI, Nace AM. Safety issues with herbal medicine. Pharmacotherapy 2000; 20: 257–69

46. Miller LG. Herbal medicinals: selected clinical considerations focusing on known or potential drug–herb interactions. Arch Intern Med 1998; 158: 2200–11

47. Krapp K, Longe JL. The Gale Encyclopedia of Alternative Medicine, Volume 2. Detroit, MI: Gale Group, 2001

48. World Health Organization. Herba Ephedra. WHO Monographs on Selected Medicinal Plants, Vol 1. Geneva: World Health Organization, 1999: 145–53

49. Blanck HM, Khan LK, Serdula MK. Use of nonprescription weight loss products: results from a multistate survey. J Am Med Assoc 2001; 286: 930–5

50. Bucci LR. Selected herbals and human exercise performance. Am J Clin Nutr 2000; 72: 624S–36S

51. Greenway FL. The safety and efficacy of pharmaceutical and herbal caffeine and ephedrine use as a weight loss agent. Obes Rev 2001; 2: 199–211

52. Blanck HM, Khan LK, Serdula MK. Use of nonprescription weight loss products: results from a multistate survey. J Am Med Assoc 2001; 286: 930–5

53. Astrup A, Breum L, Toubro S, et al. The effect and safety of an ephedrine/caffeine compound compared to ephedrine, caffeine, and placebo in obese subjects on an energy restricted diet: a double blind trial. Int J Obes 1992; 16: 269–77

54. Astrup A, Toubro S, Cannon S, et al. Thermogenic synergism between ephedrine and caffeine in healthy volunteers: a double-blind, placebo-controlled study. Metabolism 1991; 40: 323–9

55. Boozer CN, Nasser JA, Heymsfield SB, et al. An herbal supplement containing ma huang-guarana for weight loss: a randomized, double-blind trial. Int J Obes 2001; 25: 316–24

56. Bucci LR. Selected herbals and human exercise performance. Am J Clin Nutr 2000; 72: 624s–36s

57. Bell DG, Jacobs I, Zamecnik J. Effects of caffeine, ephedrine and their combination on time to exhaustion during high-intensity exercise. Eur J Appl Physiol 1998; 77: 427–33

58. Young R, Gabryszuk M, Glennon RA. Ephedrine and caffeine mutually potentiate one another's amphetamine-like stimulus effects. Pharmacol Biochem Behav 1998; 61: 169–73

59. Nightingale SL. From the Food and Drug Administration. J Am Med Assoc 1996; 275: 1534

60. Gurley BJ, Gardner SF, Hubbard MA. Content versus label claims in ephedra-containing dietary supplements. Am J Health Syst Pharm 2000; 57: 963–9

61. Hoffman BB, Lefkowitz RJ. Catecholamines, sympathomimetic drugs, and adrenergic receptor antagonists. In Hardman JG, Gilaman AG, Limbird LE, eds. Goodman and Gilman's The Pharmacological Basis of Therapeutics, 9th edn. New York, NY: McGraw-Hill, 1996: 199–248

62. White LM, Gardner SF, Gurley BJ, et al. Pharmacokinetics and cardiovascular effects of ma-huang (Ephedra sinica) in normotensive adults. J Clin Pharmacol 1997; 37: 116–22

63. Gurley BJ, Gardner SF, White LM, Wang PL. Ephedrine pharmacokinetics after the ingestion of nutritional supplements containing Ephedra sinica (ma huang). Ther Drug Monit 1998; 20: 439–45

64. Haller CA, Benowitz NL. Adverse cardiovascular and central nervous system events associated with dietary supplements containing ephedra alkaloids. N Engl J Med 2000; 343: 1833–8

65. Haller CA, Benowitz NL. Adverse cardiovascular and central nervous system events associated with dietary supplements containing ephedra alkaloids. N Engl J Med 2000; 343: 1833–8

66. Nightingale SL. From the Food and Drug Administration. J Am Med Assoc 1997; 278: 15

67. Zaacks SM, Klein L, Tan CD, et al. Hypersensitivity myocarditis associated with ephedra use. J Toxicol Clin Toxicol 1999; 37: 485–9

68. Powell T, Hsu FF, Turk J, Hruska K. Ma-huang strikes again: ephedrine nephrolithiasis. Am J Kidney Dis 1998; 32: 153–9

69. Straus SE. Herbal medicines–what's in the bottle? N Engl J Med 2002; 347: 1997–8

70. Lee MK, Cheng BW, Che CT, et al. Cytotoxicity assessment of ma-huang (ephedra) under different conditions of preparation. Toxicol Sci 2000; 56: 424–30

71. Marcus DM, Grollman AP. Botanical medicines–the need for new regulations. N Engl J Med 2002; 347: 2073–6

72. Gurley BJ, Gardner SF, Hubbard MA. Content versus label claims in ephedra-containing dietary supplements. Am J Health Syst Pharm 2000; 57: 963–9

73. FDA. Final rule declaring dietary supplements containing ephedrine alkaloids adulterated because they present an unreasonable risk. Federal Register Docket No 1995N-0304. 11 February 2004

74. Christensen NJ, Galbo H. Sympathetic nervous activity during exercise. Annu Rev Physiol 1983; 45: 139–53

75. Eisenhofer G, Rundqvist B, Friberg P. Determinants of cardiac tyrosine hydroxylase activity during exercise-induced sympathetic activation in humans. Am J Physiol 1998; 274: R626–34

76. Anastasio GD, Harston PR. Fetal tachycardia associated with maternal use of pseudoephedrine, an over-the-counter oral decongestant. J Am Board Fam Pract 1992; 5: 527–8

77. Dollery C. In Therapeutic Drugs, Volume 1. New York, NY: Churchill Livingstone, 1991

78. Koscielny J, Klussendorf D, Latza R, et al. The antiatherosclerotic effect of Allium sativum. Antherosclerosis 1999; 144: 237–49

79. Stevinson C, Pittler MH, Ernst E. Garlic for treating hypercholesterolemia: a meta-analysis of randomized clinical trials. Ann Intern Med 2000; 133: 420–9

80. Warshafsky S, Kamer RS, Sivak SL. Effect of garlic on total serum cholesterol. A meta-analysis. Ann Intern Med 1993; 119: 599–605

81. Mader FH. Treatment of hyperlipidaemia with garlic-powder tablets. Evidence from the German Association of General Practitioners' multicentric placebo-controlled double-blind study. Arzneimittelforschung 1990; 40: 1111–16

82. Gardner CD, Chatterjee LM, Carlson JJ. The effect of a garlic preparation on plasma lipid levels in moderately hypercholesterolemic adults. Atherosclerosis 2001; 154: 213–20

83. Berthold HK, Sudhop T, von Bergmann K. Effect of a garlic oil preparation on serum lipoproteins and cholesterol metabolism: a randomized controlled trial. J Am Med Assoc 1998; 279: 1900–2

84. Isaacsohn JL, Moser M, Stein EA, et al. Garlic powder and plasma lipids and lipoproteins: a multicenter, randomized, placebo-controlled trial. Arch Intern Med 1998; 158: 1189–94

85. McCrindle BW, Helden E, Conner WT. Garlic extract therapy in children with hypercholesterolemia. Arch Pediatr Adolesc Med 1998; 152: 1089–94

86. Gebhardt R. Multiple inhibitory effects of garlic extracts on cholesterol biosynthesis in hepatocytes. Lipids 1993; 28: 613–19

87. Steiner M, Lin RS. Changes in platelet function and susceptibility of lipoproteins to oxidation associated with administration of aged garlic extract. J Cardiovasc Pharmacol 1998; 31: 904–8

88. Kannar D, Wattanapenpaiboon N, Savige GS, Wahlqvist ML. Hypocholesterolemic effect of an enteric-coated garlic supplement. J Am Coll Nutr 2001; 20: 225–31

89. Ali M, Al-Qattan KK, Al-Enezi F, et al. Effect of allicin from garlic powder on serum lipids and blood pressure in rats fed with a high cholesterol diet. Prostaglandins Leukot Essent Fatty Acids 2000; 62: 253–9

90. Silagy CA, Neil HA. A meta-analysis of the effect of garlic on blood pressure. J Hypertens 1994; 12: 463–8

91. Ziaei S, Hantoshzadeh S, Rezasoltani P, Lamyian M. The effect of garlic tablet on plasma lipids and platelet aggregation in nulliparous pregnants at high risk of preeclampsia. Eur J Obstet Gynecol Reprod Biol 2001; 99: 201–6

92. Mohammad SF, Woodward SC. Characterization of a potent inhibitor of platelet aggregation and release reaction isolated from Allium sativum (garlic). Thromb Res 1986; 44: 793–806

93. Ariga T, Oshiba S, Tamada T. Platelet aggregation inhibitor in garlic [letter]. Lancet 1981; 1: 150–1

94. Boullin DJ. Garlic as a platelet inhibitor [letter]. Lancet 1981; 1: 776–7

95. Srivastava KC. Evidence for the mechanism by which garlic inhibits platelet aggregation. Prostaglandins Leukot Med 1986; 22: 313–21

96. Apitz-Castro R, Escalante J, Vargas R, Jain MK. Ajoene, the antiplatelet principle of garlic, synergistically potentiates the antiaggregatory action of prostacyclin, forskolin, indomethacin and dipyridamole on human platelets. Thromb Res 1986; 42: 303–11

97. Apitz-Castro R, Ledezma E, Escalante J, Jain MK. The molecular basis of the antiplatelet action of ajoene: direct interaction with the fibrinogen receptor. Biochem Biophys Res Commun 1986; 141: 145–50

98. Makheja AN, Bailey JM. Antiplatelet constituents of garlic and onion. Agents Actions 1990; 29: 360–3

99. Harenberg J, Giese C, Zimmerman R. Effect of dried garlic on blood coagulation, fibrinolysis, platelet aggregation and serum cholesterol levels in patients with hyperlipoproteinemia. Atherosclerosis 1988; 74: 247–9

100. Chutani SK, Bordia A. The effect of fried versus raw garlic on fibrinolytic activity in man. Atherosclerosis 1981; 38: 417–21

101. Kim-Park S, Ku DD. Garlic elicits a nitric oxide-dependent relaxation and inhibits hypoxic pulmonary vasoconstriction in rats. Clin Exp Pharmacol Physiol 2000; 27: 780–6

102. Das I, Khan NS, Sooranna SR. Potent activation of nitric oxide synthase by garlic: a basis for its therapeutic applications. Curr Med Res Opin 1995; 13: 257–63

103. Kaye AD, De Witt BJ, Anwar M, et al. Analysis of responses of garlic derivatives in the pulmonary valscular bed of the rat. J Appl Physiol 2000; 89: 353–8

104. Lawson LD, Ransom DK, Hughes BG. Inhibition of whole blood platelet-aggregation by compounds in garlic clove extracts and commercial garlic products. Thromb Res 1992; 65: 141–56

105. Dorant E, van den Brandt PA, Goldbohm RA, et al. Garlic and its significance for the prevention of cancer in humans: a critical view. Br J Cancer 1993; 67: 424–9

106. Lawson LD, Wang ZJ. Pre-hepatic fate of the organosulfur compounds derived from garlic (Allium sativum). Planta Med 1993; 59: A688–9 (abstract)

107. Lachmann G, Lorenz D, Radeck W, Steiper M. [The pharmacokinetics of S35 labeled garlic constituents alliin, allicin, and vinyldithiine]. Arzneimittelforschung 1994; 44: 734–43

108. Egen-Schwind C, Eckard R, Jekat FW, Winterhoff H. Pharmacokinetics of vinyldithiins, transformation products of allicin. Planta Med 1992; 58: 8–13

109. Rose KD, Croissant PD, Parliament CF, Levin MB. Spontaneous spinal epidural hematoma with associated platelet dysfunction from excessive garlic ingestion: a case report. Neurosurgery 1990; 26: 880–2

110. Anon. Garlic. In Blumenthal M, Goldberg A, Brinckmann J, eds. Herbal Medicine – Expanded Commission E Monographs, 1st edn. Newton, MA: Integrative Medical Communications, 2000: 139–48

111. Agarwal KC. Therapeutic actions of garlic constituents. Med Res Rev 1996; 16: 111–24

112. Le Bars PL, Katz MM, Berman N, et al. A placebo-controlled, double-blind, randomized trial of an extract of Ginkgo biloba for dementia. North American EGb Study Group. J Am Med Assoc 1997; 278: 1327–32

113. Oken BS, Storzbach DM, Kaye JA. The efficacy of Ginkgo biloba on cognitive function in Alzheimer disease. Arch Neurol 1998; 55: 1409–15

114. Kurtz A, Van Baelen B. Ginkgo biloba compared with cholinesterase inhibitors in the treatment of dementia: a review based on meta-analyses by the cochrane collaboration. Dement Geriatr Cogn Disord 2004; 18: 217–26

115. Nathan PJ, Tanner S, Lloyd J, et al. Effects of a combined extract of Ginkgo biloba and Bacopa monniera on cognitive function in healthy humans. Hum Psychopharmacol 2004; 19: 91–6

116. Cieza A, Maier P, Poppel E. Effects of Ginkgo biloba on mental functioning in healthy volunteers. Arch Med Res 2003; 34: 373–81

117. Canter PH, Ernst E. Multiple n = 1 trials in the identification of responders and non-responders to the cognitive effects of Ginkgo biloba. Int J Clin Pharmacol Ther 2003; 41: 354–7

118. Canter PH, Ernst E. Ginkgo biloba: a smart drug? A systematic review of controlled trials of the cognitive effects of ginkgo biloba extracts in healthy people. Psychopharmacol Bull 2002; 36: 108–23

119. Nathan PJ, Ricketts E, Wesnes K, et al. The acute nootropic effects of Ginkgo biloba in healthy older human subjects: a preliminary investigation. Hum Psychopharmacol 2002; 17: 45–9

120. Moulton PL, Boyko LN, Fitzpatrick JL, Petros TV. The effect of Ginkgo biloba on memory in healthy male volunteers. Physiol Behav 2001; 73: 659–65

121. Stough C, Clarke J, Lloyd J, Nathan PJ. Neuropsychological changes after 30-day Ginkgo biloba administration in healthy participants. Int J Neuropsychopharmacol 2001; 4: 131–4

122. Kennedy DO, Scholey AB, Wesnes KA. The dose-dependent cognitive effects of acute administration of Ginkgo biloba to healthy young volunteers. Psychopharmacology (Berl) 2000; 151: 416–23

123. Rigney U, Kimber S, Hindmarch I. The effects of acute doses of standardized Ginkgo biloba extract on memory and psychomotor performance in volunteers. Phytother Res 1999; 13: 408–15

124. Ernst E. [Ginkgo biloba in treatment of intermittent claudication. A systemic research based on controlled studies in the literature]. Fortschr Med 1996; 114: 85–7

125. Bartlett H, Eperjesi F. An ideal ocular nutritional supplement? Ophthal Physiol Opt 2004; 24: 339–49

126. Evans JR. Ginkgo biloba extract for age-related macular degeneration. Cochrane Database Syst Rev 2000: CD001775

127. Issing W, Klein P, Weiser M. The homeopathic preparation Vertigoheel versus Ginkgo biloba in the treatment of vertigo in an elderly population: a double-blinded, randomized, controlled clinical trial. J Altern Complement Med 2005; 11: 155–60

128. Schneider B, Klein P, Weiser M. Treatment of vertigo with a homeopathic complex remedy compared with usual treatments: a meta-analysis of clinical trials. Arzneimittelforschung 2005; 55: 23–9

129. Cesarani A, Meloni F, Alpini D, et al. Ginkgo biloba (EGb 761) in the treatment of equilibrium disorders. Adv Ther 1998; 15: 291–304

130. Ernst E, Stevinson C. Ginkgo biloba for tinnitus: a review. Clin Otolaryngol 1999; 24: 164–7

131. Wheatley D. Triple-blind, placebo-controlled trial of Ginkgo biloba in sexual dysfunction due to antidepressant drugs. Hum Psychopharmacol 2004; 19: 545–8

132. Kang BJ, Lee SJ, Kim MD, Cho MJ. A placebo-controlled, double-blind trial of Ginkgo biloba for antidepressant-induced sexual dysfunction. Hum Psychopharmacol 2002; 17: 279–84

133. Cohen AJ, Bartlik B. Ginkgo biloba for antidepressant-induced sexual dysfunction. J Sex Marital Ther 1998; 24: 139–43

134. Roncin JP, Schwartz F, D'Arbigny P. EGb 761 in control of acute mountain sickness and vascular reactivity to cold exposure. Aviat Space Environ Med 1996; 67: 445–52

135. Smith PF, Zheng Y, Darlington CL. Ginkgo biloba extracts for tinnitus: more hype than hope? J Ethnopharmacol 2005; 100: 95–9

136. Rejali D, Sivakumar A, Balaji N. Ginkgo biloba does not benefit patients with tinnitus: a randomized placebo-controlled double-blind trial and meta-analysis of randomized trials. Clin Otolaryngol Allied Sci 2004; 29: 226–31

137. Hilton M, Stuart E. Ginkgo biloba for tinnitus. Cochrane Database Syst Rev 2004; 2: CD003852

138. Schneider D, Schneider L, Shulman A, et al. Gingko biloba (Rokan) therapy in tinnitus patients and measurable interactions between tinnitus and vestibular disturbances. Int Tinnitus J 2000; 6: 56–62

139. DeBisschop M. Gingko ineffective for tinnitus. J Fam Pract 2003; 52: 766–9

140. Jung F, Mrowietz C, Kiesewetter H, Wenzel E. Effect of Ginkgo biloba on fluidity of blood and peripheral microcirculation in volunteers. Arzneimittelforschung 1990; 40: 589–93

141. Maitra I, Marcocci L, Droy-Lefaix MT, Packer L. Peroxyl radical scavenging activity of Ginkgo biloba extract EGb 761. Biochem Pharmacol 1995; 49: 1649–55

142. Hoyer S, Lannert H, Noldner M, Chatterjee SS. Damaged neuronal energy metabolism and behavior are improved by Ginkgo biloba extract (EGb 761). J Neural Transm Gen Sect 1999; 106: 1171–88

143. Huguet F, Tarrade T. Alpha 2-adrenoceptor changes during cerebral ageing. The effect of Ginkgo biloba extract. J Pharm Pharmacol 1992; 44: 24–7

144. Chung KF, Dent G, McCusker M, et al. Effect of a ginkgolide mixture (BN 52063) in antagonising skin and platelet responses to platelet activating factor in man. Lancet 1987; 1: 248–51

145. Oyama Y, Fuchs PA, Katayama N, Noda K. Myricetin and quercetin, the flavonoid constituents of Ginkgo biloba extract, greatly reduced oxidative metabolism in both resting and Ca2+ loaded brain neurons. Brain Res 1994; 635: 125–9

146. Cheung F, Siow YL, Chen WZ, O K. Inhibitory effect of Ginkgo biloba on the expression of inducible nitric oxide synthase in endothelial cells. Biochem Pharmacol 1999; 58: 1665–73

147. Lamant V, Mauco G, Braquet P, et al. Inhibition of the metabolism of platelet activating factor (PAF-acether) by three specific antagonists from Ginkgo biloba. Biochem Pharmacol 1987; 36: 2749–52

148. Kornecki E, Ehrlich YH. Neuroregulatory and neuropathological actions of the ether–phospholipid platelet-activating factor. Science 1988; 240: 1792–4

149. Akisu M, Kultursay N, Coker I, Huseyinov A. Platelet-activating factor is an important mediator in hypoxic ischemic brain injury in the newborn rat. Flunarizine and Ginkgo biloba extract reduce PAF concentration in the brain. Biol Neonate 1998; 74: 439–44

150. Birkle DL, Kurian P, Braquet P, Bazan NG. Platelet-activating factor antagonist BN 52021 decreases accumulation of free polyunsaturated fatty acid in mouse brain during ischemia and electroconvulsive shock. J Neurochem 1988; 51: 1900–5

151. Umegaki K, Shinozuka K, Watarai K, et al. Ginkgo biloba extract attenuates the development of hypertension in deoxycorticosterone acetate-salt hypertensive rats. Clin Exp Pharmacol Physiol 2000; 27: 277–82

152. Sloley BD, Urichuk LJ, Morley P, et al. Identification of kaempferol as a monoamine oxidase inhibitor and potential neuroprotectant in extracts of Ginkgo biloba leaves. J Pharm Pharmacol 2000; 52: 451–9

153. Pardon MC, Joubert C, Perez-Diaz F, et al. In vivo regulation of cerebral monoamine oxidase activity in senescent controls and chronically stressed mice by long-term treatment with Ginkgo biloba extract (EGb 761). Mech Ageing Dev 2000; 113: 157–68

154. Fowler JS, Wang GJ, Volkow ND, et al. Evidence that Ginkgo biloba extract does not inhibit MAO A and MAO B in living human brain. Life Sci 2000; 66: PL141–6

155. Watson DG, Oliveira EJ. Solid-phase extraction and gas chromatography–mass spectrometry determination of kaempferol and quercetin in human urine after consumption of Ginkgo biloba tablets. J Chromatogr B Biomed Sci Appl 1999; 723: 203–10

156. Anon. Ginkgo. In Mills S, Bone K, eds. Principles and Practice of Phytotherapy. New York, NY: Churchill Livingstone, 2000: 404–17

157. Koch E. Inhibition of platelet activating factor (PAF)-induced aggregation of human thrombocytes by ginkgolides: considerations on possible bleeding complications after oral intake of Ginkgo biloba extracts. Phytomedicine 2005; 12: 10–16

158. Destro MW, Speranzini MB, Cavalheiro Filho C, et al. Bilateral haematoma after rhytidoplasty and blepharoplasty following chronic use of Ginkgo biloba. Br J Plast Surg 2005; 58: 100–1

159. Rowin J, Lewis SL. Spontaneous bilateral subdural hematomas associated with chronic Ginkgo biloba ingestion. Neurology 1996; 46: 1775–6

160. Vale S. Subarachnoid haemorrhage associated with Ginkgo biloba. Lancet 1998; 352: 36

161. Gilbert GJ. Ginkgo biloba [letter]. Neurology 1997; 48: 1137

162. Matthews MK Jr. Association of Ginkgo biloba with intracerebral hemorrhage [letter]. Neurology 1998; 50: 1933–4

163. Rosenblatt M, Mindel J. Spontaneous hyphema associated with ingestion of Ginkgo biloba extract [letter]. N Engl J Med 1997; 336: 1108

164. Fessenden JM, Wittenborn W, Clarke L. Gingko biloba: a case report of herbal medicine and bleeding postoperatively from a laparoscopic cholecystectomy. Am Surg 2001; 67: 33–5

165. Bressler R. Herb–drug interactions: interactions between Ginkgo biloba and prescription medications. Geriatrics 2005; 60: 30–3

166. Bartlett H, Eperjesi F. Possible contraindications and adverse reactions associated with the use of ocular nutritional supplements. Ophthalmic Physiol Opt 2005; 25: 179–94

167. Ciocon JO, Ciocon DG, Galindo DJ. Dietary supplements in primary care. Botanicals can affect surgical outcomes and follow-up. Geriatrics 2004; 59: 20–4

168. Williamson EM. Drug interactions between herbal and prescription medicines. Drug Safety 2003; 26: 1075–92

169. Abebe W. Herbal medication: potential for adverse interactions with analgesic drugs. J Clin Pharm Ther 2002; 27: 391–401

170. Brekham II, Dardymov IV. New substances of plant origin which increase nonspecific resistance. Annu Rev Pharmacol 1969; 9: 419–30

171. Chong SK, Oberholzer VG. Ginseng – is there a use in clinical medicine? Postgrad Med J 1988; 64: 841–6

172. Hartz AJ, Bentler S, Noyes R, et al. Randomized controlled trial of Siberian ginseng for chronic fatigue. Psychol Med 2004; 34: 51–61

173. Wang BX, Cui JC, Liu AJ, Wu SK. Studies on the anti-fatigue effect of the saponins of stems and leaves of Panax ginseng (SSLG). J Trad Chin Med 1983; 3: 89–94

174. Yang G, Yu Y. Immunopotentiating effect of traditional Chinese drugs – ginsenoside and glycyrrhiza polysaccharide. Proc Chin Acad Med Sci Peking Union Med Coll 1990; 5: 188–93

175. Helms S. Cancer prevention and therapeutics: Panax ginseng. Altern Med Rev 2004; 9: 259–74

176. Chang YS, Seo EK, Gyllenhaal C, Block KI. Panax ginseng: a role in cancer therapy? Integr Cancer Ther 2003; 2: 13–33

177. Shin HR, Kim JY, Yun TK, et al. The cancer-preventive potential of Panax ginseng: a review of human and experimental evidence. Cancer Causes Control 2000; 11: 565–76

178. Shin HR, Kim JY, Yun TK, et al. The cancer-preventive potential of Panax ginseng: a review of human and experimental evidence. Cancer Causes Control 2000; 11: 565–76

179. Zhou W, Chai H, Lin PH, et al. Molecular mechanisms and clinical applications of ginseng root for cardiovascular disease. Med Sci Monit 2004; 10: RA187–92

180. Chen X. Cardiovascular protection by ginsenosides and their nitric oxide releasing action. Clin Exp Pharmacol Physiol 1996; 23: 728–32

181. Vuksan V, Sievenpiper JL, Koo VY, et al. American ginseng (Panax quinquefolius L) reduces postprandial glycemia in nondiabetic subjects and subject with type 2 diabetes mellitus. Arch Intern Med 2000; 160: 1009–13

182. Lieberman HR. The effects of ginseng, ephedrine, and caffeine on cognitive performance, mood and energy. Nutr Rev 2001; 59: 91–102

183. Cho YK, Sung H, Lee HJ, et al. Long-term intake of Korean red ginseng in HIV-1-infected patients: development of resistance mutation to zidovudine is delayed. Int Immunopharmacol 2001; 1: 1295–305

184. Hong B, Ji YH, Hong JH, et al. A double-blind crossover study evaluating the efficacy of Korean red ginseng in patients with erectile dysfunction: a preliminary report. J Urol 2002; 168: 2070–3

185. Choi YD, Rha KH, Choi HK. In vitro and in vivo experimental effect of Korean red ginseng on erection. J Urol 1999; 162: 1508–11

186. Bahrke MS, Morgan WP. Evaluation of the ergogenic properties of ginseng. Sports Med 1994; 18: 229–48

187. Bahrke MS, Morgan WP. Evaluation of the ergogenic properties of ginseng: an update. Sports Med 2000; 29: 113–33

188. Vogler BK, Pittler MH, Ernst E. The efficacy of ginseng. A systematic review of randomised clinical trials. Eur J Clin Pharmacol 1999; 55: 567–75

189. Anon. Ginseng. In Blumenthal M, Busse WR, Goldberg A, et al., eds. The Complete German Commission E Monographs: Therapeutic Guide to Herbal Medicines, 1st edn. Boston, MA: Integrative Medical Communications, 1998

190. Attele AS, Wu JA, Yuan CS. Ginseng pharmacology: multiple constituents and multiple actions. Biochem Pharmacol 1999; 58: 1685–93

191. Benishin CG, Lee R, Wang LCH, Liu HJ. Effects of ginsenoside Rb1 on central cholinergic metabolism. Pharmacology 1991; 42: 223–9

192. Yamaguchi Y, Haruta K, Kobayashi H. Effects on ginsenosides on impaired performance induced in the rat by scopolamine in a radial-arm maze. Psychoneuroendocrinology 1995; 20: 645–53

193. Lim JH, Wen TC, Matsuda S, et al. Protection of ischemic hippocampal neurons by ginsenoside Rb1, a main ingredient of ginseng root. Neurosci Res Suppl 1997; 28: 191–200

194. Takemoto Y, Ueyama T, Saito H, et al. Potentiation of nerve growth factor-mediated nerve fiber production in organ cultures of chicken embryonic ganglia by ginseng saponins: structure–activity relationship. Chem Pharm Bull (Tokyo) 1984; 32: 3128–33

195. Mogil JS, Shin YH, McCleskey EW, et al. Ginsenoside Rf, a trace component of ginseng root, produces antinociception in mice. Brain Res 1998; 792: 218–28

196. Nah JJ, Hahn JH, Chung S, et al. Effect of ginsenosides, active components of ginseng, on capsaicin-induced pain-related behavior. Neuropharmacology 2000; 39: 2180–4

197. Suh HW, Song DK, Huh SO, Kim YH. Modulatory role of ginsenosides injected intrathecally or intracerebroventricularly in the production of antinociception induced by kappa-opioid receptor agonist administered intracerebroventricularly in the mouse. Planta Med 2000; 66: 412–17

198. Huong NT, Matsumoto K, Yamasaki K, et al. Majonoside-R2, a major constituent of Vietnamese ginseng, attenuates opioid-induced antinociception. Pharmacol Biochem Behav 1997; 57: 285–91

199. Kimura T, Saunders PA, Kim HS, et al. Interactions of ginsenosides with ligand-bindings of GABA(A) and GABA(B) receptors. Gen Pharmacol 1994; 25: 193–9

200. Yuan CS, Attele AS, Wu JA, Liu D. Modulation of American ginseng on brainstem GABAergic effects rats. J Ethnopharmacol 1998; 62: 215–22

201. Tsang D, Yeung HW, Tso WW, Peck H. Ginseng saponins: influence of neurotransmitter uptake in rat brain synaptosomes. Planta Med 1985; 3: 221–4

202. Gillis CN. Panax ginseng pharmacology: a nitric oxide link. Biochem Pharmacol 1997; 54: 1–8

203. Siegel RK. Ginseng abuse syndrome. Problems with the panacea. J Am Med Assoc 1979; 241: 1614–15

204. Zhan Y, Xu XH, Jiang YP. [Protective effects of ginsenoside on myocardial ischemic and reperfusion injuries]. Chung Hau I Hsueh Tsa Chih 1994; 74: 626–8

205. Yun TK. Experimental and epidemiological evidence of the cancer-preventive effects of Panax ginseng C.A. Meyer. Nutr Rev 1996; 54: S71–81

206. Yun YS, Moon HS, Oh YR, et al. Effect of red ginseng on natural killer cell activity in mice with lung adenoma induced by urethane and benzo(a)pyrene. Cancer Detect Prev Suppl 1987; 1: 301–9

207. Kim JY, Germolec DR, Luster MI. Panax ginseng as a potential immunomodulator: studies in mice. Immunopharmacol Immunotoxicol 1990; 12: 257–76

208. Kenarova B, Neychev H, Hadjiivanova C, Petkov VD. Immunomodulating activity of ginsenoside Rg1 from Panax ginseng. Jpn J Pharmacol 1990; 54: 447–54

209. Scaglione F, Cattaneo G, Alessandria M, Cogo R. Efficacy and safety of the standardised Ginseng extract G115 for potentiating vaccination against the influenza syndrome and protection against the common cold. Drugs Exp Clin Res 1996; 22: 65–72

210. Chen SE, Sawchuk RJ, Staba EJ. American ginseng. III. Pharmacokinetics of ginsenosides in the rabbit. Eur J Drug Metab Pharmacokinet 1980; 5: 161–8

211. Hopkins MP, Androff L, Benninghoff AS. Ginseng face cream and unexplained vaginal bleeding. Am J Obstet Gynecol 1988; 159: 1121–2

212. Palop-Larrea V, Gonzalvez-Perales JL, Catalan-Oliver C, et al. Metrorrhagia and ginseng [letter]. Ann Pharmacother 2000; 34: 1347–8

213. Greenspan EM. Ginseng and vaginal bleeding [letter]. J Am Med Assoc 1983; 249: 2018

214. Punnonen R, Lukola A. Oestrogen-like effect of ginseng. Br Med J 1980; 281: 1110

215. Jones BD, Runikis AM. Interaction of ginseng with phenelzine [letter]. J Clin Psychopharmacol 1987; 7: 201–2

216. Ryu SJ, Chien YY. Ginseng-associated cerebral arteritis. Neurology 1995; 45: 829–30

217. Janetzky K, Morreale AP. Probable interaction between warfarin and ginseng. Am J Health-Sys Pharm 1997; 54: 692–3

218. Kimura Y, Okuda H, Arichi S. Effects of various ginseng saponins on 5-hydroxytryptamine release and aggregation in human platelets. J Pharm Pharmacol 1988; 40: 838–43

219. Kuo SC, Teng CM, Lee JC, et al. Antiplatelet components in Panax ginseng. Planta Med 1990; 56: 164–7

220. Park HJ, Lee JH, Song YB, Park KH. Effects of dietary supplementation of lipophilic fraction from Panax ginseng on cGMP and cAMP in rat platelets and on blood coagulation. Biol Pharm Bull 1996; 19: 1434–9

221. Anon. Ginseng. In Gruenwald J, Brendler T, Jaenicke C, eds. PDR for Herbal Medicines, 2nd edn. Montvale, NJ: Medical Economics Company, 2000: 346–51

222. Anon. Kava. Lancet 1988; 2: 258–9

223. Cawte J. Parameters of kava used as a challenge to alcohol. Aust N Z J Psychiatry 1986; 20: 70–6

224. Cawte J. Macabre effects of a 'cult' for kava [editorial]. Med J Aust 1988; 148: 545–6

225. Mathews JD, Riley MD, Fejo L, et al. Effects of the heavy usage of kava on physical health: summary of a pilot survey in an aboriginal community. Med J Aust 1988; 148: 548–55

226. Herberg KW. [Effect of Kava-Special Extract WS 1490 combined with ethyl alcohol on safety-relevant performance parameters.] Blutalkohol 1993; 30: 96–105

227. Ernst E. The risk–benefit profile of commonly used herbal therapies: ginkgo, St. John's wort, ginseng, echinacea, saw palmetto, and kava. Ann Intern Med 2002; 136: 42–53

228. Geier FP, Konstantinowicz T. Kava treatment in patients with anxiety. Phytother Res 2004; 18: 297–300

229. Lehrl S. Clinical efficacy of kava extract WS 1490 in sleep disturbances associated with anxiety disorders. Results of a multicenter, randomized, placebo-controlled, double-blind clinical trial. J Affect Disord 2004; 78: 101–10

230. Gastpar M, Klimm HD. Treatment of anxiety, tension and restlessness states with kava special extract WS 1490 in general practice: a randomized placebo-controlled double-blind multicenter trial. Phytomedicine 2003; 10: 631–9

231. Volz HP, Kieser M. Kava-kava extract WS 1490 versus placebo in anxiety disorders – a randomized placebo-controlled 25-week outpatient trial. Pharmacopsychiatry 1997; 30: 1–5

232. Neuhaus W, Ghaemi Y, Schmidt T, Lehmann E. [Treatment of perioperative anxiety in suspected breast carcinoma with a phytogenic tranquilizer.] Zentralbl Gynakol 2000; 122: 561–5

233. Sun J. Morning/evening menopausal formula relieves menopausal symptoms: a pilot study. J Altern Complement Med 2003; 9: 403–9

234. De Leo V, La Marca A, Morgante G, et al. Evaluation of combining kava extract with hormone replacement therapy in the treatment of postmenopausal anxiety. Maturitas 2001; 39: 185–8

235. De Leo V, La Marca A, Lanzetta D, et al. [Assessment of the association of kava-kava extract and hormone replacement therapy in the treatment of postmenopause anxiety]. Minerva Ginecol 2000; 52: 263–7

236. Witte S, Loew D, Gaus W. Meta-analysis of the efficacy of the acetonic kava-kava extract WS1490 in patients with non-psychotic anxiety disorders. Phytother Res 2005; 19: 183–8

237. Pittler MH, Ernst E. Kava extract for treating anxiety. Cochrane Database Syst Rev 2003; 1: CD003383

238. Stevinson C, Huntley A, Ernst E. A systematic review of the safety of kava extract in the treatment of anxiety. Drug Safety 2002; 25: 251–61

239. Pittler MH, Ernst E. Efficacy of kava extract for treating anxiety: systematic review and meta-analysis. J Clin Psychopharmacol 2000; 20: 84–9

240. Wheatley D. Medicinal plants for insomnia: a review of their pharmacology, efficacy and tolerability. J Psychopharmacol 2005; 19: 414–21

241. Jussofie A, Schmiz A, Hiemke C. Kavapyrone enriched extract from Piper methysticum as modulator of the GABA binding site in different regions of rat brain. Psychopharmacology (Berl) 1994; 116: 469–74

242. Keledjian J, Duffield PH, Jamieson DD, et al. Uptake into mouse brain of four compounds present in the psychoactive beverage kava. J Pharm Sci 1988; 77: 1003–6

243. Rasmussen AK, Scheline RR, Solheim E, Hansel R. Metabolism of some kava pyrones in the rat. Xenobiotica 1979; 9: 1–16

244. Bilia AR, Scalise L, Bergonzi MC, Vincieri FF. Analysis of kavalactones from Piper methysticum (kava-kava). J Chromatogr B Analyt Technol Biomed Life Sci 2004; 812: 203–14

245. Cote CS, Kor C, Cohen J, Auclair K. Composition and biological activity of traditional and commercial kava extracts. Biochem Biophys Res Commun 2004; 322: 147–52

246. Cheng D, Lidgard RO, Duffield PH, et al. Identification by methane chemical ionization gas chromatography/mass spectrometry of the products obtained by steam distillation and aqueous extraction of commercial Piper methysticum. Biomed Environ Mass Spectrom 1988; 17: 371–6

247. Klohs MW. Chemistry of kava. Psychopharmacol Bull 1967; 4; 10

248. Meyer HJ. Pharmacology of kava – 1. Psychopharmacol Bull 1967; 4: 10–11

249. Buckley JP, Furgiuele AR, O'Hara MJ. Pharmacology of kava – 2. Psychopharmacol Bull 1967; 4: 11–12

250. Hu L, Jhoo JW, Ang CY, et al. Determination of six kavalactones in dietary supplements and selected functional foods containing Piper methysticum by isocratic liquid chromatography with internal standard. J AOAC Int 2005; 88: 16–25

251. Backhauss C, Krieglstein J. Extract of kava (Piper methysticum) and its methysticin constituents protect brain tissue against ischemic damage in rodents. Eur J Pharmacol 1992; 215: 265–9

252. Heinze HJ, Munthe TF, Steitz J, Matzke M. Pharmacopsychological effects of oxazepam and kava-extract in a visual search paradigm assessed with event-related potentials. Pharmacopsychiatry 1994; 27: 224–30

253. Munte TF, Heinze HJ, Matzke M, Steitz J. Effects of oxazepam and an extract of kava roots (Piper methysticum) on event-related potentials in a word recognition task. Neuropsychobiology 1993; 27: 46–53

254. Jamieson DD, Duffield PH, Cheng D, Duffield AM. Comparison of the central nervous system activity of the aqueous and lipid extract of kava (Piper methysticum). Arch Int Pharmacodyn Ther 1989; 301: 66–80

255. Davies LP, Drew CA, Duffield P, et al. Kava pyrones and resin: studies on GABA(A), GABA(B), and benzodiazepine binding sites in rodent brain. Pharmacol Toxicol 1992; 71: 120–6

256. Friese J, Gleitz J. Kavain, dihydrokavain and dihydromethysticin non-competitively inhibit the specific binding of [3H]-batrachotoxinin-A 20-α-benzoate to receptor site 2 of voltage-gated Na$^+$ channels. Planta Med 1998; 64: 458–9

257. Magura EI, Kopanitsa MV, Gleitz J, Peters T, Krishtal OA. Kava extract ingredients, (+)-methystin and (±)-kavain inhibit voltage-operated Na(+)-channels in rat CA1 hippocampal neurons. Neuroscience 1997; 81: 345–51

258. Gleitz J, Friese J, Beile A, et al. Anticonvulsive action of (±)-kavain estimated from its properties on stimulated synaptosomes and Na$^+$ channel receptor sites. Eur J Pharmacol 1996; 315: 89–97

259. Gleitz J, Beile A, Peters T. (±)-Kavain inhibits veratridine-activated voltage-dependent Na(+) channels in synaptosomes prepared from rat cerebral cortex. Neuropharmacology 1995; 34: 1133–8

260. Baum SS, Hill R, Rommelspacher H. Effect of kava extract and individual kavapyrones on neurotransmitter levels in the nucleus accumbens of rats. Prog Neuropsychopharmacol Biol Psychiatry 1998; 22: 1105–20

261. Schelosky L, Raffauf C, Jendroska K, Poewe W. Kava and dopamine antagonism [letter]. J Neurol Neurosurg Psychiatry 1995; 58: 639–40

262. Pepping J. Kava: Piper methysticum. Am J Health-Syst Pharm 1999; 56: 957–8

263. Clouatre DL. Kava kava: examining new reports of toxicity. Toxicol Lett 2004; 150: 85–96

264. Almeida JC, Grimsley EW. Coma from the health food store: interaction between kava and alprazolam. Ann Intern Med 1996; 125: 940–1

265. Norton SA, Ruze P. Kava dermopathy. J Am Acad Dermatol 1994; 31: 89–97

266. Pittler MH, Ernst E. Efficacy of kava extract for treating anxiety: systematic review and meta-analysis. J Clin Psychopharmacol 2000; 20: 84–9

267. Russmann S, Lauterburg BH, Helbling A. Kava hepatotoxicity. Ann Intern Med 2001; 35: 68–9

268. Escher M, Desmeules J, Giostra E, Mentha G. Hepatitis associated with kava, a herbal remedy for anxiety. Br Med J 2001; 322: 139

269. Anon. Kava kava. In Gruenwald J, Brendler T, Jaenicke C, eds. PDR for Herbal Medicines, 2nd edn. Montvale, NJ: Medical Economics Company, 2000: 443–6

270. Boerth J, Strong KM. The clinical utility of milk thistle (Silybum marianum) in cirrhosis of the liver. J Herb Pharmacother 2002; 2: 11–17

271. Bean P. The use of alternative medicine in the treatment of hepatitis C. Am Clin Lab 2002; 21: 19–21

272. Tanamly MD, Tadros F, Labeeb S, et al. Randomised double-blinded trial evaluating silymarin for chronic hepatitis C in an Egyptian village: study description and 12-month results. Dig Liver Dis 2004; 36: 752–9

273. Arteel G, Marsano L, Mendez C, et al. Advances in alcoholic liver disease. Best Pract Res Clin Gastroenterol 2003; 17: 625–47

274. Giese LA. Milk thistle and the treatment of hepatitis. Gastroenterol Nurs 2001; 24: 95–7

275. Saller R, Meier R, Brignoli R. The use of silymarin in the treatment of liver diseases. Drugs 2001; 61: 2035–63

276. Ferenci P, Dragosics B, Dittrich H, et al. Randomized controlled trial of silymarin treatment in patients with cirrhosis of the liver. J Hepatol 1989; 9: 105–13

277. Lang I, Nekam K, Deak G, et al. Immunomodulatory and hepatoprotective effects of in vivo treatment with free radical scavengers. Ital J Gastroenterol 1990; 22: 283–7

278. Salmi HA, Sarna S. Effect of silymarin on chemical, functional, and morphological alterations of the liver. A double-blind controlled study. Scand J Gastroenterol 1982; 17: 517–21

279. Magliulo E, Gagliardi B, Fiori GP. [Results of a double blind study on the effect of silymarin in the treatment of acute viral hepatitis, carried out at two medical centres (author's transl).] Med Klin 1978; 73: 1060–5

280. Rambaldi A, Jacobs BP, Iaquinto G, Gluud C. Milk thistle for alcoholic and/or hepatitis B or C virus liver diseases. Cochrane Database Syst Rev 2005; 18: CD003620

281. Pares A, Planas R, Torres M, et al. Effects of silymarin in alcoholic patients with cirrhosis of the liver: results of a controlled, double-blind, randomized and multicenter trial. J Hepatol 1998; 28: 615–21

282. Bunout D, Hirsch S, Petermann M, et al. [Controlled study of the effect of silymarin on alcoholic liver disease]. Rev Med Chil 1992; 120: 1370–5

283. Trinchet JC, Coste T, Levy VG, et al. [Treatment of alcoholic hepatitis with silymarin. A double-blind comparative study in 116 patients.] Gastroenterol Clin Biol 1989; 13: 120–4

284. Saller R, Meier R, Brignoli R. The use of silymarin in the treatment of liver diseases. Drugs 2001; 61: 2035–63

285. Tasduq SA, Peerzada K, Koul S, et al. Biochemical manifestations of anti-tuberculosis drugs induced hepatotoxicity and the effect of silymarin. Hepatol Res 2005; 31: 132–5

286. Agoston M, Orsi F, Feher E, et al. Silymarin and vitamin E reduce amiodarone-induced lysosomal phospholipidosis in rats. Toxicology 2003; 190: 231–41

287. Kosina P, Kren V, Gebhardt R, et al. Antioxidant properties of silybin glycosides. Phytother Res 2002; 16(Suppl 1): S33–9

288. Dehmlow C, Murawski N, de Groot H. Scavenging of reactive oxygen species and inhibition of arachidonic acid metabolism by silibinin in human cells. Life Sci 1996; 58: 1591–600

289. Bindoli A, Cavallini L, Siliprandi N. Inhibitory action of silymarin of lipid peroxide formation in rat liver mitochondria and microsomes. Biochem Pharmacol 1977; 26: 2405–9

290. Feher J, Lang I, Nekam K, et al. Effect of silibinin on the activity and expression of superoxide dismutase in lymphocytes from patients with chronic alcoholic liver disease. Free Radic Res Commun 1987; 3: 373–7

291. Tuchweber B, Sieck R, Trost W. Prevention of silybin of phalloidin-induced acute hepatoxicity. Toxicol Appl Pharmacol 1979; 51: 265–75

292. Magliulo E, Carosi PG, Minoli L, Gorini S. Studies on the regenerative capacity of the liver in rats subjected to partial hepatectomy and treated with silymarin. Arzneimittelforschung 1973; 23: 161–7

293. Shalan MG, Mostafa MS, Hassouna MM, et al. Amelioration of lead toxicity on rat liver with Vitamin C and silymarin supplements. Toxicology 2005; 206: 1–15

294. Pepping J. Milk thistle: Silybum marianum. Am J Health-Syst Pharm 1999; 56: 1195–7

295. Riley TR 3rd, Bhatti AM. Preventive strategies in chronic liver disease: part I. Alcohol, vaccines, toxic medications and supplements, diet and exercise. Am Fam Physician 2001; 64: 1555–60

296. Jacobs BP, Dennehy C, Ramirez G, et al. Milk thistle for the treatment of liver disease: a systematic review and meta-analysis. Am J Med 2002; 113: 506–15

297. Walti M, Neftel KA, Cohen M, et al. [Radioimmunologic detection of IgE and IgG antibodies against drugs. Conclusions after experience with over 1200 patients.] Schweiz Med Wochenschr 1986; 116: 303–5

298. Gong EM, Gerber GS. Saw palmetto and benign prostatic hyperplasia. Am J Chin Med 2004; 32: 331–8

299. Berry SL, Coffey DS, Walsh PC, Ewing LL. The development of human benign prostatic hyperplasia with age. J Urol 1984; 132: 474–9

300. Buck AC. Phytotherapy for the prostate. Br J Urol 1996; 78: 325–36

301. Gerber GS, Fitzpatrick JM. The role of a lipido-sterolic extract of Serenoa repens in the management of lower urinary tract symptoms associated with benign prostatic hyperplasia. BJU Int 2004; 94: 338–44

302. Wilt T, Ishani A, Stark G, et al. Serenoa repens for benign prostatic hyperplasia. Cochrane Database Syst Rev 2000; (2) CD001423

303. Gerber GS. Saw palmetto for the treatment of men with lower urinary tract symptoms. J Urol 2000; 163: 1408–12

304. Gerber GS, Zagaja GP, Bales GT, et al. Saw palmetto (Serenoa repens) in men with lower urinary tract symptoms: effects on urodynamic parameters and voiding symptoms. Urology 1998; 51: 1003–7

305. Anon. Saw palmetto berry. In Blumenthal M, Goldberg A, Brinckmann J, eds. Herbal Medicine – Expanded Commission E Monographs, 1st edn. Newton, MA: Integrative Medical Communications, 2000: 335–40

306. Iehle C, Delos S, Guirou O, et al. Human prostatic steroid 5 alpha-reductase isoforms – a comparative study of selective inhibitors. J Steroid Biochem Mol Biol 1995; 54: 273–9

307. Plosker GL, Brogden RN. Serenoa repens (Permixon). A review of its pharmacology and therapeutic efficacy in benign prostatic hyperplasia. Drugs Aging 1996; 9: 379–95

308. Di Silverio F, D'Eramo G, Lubrano C, et al. Evidence that Serenoa repens extract displays an antiestrogenic activity in prostatic tissue of benign prostatic hypertrophy patients. Eur Urol 1992; 21: 309–14

309. Vacher P, Prevarskaya N, Skyrma R, et al. The lipidosterolic extract from Serenoa repens interferes with prolactin receptor signal transduction. J Biomed Sci 1995; 2: 357–65

310. Paubert-Braquet M, Cousse H, Raynaud JP, et al. Effect of the lipidosterolic extract of Serenoa repens (Permixon) and its major components on basic fibroblast growth factor-induced proliferation of cultures of human prostate biopsies. Eur Urol 1998; 33: 340–7

311. Vacherot F, Azzouz M, Gil-Diez-de-Medina S, et al. Induction of apoptosis and inhibition of cell proliferation by the lipodosterolic extract of Serenoa repens (LSESr, Permixon) in benign prostatic hyperplasia. Prostate 2000; 45: 259–66

312. Goepel M, Hecker U, Krege S, et al. Saw palmetto extracts potently and noncompetitively inhibit human alpha-1-adreno-ceptors in vitro. Prostate 1999; 38: 208–15

313. Brue W, Hagenlocer M, Redl K, et al. [Anti-inflammatory activity of sabal fruit extracts prepared with supercritical carbon dioxide. In vitro antagonists of cyclooxygenase and 5-lipooxygenase metabolism.] Arzneimittelforschung 1992; 42: 547–51

314. Paubert-Braquet M, Mencia Huerta JM, Cousse H, Braquet P. Effect of the lipidic lipidosterolic extract of Serenoa repens (Permixon) on the ionophore A23187-stimulated production of leukotriene B4 (LTB4) from human polymorphonuclear neutrophils. Prostaglandins Leukot Essent Fatty Acids 1997; 57: 299–304

315. Cheema P, El-Mefty O, Jazieh AR. Intraoperative haemorrhage associated with the use of extract of saw palmetto herb: a case report and review of literature. J Intern Med 2001; 250: 167–9

316. Linde K, Knuppel L. Large-scale observational studies of hypericum extracts in patients with depressive disorders – a systematic review. Phytomedicine 2005; 12: 148–57

317. Whiskey E, Werneke U, Taylor D. A systematic review and meta-analysis of Hypericum perforatum in depression: a comprehensive clinical review. Int Clin Psychopharmacol 2001; 16: 239–52

318. Kim HL, Streltzer J, Goebert D. St. John's wort for depression: a meta-analysis of well-defined clinical trials. J Nerv Ment Dis 1999; 187: 532–8

319. Linde K, Ramirez G, Mulrow CD, et al. St John's wort for depression – an overview and meta-analysis of randomised clinical trials. Br Med J 1996; 313: 253–8

320. Williams JW Jr, Mulrow CD, Chiquette E, et al. A systematic review of newer pharmacotherapies for depression in adults: evidence report summary. Ann Intern Med 2000; 132: 743–56

321. Hippius H. St. John's Wort (Hypericum perforatum) – a herbal antidepressant. Curr Med Res Opin 1998; 14: 171–84

322. Gaster B, Holroyd J. St John's wort for depression: a systematic review. Arch Intern Med 2000; 160: 152–6

323. Stevinson C, Ernst E. Hypericum for depression. An update of the clinical evidence. Eur Neuropsychopharmacol 1999; 9: 501–5

324. Josey ES, Tackett RL. St. John's wort: a new alternative for depression? Int J Clin Pharmacol Ther 1999; 37: 111–19

325. Kelly BD. St. John's wort for depression: what's the evidence? Hosp Med 2001; 62: 274–6

326. Linde K, Mulrow CD, Berner M, Egger M. St John's wort for depression. Cochrane Database Syst Rev 2005;2: CD000448

327. Linde K, Berner M, Egger M, Mulrow C. St John's wort for depression: meta-analysis of randomised controlled trials. Br J Psychiatry 2005; 186: 99–107

328. Shelton RC, Keller MB, Gelenberg A, et al. Effectiveness of St John's wort in major depression: a randomized controlled trial. J Am Med Assoc 2001; 285: 1978–86

329. Shultz V. Clinical trials with hypericum extracts in patients with depression – results, comparisons, conclusions for therapy with antidepressant drugs. Phytomedicine 2002; 9: 468–74

330. Trautmann-Sponsel RD, Dienel A. Safety of hypericum extract in mildly to moderately depressed outpatients: a review based on data from three randomized, placebo-controlled trials. J Affect Disord 2004; 82: 303–7

331. Rodriguez-Landa JF, Contreras CM. A review of clinical and experimental observations about antidepressant actions and side effects produced by Hypericum perforatum extracts. Phytomedicine 2003; 10: 688–99

332. Gupta RK, Moller HJ. St. John's Wort. An option for the primary care treatment of depressive patients? Eur Arch Psychiatry Clin Neurosci 2003; 253: 140–8

333. Vitiello B. Hypericum perforatum extracts as potential antidepressants. J Pharm Pharmacol 1999; 51: 513–17

334. Deltito J, Beyer D. The scientific, quasi-scientific and popular literature on the use of St. John's wort in the treatment of depression. J Affect Disord 1998; 51: 345–51

335. Nangia M, Syed W, Doraiswamy PM. Efficacy and safety of St. John's wort for the treatment of major depression. Public Health Nutr 2000; 3: 487–94

336. Field HL, Monti DA, Greeson JM, Kunkel EJ. St. John's wort. Int J Psychiatry Med 2000; 30: 203–19

337. Muller WE, Singer A, Wonnemann M, Hafner U, Rolli M, Schafer C. Hyperforin represents the neurotransmitter reuptake inhibiting constituent of hypericum extract. Pharmacopsychiatry 1998; 31 (Suppl 1): 16–21

338. Cott JM. In vitro receptor binding and enzyme inhibition by Hypericum perforatum extract. Pharmacopsychiatry 1997; 30 (Suppl 2): 108–12

339. Verotta L, Appendino G, Jakupovic J, Bombardelli E. Hyperforin analogues from St. John's wort (Hypericum perforatum). J Nat Prod 2000; 63: 412–15

340. Tian R, Koyabu N, Morimoto S, et al. Functional induction and de-induction of P-glycoprotein by St. John's wort and its ingredients in a human colon adenocarcinoma cell line. Drug Metab Dispos 2005; 33: 547–54

341. Calapai G, Crupi A, Firenzuoli F, et al. Serotonin, norepinephrine and dopamine involvement in the antidepressant action of Hypericum perforatum. Pharmacopsychiatry 2001; 34: 45–9

342. Franklin M, Chi J, McGavin C, et al. Neuroendocrine evidence for dopaminergic actions of hypericum extract (LI 160) in healthy volunteers. Biol Psychiatry 1999; 46: 581–4

343. Apaydin S, Zeybek U, Ince I, et al. Hypericum triquetrifolium Turra extract exhibits antinociceptive activity in the mouse. J Ethnopharmacol 1999; 67: 307–12

344. Kubin A, Wierrani F, Burner U, et al. Hypericin – the facts about a controversial agent. Curr Pharm Des 2005; 11: 233–53

345. Bladt S, Wagner H. Inhibition of MAO by fractions and constituents of hypericum extract. J Geriatr Psychiatry Neurol 1994; 7 (Suppl 1): S57–9

346. Thiede HM, Walper A. Inhibition of MAO and COMT by hypericum extracts and hypericin. J Geriatr Psychiatry Neurol 1994; 7 (Suppl 1): S54–6

347. Kerb R, Brockmoller J, Staffeldt B, et al. Single-dose and steady-state pharmacokinetics of hypericin and pseudohypericin. Antimicrob Agents Chemother 1996; 40: 2087–93

348. Biber A, Fischer H, Romer A, Chatterjee SS. Oral bioavailability of hyperforin from hypericum extracts in rats and human volunteers. Pharmacopsychiatry 1998; 31 (Suppl 1): 36–43

349. Beckman SE, Sommi RW, Switzer J. Consumer use of St. John's wort: a survey on effectiveness, safety, and tolerability. Pharmacotherapy 2000; 20: 568–74

350. Schulz V. Incidence and clinical relevance of the interaction and side effects of Hypericum preparations. Phytomedicine 2001; 8: 152–60

351. Brown TM. Acute St. John's wort toxicity [letter]. Am J Emerg Med 2000; 18: 231–2

352. Lantz MS, Buchalter E, Giambanco V. St. John's wort and antidepressant drug interactions in the elderly. J Geriatr Psychiatry Neurol 1999; 12: 7–10

353. Stevinson C, Ernst E. Can St. John's wort trigger psychoses? Int J Clin Pharmacol Ther 2004; 42: 473–80

354. Barbenel DM, Yusufi B, O'Shea D, Bench CJ. Mania in a patient receiving testosterone replacement postorchidectomy taking St. John's wort and sertraline. J Psychopharmacol 2000; 14: 84–6

355. Moses EL, Mallinger AG. St. John's wort: three cases of possible mania induction. J Clin Psychopharmacol 2000; 20: 115–17

356. Nierenberg AA, Burt T, Matthews J, Weiss AP. Mania associated with St. John's wort. Biol Psychiatry 1999; 46: 1707–8

357. Mannel M. Drug interactions with St John's wort: mechanisms and clinical implications. Drug Safety 2004; 27: 773–97

358. Bilia AR, Gallori S, Vincieri FF. St. John's wort and depression: efficacy, safety and tolerability – an update. Life Sci 2002; 70: 3077–96

359. Obach RS. Inhibition of human cytochrome P450 enzymes by constituents of St. John's wort, an herbal preparation used in the treatment of depression. J Pharmacol Exp Ther 2000; 294: 88–95

360. Ernst E. Second thoughts about safety of St. John's wort. Lancet 1999; 354: 2014–16

361. Piscitelli SC, Burstein AH, Chaitt D, et al. Indinavir concentrations and St. John's wort. Lancet 2000; 355: 547–8

362. Yue QY. Bergquist C, Gerden B. Safety of St. John's wort [letter]. Lancet 2000; 355: 576–7

363. Mai I, Stormer E, Bauer S, et al. Impact of St John's wort treatment on the pharmacokinetics of tacrolimus and mycophenolic acid in renal transplant patients. Nephrol Dial Transplant 2003; 18: 819–22

364. Ernst E. St John's Wort supplements endanger the success of organ transplantation. Arch Surg 2002; 137: 316–19

365. Turton-Weeks SM, Barone GW, Gurley BJ, et al. St John's wort: a hidden risk for transplant patients. Prog Transplant 2001; 11: 116–20

366. Moschella C, Jaber BL. Interaction between cyclosporine and Hypericum perforatum (St. John's wort) after organ transplantation. Am J Kidney Dis 2001; 38: 1105–7

367. Breidenbach T, Hoffmann MW, Becker T, et al. Drug interaction of St. John's wort with cyclosporin [letter]. Lancet 2000; 355: 1912

368. Ruschitzka F, Meier PJ, Turina M, et al. Acute heart transplant rejection due to Saint John's wort [letter]. Lancet 2000; 355: 548–9

369. Mai I, Stormer E, Bauer S, et al. Impact of St John's wort treatment on the pharmacokinetics of tacrolimus and mycophenolic acid in renal transplant patients. Nephrol Dial Transplant 2003; 18: 819–22

370. Johne A, Brockmoller J, Bauer S, et al. Pharmacokinetic interaction of digoxin with an herbal extract from St. John's wort (Hypericum perforatum). Clin Pharmacol Ther 1999; 66: 338–45

371. Anon. St. John's wort. In Blumenthal M, Goldberg A, Brinckmann J, eds. Herbal Medicine – Expanded Commission E Monographs, 1st edn. Newton, MA: Integrative Medical Communications, 2000: 359–66

372. Wheatley D. Medicinal plants for insomnia: a review of their pharmacology, efficacy and tolerability. J Psychopharmacol 2005; 19: 414–21

373. Anon. I read that the herbal supplement valerian helps people with insomnia fall asleep. Is valerian safe, and does it actually work? Mayo Clin Health Lett 2004; 22: 8

374. Shohet D, Wills RB, Stuart DL. Valepotriates and valerenic acids in commercial preparations of valerian available in Australia. Pharmazie 2001; 56: 860–3

375. Goppel M, Franz G. Stability control of valerian ground material and extracts: a new HPLC-method for the routine quantification of valerenic acids and lignans. Pharmazie 2004; 59: 446–52

376. Schumacher B, Scholle S, Holzl J, et al. Lignans isolated from valerian: identification and characterization of a new olivil derivative with partial agonistic activity at A(1) adenosine receptors. J Nat Prod 2002; 65: 1479–85

377. Wasowski C, Marder M, Viola H, et al. Isolation and identification of 6-methylapigenin, a competitive ligand for the brain GABA(A) receptors, from Valeriana wallichii. Planta Med 2002; 68: 934–6

378. Houghton PJ. The scientific basis for the reputed activity of valerian. J Pharm Pharmacol 1999; 51: 505–12

379. Mikell JR, Ganzera M, Khan IA. Analysis of sesquiterpenes in Valeriana officinalis by capillary electrophoresis. Pharmazie 2001; 56: 946–8

380. Gao XQ, Bjork L. Valerenic acid derivatives and valepotriates among individuals, varieties and species of Valeriana. Fitoterapia 2000; 71: 19–24

381. Dominguez RA, Bravo-Valverde RL, Kaplowitz BR, Cott JM. Valerian as a hypnotic for Hispanic patients. Cultur Divers Ethnic Minor Psychol 2000; 6: 84–92

382. Hendriks H, Bos R, Allersma DP, et al. Pharmacological screening of valerenal and some other components of essential oil of Valeriana officinalis. Planta Med 1981; 42: 62–8

383. Leuschner J, Muller J, Rudmann M. Characterization of the central nervous depressant activity of a commercially available valerian root extract. Arzneimittelforschung 1993; 43: 638–41

384. Sakamoto T, Mitani Y, Nakajima K. Psychotropic effects of Japanese valerian root extract. Chem Pharm Bull (Tokyo) 1992; 40: 758–61

385. Hazelhoff B, Malingre TM, Meijer DKF. Antispasmodic effects of valeriana compounds: an in-vivo and in-vitro study on the guinea-pig ileum. Arch Int Pharmacodyn Ther 1982; 257: 274–87

386. Herrera-Arellano A, Luna-Villegas G, Cuevas-Uriostegui ML, et al. Polysomnographic evaluation of the hypnotic effect of Valeriana edulis standardized extract in patients suffering from insomnia. Planta Med 2001; 67: 695–9

387. Vonderheid-Guth B, Todorova A, Brattstrom A, Dimpfel W. Pharmacodynamic effects of valerian and hops extract combination (Ze 91019) on the quantitative-topographical EEG in healthy volunteers. Eur J Med Res 2000; 5: 139–44

388. Leathwood PD, Chauffard F. Aqueous extract of valerian reduces latency to fall asleep in man. Planta Med 1985; 2: 144–8

389. Balderer G, Borbely AA. Effect of valerian on human sleep. Psychopharmacology (Berl) 1985; 87: 406–9

390. Leathwood PD, Chauffard F. Quantifying the effects of mild sedatives. J Psychiat Res 1982/83; 17: 115–22

391. Leathwood PD, Chauffard F, Heck E, Munoz-Box R. Aqueous extract of valerian root (Valeriana officinalis L.) improves sleep quality in man. Pharmacol Biochem Behav 1982; 17: 65–71

392. Donath F, Quispe S, Diefenbach K, et al. Critical evaluation of the effect of valerian extract on sleep structure and sleep quality. Pharmacopsychiatry 2000; 33: 47–53

393. Granger RE, Campbell EL, Johnston GA. (+)- And (-)-borneol: efficacious positive modulators of GABA action at human recombinant alpha1beta2gamma2L GABA(A) receptors. Biochem Pharmacol 2005; 69: 1101–11

394. Ortiz JG, Nieves-Natal J, Chavez P. Effects of Valeriana officinalis extracts on [3H]flunitrazepam binding, synaptosomal [3H]GABA uptake, and hippocampal [3H]GABA release. Neurochem Res 1999; 24: 1373–8

395. Santos MS, Ferreira F, Cunha AP, et al. Synaptosomal GABA release as influenced by valerian root extract – involvement of the GABA carrier. Arch Int Pharmacodyn Ther 1994; 327: 220–31

396. Santos MS, Ferreira F, Cunha AP, et al. An aqueous extract of valerian influences the transport of GABA in synaptosomes [letter]. Planta Med 1994; 60: 278–9

397. Garges HP, Varia I, Doraiswamy PM. Cardiac complications and delirium associated with valerian root withdrawal [letter]. J Am Med Assoc 1998; 280: 1566–7

398. Kuhlmann J, Berger W, Podzuweit H, Schmidt U. The influence of valerian treatment on 'reaction time, alertness and concentration' in volunteers. Pharmacopsychiatry 1999; 32: 235–41

399. Hadley S, Petry JJ. Valerian. Am Fam Physician 2003; 67: 1755–8

400. Anon. Valerian. In Gruenwald J, Brendler T, Jaenicke C, eds. PDR for Herbal Medicines, 2nd edn. Montvale, NJ: Medical Economics Company, 2000: 783–6

401. Andreatini R, Leite JR. Effect of valepotriates on the behavior of rats in the elevated plus-maze during diazepam withdrawal. Eur J Pharmacol 1994; 260: 233–5

Overview of selected herbs 3

L. Dey and S. M. Wicks

The preceding chapter discussed 11 of the most commonly used herbal medications, which account for over 50% of all single herb preparations among the 1500–1800 herbs sold in the USA. Table 3.1 is a brief summary of an additional 25 selected herbs commonly used in the USA.

Further reading

Barrett M, ed. The Handbook of Clinically Tested Herbal Remedies. New York, NY: The Haworth Herbal Press, 2004

Ernst E. The Desktop Guide to Complementary and Alternative Medicine: an Evidence-based Approach. London, UK: Harcourt Publishers, 2001

Foster S, Tyler VE. Tyler's Honest Herbal: a Sensible Guide to the Use of Herbs and Related Remedies. Binghamton, NY: The Haworth Herbal Press, 1999

Gruenwald J, Brendler T, Jaenicke C, eds. Physicians' Desk Reference for Herbal Medicines, 3rd edn. Montvale, NJ: Thomson PDR, 2004

Krapp K, Longe JL. The Gale Encyclopedia of Alternative Medicine, Vol 2. Detroit, MI: Gale Group, 2001

Mills S, Bone K. Principles and Practice of Phytotherapy: Modern Herbal Medicine. London, UK: Churchill Livingstone, 2000

Schulz V, Hansel R, Tyler VE. Rational Phytotherapy: a Physician's Guide to Herbal Medicine, 3rd edn. New York, NY: Springer-Verlag, 1998

Sierpina VS. Integrative Health Care: Complementary and Alternative Therapies for the Whole Person. Philadelphia, PA: FA Davis, 2001

Skidmore-Roth L. In Como D, ed. Mosby's Handbook of Herbs and Natural Supplements. St Louis, MO: Mosby, 2001

Table 3.1 An additional 26 herbs commonly used in the USA

Herb	Actions	Common uses	Daily dose	Adverse effects/warnings
Bilberry, *Vaccinium myrtillus*	antioxidant; collagen stabilizer; astringent	eye disorder; diarrhea; circulatory disorders	60–120 mg anthocyanosides; 25% extract 240–480 mg	not reported
Black cohosh, *Cimicifuga racemosa*	estrogen receptor blocker; luteinizing hormone suppressant	menopausal symptoms; menstrual disorders	standard dose 40 mg; one product contained 1 mg triterpine glycosides	GI upset; avoid during pregnancy and lactation
Cascara sagrada, *Rhamnus purshiana*	laxative	constipation	20–30 mg hydroxyanthracene (cascaroside A)	nausea; vomiting; abdominal cramps; urine discoloration; avoid during pregnancy and lactation
Cat's claw, *Uncaria tomentosa*	immune stimulant; anti-inflammatory	arthritis; cancer; HIV	20–60 mg standardized dry extract	autoimmune illness; multiple sclerosis; avoid during pregnancy and lactation
Cayenne, *Capsicum annum*	substance P blocker; decreases lipids; decreases platelet aggregation	arthritis; muscle pain; neuralgia; postmastectomy pain; psoriasis	0.025–0.075% extract; topical use	eye irritation; burning sensation; gastritis; diarrhea
Chamomile, *Matricaria recutita, Matricaria chamomilla*	antispasmodic effect; sedative effect; anti-inflammatory	GI complaints; skin inflammations; insomnia; stress and anxiety	3–4 cups of tea as needed; 0.9–2 g capsules; topical use	avoid if allergic to a member of daisy family (Asteraceae) such as ragweed, asters, chrysanthemums
Chaste tree, *Vitex agnus castus*	prolactin inhibitor; dopamine agonist; progestrogenic	menstrual disorder; promotion of lactation; infertility	30–40 mg extract; 1–5 ml diluted tincture; 1–4 ml diluted extract; 1000 mg tablets	generally not significant; avoid during pregnancy and lactation
Cranberry, *Vaccinium macrocarpon*	antibacterial action	urinary tract infections	360–960 ml liquid; 300–400 mg standardized extract	not reported
Devil's claw, *Harpagophytum procumbens*	anti-inflammatory; analgesic; antirheumatic	rheumatic and arthritic conditions	400–500 mg extract	mild GI disturbances
Dong quai, *Angelica sinensis*	phytoestrogen, antimicrobial effects; smooth muscle relaxant; IgE inhibition	dysmenorrhea; menopause symptoms; allergies	1–2 g dried root, 9–15 ml tincture	photodermatitis; uterine stimulant; contraindicated in the first trimester of pregnancy

Continued

Table 3.1   *Continued*

Herb	Actions	Common uses	Daily dose	Adverse effects/warnings
Evening primrose, *Oenothera biennis*	source of GLA	inflammation; premenstrual syndrome; menopause; fibrocystic breast; eczema	1.5–8 g	headache; GI symptoms; interaction with phenothiazines
Feverfew, *Tanacetum parthenium*	decreases platelet aggregation; smooth muscle relaxant; decreases prostaglandin from platelets and white blood cells	migraine prophylaxis and treatment	50–100 mg; 125 mg dried leaves or 2 fresh leaves	oral ulcers; rash; rebound migraine; avoid during pregnancy and lactation; interactions with warfarin
Flax seed, *Linum usitatissimum*	laxative; anticholesterolemic; anti-inflammatory	eczema; skin inflammation; hypertension; diabetes	1–6 tablespoons/day (58% standardized α-linolenic acid)	nausea; vomiting; diarrhea; hypersensitivity; avoid during pregnancy and lactation
Ginger, *Zingiber officinale*	antiemetic; positive inotropic	dyspepsia; emesis; loss of appetite; motion sickness	0.75–4.0 g extract	heartburn; avoid during pregnancy and lactation
Goldenseal, *Hidrastis canadensis*	antimicrobial	cold; diarrhea	0.75–1.5 g	mouth irritation; avoid during pregnancy and in diabetic patients
Grape seed extract, *Vitis vinifera*	antioxidant; antimutagenic; anti-inflammatory	retinopathy; allergies; prevention of atherosclerosis; cancer	40–80 mg of extract	not reported
Green tea, *Camellia sinensis*	antioxidant; stimulation of CNS; antibacterial; antimutagenic; cholesterol-lowering effect; inhibition of cell proliferation	cancer prevention; tumor progression; cardiovascular diseases; AIDS	6–10 cups; 3 capsules of standardized extract	insomnia; avoid during pregnancy and lactation
Hawthorn, *Crataegus laevigata*	cardiac glycoside effect; coronary dilatation; decrease peripheral resistance; ACE inhibition; mild diuretic; collagen stabilizer	congestive heart failure; hypertension; angina	0.9–2.3 g standardized extract	hypotension; arrhythmia
Hop, *Humulus lupulus*	sedative; antimicrobial	insomnia; nervous tension	0.5–1.0 g extract	allergic dermatitis; respiratory allergy; anaphylaxis; avoid during pregnancy and lactation

Continued

Table 3.1 *Continued*

Herb	Actions	Common uses	Daily dose	Adverse effects/warnings
Horse chestnut, *Aesculus hippo castanum*	reduces lysozomal activity; improves venous tone; inhibits capillary permeability; diuretic	chronic venous insufficiency; hematoma; varicose veins; hemorrhoids	100–150 mg extract; topical use	pruritus; nausea; stomach complaints; bleeding; nephropathy; allergic reactions; avoid during pregnancy and lactation
Licorice root, *Glycyrrhiza glabra*	laxative; expectorant; antispasmodic; anti-inflammatory; antimicrobial; estrogenic; adrenocorticotropic	gastric ulcer; catarrh; cancer prevention; inflammation; antioxidation	750–1500 mg	nausea; vomiting; hypertension; edema; headache; weakness; hypokalemia; anorexia; hypersensitivity; avoid during pregnancy and lactation
Pycnogenol, *Pinus maritima*	antioxidant and antitumor actions; inhibition of tumor necrosis factor-α; inhibition of smoking-induced platelet aggregation	cardiac and cerebral infarction; antitumor; inflammation	not specified	avoid during pregnancy, lactation and in children
Soy, *Glycine max*	phytoestrogen; anticancer; anticholesterol	postmenopausal symptoms; prevention of osteoporosis and cancer; hypercholesterolemia	25–60 g of soy protein or 60 mg of isoflavones	nausea; bloating; diarrhea; abdominal pain; hypersensitivity reaction
Willow, *Salix* spp.	antipyretic; analgesic	fever; pain; rheumatic disorders	120–140 mg salicin	avoid during pregnancy and lactation, patients with salicylate intolerance; interaction with anticoagulants
Yohimbe, *Pausinystalia yohimbe*	penile vasodilatation via peripheral α_2-adrenoreceptor antagonism	erectile dysfunction	16–18 mg of yohimbine hydrochloride	nausea and vomiting; anxiety; hypertension; tachycardia; bronchospasm; avoid during pregnancy and lactation, and in psychiatric patients

GI, gastro-intestinal; IgE, immunoglobulin E; GLA, γ-linoleic acid; CNS, central nervous system; ACE, angiotensin converting enzyme

Herbal medicine: identification, analysis, and evaluation strategies

4

C.-Z. Wang and Y. Shoyama

INTRODUCTION

Herbal medicines have been used for thousands of years. Currently, although 70 countries have national regulations on herbal medicines, the legislative control of herbal medicine lacks structure. This is due to differing definitions of medicinal herbs and products and diverse approaches to their licensing, dispensing, manufacturing, and trading[1]. According to the World Health Organization, reports of patients experiencing negative health consequences caused by the use of herbal medicines are on the rise. These cases are usually linked to the incorrect identification of plant species, the poor quality of herbal medicines, and/or inadequate labeling[1]. Thus, herbal medicine identification and analysis are very important issues in the quality assurance of herbal products.

Herbal medicine analysis or pharmacognostic analysis is the use of physics, chemistry, biology, biochemistry, and other related technologies to assay herbal medicine. The development of standardization of herbal medicine is a global subject. Many countries have established pharmacopeial or other validated criteria to help assure the quality of herbal products. However, the content of herbal medicine extracts is influenced by many factors including cultivation, harvest, storage, and extraction process. Mahady *et al.* have summarized the progress that has been made toward herbal medicine quality control, especially for the plant resources including cultivation and the production process by manufacturers[2].

In this chapter, we will introduce herbal medicine identification and commonly used analytic methods. The application of these methods is critical in the standardization of herbal extracts. Selected strategies for herbal medicine evaluation will also be discussed.

COMMONLY USED ANALYTIC METHODS

Qualitative analysis

Herbs grow in different areas, thus, the environments in which herbs are cultivated are various. The origins of medicinal plants are confused for different reasons[3]. In order to identify the origin of herbal medicines, several methods have been employed, including morphologic, chemical, spectral, chromatographic, and molecular biology techniques. In addition, other tests are necessary to ensure the quality and safety of the herbal medicine, such as assessment of moisture, ash, microbes, and toxic chemicals from the environment present within the extract.

Botanical characteristics

Macroscopic Although morphologic identification is a traditional authentication method, such description of herbal material is useful for crude drug discrimination. Description consists of the macro shapes of the herbal medicine under test. These patterns include form, size, color, surface characters, texture, cut surface, or fracture characteristics. In addition, odor and taste may sometimes be included in the botanical characteristics of a herb. For example, in the United States Pharmacopeia NF 22[4], ginkgo leaf is described as:

Dried whole, folded, or fragmented leaves, with or without attached petiole, varying from khaki green to greenish brown in color, often more brown at the apical edge, and darker on the adaxial surface. Lamina broadly obcuneate (fan-shaped), 2 to 12 cm in width and 2 to 9.5 cm in length from petiole to apical margin, mostly 1.5 to 2 times wider than long. Petiole of a similar color to leaf, channeled on the adaxial surface, 2 to 8 cm in length.

Microscopic   Microscopic observation is another method for the identification of crude herbal drugs. It refers to the observation of the characteristics of tissues and cells in sections or powders, or on the surface of drugs under the microscope. Representative samples are chosen for identification, and slides are prepared to meet the requirements of identification for each drug. Many microscopic characteristics such as pollen shape, cell size, detection of cell wall, detection of cell contents, etc. are described in the section. Figure 4.1 shows an example of the morphologic aspects of a belladonna leaf[5].

Further identification

Chemical   Chemical testing is a method with a long history and its application consists of different specific chemical reactions to identify the constituents extracted from herbal medicines. Because it deals with the compounds in the crude drug, this method is also a means for the identification of plant material. The most commonly used chemical tests are those which detect the constituents in herbal medicines, especially the representative compounds. Many test methods have been developed in pharmacopeial criteria to examine different compound series such as alkaloids, saponins, and flavonoids.

Spectral assays   Because the constituents of various medicinal plants differ, the characteristics of the spectra of their extracts will also differ. Spectrophotometry is used in qualitative analysis in which the light absorption of the substance being examined is measured at a specific wavelength. The spectral ranges involved in pharmaceutic analysis mainly consist of:

(1)   The ultraviolet region (UV, 200–380 nm);

(2)   The visible region (Vis, 380–800 nm); and

(3)   The infrared region (IR, 2.5–25 μm).

Recently, nuclear magnetic resonance (NMR) and mass spectrum (MS) techniques have been used to identify the origins of herbal medicine. These methods can also be used as quantitative assays for herbal medicines, which will be discussed in the next section. Figure 4.2 shows an example of comparative identification of *Magnolia officinalis* with its adulteration *Engelhardria roxburghiana* using UV spectral analysis[6].

Chromatographic assays   Chromatographic methods such as thin layer chromatography (TLC), gas chromatography (GC), and high performance liquid chromatography (HPLC) have been used in the identification of herbal medicines. In TLC, the adsorbent or supporter is applied to form a thin layer on a flat glass plate, plastic film, or aluminum film. After applying the sample, developing, and scanning, a chromatogram is thus recorded. In HPLC, the mobile phase, a solvent or solvent mixture of suitable polarity, is pumped through an injector, to a column containing the stationary phase, and finally to a detector. While the sample is injected into the injector and carried into the column by the mobile phase, the components are separated on the stationary phase and each component passes through the detector in succession and a chromatogram is thus recorded. In GC, the mobile phase is an inert gas, known as the carrier gas, and the chromatographic column is packed with adsorbent, porous polymer beads, or a support coated with a liquid phase. The test preparation is injected into the vaporizer with a micro-syringe and vaporized, then separated on the stationary phase, with each component passing through the detector in succession and a chromatogram is recorded. In order to identify a herbal medicine the sample chromatogram is compared to that obtained from the appropriate reference drug or substances under the same conditions. Chromatographic methods can also be used in quantitative analysis and will be discussed in the next section. Figure 4.3 shows the TLC tests of *Ipecacuanhae* radix. Lanes 1 and 2 are extracts of two botanic samples, while lane TG contains the standards cephaeline and emetine[7].

Molecular-biology related assays   Recent developments in molecular genetic markers allow for the identification of plant species through the detection of species-specific

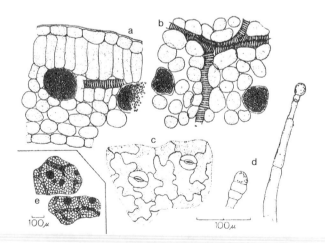

Figure 4.1   Microscopic analysis of belladonna leaf powder

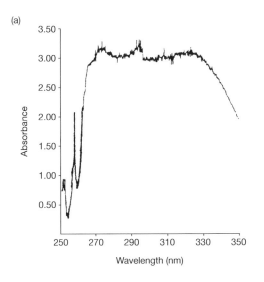
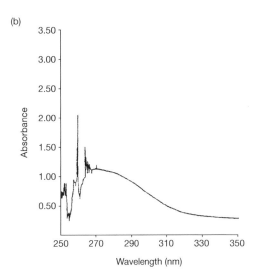

Figure 4.2 UV spectrum identification of herbal medicine. (a) is *Magnolia officinalis* and (b) is its adulteration *Engelhardria roxburghiana*

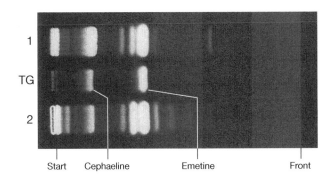

Figure 4.3 TLC test of *Ipecacuanhae* radix

alleles. Polymerase chain reaction (PCR) is the most important technique in molecular biology and was invented by Kary Mullis in 1983[8]. PCR is a method used to generate billions of copies of genomic DNA within a very short time. PCR-related techniques have been used for authentication of herbal medicines. Random amplified polymorphic DNA (RAPD) is one of the most commonly used methods. Species identification of herbal medicines has been achieved using RAPD. Diagnostic PCR or species-specific PCR is another commonly used molecular identification method for herbal medicines. This method has been used to identify ginseng and other herbs[9]. PCR-restriction fragment length polymorphism (PCR-RFLP) is a technique in which species may be differentiated by analysis of patterns derived from cleavage

of their DNA. Some herbal medicines researchers have employed this method to authenticate medicinal plant species[10,11]. Other methods, including simple sequence repeats (SSRs), amplified fragment length polymorphism (AFLP), single nucleotide polymorphs (SNPs), and DNA amplification fingerprinting (DAF), can also be operated on the same principle, and have been applied in the identification of herbal medicines[12]. Figure 4.4 shows an identification example of *Fritillaria pallidiflora* using species-specific PCR[11].

Purity tests

For the quality supervision of herbal medicines, purity tests can provide the essential quality information, and these data are important for the safety of tested herbal medicines. Basic assays include those for moisture, ash, toxic elements, herbicides and microbes[13].

Microbiologic Microbial limit tests provide an estimation of the number of viable micro-organisms present. In normal conditions, the total count of aerobic micro-organisms, the total count of fungi, and the presence of specific undesirable bacteria are investigated. Microbial counts should be determined using pharmacopeial procedures or other validated procedures.

Total ash The ash test is another necessity for herbal medicines. The percentage of total ash with reference to the air-dried drug is a factor which is defined in pharmacopeia.

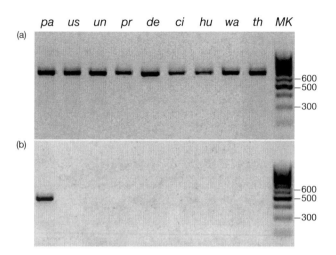

Figure 4.4 Species-specific PCR identification of *Fritillaria pallidiflora*. (a) All extracted DNA from different species are qualified; (b) only *F. pallidiflora* shows positive amplification using species-specific primers. pa, *F. pallidiflora*; us, un, pr, de, ci, hu, wa, th, other species in the genus *Fritillaria*; MK, DNA markers, and the top bp are indicated

Moisture   If a drug is known to be hygroscopic, a moisture test is important. Based on the character of various herbs, different methods have been employed to determine the moisture of crude drugs. In normal conditions, a loss on drying procedure is adequate. However, some drugs contain essential oil and, thus, other specific methods such as toluene distillation and gas chromatography are necessary.

Pesticide residues   Because herbicides and pesticides are used extensively in the cultivation of herbs, the potential for residues of herbicides and pesticides should be fully considered. Gas chromatography is usually employed to analyze pesticide residues.

Toxic elements   Since medicinal plants are grown in soil, many toxic inorganic compounds may be carried into the crude drug during the period of cultivation. The presence of these unwanted chemicals, even in small amounts, may influence the efficacy and safety of the botanic products. For this reason, heavy metals and other polluting elements must be screened for. This series of tests mainly includes limit tests for heavy metals and arsenic. Under some conditions, limit tests for chlorides and iron are required in the criteria.

Other purity tests   According to the characteristics of different herbal medicines, acid-insoluble ash, sulfated ash, water-soluble and alcohol-soluble extraction tests, as well as other tests may be necessary in order for herbal

supplements to be established in accordance with national criteria requirements.

Quantitative analysis

Determination of herbal medicines, including the quantitative analysis of certain constituents in medicinal plants or in herbal medicine extracts, is an important issue in the effective use of herbal medicines. Furthermore, for the active compounds, quantitative assay is the key factor in quality control. Although the active compounds are not recognized, assay of the marker compounds can also help to ensure commonality among different lots of extracts. Quantitative assay consists of both volumetric and equipment analysis. Titration is the classic volumetric method. Equipment assay includes spectral and chromatographic methods. Recently, immunoassay has been introduced into the analytic field of herbal medicine. In this section, we will introduce several commonly used, quantitative, analytic methods for herbal assay.

Titrimetric method

Titration is the process of gradually adjusting the dose of a medication until the desired effect is achieved. As a standard laboratory method of chemical analysis, titration can be used to determine the concentration of a known reactant which is based on some normal chemical reactions such as neutralization (acid–base titration), precipitation (precipitation titration), complex (complexometric titration), redox (redox titration), etc.[14]. A reagent, called the titrant, of known concentration and volume is used to react with a measured volume of reactant. Using a calibrated burette to add the titrant, it is possible to determine the exact amount that has been consumed when the endpoint is reached. Many methods can be used to indicate the endpoint of a reaction. Titrations often use visual indicators (the reactant mixture changes color). In simple acid–base titration, a pH indicator may be used, such as phenolphthalein, which turns (and stays) pink from colorless when a certain pH is reached or exceeded.

The procedure of titration is as follows:

- Accurately measure a volume of the reactant into a beaker or Erlenmeyer flask

- Add a suitable indicator to the flask

- Pour the titrant into the burette, read the starting point of the liquid on the burette

- Turn the tap of the burette to allow the titrant to slowly fall into the reactant

- Swirl the flask with the other hand or with a magnetic 'flea'

- The indicator should change color as the titrant is added, but then quickly return to its original color

- As the endpoint is approached, the indicator takes longer to turn back to its starting color

- Add the titrant more slowly at this point (one drop or half drop at a time)

- When the indicator remains at its end color, the reaction has reached the endpoint

- Measure the amount of titrant liquid used, as shown on the scale of the burette

- Repeat as many trials as needed, then average the volumes. Once the number of moles of reactant that have been neutralized has been determined, then it is easy to calculate the concentration in moles per liter.

For herbal medicine analysis, the titration method is more complex than that of synthetic medicine because the extraction and purification process for detected constituents is complicated. In addition, other techniques such as liquid–liquid extraction are usually employed in the titration assay process[15]. An example of titrimetric analysis of belladonna alkaloids is described below.

Approximately 50 g of the uniform well-mixed sample is powdered (0.18 mm mesh). Exactly 10.0 g powder is weighed and moistened with 5 ml ammonia solution; 10 ml 95% ethanol and 30 ml peroxide-free ether are added and the mixture is shaken vigorously. The mixture is transferred to a small percolator. If necessary, additional extractant may be used. It then stands for 4 hours and percolation proceeds with a mixture of 3 parts by volume peroxide-free ether and 1 part chloroform until the alkaloids have been completely extracted. A few ml of the extract are evaporated to dryness, and the residue is taken up in 0.5 N sulfuric acid and tested for alkaloids with potassium tetraiomercurate (II) solution. The extract is concentrated to a volume of about 50 ml by evaporation on a water bath and then transferred into a separatory funnel while rinsing with peroxide-free ether. Peroxide-free ether is added in an amount of at least 2.1 times the volume of extract so that the solution will have a density clearly below that of water. The solution is then extracted at least three times with 20 ml 0.5 N sulfuric acid and separated into two phases (if necessary by centrifuging). The acid fractions are collected in a second

separatory funnel and are treated with ammonia solution until an alkaline reaction is obtained. The alkaloids are exhaustively extracted with chloroform; the combined chloroform solutions are washed with 10 ml water and the water is discarded; the chloroform solution is then concentrated to dryness on a water bath and the residue is heated for 15 min on the water bath; the residue is taken up in a few ml chloroform, evaporated to dryness again, and the residue is again heated further for 15 min; the residue is again taken up in a few ml chloroform, 20.0 ml of 0.2 N sulfuric acid are added, the chloroform is eliminated on the water bath, and the excess acid is titrated with 0.2 N sodium hydroxide solution against methyl red as an indicator. Each ml of 0.02 N sulfuric acid is equivalent to 5.788 mg total alkaloids calculated as hyoscyamine[5].

Ultraviolet–visible spectrophotometry

Spectrophotometry is a qualitative and quantitative tool which employs the absorption of electromagnetic radiation of wavelengths between 200 and 800 nm by molecules which have π electrons or atoms possessing unshared electron pairs. This is a widely used technique, as a variety of pharmaceutical substances absorb radiation in the ultraviolet (UV, 200–380 nm) and visible (Vis, 380–800 nm) regions of the electromagnetic spectrum[16]. Qualitative assay has been introduced in the former section. In this section, we will introduce the application of UV-Vis spectrophotometry in the quantitative analysis of herbal medicine.

As they absorb radiation from the ultraviolet and visible light wave regions, bonding electrons in the spectrophotometer are set into vibration. Thus, absorption peaks are created via excitation of these valence electrons. These peaks are specific to bond type and require characteristic energy amounts which produce distinctive absorption bands. Many botanical resource constituents have certain molecular structures within UV-Vis light absorption which can be quantitatively determined using UV-Vis spectrophotometry, such as flavonoids, coumarins, lignans, cardiac glycosides, etc.[17]. Some other compounds, such as terpenoids and saccharides, are without certain molecular structures and, consequently, have no UV–Vis absorption. However, they can react with some chemical substances and then be assayed by spectrophotometry[18].

The quantitative assay of spectrophotometry is simply based on the fact that the intensity of absorption by a substance at any given wavelength is directly proportional to its concentration. The essential components of a spectrophotometer consist of a radiation source, a wavelength selector (monochromator), a photodetector, and a readout device, as illustrated in Figure 4.5[19]. The light sources and cells are different between the UV and Vis regions. For the visible range, a tungsten lamp is generally used as the light source and glass or plastic cells can be employed. In the ultraviolet range, a hydrogen lamp is used as the radiation source and generally quartz or silica cells are used, ranging from 1 mm to 1 cm in size.

A typical application of spectrophotometry in the determination of alkaloids in plant materials was reported in Journal of AOAC International[20]. The related reactions are shown below:

$$Alk + KBiI_4 \rightarrow (BiI_3)(Alk \cdot HI) \downarrow (Precipitation)$$
$$(BiI_3)(Alk \cdot HI) + HNO_3 + CS(NH_2)_2 \rightarrow \{Bi[CS(NH_2)_3]\}(NO_3)_3 \; (Yellow)$$

Briefly, alkaloids were precipitated with Dragendorff's reagent (DR, $KBiI_4$, prepared by mixing bismuth nitrate pentahydrate, acetic acid, and potassium iodide in distilled water). The precipitation $(BiI_3)(Alk \cdot HI)$ was dissolved in nitric acid and, then, bismuth reacted with thiourea in nitric acid medium to form a yellow bismuth complex $\{Bi[CS(NH_2)_3]\}(NO_3)_3$. The wavelength of maximum absorption of the bismuth complex was 435 nm. For the precipitation, because the form of alkaloid and bismuth is 1:1, the amount of alkaloid can be calculated by the amount of bismuth complex determined by a spectrophotometric method. The assay protocol was as follows:

(1) Procedure for calibration curve. The calibration curve was obtained with bismuth nitrate pentahydrate stock solution. Series dilutions of the stock solution were made by pipetting out 1, 2, 3, 4, 5, 6, 7, 8, and 9 ml stock solution into separate 10 ml standard flasks and diluting to volume with distilled water. A 1 ml amount of this solution was taken, and 5 ml thiourea solution was added to it. The absorbance value of the yellow solution was measured at 435 nm against colorless reagent blanks.

(2) Procedure for assay of alkaloid and plant extract. A 5 ml sample of alkaloid or plant extract was taken and the pH was maintained at 2–2.5 with dilute HCl. A 2 ml aliquot of DR was added to it, and the precipitate formed was centrifuged. The centrifugate was checked for complete precipitation by adding DR. After centrifugation, the centrifugate was decanted completely and meticulously. The precipitate was further washed with alcohol. The

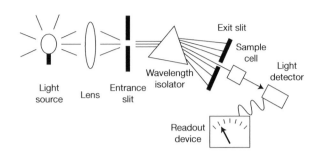

Figure 4.5   Simplified schematic diagram of spectrophotometer. Adapted from reference 19

filtrate was discarded and the residue was then treated with 2 ml disodium sulfide solution. The brownish black precipitate formed was then centrifuged. Completion of precipitation was checked by adding 2 drops of disodium sulfide. The residue was dissolved in 2 ml concentrated nitric acid, with warming if necessary. This solution was diluted to 10 ml in a standard flask with distilled water; 1 ml was then pipetted out and 5 ml thiourea solution was added to it. The absorbance was measured at 435 nm against the blank containing nitric acid and thiourea. The amount of bismuth present in the solution was calculated from the standard curve. The amount of alkaloid was then calculated by the moles of bismuth and the molecular weight of alkaloid[20].

In addition to UV spectrophotometry, other spectral methods can be used in the quantitative assay of herbal medicine, such as infrared spectrophotometry, fluorometry, and optical rotation assay. The quantitative principle of these spectral methods is similar to that of UV spectrophotometry[21].

Thin-layer chromatography

Chromatography is a concept used to encompass a range of techniques that relies on differences in partitioning behavior between a flowing mobile phase and a stationary phase to separate the components in a mixture. Thin-layer chromatography (TLC) is a chromatographic technique that is useful for separating organic compounds. Because of the simplicity and rapidity of TLC, it is often used to monitor the composition of botanical extracts and is also used in the determination of herbal medicine constituents[22].

The separation process is carried out on the TLC plate. The thin separating layer of granular material (stationary phase) is placed on a support plate of glass, metal, or a suitable film. The mixture to be separated, in the form of a solution, is applied in spots or bands (start). After the plate or film is placed into a tightly closed chamber containing a suitable solvent (mobile phase), separation takes place during capillary migration (development). When the mobile phase moves to the top of the TLC plate, the plate is taken out of the chamber and the solvent is evaporated. The separated spots or bands are then recorded (detection).

The layer, which is the stationary phase, is prepared from one of the adsorbents which are manufactured especially for TLC. Common adsorbents are silica gel, aluminum oxide, kieselguhr, cellulose, polyamide, and some reverse phase adsorbents. Silica gel is by far the most frequently used adsorbent for TLC. The mobile phase is the transport medium and consists of one or several solvents. Mobile phases are often selected by consulting literature sources to find those that were previously used for separation of the compounds of interest, or similar compounds. This is followed by a trial-and-error approach to modify the mobile phase for the particular layer and other local conditions being used, if necessary. Techniques have been expanded from linear to two-dimensional, multiple, circular, continuous, and gradient development. If the substances being separated are colored, the spots can be observed without any further effort. However, many compounds are colorless and various methods are necessary for detection of these compounds on TLC. The commonly used visualization methods are sulfuric acid/heating, iodine vapor, ceric stain, and UV light.

The development of quantitative thin layer chromatography (QTLC) was accompanied by the innovation of assay instruments and the application of high-performance TLC. High-performance TLC layers are thinner, contain adsorbent with a smaller, more uniform particle size, and are developed for a shorter distance compared to TLC layers. These factors lead to faster separations, reduced zone diffusion, better separation efficiency, and lower detection limits. QTLC is measured by direct photometric scanning. Although there are some undefined parameters, QTLC can be very powerful because of its smaller systematic error and high accuracy which can be obtained by using a large number of applications and statistical methods, thereby overcoming many of the factors that contribute to the lower reproducibility of TLC[23].

In the 1960s, Steidle first reported a quantitative TLC method for the determination of glucosides in *Linum maritimun*[24]. From then on, QTLC has been widely used in laboratories throughout the world for herbal medicine analysis and quality control. In the early years, Tyihak and Held reviewed the application of TLC for plant constituent analysis[25]. Today, progress in the TLC technique has extended its application to new fields of pharmaceutic research. For example, forced flow provides more compact zones and faster separations than capillary flow, and a significantly higher zone capacity. The varied detection methods, such as mass spectrometry, and bioactive detection, have the potential to identify and quantitatively analyze natural products[26]. Furthermore, many new techniques have been used in QTLC for the quality control of herbal medicine in recent years[27]. In this section, we give an example of the determination of E- and Z-guggulsterone in the herbal medicine *Commiphora mukul* using QTLC[28]. *Commiphora mukul* is a tree grown in northeast Africa and India, which exudes a resinous sap out of incisions that are made in its bark. E- and Z-guggulsterone are the main constituents in the resinous sap and were shown to be superior to nitroglycerin in reducing the chest pain and dyspnea associated with angina.

Analytic samples were spotted on precoated high performance silica gel aluminum plate 60F-254 (Merck, Germany) using the equipment of Camag Linomat IV (Switzerland). The plates were prewashed with methanol and activated at 60°C for 5 min prior to chromatography. The stock solutions of standard E- and Z-isomers of guggulsterone (100 µg/ml) were prepared in methanol. The standard solutions were prepared by dilution of stock solutions with methanol to 0.1–6.0 µg/ml. One microliter from each standard solution was spotted on the TLC plate. The plate was then developed with the mobile phase toluene–acetone (9 : 1, v/v). Densitometric analysis of guggulsterone was carried out in the absorbance mode at 250 nm. The calibration curves of E- and Z-guggulsterone were prepared using the quantities of the standards and their peak areas. To determine the content of E- and Z-guggulsterone in a botanical extract, 500 mg extract was made to 100 ml with methanol. The resulting solution was centrifuged at 3000 rpm for 15 min and supernatant was analyzed. Five microliters of the solution were applied to the TLC plate, followed by development and scanning in the absorbance mode at 250 nm. The content of E- and Z-guggulsterone was calculated by standard calibration. A TLC image is shown in Figure 4.6[28].

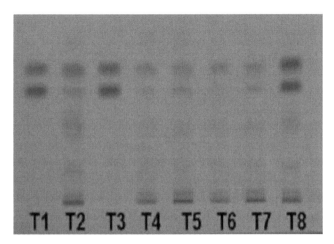

Figure 4.6   Video densitometry of guggulsterone

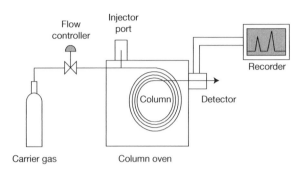

Figure 4.7   Simplified schematic diagram of a GC instrument. Adapted from reference 29

Gas chromatography

Gas chromatography (GC) is a chromatographic technique that can be used to separate volatile organic compounds. GC can be divided into two categories: gas–liquid and gas–solid chromatography. Since gas–liquid GC is widely used for pharmaceutical analysis, it will be introduced briefly in this section.

The GC equipment consists of a flowing mobile phase, an injection port, a separation column containing the stationary phase, and a detector (Figure 4.7)[29]. In the process of GC, the stationary liquid phase is confined to a long tube, the column, in which it exists as a thin film which is either distributed over an 'inert' granular support (packed columns) or supported as a thin coating on the inner surface of the capillary column (capillary columns). The column, which begins at the inlet of the GC and terminates at its detector, is adjusted to some suitable temperature and continuously swept with the mobile gas phase (carrier gas). When a mixture of volatile components is introduced at the inlet, each constituent is swept toward the detector as it ventures into the moving stream of carrier gas. The molecules of those components that are more soluble in or exhibit stronger affinities for the stationary liquid phase venture into the carrier gas less frequently, and require a longer period of time to reach the detector than do components that are less strongly oriented toward the liquid phase; hence separation is achieved.

The samples to be analyzed should be injected into the injection port. The temperature of the sample injection port is usually about 50°C higher than the boiling point of the least volatile component of the sample. Column temperature must be controlled to within tenths of a degree to maintain precision. The optimum column temperature is dependent upon the boiling point of the sample. Generally, a temperature slightly above the average boiling point of the sample results in an elution time of 2–30 min. Minimal temperatures give good resolution, but also increased elution times. If a sample has a wide boiling range, temperature programing can be useful. The column temperature is increased as separation continues.

The individual compounds are swept by the carrier gas to a detector. There are many detectors which can be used in GC. Different detectors will give different types of selectivity. Thermal conductivity detectors and flame ionization detectors are the two most common detectors on commercial gas chromatographs[30]. The detector generates a measurable electrical signal, referred to as peaks, that is proportional to the amount of analyte present. Detector response is plotted as a function of the time required for the analyte to elute from the column after injection. The resulting plot is a GC chromatogram, which is a series of peaks with each component at its own velocity. Each component is qualitatively analyzed by its retention time and quantitatively estimated by its peak area.

The mass spectrometer when used as a detector for GC, is the only universal detector capable of providing structural data for unknown identification. The mass spectrum (MS) of any substance of the distribution of matter according to atomic and molecular masses can be found when a sample of the substance is ionized into fragments (atoms or molecules) that are measured for their mass and relative population. The mass spectrometer produces a graphic depiction of the relative intensity versus the mass-to-charge ratio (m/e) of the various constituents of the sample. Comprehensive reviews of the use of the mass spectrometer as a GC detector in herbal medicine analysis have been published[31].

Chemical constituents in herbal medicine are very complex. Some of them are volatile and can be determined by GC. Since the early years, the GC method has been employed in the qualitative and quantitative assay of these constituents[32]. Essential oils, odorous and volatile products of plant constituents, have a wide application in medicine, food flavoring, and preservation, as well as in fragrance industries. For the application of GC, essential oil analysis has basically had one technical goal: to achieve the best possible separation performance by using the most effective, available technology of the day. The powerful application of GC–MS in the assay of essential oils is supported by the innovation of both separation technique and mass spectrometry detection[33].

Compared to volatile constituents, many effective compounds in herbal medicine are non-volatile. Some of them can react with certain derivative reagents and then become volatile. In an ideal derivatization, a given precursor is derivatized quantitatively and quickly. Then, without further processing, the reaction mixture is injected directly into the GC. The corresponding derivative, stable in the reaction mixture, is also stable during gas chromatography, yields a symmetrical peak, and can be separated from similar derivatives. Using the technique of derivatization, many compounds in herbal medicines have been determined such as organic acids, thiols, amines[34], phenols, flavonols[35], etc.

The following is an example of the analysis of phenolic acids and flavonoids using GC–MS. As potent antioxidants, phenolic acids and flavonoids are widely distributed in medicinal plants[36]. Before GC assay, these compounds must be reacted with certain reagents to become volatile derivatization compounds. From different potential derivative reagents, a methylization reagent is usually selected. Phenolic acids and flavonoids have been reacted with methyliodide and the methylized derivatizations prepared. These derivatizations were then identified and determined using GC–MS. The assay process was as follows[37].

In a typical procedure, a 10 ml portion of a phenolic standard solution or of a plant extract, containing 0.5 ml of phosphate buffer of pH 8.0 for the analysis of phenolic acids or of pH 10.0 for the analysis of both phenolic acids and flavonoids, was transferred to a tube with PTFE-lined screw caps. To this solution were added 1 ml of extraction solvent, 10 µl of the internal standard, and 180 mg methyl iodide. The reaction tube was sealed and vigorously stirred with a magnetic stirrer for 30 min for analyzing phenolic acids and 90 min for total analysis, at 70°C, so that the vortex formed was spread throughout

the liquid volume and the two phases were suitably in close contact. The mixture was allowed to cool down and was saturated with sodium chloride for the complete extraction of the derivatives into the organic phase. After phase separation, the organic layer was dried with anhydrous sodium sulfate and was subjected to GC analysis. A 1 µl sample was injected. The injector and detector temperatures were set at 260°C and 280°C, respectively. The oven temperature for GC analysis started at 50°C with a 5 min hold. Then temperature was programed at 5°C/min to 150°C and from 150°C to 210°C at 10°C/min with 11 min hold; the total run time was 45 min. The mass spectrometer started its run 3 min after the injection and stopped at the end of the GC run, whereby the mass areas range from 50 to 500 was recorded. The derivatives were quantified by the ratios of the areas relative to the internal standards. Figure 4.8 shows a GC–MS chromatogram from this analysis.

High-performance liquid chromatography

High-performance liquid chromatography (HPLC) was developed from traditional liquid chromatography (LC). LC is an analytic technique for separating molecules that are dissolved in a solvent. If the sample solution is in contact with a second solid or liquid phase, the different solutes will interact with the other phase to differing degrees due to differences in adsorption, or partitioning. These differences allow the mixture components to be separated from each other when the solutes pass through a column. Nearly all types of chemical structures can be analyzed using LC, including volatile and non-volatile compounds.

Compared to normal pressure LC, HPLC shares the same separation theory. Moreover, newly developed equipment has made HPLC a powerful technique in qualitative and quantitative analysis of natural products. HPLC instruments consist of reservoirs of mobile phases, pumps, an injector, a separation column, and a detector. Compounds are separated by injecting a plug of the sample mixture into the column. The different components in the mixture pass through the column at different rates due to differences in their partitioning behavior between the mobile phase and the stationary phase.

The two core portions of HPLC are the separation column and the detector. Complex natural products are separated by the column and detected when they pass through the detector. In this section, we introduce the different types of separation columns and detectors that are usually employed in natural product analysis.

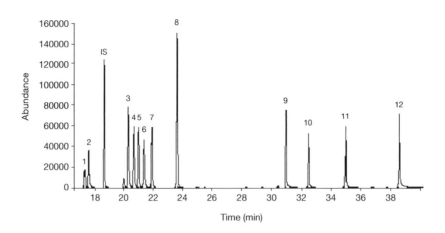

Figure 4.8   The GC–MS chromatogram of a *Mentha spicata* fortified extract

The separation columns are classified by their mechanism of elution. According to the differences in theories and the composition of stationary and mobile phases, chromatography is classified into several systems: normal phase, reverse phase, ion-exchange, and affinity chromatography. Ion-exchange chromatography is used to separate ionized compounds by changing the pH of the mobile phase. Affinity chromatography operates by using immobilized biochemicals that have a specific affinity for the compound of interest. Normal phase chromatography operates on the basis of hydrophilicity and lipophilicity by using a polar stationary phase such as non-bonded silica, and silica bonded with cyanopropyldimethylsilane, propyl-amino silane, and other groups. The mobile phase is a less polar solution and thereby hydrophobic compounds elute more quickly than do hydrophilic compounds. Each of these types of chromatography employs their own unique column. Among all the kinds of columns available, reverse phase column chromatography is normally used in natural product analysis. A variety of merchandized HPLC columns of this type are produced by many manufacturers.

For reverse phase chromatography, the stationary phase consists of silica-based packings with *n*-alkyl chains covalently bound, which provides a less polar adsorbent. The most commonly used stationary phases are C-8, signifying an octyl chain, and C-18 (or ODS), an octadecyl ligand in the matrix. The mobile phase is a polar solution such as methanol–water, or an acetonitrile–water system. The hydrophilic compounds elute more quickly than do hydrophobic compounds in the reverse phase HPLC column. Besides the few less polar constituents, nearly all types of natural products can be analyzed by reverse phase chromatography, particularly using C-18 columns[38].

As the eyes of analysis in chromatography, the online detector of HPLC is an important component that emits a response due to the eluting sample compound and subsequently signals a peak on the chromatogram. It is positioned immediately posterior to the stationary phase in order to detect the compounds as they elute from the column. The highest possible sensitivity and selectivity of detectors are required in natural product research, and this has led to the introduction of instruments with high qualitative performance. The basic mechanism is the same as that of the original instruments, but technical improvements have been made in the mechanics and electronics. The detectors normally used in HPLC are the ultraviolet/visible detector, evaporative light scattering detector, electrochemical detector, and mass spectroscopy detector.

Many natural compounds contain pi-electrons, or non-paired electrons of some functional groups. They have absorbance in the ultraviolet region (UV, 200–380 nm) and the visible region (Vis, 380–800 nm) of the electromagnetic radiation spectrum. For example, any compounds that have benzene rings will show absorbance at 205–225 and 245–265 nm. So, UV–Vis detectors make up the majority of detectors, with statistical data showing that almost 70% of published HPLC analyses are performed with these detectors[39].

Some compounds such as saccharides, terpenes, and a few alkaloids have no UV–Vis absorbance because they do not contain certain functional groups. These compounds cannot be detected using a UV–Vis detector, but can be detected by an evaporative light scattering detector (ELSD). ELSD works by measuring the light scattered from the solid solute particles remaining after nebulization and evaporation of the mobile phase. Because its response is independent of the light absorbing properties of molecules, it can reveal sample components which were missed by UV–Vis detectors[40].

The electrochemical detector is also a popular HPLC detector. It should be considered by the chromatographer because of the additional selectivity and sensitivity for some compounds. This type of detector responds to substances that are either able to be oxidized or are reducible and the electrical output is an electron flow generated by a reaction that takes place at the surface of the electrodes[41]. Some active natural products such as flavonoids, quinones, and phenolic acids can be detected by electrochemical detectors.

Mass spectrometry is used for measuring the molecular weight and structural formation of organic molecules, and is also a widely used detector in HPLC analysis. When the constituent is eluted out of the column, the detected compound or molecule is ionized, and is then passed through a mass analyzer where the ion current is detected.

The quantitative HPLC assay for herbal medicine includes two items, identification and determination of natural products. For the identification component, a comparison of the retention time of the chromatogram with standard compounds is normally the method of choice. However, because the constituents of botanical extracts are very complex, some other components may have the same retention time with certain standards. The UV–Vis spectrum obtained by the diode-array detector can be used to identify some structures of natural products. However, in normal conditions, interference compounds have similar carbon skeletons and functional groups and, consequently, the UV–Vis spectrum is similar to the standards. It is difficult to identify constituents when they have small differences using the UV–Vis spectrum. As a powerful detector, the mass spectrometer can provide much more structural information and make identification more accurate. In recent years, the developments in MS detectors have made HPLC assay more sensitive and selective. Joseph Smerma has reviewed the application of HPLC/MS in the analysis of botanical medicines and dietary supplements[42]. In this section, we introduce a typical HPLC method for the terpenoid assay of *Ginkgo biloba* (ginkgo)[43].

Ginkgo is one of most frequently used botanical dietary supplements. The bioactive constituents include the terpenoid lactones consisting of bilobalide and the

ginkgolides A, B, C, and J. The author introduced a new assay method based on HPLC/MS/MS for the measurement of terpenoid lactones in ginkgo products. The MS/MS fragmentation pathways of ginkgolides were investigated to identify abundant fragment ions that would be useful for the sensitive and selective detection of ginkgolides and bilobalide during LC/MS/MS. Sample preparation and clean-up procedures were streamlined to maximize throughput by taking advantage of the selectivity of LC/MS/MS detection. The recoveries of ginkgolides A, B, C, J, and bilobalide exceeded 90%, the intra-assay and inter-assay relative standard deviations were less than 5%, the relative error was less than 8%, and the limits of detection and quantification were 3.6–120 and 11–350 fmol, depending on the sample to be analyzed that was injected on to the LC column. Thereby, this LC/MS/MS assay facilitated the rapid quantitative analysis of ginkgolides A, B, C, and J and bilobalide in ginkgo dietary supplements with excellent recovery, reproducibility, accuracy, and sensitivity. Figure 4.9 shows analytic chromatograms[43].

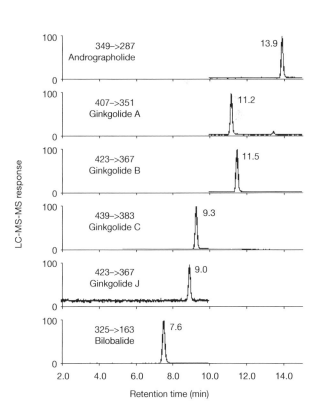

Figure 4.9 Negative ion electrospray LC/MS/MS analysis of a mixture of ginkgolides A, B, C, and J, bilobalide, and andrographolide (internal standard)

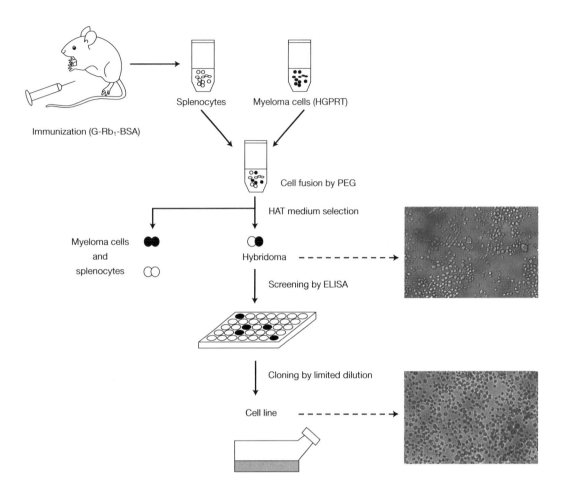

Figure 4.10   Preparation of monoclonal antibody by hybridoma fused with immunized spleen cells and myeloma cells

Enzyme-linked immunosorbent assay

Enzyme-linked immunosorbent assay (ELISA) uses antibodies or antigens coupled to an easily assayed enzyme and combines the specificity of antibodies with the sensitivity of simple enzyme assays. ELISA provides a useful measurement of antigen or antibody concentration in two ways: it can be used to detect the presence of antigens that are recognized by an antibody or it can be used to test for antibodies that recognize an antigen. The immunoassay system using monoclonal antibodies (MAbs) is not frequently used for naturally occurring bioactive compounds having smaller molecular weights. Preparation of MAbs is difficult but is one of the most important steps for the analysis of natural products[44]. As a typical assay example, we introduce the ELISA method in the determination of ginsenoside Rb$_1$.

Asian ginseng and American ginseng are popular herbal medicines in many countries. They contain more than 30 kinds of dammarane and oleanane saponins, which are considered to be pharmacologically active components. ELISA methods have been established for the determination of several ginsenosides, such as Rb$_1$, Rg$_1$, and Re.

Ginsenoside Rb$_1$ is the main saponin in both Asian ginseng and American ginseng. A hybridoma producing MAb reactive to GRb$_1$ was obtained by the general procedure indicated in Figure 4.10, and classified into IgG2b which had k light chains[45].

The reactivity of IgG type MAb, 9G7 was tested by varying antibody concentration and by performing a dilution curve. The antibody concentration (0.418 mg/ml) was selected for competitive ELISA. The free MAb following competition is bound to polystyrene microtiter plates precoated with ginsenoside Rb$_1$–HAS (Figure 4.11, left). Under these conditions, the full measuring range of the assay extends from 20 to 400 ng/ml, as indicated in Figure 4.11 (right).

Cross-reactivity is the most important factor in determining the value of an antibody. Since the ELISA

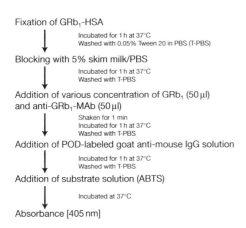

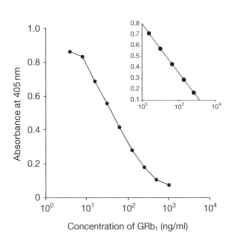

Figure 4.11   Protocol of ELISA (left) and calibration curve of ginsenoside Rb₁ (right)

for ginsenoside Rb_1 was established for phytochemical investigations involving crude plant extracts, the assay specificity was checked by determining the cross-reactivity of the MAb with various related compounds. The cross-reactivity data of MAb that were obtained were examined by competitive ELISA and calculated using picomole of ginsenoside Rb_1. The cross-reactivity of ginsenoside Rc and ginsenoside Rd, which possess a diglucose moiety attached to the C-3 hydroxy group, were weak compared to ginsenoside Rb_1 (cross-reactivity was 0.024% and 0.020%, while the reactivity of Rb_1 was 100%). Moreover, ginsenoside Re and ginsenoside Rg_1 showed no cross-reactivity (less than 0.005%). It is evident that the MAb reacted only with a small number of structurally related ginsenoside Rb_1 molecules, and very weakly, and did not react with other steroidal compounds such as glycyrrhizin, digitonin, tigogenin, tigonin, gitogenin, solamargine, solasonine, cholesterol, ergosterol, ulsolic acid, beta-sitosterol, cholic acid, and deoxycholic acid (cross-reactivity was less than 0.005%).

Since herbal medicine extracts consist of various chemical constituents in general, some pretreatment is necessary for HPLC and other chromatographic analysis. ELISA, however, can determine the concentration of ginsenoside Rb_1 directly without any pretreatment. ELISA has been used to measure the concentration of ginsenoside Rb_1 in Asian ginseng and American ginseng[46]. Compared to TLC, GC, and HPLC methods, the ELISA method was more sensitive and selective. Furthermore, no pretreatment of crude extracts was

necessary. As an outstanding determination method, it is possible to study a large number of natural products.

We have introduced some typical qualitative and quantitative methods for the analysis of herbal medicine. Many other methods have been employed in the determination of botanical constituents. They include spectral methods such as infrared (IR), nuclear magnetic resonance (NMR), and circular dichroism (CD), and other chromatographic methods such as ion chromatography, capillary electrophoresis (CE), high-speed counter current chromatography (HSCCC), etc. Each method has its advantages. Table 4.1 shows a comparison of the main assay methods commonly used in herbal medicine analysis.

QUALITY ASSURANCE AND EVALUATION STRATEGIES

The interplay of herbal medicine and human health has been documented for thousands of years. For example, herbs have been integral to Chinese medicine, which dates back about 4000 years[47]. The endurance of herbal medicines may be explained by the tendency of herbs to work slowly, often without toxic side-effects, both on the illness and its symptoms. Because quality control varies from manufacturer to manufacturer, there is uncertainty about the actual amount of active ingredients in some preparations. Most herbal companies provide data about their products and processing techniques; such information is important for the consumer.

Table 4.1   Comparison of different methods employed in herbal medicine analysis

Assay method	Quantifi-cation	Establishment	Sensitivity	Reproduc-ibility	Operation	Speed	Pollution	Cost
PCR related	no	not easy	high	good	not simple	fast	low	fairly high
Titration	yes	very easy	low	fair	simple	fast	low	very low
UV–Vis	yes	easy	low	fairly good	simple	fast	low	low
TLC	yes	fairly easy	fair	fair	fair	not fast	yes	low
GC	yes	not easy	high*	good	not simple	not fast	low	fairly high
HPLC	yes	not easy	high	good	not simple	not fast	yes	fairly high
ELISA	yes	very complex	very high	good	simple	fast	very low	low

*Limited to volatile compounds

In the overall context of quality assurance and control of herbal medicines, the World Health Organization (WHO) developed the 'Good manufacturing practices: supplementary guidelines for the manufacture of herbal medicinal products' in 1996[48]. In 1998, the WHO published a guideline for the primary tests for herbal medicine: 'Quality control methods for medicinal plant materials'[49]. Although these documents are helpful for quality assurance by manufacturers, the outlined descriptions of herbal medicine assays are not sufficient for standardization studies, especially in the development of new botanical extract products. Standardization of herbal medicine is a global subject today. Because of the diversity of sources of botanical materials, many problems must be solved before the target of standardization of herbal medicine is reached. In this section, we will discuss the current status and normal research process for the standardization of herbal medicine extracts.

Standardization of botanical extracts

Herbal medicine products are extracted from raw botanical materials. Control of the sources of botanical material is the first step in the quality assurance of herbal medicine. In the herbal market, plants may be misidentified or deliberately replaced with cheaper or more readily available alternatives. For certain species, however, the concentrations of active constituents are not stable. In addition, the extraction techniques and processing steps used by different manufacturers may vary. Many factors result in marked variability in the content and quality of commercially available herbal products[50]. The potency of herbal medications can vary from manufacturer to manufacturer and from lot to lot within a manufacturer. Some herbal manufacturers have tried to standardize

their herbal products to fixed concentrations of selected chemical constituents[51].

Standardization of herbal medicine covers many different aspects, and the emphasis of the studies varies from researcher to researcher. In the following we give an example of a study process for the standardization of herbal medicine extracts accepted by some researchers.

Due to the complexity of the herbal material market, first the species of medicinal plant should be screened and selected. In addition, even for a single species, because the chemical constituents of herbs from different geographical regions vary, the production area of certain plant species should be recognized. In this step, several species in a genus should be collected and assayed. Then, one selected herb species from a different production area should be gathered and analyzed. Many techniques have been employed in the species identification of herbs. Macroscopic and microscopic examination can be used as rapid and inexpensive identification techniques. Chemical analysis is considered the most useful method for the detection of contaminants and can be an effective method for plant identification as well. Molecular biology offers an assortment of techniques that can be very useful for authentication of medicinal plants based on differences in DNA sequences[52]. For the chemical constituent assay, qualitative and quantitative HPLC is the most commonly used method. Also, as an identification method, HPLC fingerprint is a potentially effective method for herb species authentication, even for products from compound herbal formulas[53]. Quantitative HPLC assay provides the most important information on herb extracts from different sources and its results help to determine which samples should be selected.

For the selected herbal material, after the physico-chemical characteristics of the main constituents have been considered, the extraction solvent and method should be determined. Together with quantitative analysis, the extraction method can be modified and then established. A large number of extracts should be obtained with the modified extraction method. Then, bioassay guided fractionation and isolation are used to detect the active constituents. The herb extracts should be standardized by the active constituents. Once enough samples of herbal medicine extracts from a certain species and a selected production area have been assayed, the content ranges of the active constituents should be defined. However, for many herbs the active constituents are not known. In these cases, products may be standardized on their content of certain 'marker' compounds (chemicals characteristic of the herb or present in large quantities). Based on the studies above, the quality criteria of standardized herbal extracts should be established. These criteria include not only the sources of herbal material, but also the whole treatment process of the selected herb.

Some standardized herbal extracts, which have been achieving more consistent pharmaceutical quality, have been produced by several manufacturers. The quality data provided by the manufacturers, including the content of active constituent(s) and the limitation of toxic constituents, showed the requirements of criteria for these botanical extracts. *Ginkgo biloba*, which has the highest global sales of all herbal medicine, has been standardized by many manufacturers. Van Beek reviewed the standardization and analysis studies for *Ginkgo biloba* extracts in 2002[54]. The quality control factors of *Ginkgo biloba* extracts included the general identity tests (description, chemical identification) and purity tests (loss on drying, residue on ignition or ash, heavy metals, arsenic). More importantly, the quality control criteria included the content of active constituents (flavonoid, terpene trilactone) and the limitation of toxic compounds from total extracts of *Ginkgo biloba* (such as ginkgolic acid, which is known to be allergenic). Table 4.2 gives an example of the quality requirements for the standardized *Ginkgo biloba* extract[54].

In the production process of herbal extracts by the manufacturer, standardization means adjusting the herbal drug preparation to a defined content of a constituent or a group of substances with known therapeutic activity, respectively by adding excipients or by mixing condensed fractions[55]. Because the active constituent content is influenced by many factors such as weather, harvest time, and drying conditions, the raw plant material from different lots may vary. For example, the active constituents may not reach the lower limit in some lots.

Table 4.2 Example of specifications for a standardized *Ginkgo biloba* extract

Assay items	Quality requirements
Description	brown powder with characteristic smell
Identity	green-brown color after adding FeCl3 to a 0.1% solution (g/v) in alcohol–water (1:1)
Heavy metals	not more than 20 ppm
Arsenic	not more than 2 ppm
Ginkgolic acid	not more than 10 ppm
Loss on drying	not more than 5.0 (80°C, vacuum)
Residue on ignition	not more than 1.0%
Total flavonoid content	not less than 24.0% (HPLC–UV)
Total terpene trilactone content	not less than 6.0% (HPLC–RI)

A normal protocol is to add the condensed fraction which is isolated in advance from the total extract and then to adjust the content of active constituents to match the criteria requirements.

Phytochemical research approaches for the standardization of herbal medicines

To recognize the active compound is the foundation of herbal medicine standardization. However, although some botanical extracts have been standardized, the content controlled constituents were marker compounds because the active compound was not defined in many herbs. Thus, research on active compound recognition is an important issue for the standardization of herbal medicine[56]. We introduce the normal screening process of active constituents as follows.

A standardized extract means that the manufacturer has verified that the active ingredient believed to be present in the herb is present in the preparation and that the potency and the amount of the active ingredient are assured in the preparation. However, in many conditions, because the active constituents are not defined, the quantitative constituents are the representative compounds; they may not be the active constituents. Bioassay guided fractionation and isolation of active constituents are key steps in the standardization research of herbal medicine.

The process of bioassay guided fractionation and active constituent isolation includes several steps:

(1)   Chemical extraction of material herbal medicine;

(2)   Fractionation of extract with selected method;

(3)   Test fractions with appropriate bioassay method;

(4)   Continue fractionation of positive materials;

(5)   Bioassay of new fractions;

(6)   Isolation of chemical components in active fractions;

(7)   Bioassay of individual components;

(8)   Confirmation of active compounds;

(9)   Elucidation of active compounds.

According to the different levels of screening, bioassay can be categorized into four major roles: prescreens, screens, monitorings, and secondary testings. In prescreen a bioassay is applied to large numbers of initial samples to determine whether or not they have any bioactivity of the desired type. A bioassay in a screen is used to select materials for secondary testing, whereas, in a monitoring, a bioassay is used to guide fractionation of a crude material towards isolation of the pure bioactive substances. In the secondary testing, lead compounds are evaluated in multiple models and test conditions to select candidates for development towards clinical trials[57]. The method for bioassay can be divided into two groups for screening purposes: general screening and specialized screening bioassays. Depending on the aims of the screening program, either a general screening which can pick up many different effects, or a specific assay which is directed at finding some effect against a specific disease, is performed. For the specialized screening, bioassays are classified according to the target organism which is used: lower organisms, isolated subcellular systems, isolated cellular systems, isolated organs of vertebrates, and whole animals. These *in vitro* or *in vivo* tests are more sophisticated than the primary screening bioassays[58].

The composition of herbal medicine extracts is very complex. The fractionation and isolation methods have been developed according to the characteristics of different extracts. For the fractionation, solvent fractionation and chromatographic fractionation methods were employed. Solvent fractionation is the simplest way and sometimes the most efficient for primarily separating a group of lipid-soluble constituents of interest when the others are difficult. This approach depends on the differential solubility of compounds in organic solvents. Traditional solvent fractionation methods are less adaptable to natural products due to the limitation of the

equipment. Chromatographic fractionation occupies the main position in the separation of herbal extracts because of its quick development of adsorbents and equipment. Low-pressure column chromatography, thin-layer chromatography, preparative high-performance liquid chromatography, and high-speed countercurrent chromatography are techniques normally used in the fractionation and isolation of active compounds. Focusing on the fractionation and isolation methods of active compounds, several groups of herbal medicines have been reviewed[59–61].

The fractionation process is usually divided into several steps directed by bioassay. First, herbal medicine extracts are separated by liquid–liquid extraction or classic low-pressure chromatography, which has the characteristic of low resolution, but yields high quantities from a separation. Then, the active fraction is separated by classic column chromatography, or preparative HPLC. The adsorbents of chromatography may be changed according to the different types of constituents or according to the special purpose of separation. Active fractions may be separated several times. At last, the active fraction is separated by preparative HPLC and individual compounds are obtained. After being bioassayed, the active compound is elucidated by different spectral methods, such as UV, IR, NMR, and MS, and other physical and chemical methods. Figure 4.12 shows an example of bioassay-guided fractionation and active compound isolation[62].

In the normal experimental design of bioassay-guided active compound recognition, the protocol described above is enough. However, a new point of view is that, after the above process, the constituents isolated under the guidance of biologic analysis are candidates for the real active compound or assumed active compound. It is necessary to prepare an extract from which the assumed compound is removed. This extract is called the 'knockout' extract. If a knockout extract has low biologic activity compared to the original extract, the assumed active constituent (or knockout compound) can be considered as an active constituent.

The 'knockout' concept has been widespread in genetic engineering studies from 1989[63]. Special gene knockout animals are important tools for pharmacologic research. This concept is also used to describe extracts from which the assumed active compound has been removed. To prepare the knockout extract, several chromatographic methods can be employed. The preparative protocol should be based on the chromatographic characteristic of the assumed compound and the total extract. As an example, we introduce an isolation

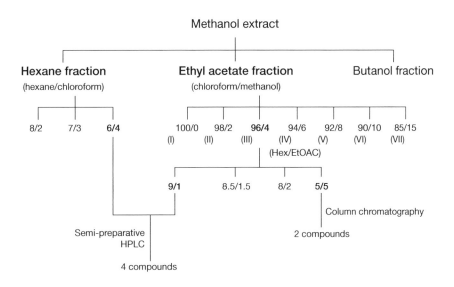

Figure 4.12   A schematic of bioassay-guided isolation (the active fractions are shown in bold)

protocol for the preparation of ginsenoside Re knockout extract.

In our antidiabetes research[64], American ginseng berry extract was found to possess antihyperglycemic activity. After screening different ginsenosides, ginsenoside Re was believed to be the active compound. For the preparation of ginsenoside Re knockout extract, column chromatography, preparative TLC or preparative HPLC methods were considered. Low-pressure column chromatography can be employed to isolate the hydrophilic constituents such as oligosaccharides, polysaccharides, and some water-soluble organic acids. Ginsenosides, the main constituents in American ginseng berry extract, should be separated by TLC or HPLC. For the TLC, a positive phase adsorbent such as silica gel is usually used. Ginsenosides have low separation resolution even in high-performance silica gel TLC, and ginsenoside Re is difficult to separate from other ginsenosides effectively (Figure 4.13b). The reverse-phase HPLC chromatogram showed that ginsenoside Re can be separated from most other ginsenosides. Only ginsenoside Rg1 cannot be separated from ginsenoside Re by HPLC (Figure 4.13a)[65].

According to the condition discussed above, the protocol of ginsenoside Re knockout extract was designed as follows. American ginseng berry extract was dissolved in water, and was loaded onto an HP-20 liquid chromatographic column. The column was eluted with water. The water elutant, which contained saccharides and water-soluble organic acids, was evaporated under vacuum and lyophilized. The column was then eluted with 95%

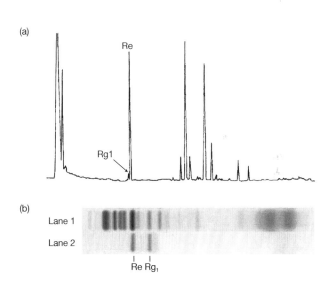

Figure 4.13   HPLC and TLC chromatograms of American ginseng root extract. (a) HPLC; (b) TLC. Lane 1, American ginseng extract; lane 2, ginsenoside standards

ethanol, and the eluate was evaporated. This 95% ethanol eluate portion was separated by reverse-phase preparative HPLC. Ginsenoside Re and Rg1 were separated and removed from the other ginsenosides. Then, ginsenoside Rg1 was added to the ginsenoside portion according to the content of ginsenoside Rg1 in the total extract. The ginsenoside portion, from which ginsenoside Re had been removed, was evaporated and

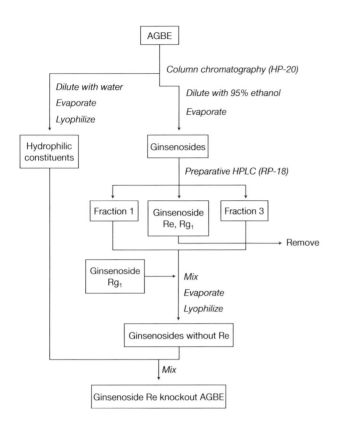

Figure 4.14 Preparation process of ginsenoside Re knockout American ginseng berry extract. AGBE, American ginseng berry extract

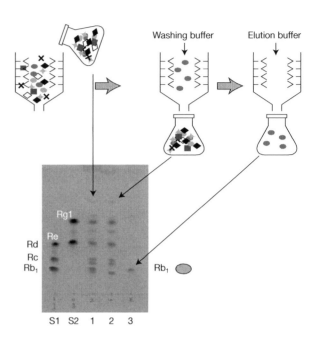

Figure 4.15 Preparation process of knockout Asian ginseng extract without ginsenoside Rb_1 using immunoaffinity chromatography. Lane S1, ginsenoside standards Rb_1, Rc, and Rd; S2, ginsenoside standards Re and Rg_1; 1, Asian ginseng extract; 2, ginsenoside Rb_1 knockout extract; 3, ginsenoside Rb_1

lyophilized. Finally, after the water eluate portion isolated from the HP-20 chromatography had been mixed with the ginsenoside portion isolated from preparative HPLC, the ginsenoside Re knockout extract was obtained (Figure 4.14). The Re knockout extract can be used for further pharmacologic tests.

Another method using MAb has been developed for the preparation of ginsenoside Rb_1 knockout extract. Since MAb has a sugar chain in the molecule, antiginsenoside Rb_1 MAb was oxidatively cleaved by sodium periodide to produce aldehyde groups. The oxidized product was treated with agarose gels conjugated with a hydrazine group to give hydrazone, resulting in an affinity gel combined with antiginsenoside Rb_1 MAb.

Asian ginseng extract was charged to the column packed with the above affinity gel, washed by phosphate buffer and then eluted by 100 mM acetate buffer containing 0.5 M KSCN and 20% methanol to give pure ginsenoside Rb_1 by a single-step purification[66]. Since the washed buffer solution contained overcharged ginsenoside Rb_1, the immunoaffinity column wash was repeated until ginsenoside Rb_1 disappeared. All washed buffer

solutions were collected and deionized. The water solution was concentrated and applied to TLC (Figure 4.15). This immunoaffinity chromatographic method can establish one-step isolation of knockout ginseng extract without ginsenoside Rb_1.

CONCLUSION

In the United States, the assurance of the quality of prescription and over-the-counter drugs is regulated under Good Manufacturing Practices (GMP) guidelines mandated by the Food and Drug Administration (FDA) regulations. For herbal medicine, however, quality control from the herb's cultivation to its harvesting, storage, extraction, and all the related processes of analysis are still under discussion[2]. Although the herbal GMP published by the WHO provide some important guidelines to the manufacturers[48], these guidelines need further improvement. In this chapter, we have introduced some commonly used analytic methods and their application in the quality assurance of botanicals, and have discussed selected herbal medicine standardization strategies. This information is necessary to the establishment process for the standardization of herbal medicine extracts.

References

1. Anon. WHO issues guidelines for herbal medicines. Bull WHO 2004; 82: 238

2. Mahady GB, Fong HHS, Farnsworth NR. Botanical Dietary Supplements: Quality, Safety and Efficacy. Tokyo: Swets and Zeitlinger Publishers, 2001: 17–25

3. Fong HH. Integration of herbal medicine into modern medical practices: issues and prospects. Integr Cancer Ther 2002; 1: 287–93

4. USPCI (United States Pharmacopeial Convention Inc.). The United States Pharmacopeia, NF 22. Toronto, ON: Webcom Limited, 2004: 2004–5

5. Stahl E. Drug Analysis by Chromatography and Microscopy. Ann Arbor, MI: Ann Arbor Science Publishers Inc., 1973: 47–50

6. Cao Y, Jiang TS, Liao L, Lin B. Comparative identification of Magnolia officinalis and its easily confusable bark of Engelhardtia roxburghiana. Chin Trad Herbal Drugs 2002; 33: 468–70

7. Wagner H, Bladt S, Zgainski EM. Plant Drug Analysis, A Thin Layer Chromatography Atlas. New York, NY: Springer-Verlag, 1983: 76–7

8. Mullis KB. The polymerase chain reaction in an anemic mode: how to avoid cold oligodeoxyribonuclear fusion. PCR Methods Appl 1991; 1: 1–4

9. Zhu S, Fushimi H, Cai S, Komatsu K. Species identification from Ginseng drugs by multiplex amplification refractory mutation system (MARMS). Planta Med 2004; 70: 189–92

10. Yang DY, Fushimi H, Cai SQ, Komatsu K. Polymerase chain reaction–restriction fragment length polymorphism (PCR–RFLP) and amplification refractory mutation system (ARMS) analyses of medicinally used Rheum species and their application for identification of Rhei Rhizoma. Biol Pharm Bull 2004; 27: 661–9

11. Wang CZ, Li P, Ding JY, et al. Identification of Fritillaria pallidiflora using diagnostic PCR and PCR-RFLP based on nuclear ribosomal DNA internal transcribed spacer sequences. Planta Med 2005; 71: 384–6

12. Techen N, Crockett SL, Khan IA, Scheffler BE. Authentication of medicinal plants using molecular biology techniques to compliment conventional methods. Curr Med Chem 2004; 11: 1391–401

13. Anon. WHO Monographs on Selected Medicinal Plant. Geneva: World Health Organization, 2002: 1–4

14. Ashworth MRF. Titrimetric Organic Analysis. New York, NY: Interscience Publishers, 1964: 1–53

15. Papariello GJ, Tishler F. Alkaloids. Encycl Ind Chem Anal 1967; 4: 587–618

16. Frost T, ed. UV Spectroscopy: Techniques, Instrumentation, Data Handling. New York, NY: Chapman & Hall, 1993: 1–15

17. Lobinski R, Marczenko Z. Recent advances in ultraviolet-visible spectrophotometry. Crit Rev Anal Chem 1992; 23: 55–111

18. Bosch Ojeda C, Sanchez Rojas F. Recent developments in derivative ultraviolet/visible absorption spectrophotometry. Anal Chim Acta 2004; 518: 1–24

19. http://microvet.arizona.edu/Courses/MIC328/Waynes%20World/AppendixDSpec.html, accessed on 18 July, 2005

20. Sreevidya N, Mehrotra S. Spectrophotometric method for estimation of alkaloids precipitable with Dragendorff's reagent in plant materials. J AOAC Int 2003; 86: 1124–7

21. Schirmer RE. Modern Methods of Pharmaceutical Analysis. Boca Raton, FL: CRC Press, 1982: 127–258

22. Sherma J. Thin-layer chromatography in food and agricultural analysis. J Chromatogr A 2000; 80: 129–47

23. Sherma J, Fried B. Handbook of Thin-layer Chromatography, 2nd edn. New York, NY: Marcel Dekker Inc., 2003: 273–306

24. Steidle VW. Quantitative Bestimmung von Scilla-Glykosiden. Planta Med 1961; 9: 435–41

25. Tyihak E, Held G. Thin-layer chromatography in pharmacognosy. In Niederwieser A, Pataki G, eds. Thin-layer Chromatography and Related Methods Vol. II. Ann Arbor, MI: Ann Arbor Science Publishers Inc., 1971: 183–234

26. Poole CF. Thin-layer chromatography: challenges and opportunities. J Chromatogr A 2003; 1000: 963–84

27. Gocan S, Cimpan G. Review of the analysis of medicinal plants by TLC: modern approaches. J Liq Chromatogr Relat Technol 2004; 27: 1377–411

28. Agrawal H, Kaul N, Paradkar AR, Mahadik KR. HPTLC method for guggulsterone. I. Quantitative determination of E- and Z-guggulsterone in herbal extract and pharmaceutical dosage form. J Pharm Biomed Anal 2004; 36: 33–41

29. www.shu.ac.uk/schools/sci/chem/tutorials/chrom/gaschrm.htm, accessed on 18 July, 2005

30. Uyanik A. Gas chromatography in anaesthesia. I. A brief review of analytical methods and gas chromatographic detector and column systems. J Chromatogr B 1997; 23: 1–9

31. Simoneit BR. A review of current applications of mass spectrometry for biomarker/molecular tracer elucidations. Mass Spectrom Rev 2004; 24: 719–65

32. Scott RPW. Recent developments in gas chromatography. II. Manufact Chem 1958; 29: 517–22

33. Marriot PJ, Shellie R, Cornwell C. Gas chromatographic technologies for the analysis of essential oils. J Chromatogr A 2001; 936: 1–22

34. Halket JM, Zaikin VV. Derivatization in mass spectrometry–3. Alkylation (arylation). Eur J Mass Spectrom 2004; 10: 1–19

35. Little JL. Artifacts in trimethylsilyl derivatization reactions and ways to avoid them. J Chromatogr A 1999; 844: 1–22

36. Haslam E, Lilley TH, Cai Y, et al. Traditional herbal medicines – the role of polyphenols. Planta Med 1989; 55: 1–8

37. Fiamegos YC, Nanos CG, Vervoort J, Stalikas CD. Analytical procedure for the in-vial derivatization-extraction of phenolic acids and flavonoids in methanolic and aqueous plant extracts followed by gas chromatography with mass-selective detection. J Chromatogr A 2004; 1041: 11–18

38. Siouffi AM. HPLC columns. Spectra Anal 1993; 22: 55–8

39. Willis FM, Felton MJ. UV detectors. Today's Chemist at Work 2004; 49–50

40. Murphy JF. The use of light scattering detectors in HPLC analysis of pharmaceuticals. Am Pharm Rev 2001; 4: 69–72

41. Rose MJ, Lunte SM, Carlson RG, Stobaugh JF. Transformation of analytes for electrochemical detection: a review of chemical and physical approaches. Adv Chromatogr 2001; 41: 203–48

42. Sherma J. High-performance liquid chromatography/mass spectrometry analysis of botanical medicines and dietary supplements: a review. J AOAC Int 2003; 86: 873–81

43. Sun Y, Li W, Fitzloff JF, van Breemen RB. Liquid chromatography/electrospray tandem mass spectrometry of terpenoid lactones in Ginkgo biloba. J Mass Spectrom 2005; 40: 373–9

44. Tanaka H, Shoyama Y. Development of ELISA-analysis methods for the quantification of bioactive natural products in plants, phytomedicines, and in humans and similar. Phytomedicine 1998; 5: 397–415

45. Tanaka H, Fukuda N, Shoyama Y. Formation of monoclonal antibody against a major ginseng component, ginsenoside Rb1 and its characterization. Cytotechnology 1999; 29: 115–20

46. Fukuda N, Tanaka H, Shoyama Y. Applications of ELISA, Western blotting and immunoaffinity concentration for survey of ginsenosides in crude drugs of Panax species and traditional Chinese herbal medicines. Analyst 2000; 125: 1425–9

47. Hadley SK, Petry JJ. Medicinal herbs: a primer for primary care. Hosp Pract 1999; 34: 105–6

48. Anon. Good manufacturing practices: supplementary guidelines for the manufacture of herbal medicinal products. WHO Technical Report Series No 863. Geneva: World Health Organization, 1996: 109–13

49. Anon. Quality control methods for medicinal plant materials. Geneva: World Health Organization, 1998: 1–122

50. Barnes J. Quality, efficacy and safety of complementary medicines: fashions, facts and the future. Part I. Regulation and quality. Br J Clin Pharmacol 2003; 55: 226–33

51. Ang-Lee MK, Moss J, Yuan CS. Herbal medicines and perioperative care. J Am Med Assoc 2001; 286: 208–16

52. Techen N, Crockett SL, Khan IA, Scheffler BE. Authentication of medicinal plants using molecular biology techniques to complement conventional methods. Curr Med Chem 2004; 11: 1391–401

53. Ohtake N, Nakai Y, Yamamoto M, et al. Separation and isolation methods for analysis of the active principles of Sho-saiko-to (SST) oriental medicine. J Chromatogr B 2004; 812: 135–48

54. Van Beek TA. Chemical analysis of Ginkgo biloba leaves and extracts. J Chromatogr A 2002; 967: 21–55

55. Van Beek TA, Bombardelli E, Morazzoni P, Peterlongo F. Ginkgo biloba L. Fitoterapia 1998; 69: 195–244

56. Loew D, Kaszkin M. Approaching the problem of bioequivalence of herbal medicinal products. Phytother Res 2002; 16: 705–11

57. Suffness M, Pezzuto JM. Assays related to cancer drug discovery. In Hostettmann K, ed. Methods in Plant Biochemistry, Vol. 6, Assays for Bioactivity. London: Academic Press, 1991: 53–71

58. Vlietinck AJ, Apers S. Biological screening methods in the search of pharmacologically active natural products. In Tringali C, ed. Bioactive Compounds from Natural Sources: Isolation, Characterization and Biological Properties. London: Taylor & Francis Inc., 2001: 1–29

59. Hazra B, Das Sarma M, Sanyal U. Separation methods of quinonoid constituents of plants used in Oriental traditional medicines. J Chromatogr B 2004; 812: 259–75

60. Wen D, Liu Y, Li W, Liu H. Separation methods for antibacterial and antirheumatism agents in plant medicines. J Chromatogr B 2004; 812: 101–17

61. Tsao R, Deng Z. Separation procedures for naturally occurring antioxidant phytochemicals. J Chromatogr B 2004; 812: 85–99

62. Fang F, Sang S, Chen KY, et al. Isolation and identification of cytotoxic compounds from bay leaf (Laurus nobilis). Food Chem 2005; 93: 497–501

63. Bernstein A, Breitman M. Genetic ablation in transgenic mice. Mol Biol Med 1989; 6: 523–30

64. Xie JT, Aung HH, Wu JA, et al. Effects of American ginseng berry extract on blood glucose levels in ob/ob mice. Am J Chin Med 2002; 30: 187–94

65. Fuzzati N. Analysis methods of ginsenosides. J Chromatogr B 2004; 812: 119–33

66. Fukuda N, Tanaka H, Shoyama Y. Isolation of the pharmacologically active saponin ginsenoside Rb1 from ginseng by immunoaffinity column chromatography. J Nat Prod 2000; 63: 283–5

Ginseng: beneficial and potential adverse effects 5

J.-T. Xie, A. S. Attele and C.-S. Yuan

INTRODUCTION

Ginseng is a slow-growing perennial herb that belongs to the family Araliaceae. It is an aromatic plant with a short rhizome with a fleshy white root and a simple aerial stem bearing one to six leaves. The root system of ginseng consists of the primary root and its branches, and some adventitious roots develop from the rhizome. The ginseng root has been used for over 2000 years, and is believed to be a panacea, promoting longevity. As described in Chinese traditional medicine textbooks, its effectiveness reaches mythical proportions. Ginseng's genus name *Panax* is derived from the Greek *pan* (all) and *akos* (cure), meaning cure-all[1-3].

Ginseng's therapeutic uses were recorded in the oldest comprehensive materia medica, *The Herbal Classic of the Divine Plowman* (Shen Nong Ben Cao Jing in Chinese), in approximately 101 BC during the West Han Dynasty of China[4]. Ginseng root has been used as a tonic to rejuvenate, revitalize, and enhance stamina and physical capacity for thousands of years. Marco Polo was aware of Chinese ginseng, and the plant was brought to Europe, possibly with the silk trade, and it is certain that the Arabs brought back ginseng from China in the ninth century[5]. Ginseng is one of the most popular herbal remedies in the USA and a number of health claims are made to support it[4,6,7]. There is a renewed interest in investigating ginseng pharmacology using biochemical and molecular biologic techniques. Pharmacologic effects of ginseng have been demonstrated in the central nervous, cardiovascular, endocrine, and immune systems. The great diversity of pharmacologic properties attributed to ginseng root suggests that it might act in a unique and fundamental way on the body. In fact, its activity often appears to be based on whole-body effects, rather than on particular organs or systems[8]. In addition, ginseng and its constituents have been ascribed antineoplastic[9], antistress[10], and antioxidant activities[11,12]. It is an herb with many active components, and there is evidence from numerous studies that ginseng has beneficial effects[13,14].

Seven major species of ginseng are distributed throughout East Asia, Central Asia, and North America. Most studies of ginseng, including those cited in this commentary, have utilized constituents from three common species, *Panax ginseng* C. A. Meyer (Asian ginseng), *Panax quinquefolius* L. (American ginseng), and *Panax japonicus* C. A. Meyer (Japanese ginseng)[4,13,15].

Active constituents found in most ginseng species include ginsenosides (or panaxosides), polysaccharides, peptides, polyacetylenic alcohols, and fatty acids[13,16,17]. There is wide variation (2–20%) in ginsenoside content in different species of ginseng. Ginsenosides belong to a chemical group called saponins, which are similar in composition and structure to steroids[4,18]. Moreover, pharmacologic differences within a single species cultivated in two different locations have been reported. For example, the potency of extracts from *Panax quinquefolius,* cultivated in the USA, for modulating neuronal activity was significantly higher than for the same species cultivated in China[19].

There is extensive literature on the beneficial and adverse effects of ginseng and its constituents. This chapter aims to review evidence-based beneficial and adverse effects of ginseng and ginsenosides, and their possible mechanisms of action.

PHARMACOLOGIC EFFECTS

Previous studies have demonstrated that ginseng and its constituents possess multiple pharmacologic actions, within the central nervous system (CNS), cardiovascular system, endocrine system, and immune system. It is also known that ginseng has antistress, antifatigue, antiviral, antifungal, antineoplastic, anti-ischemia–reperfusion, and antihyperglycemic effects. Most pharmacologic actions of ginseng are attributed to ginsenosides[4,20–22].

More than 30 ginsenosides have been isolated and identified[14,23], and novel structures continue to be reported, particularly from *Panax quinquefolius* and *Panax japonicus*[24]. Figure 5.1 illustrates the structures of some ginsenosides.

Effects on the central nervous system

Ginseng has both stimulatory and inhibitory effects on the CNS[25], and may modulate neurotransmission. Ginsenosides Rb$_1$ and Rg$_1$ play a major role in these effects[26,27].

Memory, learning and neuroprotection

Results of several animal studies have shown that Rb$_1$[28], Rg$_1$[29], and Re[30] prevent scopolamine-induced memory deficiencies. Central cholinergic systems have been implicated in mediating learning and memory processes[31]. Rb$_1$ was shown to increase the uptake of choline in central cholinergic nerve endings[27], and to facilitate the release of acetylcholine from hippocampal slices[28]. Both Rb$_1$ and Rg$_1$ appear partially to reverse scopolamine-induced amnesia by increasing cholinergic activity. Results from these investigations suggest that

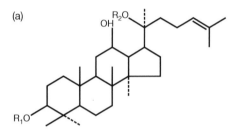

(a)

Panaxadiols

Ginsenoside	R$_1$	R$_2$
Rb$_1$	–glc (2–1) glc	–glc (6–1) glc
Rb$_2$	–glc (2–1) glc	–glc (6–1) arap
Rc	–glc (2–1) glc	–glc (6–1) araf
Rd	–glc (2–1) glc	–glc
Rg$_3$	–glc (2–1) glc	–H
Rh$_2$	–glc	–H
Rh$_3$	–glc	

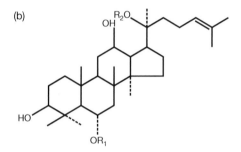

(b)

Panaxatriols

Ginsenoside	R$_1$	R$_2$
Rb$_1$	–glc (2–1) glc	–glc (6–1) glc
Rb$_2$	–glc (2–1) glc	–glc (6–1) arap
Rc	–glc (2–1) glc	–glc (6–1) araf
Rd	–glc (2–1) glc	–glc
Rg$_3$	–glc (2–1) glc	–H
Rh$_2$	–glc	–H
Rh$_3$	–glc	

(c)

Oleanic acid

Ginsenoside	R$_1$	R$_2$
Rb$_1$	–glcUA (2–1)	–glc

Figure 5.1   Structures of ginsenosides discussed in the text. Based on chemical structure, there are two major groups, panaxadiols (a) and panaxatriols (b). Rh$_3$, as shown in the lower part of (a), differs from other panaxadiols at the side chain. Ginsenoside Ro, a non-steroidal saponin, is shown in (c)

ginsenosides may facilitate learning and memory and are able to enhance nerve growth[32,33]. In fact, the total effect of the ginseng root is stimulatory, but diols, such as Rb_1, are sedative, and triols, such as Rg_1, are stimulatory. A previous study showed that, with the 'shuttle-box' method for active avoidance, the most pronounced effect on learning and memory was obtained by 10 mg/kg. With the 'step-down' method for passive avoidance, the dose of 30 mg/kg significantly improved retention. These results show that ginseng at appropriate doses improves learning, memory, and physical capabilities[8].

Ginsenosides may also possess the ability to protect neurons from ischemic damage. Rb_1 was shown to rescue hippocampal neurons from lethal ischemic damage[34], and to delay neuronal death from transient forebrain ischemia *in vitro*[35]. In another *in vivo* experiment, total saponins of ginseng were shown to possesses protective effects against ischemia–reperfusion in the rat brain[36]. In addition, Rg_1 was shown to increase the membrane fluidity of cortical cells from 27-month-old rats[37]. Rb_1 increased the fluidity of synaptosomal membranes impaired by $FeSO_4$–cystein[38]. Both Rb_1 and Rg_1 significantly decreased the hippocampal $[Ca^{2+}]_i$ level that was found to increase in aged rats[39].

Neurotransmitter modulation

Results of *in vitro* studies have shown that ginsenosides may modulate nerve transmission by decreasing the availability of neurotransmitters. Tsang and colleagues[26] demonstrated that ginseng extract concentration-dependently inhibited the uptake of γ-aminobutyric acid (GABA), glutamate, dopamine, noradrenaline (norepinephrine), and serotonin in rat brain synaptosomes. Ginsenosides competed with agonists for binding to $GABA_A$ and $GABA_B$ receptors[40]. Yuan and co-workers[41] demonstrated that *Panax quinquefolius* extracts interact with the ligand binding of $GABA_A$ receptors in brainstem neurons, which suggests that regulation of GABA-ergic neurotransmission may be an important action of ginseng.

Other central nervous system effects

An *in vivo* study that explored the effects of ginsenosides on drug-induced sleep showed that a mixture of Rb_1, Rb_2, and Rc prolonged the hexobarbital sleeping time in mice and decreased exploratory activity[42], suggesting a CNS-depressing effect. Other studies demonstrated that ginseng may ameliorate some adverse effects of morphine. Rats sensitized to morphine developed dopaminergic hyperfunction[43]. Kim and associates[44] showed that total saponin of ginseng prevented the development of dopamine receptor supersensitivity induced by the chronic administration of morphine. Ginsenosides may also possess antinociceptive properties. Ginseng total extract and Rf were shown to inhibit Ca^{2+} channels on primary sensory neurons to the same degree as opioids[45]. In addition, pretreatment of rats with ginsenosides inhibited substance P-induced pain behaviors[46].

Ginseng effects on actions induced by opioids and psychostimulants were evaluated. Analgesic effects of opioids, such as morphine and U-50, 488H, were blocked by ginseng in a non-opioid-dependent manner. Ginseng inhibited the tolerance to and dependence on morphine, and prevented the suppressive effect on the development of morphine tolerance caused by co-exposure to foot-shock stress but not psychologic stress. These results provide evidence that ginseng may be useful clinically for the prevention of abuse of and dependence on opioids and psychostimulants[47]. In addition, oral administration of *Panax notoginseng* reduced grooming episode duration and number and increased inner crossing in open field. The experiments suggested that notoginsenosides can modulate emotional responses in rats[48].

Ca^{2+} is an important regulator for many neuronal functions, including exocytosis and excitability. Voltage-dependent Ca^{2+} channels play a key role in the control of free cytosolic Ca^{2+}. It is also known that there are at least more than five different subtypes of voltage-dependent Ca^{2+} channels in the nervous system, such as L-, N-, P-, O-, and T-type of Ca^{2+} channels. Data showed that ginsenosides are negatively coupled to three types of Ca^{2+} channel in bovine adrenal chromaffin cells. Thus, the selective regulation of voltage-dependent Ca^{2+} channel subtypes by ginsenosides in bovine adrenal chromaffin cells could be the cellular basis of the anti-stress effect by ginseng[45,49].

Data from our laboratory indicated that American ginseng aqueous extract tonically and reversibly blocked the Na^+ channels in a concentration- and voltage-dependent manner using whole-cell patch clamp techniques. Ginsenoside Rb_1, a major constituent of the American ginseng extract, produced a similar effect. The data suggest that Na^+ channels are blocked by ginseng extract and Rb_1, primarily owing to interaction with the inactive state of the channel. Inhibition of Na^+ channel activity by American ginseng extract may contribute to its neuroprotective effect during ischemia[50].

Effects on the cardiovascular system

Effects on blood pressure

Cardiovascular effects of ginseng root and individual ginsenosides have been studied extensively. Human studies suggested that ginseng may decrease systolic blood pressure[51] and enhance the efficacy of digoxin in class IV heart failure[52], and that the prolonged hypotensive effect is probably due to a Ca^{2+} channel blocking effect and interference with Ca^{2+} mobilization into vascular smooth muscle cells[4]. Ginsenoside Rb_1 decreased blood pressure in animal experiments[53], perhaps owing to relaxation of smooth muscle. However, ginsenoside Rb_1 has also been reported to have hypertensive effects[54]. Sung and associates[55] noted that, in hypertensive subjects treated with Korean red ginseng, forearm blood flows after infusion of acetylcholine or bradykinin were higher than those of non-treated hypertensive subjects. Similar results have been reported in *in vivo* animal studies. A crude saponin fraction of Korean red ginseng decreased systolic blood pressure in hypertensive rats[56], while the hypotensive effect of the saponin-free fraction was minimal. Lee and co-workers[57], working with anesthetized dogs, noted that intravenous administration of an ethanol or ether extract of ginseng (40 mg/kg) decreased total peripheral resistance and caused vasodilatation and bradycardia, while a similar dose of an aqueous extract increased total peripheral resistance. These discrepancies of 'Yin' and 'Yang' in ginseng could reflect differences in ginsenoside content due to the method of extraction[58]. On the other hand, it was shown that ginsenoside potentiated nitric oxide (NO)-mediated neurogenic vasodilatation of monkey cerebral arteries[59].

Anti-ischemia–reperfusion effects

The preventive effects of ginseng and ginsenoside on myocardial ischemia and reperfusion damage have been shown in both animal experiments and clinical trials[60–62]. *Panax ginseng* extract significantly limited the increase in left ventricular end-diastolic pressure and coronary perfusion pressure in rats responding to hyperbaric oxygen compared to untreated rats. The results indicated that ginseng prevented myocardial ischemia–reperfusion injury and impairment of endothelial function induced by reactive oxygen species arising from hyperbaric oxygen exposure, through an antioxidant intervention. In a clinical trial, both total ginsenosides and ginsenoside Rb showed protective effects on myocardial ischemic and reperfusion injuries

in open heart surgery. In addition, ginsenosides possess protective effects against cultured vascular endothelial cell damage induced by oxygen free radicals *in vitro*.

Nitric oxide-related activities

Many reports have described vasodilator actions mediated by NO release. Results of *in vitro* studies using vascular ring preparations suggested that the vasodilator actions of ginseng reflect the interaction of ginseng with an endogenous vasoactive substance[63], subsequently identified as NO. Total ginseng root extract did not alter basal vascular tone in ring preparations of vessels from rabbits, dogs, and humans, but relaxed vessels precontracted with norepinephrine or prostaglandin $F_2\alpha$[63]. Endothelium-dependent relaxation of the isolated rat aorta by ginsenoside Rg_3 was 100-fold more potent than by ginsenoside Rg_1[64].

Other studies reported that the NO-mediated vasorelaxation induced by ginsenosides may involve Ca^{2+}-activated K^+ channels[65] and tetraethylammonium-sensitive K^+ channels[64]. The ability of ginseng to release NO from the corpus cavernosum and cause concentration-dependent relaxation may contribute to the mechanism of penile erection[66]. The adrenergic nervous system has also been implicated in the complex cardiovascular effects of ginseng[67]. It was reported that panaxatriols, particularly Rg_2, reduced acetylcholine-evoked release of catecholamines from adrenal chromaffin cells[68].

Much evidence points to a close link between damaging action, oxygen free radicals, and many forms of human disease[69,70], including cardiopulmonary pathology and reperfusion ischemia in the heart and lung. It is interesting that ginseng, an important component of a traditional Chinese mixture of herbs used to treat coronary artery disease and myocardial infarction[71], has well-recognized antioxidant actions[72,73]. Antioxidant effects have been demonstrated in neonatal rat cardiomyocyte preparations in which ginseng reduced lactic acid dehydrogenase release[71]. In an *in vivo* animal experiment, *Panax ginseng* extract prevented myocardial ischemia–reperfusion damage and impairment of endothelial function induced by reactive oxygen species arising from hyperbaric oxygen exposure through an antioxidant intervention[61,74].

The vascular endothelial cell of the circulatory system is an early target of free radical injury. The protective action of ginseng against endothelial cell injury caused by a variety of reduced oxygen species generated by brief electrolysis of the medium was reported in a pulmonary model[14,75]. Such treatment decreases the synthesis of

NO and reverses the normal vasodilator response to acetylcholine in lungs precontracted with a thromboxane analog U46619[75,76]. Ginsenoside prevented these vascular effects and reduced the pulmonary edema that followed free radical injury[77]. Ginsenoside-induced vascular effects were reversed by nitro-L-arginine, an inhibitor of NO release. An aqueous extract of ginseng root inhibited iron-mediated peroxidation of arachidonic acid, and hydroxyl radical formation from added hydrogen peroxide[78].

Red ginseng was found to promote the proliferation of vascular endothelial cells, and inhibit the production and promote the decomposition of endothelin, which is known to constrict blood vessels and raise blood pressure[79].

Oxidized low-density lipoprotein is believed to be involved in the pathogenesis of atherosclerosis. *Panax quinquefolius* saponins were reported to reduce lipid peroxide levels in cultured rat cardiomyocytes[80]. The cardioprotective action of ginseng against ischemia–reperfusion injury has been demonstrated in patients undergoing cardiopulmonary bypass for mitral valve surgery. Total ginseng extract enhanced recovery of cardiac hemodynamic performance and significantly lowered mitochondrial swelling during the period of ischemia[61]. Treatment of rats with a standardized ginseng extract for 7 days resulted in cardioprotective effects. After exposure to hyperbaric hypoxia, the hearts of rats in the ginseng-treated group showed less coronary vasoconstriction in response to angiotensin II.

It is recognized that NO, as well as being an important cell-signaling molecule, is an antioxidant[81]. NO-releasing agents protected lung fibroblasts from oxygen-radical damage caused by hypoxanthine/xanthine oxidase[82]. Several observations have suggested that release of NO by ginseng may underlie its antioxidant effects. In bovine aortic endothelial cells, ginseng extract and Rg_1 enhanced the conversion of $[^{14}C]$L-arginine to $[^{14}C]$L-citrulline[77]. Under conditions that simulated oral ingestion, ginseng extract dilated preconstricted perfused lung and preserved acetylcholine dilatation following free radical injury[76]. Superoxide dismutase converts superoxide radical to hydrogen peroxide, which, in turn, is broken down to water and oxygen by catalase. Thus, superoxide dismutase and catalase constitute the first co-ordinated unit of defense against oxygen free radicals. Reports[83,84] indicate that Rb_1 and Rb_2 enhanced expression of the Cu, Zn-superoxide dismutase gene, probably mediated by the AP2 transcription factor. Rb_2 was reported to be the major inducer of the catalase gene[84]. If demonstrated to occur in vascular endothelial cells,

this effect may be thought to contribute to the antioxidant activity of ginseng.

Antineoplastic and immunomodulatory effects

Considerable interest has been shown by researchers in how ginseng might prevent or assist in the treatment of cancer. Ginsenosides have been shown to exert anticarcinogenic effects *in vitro* through different mechanisms. Several ginsenosides show direct cytotoxic and growth inhibitory effects against tumor cells[8,85,86]. Others have been shown to induce differentiation and inhibit metastasis[87,88].

Tumor cell growth inhibition and apoptosis

Ginsenoside Rh_2 inhibited growth and stimulated melanogenesis[85], and arrested cell cycle progression at the G_1 stage[89] in B16–BL6 melanoma cells. In association with G_1 arrest, there was a suppression of cyclin-dependent-kinase-2 (Cdk2) activity. Ginsenosides Rb_1, Rb_2, and Rc are metabolized by intestinal bacteria after oral administration to a modified ginsenoside named M1[90,91]. Wakabayashi and associates[86] reported that M1 inhibited the proliferation of B16–BL6 mouse melanoma cells, and at a higher concentration induced cell death within 24 h by regulating apoptotis-related proteins. Ginsenosides from *Panax notoginseng* (Sanchi ginseng) also showed effects in a two-stage mouse skin model with 7,12-dimethylbenz[a]anthracene (DMBA) and in lung carcinogenesis induced by 4-nitroquinilin-1-oxide. Anticarcinogenic effects of majonoside from Vietnamese ginseng have also been shown in two-stage tests of mouse skin[3].

It has been reported that orally administered and subcutaneously injected Rh_2 inhibited the growth of human ovarian cells transplanted into nude mice, and significantly prolonged their survival times[92,93]. Intravenously or orally administered Rg_3 led to a decrease in lung metastasis of B16–BL6 melanoma cells[93]. Several studies which utilized medium-term and long-term anticarcinogenesis models of mice showed that ginseng extracts had a tumor inhibitory effect in mice that were exposed to chemical carcinogens[94,95]. Results of a cohort study showed that ginseng consumers had a lower risk for gastric and lung cancers, suggesting that ginseng may have a non-organ-specific anticarcinogenic effect[96]. It seems that a large-scale, controlled clinical study is needed to validate this result.

Antimitogenic activity

Sister chromatid exchange is regarded as a sensitive indicator of DNA damage[97], and significantly correlates with the mutagenic activities of many chemicals[98]. Rh_2 significantly suppressed both the baseline and induced sister chromatid exchanges in human lymphocytes[99]. In addition, ginseng may enhance the proofreading activity of eukaryotic DNA polymerase. Cho *et al.*[100] showed that total ginseng extracts activated both polymerase and exonuclease activities of DNA polymerase δ.

Differentiation and inhibition of metastasis

In vitro studies have demonstrated that Rh_2 and Rh_3 induced differentiation of promyelocytic leukemia HL-60 cells into granulocytes, possibly by modulating protein kinase-C isoforms[88]. Total ginseng extract was shown to induce differentiation of cultured Morris hepatoma cells. In addition, Mochizuki *et al.* showed that Rg_3 significantly inhibited the adhesion and invasion of B16–BL6 cells into reconstituted basement membranes, and inhibited pulmonary metastasis.

Immunomodulatory effects

In general, immunomodulatory and anticarcinogenic activities of ginsenosides are discussed together. However, few investigations have viewed these two events as sequential steps. Yun and co-workers[101] followed the natural killer (NK) cell activity and the incidence of lung adenoma in mice treated with urethane or benzopyrenes. In mice administered ginseng, the NK activity was depressed for 4–24 weeks, and then returned to control levels. Concurrently, in animals treated with ginseng, a lower incidence of lung adenoma was reported. Kim *et al.*[102] evaluated multiple immune system components in mice subchronically exposed to cyclophosphamide. This study also revealed that ginseng possesses some immunomodulatory properties, primarily associated with NK cell activity. In fact, ginseng may also prevent cancer through effects on the immune system. The effects of long-term oral administration of ginseng extract on levels of immunoglobulin types were studied in mice. Serum levels of γ-globulin decreased dose-dependently after ginseng administration. Among the immunoglobulin isotypes, only serum IgG_1 decreased. The researchers suggested that, since IgG_1 is rarely involved in killing cancer cells and can act as a blocking antibody, this effect of ginseng may be beneficial for the prevention and inhibition of cancer. Experiments have also shown that the anticarcinogenic activity of ginseng may be related to the augmentation of NK cell activity[8].

An experiment *in vivo* showed that oral administration of ginseng extract for 4 consecutive days enhanced the activities of B and T lymphocytes and NK cells in mice and increased production of interferon following an interferon inducer. In another animal experiment, ginseng extract was found to be effective against Semliki forest viral infection in mice[8]. Ginsenoside Rg_1 was shown to increase both humoral and cell-mediated immune responses. Kenarova and co-workers[103] reported that spleen cells, recovered from ginsenoside-treated mice injected with sheep red cells as the antigen, showed a significantly higher plaque-forming response and hemagglutinating antibody titers. In addition, Rg_1 increased the number of antigen-reactive T helper cells, T lymphocytes, and NK cells. Park and associates[104] observed that the acidic polysaccharide isolated from *Panax ginseng* possesses immunomodulating activities, mediated by the production of NO.

As described above, ginseng extracts and several ginsenosides have been shown to possess some anticarcinogenic and immunomodulatory effects. It would be interesting to see whether their efficacy could be observed in double-blind, randomized, placebo-controlled clinical studies.

Effect on human immunodeficiency virus

Cho and colleagues[105] observed that $CD4^+$ T-cell counts in human immunodeficiency virus (HIV)-1-infected patients treated with Korean red ginseng were maintained or even increased during 24 months of therapy. Their data also suggested that the maintenance of $CD4^+$ T-cell counts by zidovudine and Korean red ginseng intake for a prolonged period might be indirectly associated with delayed development of resistance to zidovudine by the ginseng intake.

Antihyperglycemic effects

Historic records reveal that, in traditional medical systems, a disease corresponding to type 2 diabetes was treated with plant extracts[106]. Pharmacologic activity evaluations of ginseng root on blood sugar levels started early last century[107]. Between 1921 and 1932, Japanese scientists reported that ginseng root decreased baseline blood glucose and reduced hyperglycemia caused by adrenaline (epinephrine) or high-concentration glucose administration[108,109]. Ginseng root has since been used to treat diabetic patients[2,4,110]. Since the 1980s, the number of published studies on ginseng root in treating diabetes increased remarkably, including both *in vitro* studies and *in vivo* experiments[111–117]. Ginseng root has been shown in clinical studies to have beneficial effects in both insulin-dependent and non-insulin-dependent diabetic patients. Oral administration of ginseng tablets (2000 mg daily for 8 weeks) to 36 non-insulin-dependent patients elevated mood, improved physical performance, reduced fasting blood glucose and serum aminoterminal propeptide of type III procollagen concentrations, and lowered glycated hemoglobin level[118–120]. Other clinical trials have also supported the notion that ginseng root possesses antihyperglycemic activity[121,122].

Recently, we have observed that Chinese and American ginseng berry extract and American ginseng leaf extract, which have a distinct ginsenoside profile compared to the profile of the root, have the ability to reduce hyperglycemia and body weight in C57BL/6J (*ob/ob*) mice and in C57BL/KsJ (*db/db*) mice as well[123–126]. Furthermore, the data also demonstrated that ginsenoside Re, a major constituent of the ginseng berry, plays a significant role in antihyperglycemic action. This antidiabetic effect of ginsenoside Re was not associated with body weight changes, suggesting that other constituents in the berry extract have distinct pharmacologic mechanisms on energy metabolism. In addition, we also observed that another constituent, the polysaccharide fraction, obtained from American ginseng berry extract, possesses an antihyperglycemic effect in both adult *ob/ob* and *db/db* mice[127]. The polysaccharide fraction, however, did not affect body weight changes in diabetic mice. More interestingly, we compared the antihyperglycemic effects of *Panex ginseng* root and berry extracts[128]. These results suggested that ginseng berry exhibits significantly more potent antihyperglycemic and anti-obese effects than ginseng root.

WHY ARE THERE SO MANY DIVERSE EFFECTS?

Ginseng contains over 30 ginsenosides, and single ginsenosides have been shown to produce multiple effects in the same tissue. Furthermore, the variety of ginsenosides may produce diverse pharmacologic effects[23,26,129,130], even opposing activities on the vascular system[58]. A study showed the influence of centrally administered ginsenoside by *in situ* hybridization histochemistry in the rat brain on the regulation of mRNA levels of the family of *N*-methyl-D-aspartate (NMDA) receptor subtypes. The ginsenosides Rc and Rg_1, the major components of ginseng saponin, differentially modulate NMDA receptor

subunit mRNA levels. The results show that structure differences of ginsenosides may diversely affect the modulation of expression of NMDA receptor subunit mRNA after infusion into the cerebroventricle in rats[130]. In addition, non-ginsenoside constituents of ginseng also exert pharmacologic effects. Thus, it is not surprising that the overall activity of the herb is complex.

Ginsenosides and steroids

Ginsenosides (except Ro) belong to a family of steroids called steroidal saponins[85,88,131]. They have been named ginsenoside saponins, triterpenoid saponins, or dammarane derivatives under previous classifications[132,133]. Ginsenosides possess a rigid four *trans*-ring steroid skeleton, with a modified side chain at C-20[134]. The classic steroid hormones have a truncated side chain (progesterone, cortisol, and aldosterone) or no side chain (estradiol and testosterone)[131,135]. Many steroids have a β-OH group at C-3; ginsenosides (Rb_1, Rb_2, Rc, and Rd, etc.) usually have a sugar residue attached to the same site[4,134]. Sugar moities are cleaved by acid hydrolysis during extraction, or by endogenous glycosidases to give the aglycone[4,131,134]. Steroidal saponins, which share structural features with steroid hormones, have been used in the industrial synthesis of progesterone and pregnanolone[131].

Steroids possess numerous physiologic activities, partly due to the nature of the steroid skeleton. The *trans*-ring junctions of the skeleton allow substituent groups, which interact with receptors, to be held in rigid, stereochemically defined orientations[131]. In addition, the steroid skeleton endows a favored structure for the whole molecule to allow, for example, insertion into membranes[136]. Reports showed that Rg_1 is a functional ligand of the nuclear glucocorticoid receptor (GR)[137,138].

Structural diversity of ginsenosides

As illustrated in Figure 5.1, ginsenosides exhibit considerable structural variation. They differ from one another by the type of sugar moiety, their number, and site of attachment. The sugar moieties present are glucose, maltose, fructose, and saccharose. They are attached to C-3, C-6 or C-20. The binding site of the sugar has been shown to influence biologic activity. Rh_1 and Rh_2 are structurally similar, except for the binding site of the β-D-glucopyranosyl group. In Rh_1 the sugar is at C-3, and in Rh_2, at C-6. Ginsenoside Rh_2 decreased growth of B16–BL6 melanoma cells, and stimulated melanogenesis and cell-to-cell adhesiveness. In contrast, Rh_1 had no effect on cell growth and cell-to-cell adhesiveness, but stimulated melanogenesis[129]. Significantly, only Rh$_2$ was incorporated in the lipid fraction of the B16–BL6 melanoma cell membrane.

Ginsenosides also differ in their number and site of attachment of hydroxyl groups. Polar substituents interact with phospholipid head groups in the hydrophilic domain of the membrane. Consequently, the insertional orientation of ginsenosides into membranes would be influenced by the number and site of polar OH groups. Differences in the number of OH groups were shown to influence pharmacologic activity. Ginsenosides Rh$_2$ and Rh$_3$ differ only by the presence of an OH group at C-20 in Rh$_2$. Although both Rh$_2$ and Rh$_3$ induced differentiation of promyelocyte leukemia HL-60 cells into morphologic and functional granulocytes, the potency of Rh$_2$ was higher[88].

Another factor that contributes to structural differences between ginsenosides is stereochemistry at C-20. Most ginsenosides that have been isolated are naturally present as enantiomeric mixtures[131,139]. Since the modules with which they react in biologic systems are also optically active, stereoisomers are considered to be functionally different chemical compounds[140]. Consequently, they often differ considerably in potency, pharmacologic activity, and pharmacokinetic profile. Both 20(S) and 20(R) ginsenoside Rg$_2$ inhibit acetylcholine-evoked secretion of catecholamines from cultured bovine adrenal chromaffin cells[141]. However, the 20(S) isomer showed a greater inhibitory effect.

(S)-Ganodermic acids are steroidal saponins which share structural features with ginsenosides[142]. Twelve compounds of (S)-ganodermic acid are either paired stereo or positional isomers, and show differential activation of human phospholipase C and A$_2$ by infiltrating into platelet membranes[143]. In this regard, the stereochemistry of the substituent was found to be the most important structural characteristic.

Structural alterations in the gut after oral administration also contribute to diversity. Certain ginsenosides, such as Rb$_1$ and Rg$_1$, are poorly absorbed after ingestion[144]. Rb$_1$ was hydrolyzed to compound K by intestinal flora; this was shown to increase the cytotoxicity of antineoplastic drugs[145] and induce apoptosis in B16–BL6 melanoma cells[86].

WHAT ARE THE UNDERLYING MECHANISMS OF ACTION?

Ginsenosides are amphiphilic in nature[131], and have the ability to intercalate into the plasma membrane. This leads to changes in membrane fluidity, and thus affects membrane function, eliciting a cellular response. There is evidence to suggest that ginsenosides interact directly with specific membrane proteins. Moreover, like steroid hormones, they are lipid-soluble signaling molecules, which can traverse the plasma membrane and initiate genomic effects. Figure 5.2 illustrates possible sites of action of ginsenosides, which are discussed below.

Ginsenosides and the plasma membrane

Cellular membranes may exist under conditions of curvature stress, being close to the hexagonal phase transition[146]. Consequently, the physicochemical properties of these membranes are sensitive to changes in membrane components and lipophilic agents, which may modulate curvature stress[147].

It has become increasingly evident that the lipid environment of membrane proteins, including ion channels, transporters, and receptors, plays an important role in their function[136]. In artificial and biologic membranes, cholesterol, a major membrane lipid, is organized into structural and kinetic domains or pools[148]. Membrane proteins are thought to be selectively localized in cholesterol-rich domains (acetylcholine receptor) or in cholesterol-poor domains (the sarcoplasmic Ca^{2+}-ATPase)[148]. Therefore, the biophysical properties of the different domains, rather than the bulk lipid, may selectively influence transmembrane protein function and mimic specificity at the effector level.

Ginsenosides may interact with the polar heads of membrane phospholipids and the β-OH of cholesterol through their OH groups. Moreover, their hydrophobic steroid backbone could intercalate into the hydrophobic interior of the bilayer. Both of these effects may contribute to altering the lipid environment around membrane proteins. Cholesterol is an intrinsic membrane lipid, which shares the steroid backbone and amphipathic nature of ginsenosides. Cholesterol enrichment has an inhibitory effect on the function of many membrane ATPases[136], and it may directly interact with the boundary lipids of ATPase and alter the intermolecular hydrogen bonds of the protein[149]. In contrast, ginsenoside Rb$_1$ has been shown to increase Na$^+$–K$^+$-ATPase and Ca^{2+}–Mg^{2+}-ATPase activity in neurons[38]. It is possible that some ginsenosides interact with membrane cholesterol and displace it from the immediate environment of ATPases. Since removal of cholesterol will lead to an increase in membrane fluidity[150], conformational changes that ATPases undergo during their transport cycle[151] may be facilitated.

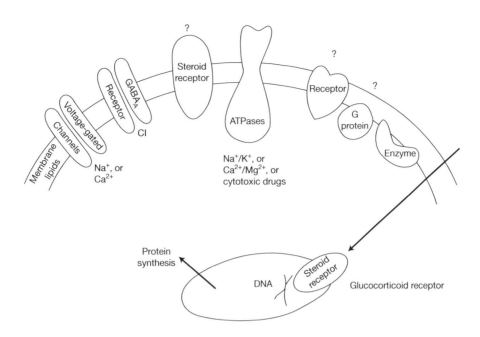

Figure 5.2 Drawing to illustrate potential sites of action of ginsenosides on plasma membrane and nuclear membrane. The question mark, '?' indicates hypothetical sites

Non-genomic action by steroids has only recently been widely recognized. Evidence for these rapid effects is now available for steroids of all classes[152]. In many of these cases, the steroid effect occurs at the membrane level and is not associated with entry into the cell. Several mechanisms for these effects have been proposed, including changes in membrane fluidity and activity of steroid hormones on plasma membrane receptors[153]. Ginsenosides may also modify membrane protein structure by changing membrane dynamics and modulating the activity of ion channels, membrane-bound receptors, and enzymes. Consequently, a single ginsenoside may be capable of interacting with multireceptor systems.

Ginsenosides and membrane channels

Ginsenoside effects on membrane channels show similarities to those of steroid hormones including progesterone, estrogen, and vitamin D metabolites, which modulate rapid Ca^{2+} influx in several tissues[153]. Several ginsenosides inhibit Ca^{2+} influx through voltage-gated Ca^{2+} channels in adrenal chromaffin cells[88]. Of the five ginsenosides that were tested (Rb_1, Re, Rf, Rg_1, and Rc), the inhibitory potency was highest for Rc. Tachikawa and associates[68] showed that, in bovine adrenal chromaffin cells, Rg_2 inhibited Na^+ influx through nicotinic receptor-gated cation channels, possibly by binding to the receptor-operated Na^+ channel. It is likely that the resulting decrease in catecholamine secretion may contribute to the antistress effects of *Panax ginseng*. Ginsenosides can also regulate Na^+ channels on nerve cells. Using standard patch clamp techniques, we observed that extracts of *Panax quinquefolius* and ginsenoside Rb_1 reversibly inhibited Na^+ channels in a concentration- and voltage-dependent manner[50], and caused partial inhibition of neuronal Na^+ channels during activation and inactivation states (unpublished data).

Ginsenoside activity on membrane pumps is not limited to ion transporters. P-glycoprotein is a membrane ATPase pump that actively exports cytotoxic compounds, and contributes to anticancer multi-drug resistance[154]. Several ginsenosides, including 20(*S*)Rh_2, inhibit the transport function of P-glycoprotein and increase sensitivity to cancer chemotherapeutics in resistant cells[145].

Ginsenosides and GABA receptors

Several ginsenosides (Rb_1, Rb_2, Rc, Re, Rf, and Rg_1)[40] and total ginseng extracts[41] modulated the binding of the $GABA_A$ agonist muscimol. Ginseng extract and Rc decreased the affinity of $GABA_B$ agonist baclofen binding[40]. Like ginsenosides, steroidal compounds regulate GABA-ergic neurotransmission in the brain. Several endogenous steroids such as progesterone, androsterone, neurosteroids, and their metabolites stimulate GABA$_A$-mediated chloride ion flux[152].

Ginsenosides and other membrane proteins

Agents that modify the physical properties of the phospholipid bilayer, such as its fluidity, can modulate the activity of membrane-bound G proteins in the absence of the receptors[155]. Some Ca^{2+} channels in sensory neurons are linked to G protein-coupled receptors[45]. Ginsenoside Rf was shown to produce antinociception by inhibiting Ca^{2+} channels on sensory neurons through a pertussis toxin-sensitive G protein[156]. However, whether Rf binds to the receptor or directly modulates G protein activity is not known.

One target molecule that may account for the anticancer effects of ginsenoside Rh$_2$ is Cdk2[89], an intracellular cell cycle regulating enzyme. It is not known whether Rh$_2$ directly inhibits Cdk2 activity. However, Cdk2 can also be indirectly suppressed via modulating signaling cascades originating at the cell membrane[157]. Rh$_2$ was shown to be incorporated in membranes to a level comparable to that of steroids[85]. Its ability to change membrane fluidity, adhesiveness, and cell-surface sugar structures further demonstrates that Rh$_2$ targets membrane components[85].

Some pharmacologic effects of ginsenosides may be mediated by binding to steroid hormone receptors. Both neural and non-neural membrane steroid receptors have been reported and, in most cases, steroids bind to membrane receptors with specificity and modest affinity[153]. The differential effects of various ginsenosides on the lipid bilayer argue against a non-specific activity. In contrast, these effects suggest a specific interaction between the ginsenoside and specific membrane proteins.

Membrane-associated enzymes sensitive to curvature strain such as protein kinase C (PKC) are highly responsive to perturbations of membrane structure[158]. A study has shown that the synergism exhibited by diacylglycerol and fatty acids in activating PKC is due to the synergistic effect of these molecules in inducing curvature strain in bilayers[147]. It was shown that ginsenosides Rh$_2$ and Rh$_3$ induced differentiation of human promyelocytic leukemia HL-60 cells into morphologic and functional granulocytes by modulating PKC activity[88]. PKCs directly phosphorylate a number of intracellular proteins and regulate important cellular functions, including cell growth and cell differentiation[159]. Coincidently, with the differentiation of HL-60 cells by ginsenoside Rh$_2$ there was an increase in PKC activity[88]. It is possible that gin-senosides Rh$_2$ and Rh$_3$ modulate PKC activity by altering curvature strain of the lipid bilayer. The ability of ginsenosides independently to target multiple plasma membrane-anchored proteins may account for the variety of responses that can be triggered.

Genomic effects of ginsenosides

As discussed earlier, ginsenosides belong to a family of steroids and share their structural characteristics[131]. Like steroids, they can freely traverse cell membranes. Moreover, their presence has been demonstrated within cells, particularly in the nucleus[86]. According to the classic theory of steroid hormone action, steroids, which bind nuclear receptors, are thought primarily to affect the transcription of mRNA and subsequent protein synthesis[152]. Intracellular steroid-binding proteins present possible attractive targets for ginsenosides.

A study showed the biologic effects resulting from structural similarities between ginsenosides and steroids. Lee and co-workers[137] showed that Rg$_1$ is a functional ligand of the GR. In this regard, the binding of the synthetic glucocorticoid dexamethasone to the GR was competitively inhibited by Rg$_1$, although the affinity of Rg$_1$ for the GR was lower than for dexamethasone. Ligand-occupied GR, when complexed with specific DNA sequences named glucocorticoid response elements (GREs), regulated the transcription of target genes[160]. Subsequent to ligand binding, Rg$_1$ activated GRE-containing reporter plasmids in a dose-dependent manner. Moreover, the GR-mediated transactivation and growth inhibition of FTO2B cells by dexamethasone and Rg$_1$ were inhibited by the specific glucocorticoid antagonist RU486. Rg$_1$ exhibits many other features of a glucocorticoid, such as synergistic activation of gene transcription by cAMP and the ability to down-regulate the GR content of cells[138].

After oral administration, ginsenosides Rb$_1$ and Rb$_2$ are metabolized by intestinal bacteria to compound K, also known as M1[91], which induces apoptosis of tumor cells[86]. Compound K was shown to have a nucleosomal distribution[86]. This, together with the observation of up-regulation of the CDK inhibitor p27 and the down-regulation of c-Myc and cyclin D1, suggests that the modification of apoptosis-related proteins by compound K is induced by transcriptional regulation[86]. Another investigation showed the binding of Rb$_2$ to transcription factor AP2[161]. The subsequent genomic event was shown to be the induction of the *SOD1* gene (Cu–Zn superoxide dismutase), a key enzyme in the metabolism of oxygen free radicals.

Summary

Ginseng is a highly valued herb in the Far East, and has gained popularity in the West during the past decade. The major active components of ginseng are ginsenosides, a diverse group of steroidal saponins, which demonstrate the ability to target a myriad of tissues, producing an array of pharmacologic responses. However, many mechanisms of ginsenoside activity still remain unknown. Since ginsenosides and other constituents of ginseng produce effects that are different from one another, and a single ginsenoside initiates multiple actions in the same tissue, the overall pharmacology of ginseng is complex. The ability of ginsenosides independently to target multi-receptor systems at the plasma membrane, as well as activate intracellular steroid receptors, may explain some pharmacologic effects.

After the discussion of the structural variability of ginsenosides, structural and functional relationship to steroids, and potential targets of action, it seems that effects of the ginsenosides may be initiated at the cell membrane, as well as via intracellular protein binding. Consequently, ginsenosides may follow a dual model of action.

One pathway of ginsenoside activity involves binding to membrane receptors that trigger changes in electrolyte transport systems and activation of signaling pathways. In this regard, differences in lipophilicity between the ginsenosides, and the cholesterol content of membrane domains, may be important. Future studies should be carried out to demonstrate the partitioning of ginsenosides in membranes, and to determine whether they induce changes in the structure of membrane proteins. Another possible mechanism by which ginsenosides produce pharmacologic effects is by binding to plasma membrane steroid receptors. Research in this area is still in its infancy, although there is growing interest in nongenomic signaling by steroids.

The second pathway of ginsenoside activity involves binding to intracellular steroid receptors, where the ligand–receptor complex acts as a transcription factor in the nucleus. The demonstration of ginsenoside Rg_1 as a functional ligand of the nuclear glucocorticoid receptor[137,138] supports this view. More studies should be directed to show that other ginsenosides may function as steroid receptor agonists, and to quantitate their binding. In this regard, computer-based images of functional groups on ginsenosides for the construction of pharmacophore models[162] would be useful. Future research should also focus on whether there is interaction between the two pathways of ginsenoside action, both of which may occur in the same cell. Therefore, the initial rapid response via membrane phenomena may be augmented by the delayed genomic response.

Two factors may contribute to the multiple pharmacologic effects of ginseng. The first is the structural and stereoisomerism exhibited by ginsenosides, which increases their diversity. The second is the ability of ginsenosides to target membrane-anchored receptors and ion channels, as well as nuclear receptors. Certainly, the argument can be raised that evidence for most pharmacologic effects of ginseng has been obtained from *in vitro* studies, many of which have not been confirmed *in vivo*. Nevertheless, the view that ginsenosides may initiate effects at the plasma membrane by interacting with multi-receptor systems, and that they also freely traverse the membrane and produce genomic effects, complements the intriguing pharmacology of ginseng.

POTENTIAL ADVERSE EFFECT OF GINSENG

As described above, a number of research data have demonstrated that ginseng and its major active components, ginsenosides, have a multiple constitution and multi-faceted pharmacologic actions[163]. Ginseng and ginsenosides influence the CNS (including learning, memory, and behavior), as well as cardiovascular, gastrointestinal, endocrine, and immune systems[163–165]. According to previous studies, it is commonly accepted that ginseng administration, in general, is safe when used appropriately[166–168]. However, is ginseng free from adverse effects? Like all other herbal medications, there is no doubt that ginseng contains a number of identified and unidentified chemical constituents with or without pharmacologic activities. Therefore, ginseng can have adverse effects, if consumed inappropriately or abused (e.g. ginseng abuse syndrome), or due to the lack of quality control in ginseng products[15,168–176].

Toxic effects in animal studies

Acute toxic effects

Acute toxicity studies have been performed in mice and rats[177]. The LD_{50} of ginseng root extract in mice was 5 g/kg after oral administration[4]. In another report, the LD_{50} of the root was 10–30 g/kg in mice[178]. The LD_{50} of ginseng leaf and stem extract was approximately 625 mg/kg with intraperitoneal injection in mice[179], and the LD_{50} values of the crude saponin fraction and saponins of ginseng leaf were 381 and 299 mg/kg, respectively, after intravenous injection. Behavioral changes observed after intraperitoneal administration of lethal doses showed that the crude saponin fraction produced extended posture, with the abdomen of the mice touching the floor and abnormal gait after a few minutes. Approximately 10 min later, swimming convulsions appeared and the mice died after 15–25 min. The LD_{50} was approximately 300 mg/kg[180]. Variable ginseng extracts contribute to the inconsistent LD_{50} data, making direct comparison impossible.

Our laboratory also evaluated the acute toxicity of ginseng berry extract in *ob/ob* mice. No adverse effects were observed in six animals that received 500 mg/kg daily by intraperitoneal injection for 12 days, while the maximum daily therapeutic dose used in other studies was 150 mg/kg[124,125]. However, all four *ob/ob* mice died within 24 h after receiving a single intraperitoneal dose of the extract at 1500 mg/kg (Yuan and colleagues, unpublished data).

Subacute toxic effects

In rats, ginseng leaf and stem extract at intraperitoneal doses up to 80 mg/kg for 21 days did not affect blood cells, hemoglobin levels, or renal function. In another subacute study, there were significant increases in body weight and food consumption in rats, while the brain, heart, lung, liver, spleen, kidneys, stomach, and testes/ovaries were normal in both gross and histopathologic examination[181].

Chronic toxic effects

No toxic effects were noted in rats following ingestion of ginseng extract at a daily dose of 105–210 mg/kg for 25 weeks[182]. Aphale and co-workers[181] found no toxicity after 90 days of ginseng administration. Chronic treatment of mice, rats, rabbits, and dogs has shown very few observable signs of toxicity. No evidence of toxicity was observed in male and female beagle dogs fed ginseng extract for 90 days at daily doses up to 15 mg/kg. The study showed that there were no treatment-related changes in body weight or blood chemistry[183]. A long-term safety investigation of ginseng product was performed in rats. Intake of the product during a 6-month period at a dose of 0.75 ml/kg did not show any unfavorable effects on integral, morphologic, biochemical, or hematologic parameters. In addition, two generations of rats that received ginseng product did not

exhibit embryotoxic, gonadotoxic, or teratogenic effects, nor a negative effect on the growth and development of their offspring[184].

Adverse effects in humans

General consideration

No significant adverse effects have been reported in ginseng clinical trials. However, several studies have observed that ginseng's side-effect profile includes insomnia, headache, nausea and vomiting, diarrhea, epistaxis, and skin eruption. Although the incidence of the individual symptoms was not clear, these symptoms usually occurred after inappropriate ginseng dose and its long-term use[167,185,186]. In addition, nervousness and gastrointestinal upset have also been reported after prolonged high doses of ginseng (e.g. up to 15 g/day for 2 years)[14]. Clinically, 'ginseng abuse syndrome' was described by Siegel[169]; 10% of subjects experienced hypertension together with nervousness, sleeplessness, skin eruption, and morning diarrhea. Edema was also seen in five subjects[169,172]. However, since this study did not differentiate between the species of ginseng used, its reliability was questioned by Mills *et al*.[8]. Moreover, symptoms described in the study may also be attributable to significant caffeine intake in most of the subjects[187].

Significant ginseng adverse effects can be found in a limited number of cases. Stevens–Johnson syndrome was noted in a 27-year-old man following the intake of two ginseng tablets for 3 days, resulting in moderate infiltration of the dermis by mononuclear cells. The patient recovered completely after 30 days[15,170]. More seriously, agranulocytosis was induced in a patient who took a Chinese ginseng product for relief of arthritis and back pain[182]. It is possible that some patients are very sensitive to ginseng administration.

Cardiovascular effects

Several clinical reports have demonstrated that ginseng and its products may cause cardiovascular adverse effects. A 39-year-old Czech man who had taken various ginseng products for 3 years manifested hypertension, dizziness, a loud palpable fourth heart sound, and 'thrusting' apical pulse. Shortness of breath and inability to concentrate were also noted[15,170,188]. Another report showed that hypertension is a contraindication to ginseng administration[189]. Therefore, use of ginseng requires caution in patients with cardiovascular conditions, agitation, diabetes, and psychosis[18]. In contrast, animal studies have shown that ginseng has a hypotensive effect and this effect may be related to the ginseng saponin fraction. Future studies are needed to address the inconsistent cardiovascular effects of ginseng.

Endocrine effects

There have been several clinical reports concerning adverse endocrine effects induced by high-dose ginseng or ginseng preparations. Several of ginseng's estrogen-like effects were reported. A postmenopausal woman who had used pills and topical creams containing ginseng experienced an estrogen-like effect of mastalgia and vaginal bleeding[190]. Another case reported that swelling and tenderness of the breasts were induced by ginseng in a menopausal woman. Likewise, another clinical case indicated postmenopausal bleeding in a 44-year-old woman who applied a topical ginseng face cream[191]. Oshima and colleagues[192] believed that the estrogen-like effects were not unexpected, since small quantities of estrone, estradiol, and estriol are present in ginseng root. However, the major active constituents of ginseng are ginsenosides, which are structurally similar to steroids such as testosterone, estrogen, and adrenocorticotropic hormone (ACTH)[18].

Based on the cases described above, pregnant, menopausal, and elderly women should be advised to use ginseng prudently, and patients receiving hormonal therapy should avoid ginseng completely[5,18,185,187]. Additionally, patients who have spontaneous nose bleeding and excessive menstrual bleeding should take ginseng prudently.

Other adverse effects

Ginseng may induce diuretic resistance in some patients[193], although the possible ginseng–drug interaction mechanism is unknown. Ginseng may also interact with warfarin, an anticoagulant with a narrow therapeutic index[175]. A case report showed that a man with a mechanical heart valve, stabilized with warfarin administration over 5 years, became destabilized following administration of a ginseng product[194]. The patient's international normalized ratio (INR) decreased from 3.1 to 1.5 after 2 weeks of ginseng intake. Following the discontinuation of ginseng therapy, the INR returned to 3.3 within 2 weeks. In this patient, ginseng use appeared to be associated with a significant decrease in warfarin anticoagulation since no other changes in medicine and foods could be found to be responsible.

Biochemical analysis did not detect vitamin K in ginseng[195]. The mechanism for this interaction has not been identified.

Although only one case report of ginseng–warfarin interaction has been reported to date, its impact on clinical medicine cannot be overestimated. In a number of recently published drug handbooks[196], and the publications Drug Interaction Facts[197] and Handbook of Herbs and Natural Supplements[198] as well as herbal review articles published in widely-read medical journals[167,173], a possible ginseng–warfarin interaction has been discussed, indicating that the issue has received the medical community's attention. Recently, we conducted a randomized, double-blind, placebo-controlled trial to evaluate the potential interactions between American ginseng and warfarin[175]. The clinical trial demonstrated that American ginseng reduces warfarin's anticoagulant effect. Thus, when prescribing warfarin, physicians should ask patients about ginseng use.

In addition, ginseng can inhibit platelet aggregation, as seen in *in vivo* and *in vitro* animal experiments. Furthermore, potential bleeding caused by ginseng is a concern for surgical patients[173].

To date, most adverse effects of ginseng have been reported from animal study data and individual clinical case reports. Controlled clinical studies are urgently needed to determine ginseng's potential adverse effects. Because long-term, high-dose ginseng use may be responsible for the reported adverse events, it is recommended that the daily ginseng dose should be 0.5–2.0 g dry root, or the equivalent extract, for short-term treatment[167]. Ginseng should not be used in children under the age of 2 years.

Possible reasons for the adverse effects

The possible reasons or mechanisms for the adverse effects of ginseng and its products may be multi-faceted, but are so far still unclear. According to previous studies, there are several plausible hypotheses that may be generally accepted. For example, high-dose administration may cause insomnia, headaches, diarrhea, sleeplessness, depression, as well as cardiovascular, endocrine, and nervous system disorders. Although the daily recommended ginseng dose is not over 2 g[167], a daily dose of 59 g was reported to achieve behavioral stimulation[169]. Other factors that may contribute to adverse effects of ginseng include the variety of ginseng species, variability in commercial ginseng preparations[16,199], different ginseng species[5,200], and potential ginseng–drug interactions[173,175,201]. To minimize possible adverse effects of ginseng, consumers should be advised to use it appropriately, and the herbal industry has a responsibility to provide standardized ginseng preparations. Future

investigations are needed to clarify both the beneficial and the adverse effects of ginseng, and their underlying mechanisms of action.

References

1. Hu SY. A contribution to our knowledge of ginseng. Am J Chin Med 1977; 5: 1–23
2. Blumenthal M, Goldberg A, Brinckmann J. Ginseng root, Newton, MA: Integrative Medicine Communications, 2000: 170–7
3. Yun T. Panax ginseng – a non-organ-specific cancer preventive? Lancet Oncol 2001; 2: 49–55
4. Huang KC. The Pharmacology of Chinese Herbs. Boca Raton, FL: CRC Press, 1999: 17–51
5. Phillipson JD, Anderson LA. Ginseng-quality, safety and efficacy? Pharmacol J 1984; 232: 161–5
6. Vogler BK, Pittler MH, Ernst E. The efficacy of ginseng. A systematic review of randomised clinical trials. Eur J Clin Pharmacol 1999; 55: 567–75
7. Barnes AS, Powell-Griner E, McFann K, Nahin RL. Complementary and alternative medicine use among adults. Adv Data 2004; 343: 1–19
8. Mills S, Bone K, Corrigan D, et al. Principles and practice of phytotherapy. Modern herbal medicine. In Ginseng (Panax ginseng C Meyer). Edinburgh: Churchill Livingstone, 2000: 418–32
9. Chang YS, Seo EK, Gyllenhaal C, Block KI. Panax ginseng: a role in cancer therapy (review). Integr Cancer Ther 2003; 2: 13–33
10. Kaneko H, Nakanishi K. Proof of the mysterious efficacy of ginseng: basic and clinical trials: clinical effects of medical ginseng, Korean red ginseng: specifically, its anti-stress action for prevention of disease. J Pharmacol Sci 2004; 95: 158–62
11. Shao ZH, Xie JT, Vanden Hoek TL, et al. Antioxidant effects of American ginseng berry extract in cardiomyocytes exposed to acute oxidant stress. Biochim Biophys Acta 2004; 1670: 165–71
12. Bae JW, Lee MH. Effect and putative mechanism of action of ginseng on the formation of glycated hemoglobin in vitro. J Ethnopharmacol 2004; 90: 137–40
13. Lee FC. Facts about Ginseng. Elizabeth, NJ: Hollyn International Corp, 1992
14. Gillis CN. Panax ginseng pharmacology: a nitric oxide link? Biochem Pharmacol 1997; 54: 1–8
15. Morgan A, Cupp MJ. Panax ginseng. In Cupp MJ, ed. Toxicology and Clinical Pharmacology of Herbal Products. Totowa, NJ: Humana Press, 2002: 141–53
16. Harkey MR, Henderson GL, Gershwin ME, et al. Variability in commercial ginseng products: an analysis of 25 preparations. Am J Clin Nutr 2001; 73: 1101–6
17. Li W, Fitzloff JF. Determination of 24 (R)-pseudoginsenoside F11 in North American ginseng using high performance liquid chromatography with evaporative light scattering detection. J Pharm Biomed Anal 2001; 25: 257–65
18. Sierpina VS. Ginseng. In Integrative Health Care, Complementary and Alternative Therapies for the Whole Person. Philadelphia, PA: F. D. Davis Company, 2001: 134–5
19. Yuan CS, Wu JA, Lowell T, Gu M. Gut and brain effects of American ginseng root on brainstem neuronal activities in rats. Am J Chin Med 1998; 26: 47–55
20. Ng TB, Wang H. Panaxagin, a new protein from Chinese ginseng possesses anti-fungal, anti-viral, translation-inhibiting and ribonucease activities. Life Sci 2001; 68: 739–49
21. Nishijo H, Uwano T, Zhong YM, Ono T. Proof of the mysterious efficacy of ginseng: basic and clinical trials: effects of red ginseng on learning and memory deficits in an animal model of amnesia. J Pharmacol Sci 2004; 95: 145–52
22. Qiao C, Den R, Kudo K, et al. Ginseng enhances contextual fear conditioning and neurogenesis in rats. Neurosci Res 2005; 51: 31–8
23. Tachikawa E, Kudo K. Proof of the mysterious efficacy of ginseng: basic and clinical trials: suppression of adrenal medullary function in vitro by ginseng. J Pharmacol Sci 2004; 95: 140–4
24. Yoshikawa M, Murakami T, Yashiro K, et al. Bioactive saponins and glycosides. XI. Structures of new dammarane-type triterpene oligoglycosides, quinquenosides I, II, III, IV, and V, from American ginseng, the roots of Panax quinquefolium L. Chem Pharm Bull (Tokyo) 1998; 46: 647–54
25. Saito H, Tsuchiya M, Naka S, Takagi K. Effects of Panax ginseng root on conditioned avoidance response in rats. Jpn J Pharmacol 1977; 27: 509–16
26. Tsang D, Yeung HW, Tso WW, Peck H. Ginseng saponins: influence on neurotransmitter uptake in rat brain synaptosomes. Planta Med 1985; 3: 221–4
27. Benishin CG. Actions of ginsenoside Rb₁ on choline uptake in central cholinergic nerve endings. Neurochem Int 1992; 21: 1–5
28. Benishin CG, Lee R, Wang LC, Liu HJ. Effects of ginsenoside Rb₁ on central cholinergic metabolism. Pharmacology 1991; 42: 223–9
29. Yamaguchi Y, Haruta K, Kobayashi H. Effects of ginsenosides on impaired performance induced in the rat by scopolamine in a radial-arm naze. Psychoneuroendocrinology 1995; 20: 645–53
30. Yamaguchi Y, Higashi M, Kobayashi H. Effects of oral and intraventricular administration of ginsenoside Rg₁ on the performance impaired by scopolamine in rats. Biomed Res 1996; 17: 487–90
31. Perry EK. The cholinergic hypothesis – ten years on. Br Med Bull 1986; 42: 63–9
32. Takemoto Y, Ueyama T, Saito H, et al. Potentiation of nerve growth factor-mediated nerve fiber production in organ

cultures of chicken embryonic ganglia by ginseng saponins: structure–activity relationship. Chem Pharm Bull (Tokyo) 1984; 32: 3128–33

33. Salim KN, McEwen BS, Chao HM. Ginsenoside Rb₁ regulates ChAT, NGF and trkA mRNA expression in the rat brain. Brain Res Mol Brain Res 1997; 47: 177–82

34. Lim JH, Wen TC, Matsuda S, et al. Protection of ischemic hippocampal neurons by ginsenoside Rb₁, a main ingredient of ginseng root. Neurosci Res 1997; 28: 191–200

35. Wen TC, Yoshimura H, Matsuda S, et al. Ginseng root prevents learning disability and neuronal loss in gerbils with 5-minute forebrain ischemia. Acta Neuropathol (Berl) 1996; 91: 15–22

36. Zhang Y, Liu T. Protective effects of total saponins of P ginseng on ischemia–reperfusion injury in rat brains. Chin J Pharmacol Toxicol 1994; 8: 7–12

37. Li JQ, Zhang JT. Effects of age and ginsenoside Rg₁ on membrane fluidity of cortical cells in rats. Acta Pharm Sin 1997; 32: 23–7

38. Jiang XY, Zhang JT, Shi CZ. Mechanism of action of ginsenoside Rb₁ in decreasing intracellular Ca²⁺. Yao Xue Xue Bao 1996; 31: 321–6

39. Liu M, Zhang JT. Protective effects of ginsenoside Rb₁ and Rg₁ on cultured hippocampal neurons. Yao Hsueh Hsueh Pao – Acta Pharmaceutica Sinica 1995; 30: 674–8

40. Kimura T, Saunders PA, Kim HS, et al. Interactions of ginsenosides with ligand-bindings of GABAA and GABAB receptors. Gen Pharm 1994; 25: 193–9

41. Yuan CS, Attele AS, Wu JA, Liu D. Modulation of American ginseng on brainstem GABAergic effects in rats. J Ethnopharmacol 1998; 62: 215–22

42. Takagi K, Saito H, Tsuchiya M. Pharmacological studies of Panax ginseng root: pharmacological properties of a crude saponin fraction. Jpn J Pharmacol 1972; 22: 339–46

43. Bhargava HN. Inability of cyclo (LEU-GLY) to facilitate the development of tolerance to and physical dependence on morphine in the rat. Life Sci 1980; 27: 117–23

44. Kim HS, Kang JG, Oh KW. Inhibition by ginseng total saponin of the development of morphine reverse tolerance and dopamine receptor supersensitivity in mice. Gen Pharmacol 1995; 26: 1071–6

45. Nah SY, Park HJ, McCleskey EW. A trace component of ginseng that inhibits Ca²⁺ channels through a pertussis toxin-sensitive G protein. Proc Natl Acad Sci USA 1995; 92: 8739–43

46. Yoon SR, Nah JJ, Shin YH, et al. Ginsenosides induce differential antinociception and inhibit substance P induced-nociceptive response in mice. Life Sci 1998; 62: PL 319–25

47. Tokuyama S, Takahashi M. Pharmacological and physiological effects of ginseng on actions induced by opioids and psychostimulants. Jpn J Pharmacol 2001; 117: 195–201

48. Cicero AFG, Bandieri E, Arletti R. Orally administered Panax notoginseng influence on rat spontaneous behaviour. J Ethnopharmacol 2000; 73: 387–90

49. Choi S, Jung S, Kim C, et al. Effect of ginsenosides on voltage-dependent Ca²⁺ channel subtypes in bovine chromaffin cells. J Ethnopharmacol 2001; 74: 75–81

50. Liu D, Li B, Liu Y, et al. Voltage-dependent inhibition of brain Na⁺ Channels by American ginseng. Eur J Pharmcol 2001; 413: 47–54

51. Han KH, Choe SC, Kim HS, et al. Effect of red ginseng on blood pressure in patients with essential hypertension and white coat hypertension. Am J Chin Med 1998; 26: 199–209

52. Ding DZ, Shen TK, Cui YZ. Effects of red ginseng on the congestive heart failure and its mechanism. Zhongguo Zhong Xi Yi Jie He Za Zhi 1995; 15: 325–7

53. Kaku T, Miyata T, Uruno T, et al. Chemico-pharmacological studies on saponins of Panax ginseng C. A. Meyer. II. Pharmacological part. Arzneimittelforschung 1975; 25: 539–47

54. Awang DVC. The anti-stress potential of North American ginseng (Panax quinquefolius L.). J Herbs Spices Med Plants 1998; 6: 87–91

55. Sung J, Han KH, Zo JH, et al. Effects of red ginseng upon vascular endothelial function in patients with essential hypertension. Am J Chin Med 2000; 28: 205–16

56. Jeon BH, Kim CS, Kim HS, et al. Effect of Korean red ginseng on blood pressure and nitric oxide production. Acta Pharmacol Sinica 2000; 21: 1095–100

57. Lee DC, Lee MO, Kim CY, Clifford DH. Effect of ether, ethanol and aqueous extracts of ginseng on cardiovascular function in dogs. Can J Comp Med 1981; 45: 182–7

58. Sengupta S, Toh SA, Sellers LA, et al. Modulating angiogenesis: the yin and the yang in ginseng. Circulation 2004; 110: 1219–25

59. Toda N, Kazuhide A, Fujioka H, Okamura T. Ginsenoside potentiates NO-mediated neurogenic vasodilatation of monkey cerebral arteries. J Ethnopharmacol 2001; 76: 109–13

60. Facino RM, Carini M, Aldini G, et al. Panax ginseng administration in the rat prevents myocardial ischemia–reperfusion damage induced by hyperbaric oxygen: evidence for an antioxidant intervention. Planta Med 1999; 65: 614–19

61. Zhan Y, Xu XH, Jiang YP. Effects of ginsenosides on myocardial ischemia/reperfusion damage in open-heart surgery patients. Med J China 1994; 74: 626–8

62. Mei B, Wang YF, Wu JX, Chen WZ. Protective effects of ginsenosides on oxygen free radical induced damages of cultured vascular endothelial cells in vitro. Yao Xue Xue Bao 1994; 29: 801–8

63. Chen X, Gillis CN, Moalli R. Vascular effects of ginsenosides in vitro. Br J Pharmacol 1984; 82: 485–91

64. Kim ND, Kang SY, Park JH, Schini-Kerth VB. Ginsenoside Rg₃ mediates endothelium-dependent relaxation in response to ginsenosides in rat aorta: role of K⁺ channels. Eur J Pharmacol 1999; 367: 41–9

65. Li Z, Chen X, Niwa Y, et al. Involvement of Ca²⁺-activated K⁺ channels in ginsenosides-induced aortic relaxation in rats. J Cardiovasc Pharmacol 2001; 37: 41–7

66. Chen X, Lee TJ. Ginsenosides-induced nitric oxide-mediated relaxation of the rabbit corpus cavernosum. Br J Pharmacol 1995; 115: 15–18

67. Zhang FL, Chen X. Effects of ginsenosides on sympathetic neurotransmitter release in pithed rats. Acta Pharmacol Sin 1987; 8: 217–20

68. Tachikawa E, Kudo K, Kashimoto T, Takahashi E. Ginseng saponins reduce acetylcholine-evoked Na⁺ influx and catecholamine secretion in bovine adrenal chromaffin cells. J Pharmacol Exp Ther 1995; 273: 629–36

69. Cross CE, Halliwell B, Borish ET, et al. Oxygen radicals and human disease. Ann Intern Med 1987; 107: 526–45

70. Das DK. Cellular, biochemical, and molecular aspects of reperfusion injury. Ann NY Acad Sci 1994; 723: 116–27

71. Chen X. Cardiovascular effects of ginsenosides and their nitric-oxide mediated antioxidant actions. In Packer L, MG Traber W Xin, eds. Proceedings of the International Sympo-

sium on Natural Antioxidants. Champaign, IL: AOCS, 1996: 485–98

72. Han BH, Han YN, Park MH. Chemical and biochemical studies on antioxidant components of ginseng. In Chang HM, HW Yeung, WW Tso A Koo, eds. Advances in Chinese Medicinal Materials Research. Singapore: World Scientific Press, 1995: 485–98

73. Kitts DD, Wijewickreme AN, Hu C. Antioxidant properties of a North American ginseng extract. Mol Cell Biochem 2000; 203: 1–10

74. Maffei Facino R, Carini M, Aldini G, et al. Panax ginseng administration in the rat prevents myocardial ischemia–reperfusion damage induced by hyperbaric oxygen: evidence for an antioxidant intervention. Planta Med 1999; 65: 614–19

75. Chen X, Gillis CN. Effect of free radicals on pulmonary vascular response to acetylcholine. J Appl Physiol 1991; 71: 821–5

76. Rimar S, Gillis CN. Nitric oxide and experimental lung injury. In Zapol WM KD Bloch, eds. Nitric Oxide and the Lung. New York, NY: Marcel Dekker, 1997: 165–83

77. Kim H, Chen X, Gillis CN. Ginsenosides protect pulmonary vascular endothelium against free radical-induced injury. Biochem Biophys Res Commun 1992; 189: 670–6

78. Zhang D, Yasuda T, Yu Y, et al. Ginseng extract scavenges hydroxyl radical and protects unsaturated fatty acids from decomposition caused by iron-mediated lipid peroxidation. Free Radical Biol Med 1996; 20: 145–50

79. Nakagima S, Uchiyama Y, Yoshida K, et al. The effects of ginseng radix rubra on human vascular endothelial cells. Am J Chin Med 1998; 26: 365–73

80. Li J, Huang M, Teoh H, Man RY. Panax quinquefolium saponins protect low density lipoproteins from oxidation. Life Sci 1999; 64: 53–62

81. Patel RP, McAndrew J, Sellak H, et al. Biological aspects of reactive nitrogen species. Biochim Biophys Acta 1999; 1411: 385–400

82. Wink DA, Hanbauer I, Krishna MC, et al. Nitric oxide protects against cellular damage and cytotoxicity from reactive oxygen species. Proc Natl Acad Sci USA 1993; 90: 9813–17

83. Kimata H, Sumida N, Matsufuji N, et al. Interaction of saponin of bupleuri radix with ginseng saponin: solubilization of saikosaponin-a with chikusetsusaponin V (= ginsenoside-Ro). Chem Pharm Bull (Tokyo) 1985; 33: 2849–53

84. Chang MS, Lee SG, Rho HM. Transcriptional activation of Cu/Zn superoxide dismutase and catalase genes by panaxadiol ginsenosides extracted from Panax ginseng. Phytother Res 1999; 13: 641–4

85. Ota T, Fujikawa-Yamamoto K, Zong ZP, et al. Plant-glycoside modulation of cell surface related to control of differentiation in cultured B16 melanoma cells. Cancer Res 1987; 47: 3863–7

86. Wakabayashi C, Murakami K, Hasegawa H, et al. An intestinal bacterial metabolite of ginseng protopanaxadiol saponins has the ability to induce apoptosis in tumor cells. Biochem Biophys Res Commun 1998; 246: 725–30

87. Mochizuki M, Yoo YC, Matsuzawa K, et al. Inhibitory effect of tumor metastasis in mice by saponins, ginsenoside-Rb$_2$, 20(R)- and 20(S)-ginsenoside-Rg$_3$, of red ginseng. Biol Pharm Bull 1995; 18: 1197–202

88. Kim YS, Kim DS, Kim SI. Ginsenoside Rh$_2$ and Rh$_3$ induce differentiation of HL-60 cells into granulocytes: modulation of protein kinase C isoforms during differentiation by ginsenoside Rh$_2$. Int J Biochem Cell Biol 1998; 30: 327–38

89. Ota T, Maeda M, Odashima S, et al. G1 phase-specific suppression of the CdK2 activity by ginsenoside Rh$_2$ in cultured murine cells. Life Sci 1997; 60: 39–44

90. Hasegawa H, Sung JH, Matsumiya S, Uchiyama M. Main ginseng saponin metabolites formed by intestinal bacteria. Planta Med 1996; 62: 453–7

91. Karikura M, Miyase T, Tanizawa H, et al. Studies on absorption, distribution, excretion and metabolism of ginseng saponins. VII. Comparison of the decomposition modes of ginsenoside-Rb$_1$ and -Rb$_2$ in the digestive tract of rats. Chem Pharm Bull (Tokyo) 1991; 39: 2357–61

92. Tode T, Kikuchi Y, Kita T, et al. Inhibitory effects by oral administration of ginsenoside Rh2 on the growth of human ovarian cancer cells in nude mice. J Cancer Res Clin Oncol 1993; 120: 24–6

93. Kim HS, Lee EH, Ko SR, et al. Effects of ginsenosides Rg$_3$ and Rh$_2$ on the proliferation of prostate cancer cells. Arch Pharm Res 2004; 27: 429–35

94. Yun TK, Kim SH, Lee YS. Trial of a new medium-term model using benzo(a)pyrene induced lung tumor in newborn mice. Anticancer Res 1995; 15: 839–45

95. Yun TK. Experimental and epidemiological evidence of the cancer preventive effects of Panax ginseng C. A. Meyer. Nutrition Rev 1996; 54: S71–S81

96. Yun T, Choi S. Preventive effect of ginseng intake against various human cancers: a case study on 1987 pairs. Cancer Epidem Biomarker Prev 1995; 4: 401–8

97. Perry P, Evans HJ. Cytological detection of mutagen-carcinogen exposure by sister chromatid exchange. Nature 1975; 258: 121–5

98. Nitta H, Matsumoto K, Shimizu M, et al. Panax ginseng extract improves the performance of aged fischer 344 rats in radial maze task but not in operant brightness discrimination task. Biol Pharm Bull 1995; 18: 1286–8

99. Zhu JH, Takeshita T, Kitagawa I, Morimoto K. Suppression of the formation of sister chromatid exchanges by low concentrations of ginsenoside Rh$_2$ in human blood lymphocytes. Cancer Res 1995; 55: 1221–3

100. Cho SW, Cho EH, Choi SY. Ginsenosides activate DNA polymerase from bovine placenta. Life Sci 1995; 57: 1359–65

101. Yun YS, Moon HS, Oh YR, et al. Effect of red ginseng on natural killer cell activity in mice with lung adenoma induced by urethane and benzo(a)pyrene. Cancer Detection Prev 1987; 1: 301–9

102. Kim JY, Germolec DR, Luster MI. Panax ginseng as a potential immunomodulator: studies in mice. Immunopharmacol Immunotoxicol 1990; 12: 2578

103. Kenarova B, Neychev H, Hadjiivanova C, Petkov VD. Immunomodulating activity of ginsenoside Rg$_1$ from Panax ginseng. Jpn J Pharmacol 1990; 54: 447–54

104. Park KM, Kim YS, Jeong TC, et al. Nitric oxide is involved in the immunomodulating activities of acidic polysaccharide from Panax ginseng. Planta Med 2001; 67: 122–6

105. Cho YK, Sung H, Lee HJ, et al. Long-term intake of Korean red ginseng in HIV-1-infected patients: development of resistance mutation to zidovudine is delayed. Int Immunopharmacol 2001; 1: 1295–305

106. Ackerknecht EH. A Short History of Medicine, Baltimore/London: Johns Hopkins University Press, 1982

107. Xie JT, Mehendale S, Yuan CS. Ginseng and diabetes. Am J Chin Med 2005; 33: 397–404

108. Wang C. Advances in study of pharmacology of ginseng. Acta Pharmaceut Sin 1965; 12: 477–586

109. Wang C. Recent advances in study of pharmacology of ginseng. Acta Pharmaceut Sin 1980; 15: 312–20

110. Bensky D, Gamble A. Ginseng. In Chinese Herbal Medicine, Materia Medica. Seattle, WA: Eastland Press, 1993: 314–17

111. Kimura M. Hypoglycemic component in ginseng radix and its insulin release. In Proceedings of the 3rd International Ginseng Symposium. Korean Ginseng Research Institute, Seoul, Korea, 1980: 37–8

112. Kimura M, Waki I, Tanaka O, et al. Pharmacological sequential trials for the fractionation of components with hypoglycemic activity in alloxan diabetic mice from ginseng radix. J Pharmacobio-Dyn 1981; 4: 402–9

113. Kimura M, Suzuki J. The pattern of action of blended Chinese traditional medicines to glucose tolerance curves in genetically diabetic KK-CAy mice. J Pharmacobio-Dyn 1981; 4: 907–15

114. Kimura M, Suzuki J, Koizumi T. Glucose tolerance curves in genetically diabetic KK-CAy mice: the pharmacokinetic analysis for humping effect. J Pharmacobio-Dyn 1981; 4: 149–61

115. Kimura M, Waki I, Chujo T, et al. Effects of hypoglycemic components in ginseng radix on blood insulin level in alloxan diabetic mice and on insulin release from perfused rat pancreas. J Pharmacobio-Dyn 1981; 4: 410–17

116. Yokozawa T, Kobayashi T, Oura H, Kawashima Y. Studies on the mechanism of the hypoglycemic activity of ginsenoside-Rb2 in streptozotocin-diabetic rats. Chem Pharm Bull (Tokyo) 1985; 33: 869–72

117. Kimura I, Nakashima N, Sugihara Y, et al. The antihyperglycaemic blend effect of traditional chinese medicine byakko-kaninjinto on alloxan and diabetic KK-CA(y) mice. Phytother Res 1999; 13: 484–8

118. Kwan HJ, Wan JK. Clinical study of treatment of diabetes with power of the steamed insam (ginseng) produced in Kaesong, Korea. Tech Inf 1994; 6: 33–5

119. Sotaniemi EA, Haapakoski E, Rautio A. Ginseng therapy in non-insulin-dependent diabetic patients. Diabetes Care 1995; 18: 1373–5

120. World Health Organization. Radix ginseng. In WHO Monographs on Selected Medicinal Plants (Volume 1). Malta, Geneva, 1999: 168–82

121. Vuksan V, Sievenpiper JL, Koo VY, et al. American ginseng (Panax quinquefolius L) reduces postprandial glycemia in nondiabetic subjects and subjects with type 2 diabetes mellitus. Arch Intern Med 2000; 160: 1009–13

122. Vuksan V, Stavro MP, Sievenpiper JL, et al. Similar postprandial glycemic reductions with escalation of dose and administration time of American ginseng in type 2 diabetes. Diabetes Care 2000; 23: 1221–6

123. Attele AS, Zhou YP, Xie JT, et al. Antidiabetic effects of Panax ginseng berry extract and the identification of an effective component. Diabetes 2002; 51: 1851–8

124. Xie JT, Aung HH, Wu JA, et al. Effects of American ginseng berry extract on blood glucose levels in ob/ob mice. Am J Chin Med 2002; 30: 187–94

125. Xie JT, Zhou Y-P, Dey L, et al. Ginseng berry reduces blood glucose and body weight in db/db mice. Phytomedicine 2002; 9: 254–8

126. Xie JT, Mehendale A, Wang A, et al. American ginseng leaf: ginsenoside analysis and hypoglycemic activity. Pharmacol Res 2004; 49: 113–17

127. Xie JT, Wu JA, Mehendale S, et al. Anti-hyperglycemic effect of the polysaccharides fraction from American ginseng berry extract in ob/ob mice. Phytomedicine 2004; 11: 182–7

128. Dey L, Xie JT, Wang A, et al. Anti-hyperglycemic effects of ginseng: comparison between root and berry. Phytomedicine 2003; 10: 600–5

129. Odashima S, Ohta T, Kohno H, et al. Control of phenotypic expression of cultured B16 melanoma cells by plant glycosides. Cancer Res 1985; 45: 2781–4

130. Kim HS, Hwang SL, Oh S. Ginsenoside Rc and Rg₁ differentially modulate NMDA receptor subunit mRNA levels after intracerebroventricular infusion in rats. Neurochem Res 2000; 25: 1149–54

131. Banthorpe DV. Terpenoids. In Natural Products. Essex: Longman Scientific and Technical, 1994: 331–9

132. Ourisson G, Crabbe P, Rodic OR. Tetracyclic Triterpenes. San Francisco, CA: Holden-Day Publisher, 1964

133. Boar RB. Terpenoids and Steroids. Dorking, UK: Bartholomew Press, 1983

134. Shibata S, Tanaka O, Shoji J, Saito H. Chemistry and pharmacology of Panax. Econ Medicin Plant Res 1985; 1: 217–83

135. Heftmann E, Mosetting E. Biochemistry of Steroids. London: Reinhold Publishing Corporation, 1960

136. Bastiaanse EM, Hold KM, Van der Laarse A. The effect of membrane cholesterol content on ion transport processes in plasma membranes. Cardiovasc Res 1997; 33: 272–83

137. Lee YJ, Chung E, Lee KY, et al. Ginsenoside-Rg₁, one of the major active molecules from Panax ginseng, is a functional ligand of glucocorticoid receptor. Mol Cell End 1997; 133: 135–40

138. Chung E, Lee KY, Lee YJ, et al. Ginsenoside Rg₁ down-regulates glucocorticoid receptor and displays synergistic effects with cAMP. Steroids 1998; 63: 421–4

139. Soldati F, Sticher O. HPLC separation and quantitative determination of ginsenosides from Panax ginseng, panax quinquefolium and from ginseng drug preparations. Planta Med 1980; 38: 348–57

140. Islam MR, Mahdi JG, Bowen ID. Pharmacological importance of stereochemical resolution of enantiomeric drugs. Drug Safety 1997; 17: 149–65

141. Kudo K, Tachikawa E, Kashimoto T, Takahashi E. Properties of ginseng saponin inhibition of catecholamine secretion in bovine adrenal chromaffin cells. Eur J Pharmacol 1998; 341: 139–44

142. Shiao MS, Lin LJ. Two new triterpenes of the fungus Ganoderma lucidum. J Nat Prod 1987; 50: 886–91

143. Wang CN, Chen JS, Shiao MS, Wang CT. Activation of human platelet phospholipases C and A2 by various oxygenated triterpenes. Eur J Pharmacol 1994; 267: 33–42

144. Odani T, Tanizawa H, Takino Y. Studies on the absorption, distribution, excretion and metabolism of ginseng saponins. III. The absorption, distribution and excretion of ginsenoside Rb1 in the rat. Chem Pharm Bull (Tokyo) 1983; 31: 1059–66

145. Hasegawa H, Sung JH, Matsumiya S, et al. Reversal of daunomycin and vinblastine resistance in multidrug-resistant P388 leukemia in vitro through enhanced cytotoxicity by triterpenoids. Planta Med 1995; 61: 409–13

146. Rilfors L, Hauksson JB, Lindblom G. Regulation and phase equilibria of membrane lipids from Bacillus megaterium and Acholeplasma laidlawii strain A containing methyl-branched acyl chains. Biochemistry (Mosc) 1994; 33: 6110–20

147. Goldberg EM, Zidovetzki R. Synergistic effects of diacylglycerols and fatty acids on membrane structure and protein kinase C activity. Biochemistry (Mosc) 1998; 37: 5623–32

148. Schroeder F, Jefferson JR, Kier AB, et al. Membrane cholesterol dynamics: cholesterol domains and kinetic pools. Proc Soc Exp Biol Med 1991; 196: 235–52

149. Mas-Oliva J, Santiago-Garcia J. Cholesterol effect on thermostability of the (Ca^{2+}, Mg^{2+})-ATPase from cardiac muscle sarcolemma. Biochem Int 1990; 21: 233–41

150. Kirkwood A, Pritchard JR, Schwarz SM, et al. Effect of low-density lipoprotein on endothelial cell membrane fluidity and mononuclear cell attachment. Am J Physiol 1991; 260: C43–9

151. Pederson PL, Carafoli E. Ion motive ATPases. Ubiquity, properties, and significance to cell function. Trends Biochem Sci 1987; 12: 146–50

152. Wehling M. Specific, nongenomic actions of steroid hormones. Annu Rev Physiol 1997; 59: 365–93

153. Brann DW, Hendry LB, Mahesh VB. Emerging diversities in the mechanism of action of steroid hormones. J Steroid Biochem Mol Biol 1995; 52: 113–33

154. Pastan I, Gottesman MM. Multidrug resistance. Annu Rev Med 1991; 42: 277–86

155. Gudi R, Nolan JP, Frangos JA. Modulation of GTPase activity of G proteins by fluid shear stress and phospholipid composition. Proc Natl Acad Sci USA 1998; 95: 2515–19

156. Mogil JS, Shin YH, McCleskey EW, et al. Ginsenoside Rf, a trace component of ginseng root, produces antinociception in mice. Brain Res 1998; 792: 218–28

157. Sherr CJ. G1 phase progression: cycling on cue. Cell 1994; 79: 551–5

158. Zidovetzki R, Lester DS. The mechanism of activation of protein kinase C: a biophysical perspective. Biochim Biophys Acta 1992; 1134: 261–72

159. Nishizuka Y. The role of protein kinase C in cell surface signal transduction and tumour promotion. Nature 1984; 308: 693–8

160. McEwan IJ, Almlof T, Wikstrom AC, et al. The glucocorticoid receptor functions at multiple steps during transcription initiation by RNA polymerase II. J Biol Chem 1994; 269: 25629–36

161. Kim YH, Park KH, Rho HM. Transcriptional activation of the Cu, Zn-superoxide dismutase gene through the AP2 site by ginsenoside Rb_2 extracted from a medicinal plant, Panax ginseng. J Biol Chem 1996; 271: 24539–43

162. Rohrer DC. 3D molecular similarity methods: in search of a pharmacophore. In Codding PW, ed. Structure-based Drug Design. Norwell, MA: Kluwer Academic Publishers, 1998: 65–76

163. Attele AS, Wu JA, Yuan CS. Ginseng pharmacology: multiple constituents and multiple actions. Biochem Pharmacol 1999; 58: 1685–93

164. Kim YK, Guo Q, Packer L. Free radical scavenging activity of red ginseng aqueous extracts. Toxicology 2002; 172: 149–56

165. Yuan CS, Wang X, Wu JA, et al. Effect of Panax quinquefolius L. on brainstem neuronal activities: comparison between Wisconsin-cultivated and Illinois-cultivated roots. Phytomedicine 2001; 8: 178–83

166. Singh B, Saxena AK, Chandan BK, et al. Adaptogenic activity of a novel, withanolide-free aqueous fraction from the roots of Withania somnifera Dun. Phytother Res 2001; 15: 311–18

167. Ernst E. The risk–benefit profile of commonly used herbal therapies: ginkgo, St. John's wort, ginseng, echinacea, saw palmetto, and kava. Ann Intern Med 2002; 136: 42–53

168. Bent S, Ko R. Commonly used herbal medicines in the United States: a review. Am J Med 2004; 116: 478–85

169. Siegel RK. Ginseng abuse syndrome. Problems with the panacea. J Am Med Assoc 1979; 241: 1614–15

170. Dega H, Laporte JL, Frances C, et al. Ginseng as a cause for Stevens–Johnson syndrome. Lancet 1996; 347: 1344

171. Faleni R, Soldati F. Ginseng as cause of Stevens–Johnson syndrome? Lancet 1996; 348: 267

172. Nocerino E, Amato M, Izzo A. The aphrodisiac and adaptogenic properties of ginseng. Fitoterapia 2002; 71: S1–S5

173. Ang-Lee MK, Moss J, Yuan CS. Herbal medicines and perioperative care. J Am Med Assoc 2001; 286: 208–16

174. Yuan CS, Wu JA, Osinski J. Ginsenoside variability in American ginseng samples [Comment]. Am J Clin Nutr 2002; 75: 600–1

175. Yuan CS, Wei G, Dey L, et al. Brief communication: American ginseng reduces warfarin's effect in healthy patients: a randomized, controlled trial. Ann Intern Med 2004; 141: 23–7

176. Izzo AA, Di Carlo G, Borrelli F, Ernst E. Cardiovascular pharmacotherapy and herbal medicines: the risk of drug interaction. Int J Cardiol 2005; 98: 1–14

177. Schulz V, Hansel R, Tyler VE. Rational Phytotherapy – A Physicians' Guide to Herbal Medicine, Berlin: Springer-Verlag, 1998

178. Brekhman II, Dardymov IV. New substances of plant origin which increase nonspecific resistance. Annu Rev Pharmacol 1969; 9: 419–30

179. Wang BX, Cui JC, Liu AJ. The action of ginsenosides extracted from the stems and leaves of Panax ginseng in promoting animal growth. Yao Hsueh Hsueh Pao – Acta Pharmaceut Sin 1982; 17: 899–904

180. Saito H, Morita M, Takagi K. Pharmacological studies of Panax ginseng leaves. Jpn J Pharmacol 1973; 23: 43–56

181. Aphale AA, Chhibba AD, Kumbhakarna NR, et al. Subacute toxicity study of the combination of ginseng (Panax ginseng) and ashwagandha (Withania somnifera) in rats: a safety assessment. Ind J Physiol Pharmacol 1998; 42: 299–302

182. Popov IM, Goldwag WJ. A review of the properties and clinical effects of ginseng. Am J Chin Med 1973; 1: 263–70

183. Hess FG Jr, Parent RA, Stevens KR, et al. Effects of subchronic feeding of ginseng extract G115 in beagle dogs. Food Chem Toxicol 1983; 21: 95–7

184. Sorokina E, Aksiuk IN, Kirpatovskaia NA, Levitskaia AB. Experimental animal study of the safety of biologically active food supplement obtained from ginseng root. Vopr Pitan 2000; 69: 53–6

185. Miller LG. Herbal medicinals: selected clinical considerations focusing on known or potential drug–herb interactions. Arch Intern Med 1998; 158: 2200–11

186. Awang DVC. Clinical trial of ginseng. Altern Therap Women's Health 2002; 4: 17–24

187. Bucci LR. Selected herbals and human exercise performance. Am J Clin Nutr 2000; 72: 624S–36S

188. Hammond TG, Whitworth JA. Adverse reactions to ginseng. Med J Aust 1981; 1: 492

189. Carabin IG, Burdock GA, Chatzidakis C. Safety assessment of Panax ginseng. Int J Toxicol 2000; 19: 293–301

190. Greenspan EM. Ginseng and vaginal bleeding. J Am Med Assoc 1983; 249: 2018

191. Hopkins MP, Takahashi M, Otake K. Isolation and hypoglycemic activity of eleutherans A, B, C, D, E, F, and G: glycans of Eleutherococcua senticosus roots. J Nat Prod 1986; 49: 293–7

192. Oshima Y, Sato K, Hikino H. Isolation and hypoglycemic activity of quinquefolans A, B, and C, glycans of Panax quinquefolium roots. J Nat Prod 1987; 50: 188–90

193. Becker BN, Greene J, Evanson J, et al. Ginseng-induced diuretic resistance. J Am Med Assoc 1996; 276: 606–7

194. Janetzky K, Morreale AP. Probable interaction between warfarin and ginseng. Am J Health Syst Pharm 1997; 54: 692–3

195. Zhang GD. Progress in the chemical constituents and analytical methods of Panax ginseng (author's transl). Yao Xue Xue Bao 1980; 15: 375–84

196. Mosby's Drug Guide, 4th edn. Philadelphia, PA: Mosby, 2001

197. Tatro DS. Drug Interaction Facts. St Louis, MO: Wolters Kluwer Company, 2001

198. Skidomore-Roth L. Handbook of Herbs and Natural Supplements. St. Louis, MO: Mosby, 2001

199. Cui J, Garle M, Eneroth P, Bjørkhem I. What do commercial ginseng preparations contain? Lancet 1994; 344: 134

200. Awang DVC. Maternal use of ginseng and neonatal androgenization. J Am Med Assoc 1991; 265: 1828

201. Windrum P, Hull DR, Morris TCM. Herb–drug interactions. Lancet 2000; 355: 1019–20

Green tea

6

D. D. McFadden

Better to be deprived of food for three days, than tea for one.   Ancient Chinese Proverb

INTRODUCTION

According to Chinese legend, Shen Nong, a famous Chinese emperor who was also a 'creative scientist', discovered tea nearly 5000 years ago in 2737 BC. His far-reaching edicts required that all drinking water be boiled as a hygienic precaution. One summer day when he was visiting a distant region of his realm he and his court stopped to rest. As the servants began to boil water, dried leaves from a nearby bush fell into the boiling water, producing a brown liquid. The Emperor drank some and found it very refreshing. Thus tea was created and Shen Nong earned the title of 'father of tea'. His intriguing description of tea has some validity even today; he credited tea with being 'good for tumors or abscesses that come about the head, or for ailments of the bladder. It dissipates heat caused by the phlegm, or inflammation of the chest. It quenches thirst, lessens the desire for sleep and gladdens and cheers the heart'[1].

Although tea was discovered in China and is often considered an 'Oriental' beverage, it has become increasingly popular in the West. After water, tea is the most consumed beverage in the world[2]. During the 13 years I lived and worked in China, I noted that, for the Chinese, tea is an integral part of their daily life and culture. Oriental tradition mandates the serving of tea to all guests. Even at hospital committee meetings, it was the tradition for the secretarial staff to juggle the recording of minutes with serving and 'refilling' teacups for each committee member.

Over the past several decades, there has been increasing interest in the potential health benefits of tea. Numerous scientific abstracts note its antiviral and antibacterial properties, its effects on prevention of cancer and cardiovascular disease (CVD), as well as its use as a possible adjunct treatment for hypertension, hyperlipidemia, and obesity. Other studies have noted possible benefits for allergy, asthma, arthritis, diabetes, memory loss, tooth decay, and osteoporosis[3].

In this chapter, we will examine some of the medical literature that supports these concepts. The proposed health benefits of tea will be considered under the following headings: adjunct supplement for HIV infection, cancer prevention, CVD prevention, hyperlipidemia, and obesity treatment.

TYPES OF TEA

There are many different types of tea, which may well differ in their health effects.

Green tea is prepared by heating leaves of the plant *Camelia sinensis* in hot water. Green tea accounts for approximately 20% of the tea that is consumed worldwide[4]. Black tea is consumed by more than 80% of the world's population. Black tea is made by allowing the green tea leaves to 'ferment' or 'auto-oxidize' enzymatically. This allows the conversion of green tea catechins to theaflavins. The catechins are compounds that include epigallocatechin gallate (EGCG), the most potent antioxidant in tea[5].

There are three categories of tea, depending on fermentation level; green tea (unfermented), oolong tea (partially fermented), and black tea (fermented). Although this process is often termed 'fermentation', this is incorrect as fermentation usually implies additives.

The more correct term should be oxidation, which involves exposure to air while drying. In general, green tea has been found to be superior to black tea for health benefits as it has a higher content of epigallocatechin gallate, a potent antioxidant. However, when Hirata et al.[6] compared the effects of black tea with caffeine on coronary circulation, they found it to be superior to caffeine in improving coronary function although there was no comparison with green tea[7].

A brief history

During the Sui dynasty (AD 518–617), tea was consumed more for its taste than for its health benefits. It was also during this period that tea began to be used as currency. During the Tang dynasty (AD 618–907), tea drinking evolved into a form of art. It spread throughout Chinese culture, reaching into every aspect of the society. It was given to nomads from Tibet and Mongolia.

In AD 800, Lu Yu wrote the first book on tea, the *Ch'a Ching* (the Holy Scripture of Tea.) His book classified the various methods of tea cultivation and preparation. As a poet, Lu Yu saw the harmony and order that reigned through all things in the tea service. After writing his great book, he attracted many students and became a friend of the Emperor.

According to the *Ch'a Ching*, tea should be prepared in the following manner:

> *After being plucked on a sunny day, the tea leaves must be baked over an even fire, with no wind. After baking they should be placed in a paper bag to cool. When completely cold the leaves can be ground. Then spring water should be heated to just under the boiling point and a pinch of salt added. Then bring it to a second boil, and stir in the middle portion of the liquid. Steep the ground tea leaves in this water in each cup individually and drink before it cools. The first and second cups taste the best, and more than four or five cups should not be consumed.*

Even though milk and sugar were available, they were never added to tea. Different teas held different medicinal purposes, although by this time tea was primarily considered a beverage rather than a medicine. The tea was typically drunk from bowls or cups that had been glazed blue on the inside, which was thought to bring out the greenness of the tea[8].

During the Song dynasty (AD 690–1279), tea rooms and houses were built in order for tea to be enjoyed in a social setting. Teahouses sprang up in towns and cities all over China and remain popular even today in China. Tea was originally made in bowls, but teapots were introduced during this period. A whole tea culture was created which included listening to music, gossiping with friends, and enjoying fine works of art while sipping tea in a popular tea house[8].

Current tea consumption

Even today in modern China, teahouses attract many local as well as foreign tourists. The tea is often served with a buffet of dried fruits, nuts, and numerous other snacks. Graceful, young Chinese xiaojies (waitresses) dressed in traditional colorful chipaos (Chinese dress) re-enact ancient tea ceremonies. Soft background Chinese music adds to the unique Oriental atmosphere. Often teahouses are perched lakeside, overlooking a serene body of water shrouded in a rising thin mist that adds a meditative, reflective atmosphere to the scene.

The popularity of tea consumption is growing rapidly in Western countries. In the USA, there are now more than 1200 teashops where there were almost none 15 years ago. Tea sales have almost doubled to $5 billion[8].

Reports of the health benefits of green tea have been intriguing, but difficult to interpret. Although, several confounding factors such as variations in diets, environmental conditions, socioeconomic factors, and habits such as smoking and alcohol consumption may influence study results, the most serious problem is a lack of large-scale, well-designed, prospective human studies. Further, although many health benefits of green tea catechins have been noted at the molecular and cellular levels, these *in vitro* studies use concentrations of catechins that are difficult to obtain by human consumption[10].

GREEN TEA AS MEDICINE

Green tea and infectious disease

Does tea possess antimicrobial effects? *In vitro* studies have demonstrated that both green and jasmine teas suppressed growth of *Staphylococcus aureus* and *Listeria monocytogenes* on selective agar. However, when they were individually evaluated for antimicrobial activity in a food model (ground beef), there was no significant difference between the tea and the control[11].

What about green tea for treatment of HIV? The active compounds of green tea are the polyphenolic catechins which includes epigallocatechin gallate (EGCG). This catechin accounts for about 50% of the total catechins in tea. EGCG binds strongly to many biologic molecules and affects a variety of enzyme activities. It is this specific component of green tea that is likely responsible for the many presumed health benefits. Kawai *et al.*[12] published the results of an *in vitro* study in which they noted that EGCG has antiviral properties. It inhibits HIV-1 replication *in vitro* by inhibiting the activity of HIV-1 reverse transcriptase, which leads to a decrease in HIV p24 antigen concentration. They reported that EGCG prevents the attachment of HIV-1 virion, gp120, to CD4 molecules on T-helper cells.

However, a crucial aspect of extrapolating *in vitro* results to clinically relevant strategies is the requirement to achieve 'physiologically relevant concentrations' of EGCG in the blood. Current phase I clinical trials involving pharmacokinetic studies of EGCG showed that only a small percentage of the orally administered catechin appeared in the blood. Drinking the equivalent of two cups of tea resulted in a mean plasma level of 0.17 μmol/l. In the *in vitro* studies just mentioned, EGCG levels were 25 to 250 μmol/l. Thus, although 'provocative', the Kawai paper does not yet prove the benefit of green tea, either for the treatment or prevention of human HIV infection[13].

Green tea and cancer

Tea consumption has been associated with a possible decreased prevalence of cancer. One potential mechanism is the protective effect of strong antioxidants such as tea polyphenols. In one phase II, randomized, controlled tea intervention trial[14], a total of 143 heavy smokers were randomized to drink either decaffeinated green or black tea or water, four cups daily for 4 months. Measurement of delta-hydroxydeoxyguanosine (δ-OHdG) was done to assess oxidative DNA damage. After 4 months there was a highly significant 31% decrease ($p = 0.002$) in urinary δ-OHdG in green tea drinkers. No change was noted in the black tea group. Green tea may protect smokers from oxidative damage and could reduce cancer and CVD risk caused by free radicals.

Animal studies involving rats, mice, and hamsters showed that tea consumption protects against lung, stomach, esophagus, duodenum, pancreas, liver, breast, colon, and skin cancers[15]. But what about human studies?

There has been much interest concerning the possible protective effect of green tea against prostate cancer. A case–control study in China noted that the adjusted OR of prostate cancer in tea drinkers relative to non-tea drinkers ranged from 0.09 to 0.28, depending on volume consumed and duration of consumption[16].

In Japan and China – areas where tea consumption is very high – the prevalence of prostate cancer is one of the lowest in the world. In contrast, the high-fat diet typical of Western countries is associated with high incidence rates. Migratory studies of Asian men who move to the USA show that these men acquire a higher prevalence of prostate cancer and eventually the incidence in this population is similar to that in the indigenous American male population. These studies suggest that changes in dietary habits may have major impacts on prostate cancer risk. Animal studies have shown that EGCG, the most prevalent polyphenol in green tea, may decrease PSA levels. Prostate cancer is a complex, heterogeneous malignancy. It has been challenging to provide satisfactory treatment options. Chemoprevention seems to be an ideal strategy, especially since prostate cancer is highly prevalent in elderly men and even a modest delay in neoplastic development could result in a substantial decrease in prevalence. However, more and larger prospective human studies need to be performed to confirm the protective effect of green tea for prostate cancer[17].

There is also some evidence that green tea is one of the chemicals that may have chemoprotective effects against bladder cancer. Other chemicals noted to have similar protective effects include vitamins A, B_6, C, and E. However, these data, although highly supportive, are far from definitive as epidemiologic studies have widely variable results[18].

Although some case–control studies have noted reduced cancer rates among tea drinkers, such studies are often subject to 'recall' bias, especially when reporting the amount of tea consumed. In one study designed to guard against this problem a biomarker – a tea polyphenol, urinary epigallocatechin (EGC) – was used to assess tea exposure. Mimi Yu at the University of Southern California and a US–Chinese collaboration reported a prospective cohort study of 18 244 men aged 45–64 followed up since 1986 in Shanghai, China. They identified 190 men who developed gastric cancer, 42 men with esophageal cancer, and 772 controls. In each study, participants had urinary polyphenols and their metabolites measured. Findings were adjusted for smoking, alcohol intake, blood carotene levels, and presence of *H. pylori*. They found urinary EGC was associated with a lower risk of both cancers. Protective effects were noted mainly in people who had below-average levels of carotenes–antioxidants commonly found in fruits and vegetables that are also thought to reduce cancer risk. They noted that 'the action of tea polyphenols is multifactoral', including antioxidant activity and apoptotic induction. Also, because of processing methods, 'the levels of polyphenols such as EGC in green tea may be ten times greater than those in black tea'[19].

However, in a pooled analysis of two prospective cohort studies in Northern Japan involving over 88 000 subjects, no association was noted between green tea consumption and risk of gastric cancer. The results disagree with most of the eight case–control studies, but agree with the five other prospective studies[20]. Thus, in summary, the evidence for green tea's protective effect against gastric cancer is inconclusive.

What about green tea and breast cancer? In a pooled analysis of two prospective studies involving 35 000 Japanese women, green tea was not associated with a lower risk of breast cancer (RR = 0.84) for women drinking at least five cups compared with less than one cup per day[21].

In 1998, a literature review looked at 31 human studies and four review studies investigating green tea as chemoprevention for cancer. Three studies reported an inverse association with colon cancer and one reported a positive association. For rectal cancer, only one of four studies reported an inverse association; increased risks were noted in two studies. An inverse association was noted for urinary bladder cancer in two studies. Of ten studies examining green tea and stomach cancer, six suggested an inverse association and three a positive association. In pancreatic cancer, two out of three studies showed an inverse association. A strong inverse effect was noted with green tea and esophageal cancer. Lung cancer studies have shown an inverse effect with Okinawan tea, but an increased risk was noted in another study[22].

In another more recent literature review, Borelli[23] identified 21 epidemiologic investigations of the relationship of GI cancers and preneoplastic lesions to green tea consumption. Overall these studies seemed to suggest a protective effect of green tea for adenomatous polyps and chronic atrophic gastritis, but there was no clear evidence for prevention of gastric and intestinal cancer.

By what mechanism might green tea be protective against cancer? Some studies have suggested that green tea may offer some protection against UV-induced DNA damage in human cell cultures as well as in human peripheral blood cells[24]. In an animal study, green tea polyphenol supplementation enhanced the cellular thiol levels (glutathione) that are depleted by a high flux of oxidants. This mechanism may allow green tea polyphenols to be protective against oral cancer[25].

Although most studies have looked at the chemoprotective effect of green tea extract (GTE), one study looked at GTE as a potential treatment for advanced lung cancer. GTE taken by 17 patients with advanced lung cancer had very limited activity. Although this study is very small, it suggests that it may be more appropriate to continue to pursue studies looking at the chemopreventive effect of green tea[26].

Overall, the evidence supporting green tea for chemoprevention of cancer is considerable and consequently the Chemoprevention Branch of the National Cancer Institute has plans to study tea compounds as cancer-chemopreventive agents in human trials[27].

Green tea and cardiovascular disease

In a study of 393 Japanese patients who had coronary angiography for suspected coronary artery disease (CAD), Hirano and Momiyama[28] investigated the association of green tea intake and CAD. There was no difference in intake of tea between patients with or without CAD. However, between CAD patients with and without myocardial infarction (MI), there was a significant difference between green tea drinkers and non-drinkers (14% vs 27%; $p < 0.025$). A green tea intake of one cup or more per day was found to be inversely associated with an MI and thus protective[28].

Smoking is known to be a major CAD risk factor that induces vascular injury by platelet aggregation and oxidative stress. Green tea is known to have both antioxidant and antiplatelet effects. A study was designed to assess the chemoprotective effect of green tea on atherosclerotic biologic markers in smokers. Twenty adult male smokers in Japan ingested 600 ml of green tea for 4 weeks, after which plasma levels of oxidized LDL and soluble P-selectin decreased significantly ($p < 0.05$ and $p < 0.001$, respectively)[29].

At a molecular level, EGCG was noted to be beneficial for the treatment of reperfusion-induced myocardial damage in rats. The mechanism appeared to be the inhibition of NFκB and the AP-1 pathway[30].

Cigarette smoke contains nicotine and large amounts of free radicals that may result in endothelial injury. In the above-mentioned Japanese study, 20 healthy smokers were randomized to consume green tea or hot water in a cross-over design. Green tea consumption was associated with significantly less urinary 8-iso-PGF2α, a specific product of lipid peroxidation. Thus it appears green tea consumption attenuates oxidative stress in healthy smokers through the antioxidant effects of catechins. This resulted in increased free blood flow during reactive hyperemia in smokers and reversal of endothelial dysfunction[31].

There have been a few studies examining the association of green tea and cerebrovascular disease. In a study involving Wistar rats, Suzuki *et al.*[32] demonstrated a protective effect of green tea catechin after right middle cerebral artery occlusion. Brain infarct areas and volume were reduced. Infarct volume was inversely correlated with plasma EGCG concentration. Their conclusion: green tea catechins protect the penumbra from irreversible damage due to cerebral ischemia.

In 1998 Chen *et al.*[33] conducted a cross-sectional study in 12 provinces of China involving over 14 000 subjects. Data regarding tea drinking and stroke were collected. After adjusting for other risk factors, there was a strong inverse correlation between tea drinking and stroke ($p < 0.05$). The odds ratio of stroke was 0.6 for tea-drinkers vs non-tea-drinkers. The association for tea consumption over 150 g per month and stroke was statistically significant ($p < 0.05$), with an OR = 0.56 for black tea, OR = 0.35 for green tea, and 0.75 for jasmine tea. Their conclusion: tea drinking was independently associated with stroke prevalence and might play a preventive role.

In a rat model, green tea catechins may also prevent hypertension. Hara *et al.*[34] demonstrated that tea catechins can limit the increase in rat blood pressure in a spontaneously hypertensive rat model by impeding the action of angiotensin converting enzyme and suppressing production of angiotensin II. However, if the amount of tea catechin used in the rat model is converted to the equivalent amount needed for humans it would equal ten moderately large cups of tea per day!

Some epidemiologic studies suggest that drinking multiple cups of tea daily lowers LDL-cholesterol. In a double-blind, randomized, placebo-controlled trial, 240 men and women with mild to moderate hypercholesterolemia were recruited from outpatient clinics in six urban hospitals in China. They were randomly assigned to receive theaflavin-enriched green tea extract (375 mg) or placebo for 12 weeks. Outcome measures included measurement of total HDL- and LDL-cholesterol and triglycerides. After 12 weeks in the green tea group, the mean total cholesterol decreased by 11.3% from baseline ($p < 0.01$), LDL decreased by 16.4% ($p < 0.01$), HDL increased by 2.3%, and triglycerides by 2.6% (both non-significant changes). In the placebo group there was no significant change. No significant adverse event was noted[35].

Green tea and obesity

In a study performed at the University of Geneva, researchers noted that men who were given a combination of caffeine and green tea extract burned more calories that those given only caffeine or placebo[36]. A randomized controlled trial examined energy expenditure of 11 normal weight Japanese females (BMI 21.2) who each consumed either water, oolong tea, or green tea in a cross-over design. Cumulative increases in energy expenditure were significantly increased after both oolong and green tea[37]. In a small Japanese study, a 12-week, double-blind study was performed in 35 men who ingested either one bottle of oolong tea per day containing 690 mg catechins (green tea extract group; $n = 17$) or one bottle of oolong tea per day containing just 22 mg catechins (control group; $n = 18$). Body weight, BMI, waist circumference, body fat mass, and subcutaneous fat area were significantly lower in the green tea extract group[38].

Green tea may also have a beneficial effect on glucose metabolism. In an animal study performed in Sprague–Dawley rats, Taiwanese researchers at the National Taiwan University noted the following effects of 12 weeks of green tea supplementation compared to control rats: lower fasting plasma glucose, insulin, triglyceride, and free fatty acids. Insulin-stimulated glucose uptake of adipocytes was significantly increased. Results indicated green tea polyphenols significantly increased insulin sensitivity in Sprague–Dawley rats[39].

Are there any negative effects from drinking green tea? It may cause insomnia because of its caffeine content. However, green tea contains significantly less caffeine than coffee: 30–60 mg in 170–227 g of tea vs 100 mg in 227 g of coffee[40].

Space will not permit us to consider the possible association of green tea consumption with other health benefits such as its effect on allergy, asthma, arthritis, memory loss, tooth decay, and osteoporosis. In general, there are fewer data to support such associations than for the diseases mentioned above, especially chemoprevention of cancer.

CONCLUSION

We have explored the potential health benefits of green tea consumption looking at animal studies, human epidemiologic cross-sectional surveys, a few case–control studies, and a few small experimental human studies. Although there have been hundreds of studies examining tea's potential health benefits, most are very small studies and many are *in vitro* or animal studies. Many of the studies were performed in rats; one researcher aptly stated, if we were talking about rats, 'I would strongly advise them to consume green tea regularly!'[41]. Thus, given the lack of large-scale, well-designed prospective human studies, definitive conclusions about tea's health benefits must await future study.

Nevertheless, to date, very few negative effects of green tea consumption have been noted and, thus, although it may be prudent to not proclaim green tea a 'magic potion' to prevent all diseases, likewise it would be illogical to discourage tea consumption in those who enjoy its taste and appreciate the social context of the 'tea culture'. Health benefits may indeed exist. Better-designed, large-scale prospective human studies are needed. When giving advice to our patients concerning green tea consumption, an honest, open discussion about the significance and limitations of the current data would seem most appropriate.

References

1. History of tea: China, www.gol127.com/HistoryTeaChina.html
2. Rietveld A. Antioxidant effects of tea. J Nutr 2003; 133: 3285S
3. Liao S, Dang MT, Hiipakka RA. Evidence-based medicinal action of male hormones and green tea catechins, In Yuan CS, Bieber EJ, eds. Textbook of Complementary and Alternative Medicine. London: Parthenon, 2003: 59
4. Siddiqui IA. Antioxidants of the beverage tea in promotion of human health. Antioxid Redox Signal 2004; 6: 571
5. Heber D. Herbal preparations for obesity: are they useful? Prim Care Clin Office Pract 2003; 30: 441–63
6. Hirata K, Shimada K, Watanabe H. Black tea increases coronary flow velocity reserve in healthy male subjects. Am J Cardiol 2004; 93: 1384–8
7. Cheng TO. Will green tea be even better than black tea to increase coronary flow velocity reserve? Am J Cardiol 2004; 94: 1223
8. www.gol127.com/HistoryTeaChina.html
9. Fields H. Take two tea bags and call me. US News World Report 24 January 2005: 58–9
10. Yuan CS, Bieber EJ, eds. Textbook of Complementary and Alternative Medicine. London: Parthenon, 2003
11. Kim S. Antibacterial effect of water-soluble tea extracts. J Food Prot 2004; 67: 2608–12
12. Kawaii KN, Tsuno N, Kitayama J, et al. Epigallocatechin gallate, the main component of tea polyphenol, binds to CD4 and interferes with gp120 binding. J Allergy Clin Immunol 2003; 134: 49–54
13. Nance C, Shearer WT. Is green tea good for HIV-1 infection? J Allergy Clin Immunol 2003; 112: 851–3
14. Rietveld A. Antioxidant effects of tea. J Nutr 2003; 133: 3285S
15. Mukhtar H, Ahmad N. Tea polyphenols: prevention of cancer and optimizing health. Am J Clin Nutr 2000; 71(6 Suppl): 1698S–702S
16. Jian L. Protective effect of green tea against prostate cancer: a case–control study in southeast China. Int J Cancer 2004; 108: 130–5
17. Kamat AM. Chemoprevention of bladder cancer. Urol Clin N Am 2002; 29: 157–68
18. Gupta S, Mukhtar H. Green tea and prostate cancer. Urol Clin N Am 2002; 29: 49–57
19. Morris K. Tea chemicals confirmed as cancer-busting compounds. Lancet Oncol 2002; 3: 262
20. Koizumi Y, Tsubono Y, Nakay N. No association between green tea and risk of gastric cancer. Cancer Epidemiol Biomarkers Prev 2003; 12: 472–3
21. Suzuki Y, Tsubono Y. Green tea and the risk of breast cancer. Br J Cancer 2004; 90: 1361
22. Bushman JL. Green tea and cancer in humans: a review of the literature. Nutr Cancer 1998; 31: 151
23. Borelli F. Green tea and gastrointestinal cancer risk. Aliment Pharmacol Ther 2004; 19: 497
24. Morley N, Clifford T, Salter L. The green tea polypheno (-)-epigallocatechin gallate and green tea can protect human cellular DNA from ultraviolet and visible radiation-induced damage. Photodermatol Photoimmunol Photomed 2005; 21: 15–22
25. Srinivasan P, Sabitha KE. Therapeutic efficacy of green tea polyphenos on cellular thiols in 4-nitroquinoline 1-oxide-induced oral carcinogenesis. Chemico Biol Interact 2004; 149: 81–7
26. Laurie SA, Miller VA. Phase I study of green tea extract in patients with advanced lung cancer. Cancer Chemother Pharmacol 2005; 55: 33–8
27. Siddiqui IA, Afaq F. Antioxidants of the beverage tea in promotion of human health. Antioxid Redox Signal 2004; 6: 571–82
28. Hirano R, Momiyama Y. Comparison of green tea intake in Japanese patients with and without angiographic coronary artery disease. Am J Cardiol 2002; 90: 1150–3
29. Lee W, Min WK, Chun S, Lee YW. Long-term effects of green tea ingestion on atherosclerotic biological markers in smokers. Clin Biochem 2005; 38: 84–7
30. Aneja R, Hake PW, Burroughs TJ. Epigallocatechin, a green tea polyphenol, attenuates myocardial ischemia reperfusion injury in rats. Mol Med 2004; 10: 55–62
31. Nagaya N, Yamamoto H, Uematsu M, et al. Green tea reverses endothelial dysfunction in healthy smokers. Br Heart J 2004; 90: 1485
32. Suzuki M, Tabuchi M, Ikeda M, et al. Protective effects of green tea catechins on cerebral ischemic damage. Med Sci Monitor 2004; 10: BR166
33. Chen Z, Li Y, Zhao LC, et al. A study on the association between tea consumption and stroke (in Chinese). Zhonghau Liu Xing Bing Xue Za Zhi 2004; 25: 66
34. Hara Y, Matsuzaki T, Suzuki T. Green tea controls high blood pressure. Nippon Nogeikagaku Kaishi 1987; 61: 803

35. Maron DJ, Lu GP, Cai NS, Wu ZG. Cholesterol-lowering effect of a theaflavin-enriched green tea extract. Arch Intern Med 2003; 163: 1448–53

36. Dulloo AG, Duret C. Efficacy of a green tea extract rich in catechin polyphenols and caffeine in increasing 24 hr energy expenditure and fat oxidation in humans. Am J Clin Nutr 1999; 70: 1040–5

37. Komatsu T, Nakamori M. Oolong tea increases energy metabolism in Japanese females. J Med Investigat 2003; 50: 170–5

38. Nagao T, Komine Y. Ingestion of a tea rich in catechins leads to a reduction in body fat and malondialdehyde-modified LDL in men. Am J Clin Nutr 2005; 81: 122–9

39. Wu LY. Effect of green tea supplementation on insulin sensitivity in Sprague–Dawley rats. J Agric Food Chem 2004; 52: 643–8

40. Chinese cuisine, the miracle of green tea. www.About. com

41. Fields H. Take two tea bags and call me. US News World Report 25 January 2005: 58

Herbal, food, and drug interactions 7

J. Moss

INTRODUCTION

Although potential interactions between drugs and foods have long been appreciated by pharmacologists, several highly publicized interactions between the two, and a trend toward the use of herbal medications, have made the subject a matter for public concern and discussion.

One example of a drug–food interaction is that between the monoamine oxidase inhibitors (MAOIs) and foods containing tyramine. Some 40 years ago, the interaction of tyramine with MAOIs was recognized as one of the most lethal adverse reactions in medicine. Tyramine, which is present in many foods including beer, wine, and cheese, is usually degraded by intestinal monoamine oxidase (MAO). When an MAOI is administered, tyramine is absorbed systemically and transported into the presynaptic sympathetic nerve terminals[1], where it is converted to octopamine. The expected long-term consequence of the storage and release of octopamine is sympathetic inhibition. Because of the release of this relatively inactive biogenic amine, acute tyramine uptake or release can cause sympathetic excess. When MAO in the gut and liver is inhibited, excess dietary tyramine enters the circulation, causing precipitous release of norepinephrine with potential catastrophic cardiovascular consequences. Such a reaction was widely publicized in the Libby Zion case[2]. After Ms Zion, who was taking the MAOI phenalzine, was given meperidine by the resident who treated her, she suffered respiratory arrest and died. The development of linezolid antibiotics and selegiline-based anti-epileptics has refocused interest on such interactions[3].

Although the interaction between tyramine and MAOIs is well recognized by both physicians and patients, the extent to which other dietary factors contribute to variability in patient response to drugs is less well appreciated. Most physicians in clinical practice acknowledge clinically important interpatient variability in responsiveness to drugs. Traditionally, the causes have been explained as pharmacokinetic, pharmacodynamic, or pharmacogenetic. There is evidence, however, that some variability in response may be attributed to dietary factors. Two examples of the interaction between food and drugs reported in the literature are the effect of grapefruit juice on cytochrome P450 3A4 and the effect of solanaceous plants (potato, eggplant, and tomato) on butyrylcholinesterase. Because of these interactions, several approved drugs have been withdrawn from the marketplace, and the strategy behind drug development has changed.

CYTOCHROME P450 3A4

Cytochrome P450 3A4, located in the small bowel and the liver, affects the metabolism of oral and parenteral drugs. Cytochrome P450 enzymes are the major degradative pathways for many drugs including alfentanil[4], midazolam, lidocaine, and numerous antibiotics. The pharmacokinetic and pharmacodynamic effects of inhibition of cytochrome P450 3A4 have been reviewed by Dresser et al[5]. Although the effect of inhibition may initially appear to be of academic interest only (extending half-lives of drugs, for example), inhibition of this enzyme has resulted in prolonged sedation or serious arrhythmias and rhabdomyolysis. Drugs like cimetidine, which inhibits P450-mediated metabolism, also inhibit the breakdown of opiates such as morphine or fentanyl. In animals treated with cimetidine before they were given fentanyl, the half-life of fentanyl increased from 155 to 340 minutes[6]. In this instance, excessive sedation resulted from the drug interaction[7]. Ventricular arrhythmias (torsades de pointes) are other manifestations of the interaction when cisapride, astemizole, or terfenidine are co-administered with ketaconazole or erythromycin, potent cytochrome P450 inhibitors. Hypotension is associated with the interaction between the isoenzyme CYP 3A4 and the calcium channel antagonists or sildenifil. Finally, fatal rhabdomyolysis has been associated with co-administration of some of the co-enzyme A reductase inhibitors (statins) and some cytochrome 3A4 inhibitors. Drug-induced inhibition of cytochrome P450 is so well documented that there have been attempts to exploit inhibition of this pathway to reduce the dosage (and thereby decrease the cost) of concomitantly administered drugs such as cyclosporin.

Natural products in the diet may have the same effect as drug–drug interaction on cytochrome P450 3A4[8]. The inhibitory effect of grapefruit juice on drug metabolism was discovered accidentally during studies of the calcium channel receptor antagonist felodipine. After grapefruit juice was added to mask the taste of the drug, investigators noticed a doubling of the drug's peak concentration in plasma[9]. In a subsequent trial, drinking 200 ml of grapefruit juice or double-strength grapefruit juice increased the felodipine mean area under the plasma concentration–time curve by 185% and 234%, respectively[10]. The interaction was tested with similar and then with other drugs also dependent on this route for metabolism[11–14]. That grapefruit juice could alter drug concentrations became widely known during the phase IV monitoring studies of the best-selling antihistamines terfenadine and astemizole, which ultimately led to their removal from the marketplace. Sudden death (defined by prolonged Q–T interval) or torsades de pointes in patients were associated with taking both the antihistamines and antifungal drugs or erythromycin. The mechanism for this unusual arrhythmia was inhibition of the cytochrome P450 isozyme CYP 3A4. Recently, an article and series of letters in the *New England Journal of Medicine* focused attention on this issue[15,16]. Normally, the presystemic metabolism of oral terfenedine (Seldane®) by CYP 3A4 is so efficient that unmetabolized terfenedine is not detectable in plasma, protecting the patient against its potentially cardiotoxic effects (prolonged Q–T interval, torsades de pointes). In a study of six subjects in whom unmetabolized terfenedine had accumulated, grapefruit juice increased plasma terfenedine concentrations and aggravated Q–T prolongation[17]. In a follow-up study, when 11 healthy volunteers received a single dose of amiodarone along with three glasses of grapefruit juice on the same day, metabolism was inhibited completely and PR and QTc intervals changed[18]. A recent review of interactions between grapefruit juice and cardiovascular drugs has highlighted the problem[19].

CYP 3A4 inhibition is more important with drugs taken orally rather than administered intravenously. Although CYP 3A4 is predominantly found in the liver and intestine, its clinically important inhibition occurs in the small bowel. In a study of the interaction between grapefruit juice and midazolam in humans, subjects received either intravenous or oral midazolam (5 and 15 mg, respectively) after pretreatment with water or grapefruit juice. The investigators hypothesized that because midazolam does not undergo significant enterohepatic circulation, some of the oral midazolam might be metabolized by the intestinal enzyme during the absorption phase. With inhibition of the intestinal enzyme, a higher level of midazolam would reach the circulation. The pharmacokinetics and pharmacodynamics of intravenous midazolam were unchanged by ingestion of grapefruit juice, but oral midazolam with grapefruit juice versus water increases peak plasma concentration by 56%[20]. Similar effects of grapefruit juice on triazolam (Halcion®) concentrations were found in 10 young subjects[21]. The altered pharmacokinetics were manifested by increased drowsiness.

In addition to interaction with prescription medications, foods can also interact with over-the-counter or herbal medications. For example, drinking grapefruit juice may make caffeine levels rise. Grapefruit juice decreased the metabolism and increased the area under the plasma concentration–time curve of caffeine by 28% and prolonged its half-life by 31%. On the other hand, when herbals (St John's wort) induce the cytochrome P450 3A4 enzyme, peak levels of a drug are decreased. Decrease in peak levels has been demonstrated for warfarin, theophylline, cyclosporine, birth control pills, and other drugs[22–25].

Although the effects of grapefruit juice on CYP 3A4 are known, the component in it and the mechanism that produces inhibition are unknown. The first candidate studied for inhibition was naringin, a bioflavonoid that gives grapefruit juice its bitterness. Several studies demonstrated that naringonen, the human metabolite of naringen, inhibits the CYP 3A4 enzyme. Recently, however, another candidate for the natural inhibitor in grapefruit juice has emerged[26]. Bergamottin, a citrus psoralen[27], inactivates cytochrome P450 3A4[28] and increases P-glycoprotein-mediated ATP hydrolysis more than two-fold. In animals, bergamottin inhibited metabolism of nifedipine[29]. In healthy volunteers who received 40 mg of simvastatin, inhibition dissipated 3–7 days after ingestion of the last dose of grapefruit juice.

BUTYRYLCHOLINESTERASE

Acetylcholinesterase and butyrylcholinesterase are closely related enzymes. Acetylcholinesterase is predominant in the neuromuscular junction and terminates the action of cholinergic transmission. Butyrylcholinesterase, which is present in plasma, has an unknown action[30]. A desire to minimize paralysis time in patients undergoing surgical procedures was the impetus for the development of short-acting drugs degraded by endogenous enzymes. Drugs such as succinylcholine and mivacurium are highly dependent upon butyrylcholinesterase for their metabolism[31,32].

Although the natural role of butyrylcholinesterase is unknown, the mutation that substitutes glycine for aspartate at position 70 'pseudocholinesterase' prevents hydrolysis of succinylcholine and a variety of other drugs. In individuals expressing the genetic mutation for butyrylcholinesterase, the action of these drugs is prolonged. The genetic mutation is rare enough that drugs such as mivacurium were designed with this enzyme as a specific metabolic pathway. Variation of the butyrylcholinesterase gene has been explored[33]. While the true biologic function of butyrylcholinesterase remains unknown[30], studies in Israel suggest that the perpetuation of the ASP 70 mutation in humans is based on diet. Many naturally occurring butyrylcholinesterase mutants exist, but few are of clinical importance.

As with cytochrome P450, there is an important drug–drug interaction with butyrylcholinesterase. That non-depolarizing muscle relaxants inhibit cholinesterase has been known since the 1950s. In a more recent study, inhibition of butyrylcholinesterase by the neuromuscular antagonist pancuronium prolonged neuromuscular block by mivacurium[34].

We and others have focused on a possible interaction of the enzyme with diet. The interaction between food and butyrylcholinesterase is a complex one. Naturally occurring cholinesterase inhibitors, solanadine and chaconine, are found in solanaceae – plants such as potato, eggplant, and tomato. It is believed that they developed as natural insecticides. The ASP 70 mutation in butyrylcholinesterase confers resistance to these natural insecticides[35]. Solanaceous glycoalkaloids inhibit butyrylcholinesterase *in vitro*, and the atypical enzyme is much less sensitive to this inhibition. This hypothesis is confirmed by the geographic overlap between the frequency of the mutation and the distribution of solanaceous plants.

The function and inhibition of acetylcholinesterase have also been studied. The history of direct toxicity from potatoes and solanaceous plants is significant[36–38]. The symptoms of toxicity are consistent with cholinergic overdose (acetylcholinesterase inhibition), and sometimes toxicity has resulted in fatalities. Symptoms appear

approximately 2–24 hours after ingestion of potatoes[37]. In a well-documented outbreak of potato poisoning that involved 78 British school children, the most severely affected child recovered only after 1 week of hospitalization. Butyrylcholinesterase concentrations in 10 of 17 children analyzed were abnormally low 6 days after exposure. In all but one child, levels had returned to normal after 4–5 weeks, suggesting that solanaceous glycoalkaloids persist in the body. The level of circulating glycoalkaloids associated with an ordinary serving of potatoes can significantly alter butyrylcholinesterase activity in plasma.

To ascertain the interaction between solanaceous glycoalkaloids and certain anesthetic drugs, we demonstrated that solanaceous glycoalkaloids inhibit human butyrylcholinesterase at concentrations similar to those found in the serum of individuals who have eaten a serving of potatoes (Figure 7.1)[39]. After co-application of anesthetic drugs with neuromuscular blocking drugs and cholinesterase inhibitors, inhibition of cholinesterase was additive. When rabbits treated with solanaceous glycoalkaloids were paralyzed with mivacurium, which

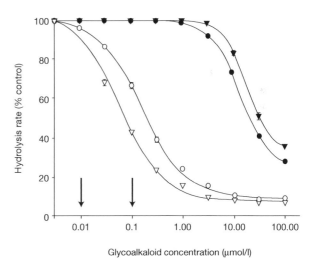

Figure 7.1 Solanaceous glycoalkaloids (SGAs) inhibit human acetylcholinesterase (AChE) and butyrylcholinesterase (BuChE). The effects of varied SGA concentrations on the hydrolytic activity of human AChE (solid symbols) and BuChE (open symbols) are shown. Substrate hydrolysis activity was normalized and is presented as percentage of control. Inhibition by both α-solanine (circles) and α-chaconine (triangles) was concentration-dependent. Arrows denote the range of serum SGA levels after potato consumption. Data points are mean ± SEM of at least five experiments for each concentration. Determinations within each experiment were carried out in triplicate. Error bars not visible are within symbol size. Reprinted with permission from reference 39

(a)

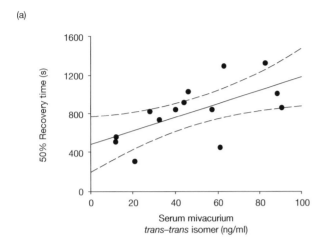

(b)

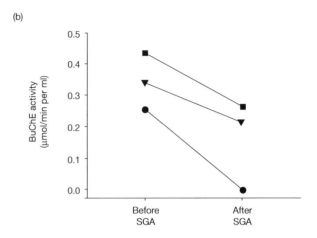

(c)

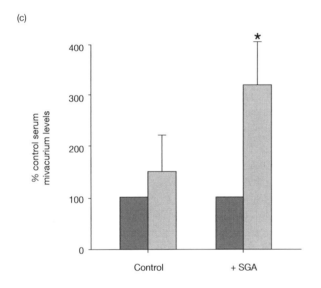

Figure 7.2 Serum mivacurium levels correlate with neuromuscular blockade. Solanaceous glycoalkaloid (SGA) administration inhibits serum cholinesterase and increases serum mivacurium levels. (a) Levels of the *trans–trans* isomer of mivacurium were determined in 14 rabbits. Each value is the mean of triplicate determinations. Mivacurium levels are plotted versus the time needed for 50% recovery of twitch amplitude after mivacurium administration. Animals with higher mivacurium levels showed longer recovery times ($r^2 = 0.39$; dashed line is 95% confidence interval; $p < 0.05$). (b) Three animals with measurable serum cholinesterase activity showed decreases after SGA administration. Blood samples from two other animals had basal cholinesterase activity near the lower limit of detection (not shown). (c) Mivacurium *trans–trans* isomer levels were determined in blood samples collected after two consecutive mivacurium administrations (10 min after each mivacurium infusion). All data were normalized to the serum levels after the first mivacurium administration. Light gray bars indicate the percentage change in mivacurium levels after the second administration under control conditions (left) and with coadministration of SGA (right; *$p < 0.05$ relative to initial determinations, paired *t* test; $n = 7$ animals). Reprinted with permission from reference 39

depends upon butyrylcholinesterase for its metabolism, mivacurium levels persisted. Because mivacurium metabolism had been inhibited, time for recovery from mivacurium-induced paralysis was prolonged (149 ± 12% of control, Figure 7.2). Our *in vivo* and *in vitro* findings suggest that solanaceous glycoalkaloids in a normal diet could significantly impair the metabolism of anesthetic drugs.

CONCLUSION

The effect on drug metabolism of common foods such as cheese, grapefruit juice, and potatoes has been demon-

strated in a variety of preclinical and clinical studies. Patients recognize food–drug interactions immediately. Increasingly, pharmaceutical companies have become aware of the potential drug interactions such as the ones described above, both because of safety issues and the economic impact these interactions cause. There is already evidence that food–drug interactions have altered the process for the development of new entities. For example, new muscle relaxants under development do not utilize butyrylcholinesterase to facilitate rapid and predictable metabolism but rather rely on organic degradation. Similarly, drugs that bypass cytochrome P450 metabolism have already replaced older drugs that utilize the pathway. While physicians and consumers ultimately bear the responsibility for recognition of potential interactions, the downstream effects will be keenly perceived by pharmaceutical manufacturers in the development of new drugs.

References

1. Brown C, Taniguchi G, Yip K. The monoamine oxidase inhibitor–tyramine interaction. J Clin Pharmacol 1989; 29: 529–32

2. Asch DA, Parker RM. The Libby Zion case. One step forward or two steps backward? N Engl J Med 1988; 318: 771–5

3. Humphrey SJ, Curry JT, Turman CN, Stryd RP. Cardiovascular sympathomimetic amine interactions in rats treated with monoamine oxidase inhibitors and the novel oxazolidinone antibiotic linezolid. J Cardiovasc Pharmacol 2001; 37: 548–63

4. Yun CH, Wood M, Wood AJ, Guengerich FP. Identification of the pharmacogenetic determinants of alfentanil metabolism: cytochrome P-450 3A4. An explanation of the variable elimination clearance. Anesthesiology 1992; 77: 467–74

5. Dresser GK, Spence JD, Bailey DG. Pharmacokinetic– pharmacodynamic consequences and clinical relevance of cytochrome P450 3A4 inhibition. Clin Pharmacokinet 2000; 38: 41–57

6. Borel JD, Bentley JB, Nenad RE, Sipes IG. Cimetidine alteration of fentanyl pharmacokinetics in dogs. Proceedings of the International Anesthesia Research Society 56th Congress, San Francisco, CA, 1982: 149

7. Hiller A, Olkkola KT, Isohanni P, Saarnivaara L. Unconsciousness associated with midazolam and erythromycin. Br J Anaesth 1990; 65: 826–8

8. Fujita K. Food–drug interactions via human cytochrome P450 3A (CYP3A). Drug Metab Drug Interact 2004; 20: 195–217

9. Bailey DG, Spence JD, Munoz C, Arnold JM. Interaction of citrus juices with felodipine and nifedipine. Lancet 1991; 337: 268–9

10. Edgar B, Bailey D, Bergstrand R, et al. Acute effects of drinking grapefruit juice on the pharmacokinetics and dynamics of felodipine – and its potential clinical relevance. Eur J Clin Pharmacol 1992; 42: 313–17

11. Fuhr U, Harder S, Lopez-Rojas P, et al. Increase of verapamil concentrations in steady state by coadministration of grapefruit juice (abstract). Naunyn Schmiedebergs Arch Pharmacol 1994; 349 (Suppl): R134

12. Soons PA, Vogels BA, Roosemalen MC, et al. Grapefruit juice and cimetidine inhibit stereoselective metabolism of nitrendipine in humans. Clin Pharmacol Ther 1991; 50: 394–403

13. Fuhr U, Maier A, Blume H, et al. Grapefruit juice increases oral nimodipine bioavailability (abstract). Eur J Clin Pharmacol 1994; 47: A100

14. Bailey DG, Arnold JM, Strong HA, et al. Effect of grapefruit juice and naringin on nisoldipine pharmacokinetics. Clin Pharmacol Ther 1993; 54: 589–94

15. Kaplan EL, Winston AP, Schoenholtz JC, et al. Oral erythromycin and the risk of sudden death [letter]. N Engl J Med 2005; 352: 301–4

16. Roden DM. Drug-induced prolongation of the QT interval. N Engl J Med 2004; 350: 1013–22

17. Honig P, Wortham D, Lazarev A, Cantilena LR. Pharmacokinetics and cardiac effects of terfenadine in poor metabolizers receiving concomitant grapefruit juice (abstract). Clin Pharmacol Ther 1995; 57: 185

18. Libersa CC, Brique SA, Motte KB, et al. Dramatic inhibition of amiodarone metabolism induced by grapefruit juice. Br J Clin Pharmacol 2000; 49: 373–8

19. Bailey DG, Dresser GK. Interactions between grapefruit juice and cardiovascular drugs. Am J Cardiovasc Drugs 2004; 4: 281–97

20. Kupferschmidt HH, Ha HR, Ziegler WH, et al. Interaction between grapefruit juice and midazolam in humans. Clin Pharmacol Ther 1995; 58: 20–8

21. Hukkinen SK, Varhe A, Olkkola KT, Neuvonen PJ. Plasma concentrations of triazolam are increased by concomitant ingestion of grapefruit juice. Clin Pharmacol Ther 1995; 58: 127–31

22. Barone GW, Gurley BJ, Ketel BL, et al. Drug interaction between St. John's wort and cyclosporine. Ann Pharmacother 2000; 34: 1013–16

23. Moore LB, Goodwin B, Jones SA, et al. St. John's wort induces hepatic drug metabolism through activation of the pregnane X receptor. Proc Natl Acad Sci USA 2000; 97: 7500–2

24. Izzo AA, Ernst E. Interactions between herbal medicines and prescribed drugs: a systematic review. Drugs 2001; 61: 2163–75

25. Wang Z, Gorski JC, Hamman MA, et al. The effects of St. John's wort (Hypericum perforatum) on human cytochrome P450 activity. Clin Pharmacol Ther 2001; 70: 317–26

26. Wang EJ, Casciano CN, Clement RP, Johnson WW. Inhibition of P-glycoprotein transport function by grapefruit juice psoralen. Pharm Res 2001; 18: 432–8

27. He K, Iyer KR, Hayes RN, et al. Inactivation of cytochrome P450 3A4 by bergamottin, a component of grapefruit juice. Chem Res Toxicol 1998; 11: 252–9

28. Kane GC, Lipsky JJ. Drug–grapefruit juice interactions. Mayo Clin Proc 2000; 75: 933–42

29. Mohri K, Uesawa Y. Effects of furanocoumarin derivatives in grapefruit juice on nifedipine pharmacokinetics in rats. Pharm Res 2001; 18: 177–82

30. Cooper JR. Unsolved problems in the cholinergic nervous system. J Neurochem 1994; 63: 395–9

31. Savarese JJ, Ali HH, Basta SJ, et al. The clinical neuromuscular pharmacology of mivacurium chloride (BW B1090U). A short-acting nondepolarizing ester neuromuscular blocking drug. Anesthesiology 1988; 68: 723–32

32. Cook DR, Freeman JA, Lai AA, et al. Pharmacokinetics of mivacurium in normal patients and in those with hepatic or renal failure. Br J Anaesth 1992; 69: 580–5

33. Whittaker M. Cholinesterase. In Beckman L, ed. Monographs in Human Genetics, Vol. 11. Basel: Karger, 1986: 45–85

34. Erkola O, Rautoma P, Meretoja OA. Mivacurium when preceded by pancuronium becomes a long-acting muscle relaxant. Anesthesiology 1996; 84: 562–5

35. Neville LF, Gnatt A, Loewenstein Y, et al. Intramolecular relationships in cholinesterases revealed by oocyte expression of site-directed and natural variants of human BCHE. EMBO J 1992; 11: 1641–9

36. Harris FW, Cockburn T. Alleged poisoning by potatoes. Analyst 1918; 43: 133–7

37. Morris SC, Lee TH. The toxicity and teratogenicity of Solanaceae glycoalkaloids, particularly those of the potato (Solanum tuberosum): a review. Food Technol Aust 1984; 36: 118–24

38. Hansen A. Two fatal cases of potato poisoning. Science 1925; 61: 340–1

39. McGehee DS, Krasowski MD, Fung DL, et al. Cholinesterase inhibition by potato glycoalkaloids slows mivacurium metabolism. Anesthesiology 2000; 93: 510–19

Risks of ephedra-containing supplements　　8

S. R. Mehendale, B. A. Bauer and C.-S. Yuan

INTRODUCTION

Ephedra-containing products were available to consumers in the USA as dietary supplements following the enactment of the Dietary Supplement Health and Education Act (DSHEA, 1994)[1] for almost a decade. These supplements, which were claimed to promote weight loss[2,3] and to enhance physical performance[4], were aggressively marketed. However, numerous, severe adverse event reports associated with the use of ephedra were received by the FDA during this period. A resulting in-depth review of all data by the FDA led to the conclusion that ephedra use presented an unreasonable risk of illness or injury to the consumer and ultimately led to the prohibition of sale of ephedra supplements in accordance with the DSHEA[5] (Table 8.1). Although a few controlled clinical studies did report a short-term weight loss with supervised ephedra use (alone or in combination with caffeine)[6,7], the risks of keeping ephedra on the market were considered to far outweigh any benefits. This chapter reviews the probable reasons that made ephedra-containing supplements hazardous and discusses possible measures that can be undertaken to make dietary supplements safer.

ADVERSE EVENTS WITH EPHEDRA USE

Adverse events associated with ephedra/ephedrine alkaloids coincide with the known effects of sympathomimetic agents, particularly presenting as cardiovascular, autonomic, or psychiatric effects[8]. Adverse event reports from selected sources are summarized here to describe the spectrum of adverse effects.

Data collected by the FDA

There were 3308 adverse events reported in the FDA's Center for Food Safety and Applied Nutrition's Special Nutritional Adverse Event Monitoring System for all dietary supplements between 1993 and 2001, of which 1398 or 42% were associated with ephedra-containing dietary supplements[9]. Of those, 405 or 30% of the cases were serious or major adverse events such as chest pain, hypertension, arrhythmia, myocardial infarction, stroke, or death.

Summary of adverse event reports by a company

Reports of adverse events (compiled from 1997 to 2002 by a leading manufacturer of ephedra) were submitted to the FDA in 2002 and were analyzed by the US House of Representatives[10]. Of the 13000 adverse event reports, 1985 (15%) were considered significant and included 465 with chest pain, 336 with high blood pressure, 966 with rhythm disturbances, 20 with myocardial infarction, 24 with stroke, 321 with psychiatric events, and 3 deaths. The report indicated that many of the patients with significant adverse events were young, healthy, non-obese, and without predisposing medical conditions, who used ephedra supplements according to the recommendations of the manufacturer.

Adverse events in clinical trials of ephedra

A search was conducted in PubMed using keywords, 'ephedra' and 'clinical trials'. Twelve clinical studies were identified in which ephedra (or ephedra in combination with caffeine and other ingredients), was administered to an aggregate total of 378 subjects (including subject number corrected for cross-over design). Of these, 142 subjects were enrolled in studies in which ephedra was administered acutely[11–18] and 236 subjects were enrolled in studies in which ephedra was administered for 2 to 24 weeks[6,7,13,19,20]. The commonly encountered adverse events included mild but significant increase in heart rate and blood pressure, palpitations, dryness of mouth, insomnia, headache, nausea, irritability, anxiety, and loss

Table 8.1   Timeline: ephedra use and FDA intervention

2500 years ago	ephedra is used in China and other Asian countries as a medicinal herb[21]
1972	Danish physician notes weight loss in asthma patients treated with a combination product containing ephedrine, caffeine and phenobarbital. Ephedra rapidly becomes a popular obesity treatment in Europe[3]
1994	ephedra is classified and marketed as a dietary supplement under the Dietary Supplement Health and Education Act (DSHEA)[1]
1995–96	several hundred adverse effects from ephedra use are reported to FDA[22]. FDA convened a meeting of the Food Advisory Committee, which recommended that doses should be established to ensure safety[23]
4 June 1997	FDA's proposed rule on dietary supplements containing ephedra alkaloids. The rule would have classified a dietary supplement as misbranded if it contained 8 mg or more of ephedrine alkaloids per serving or a total daily dose recommendation of 24 mg or more of ephedra alkaloids. It further would have required labeling to state that the product was not to be used for more than 7 days[24]
1998	Metabolife, a company marketing ephedra-containing supplements, states that the company 'has never received one notice from a consumer that any adverse health event has occurred with the use of Metabolife'[25]
4 August 1999	Government Accounting Office (GAO) releases report in response to a directive from the House Committee on Science. GAO determines that the number of adverse events with ephedra merits FDA attention and the need for steps to address safety issues, but 'expressed concerns about the use of the adverse events in supporting the proposed dosing level and limits on duration of use'. GAO concludes that FDA needs additional evidence to support the restrictions[26]
July 2002	FDA asks Department of Justice to pursue criminal investigation against Metabolife regarding the false statements about ephedra-related adverse events[23]
16 August 2002	Metabolife reveals that the company has received 13 000 consumer complaints related to ephedra use during the previous 5 years, including those of severe adverse effects such as seizures, myocardial infarction, stroke, or death[27]
8 October 2002	FDA requests strict warning labels and a requirement for GMP (good manufacturing practices) regulations for ephedra dietary supplements[28]
9 October 2002	AMA urges FDA to remove ephedra-containing dietary supplements from the market because 'the risk/benefit ratio for these products is unacceptable'[29]
February 2003	FDA-sponsored meta-analysis by Rand Corporation concludes ephedra use associated with significantly increased risk of adverse events, although may have some efficacy for weight loss (as observed in controlled clinical trials)[22]
30 December 2003	FDA advises consumers to stop using ephedra supplements[30] following an in-depth review of all available data
12 April 2004	FDA's final rule goes into effect prohibiting the sale of dietary supplements containing ephedrine alkaloids (ephedra)[5], which are determined to present an unreasonable risk of illness or injury to consumers

of appetite. The increased cardiovascular stimulation was also confirmed in two studies measuring electrocardiographic changes[14,15]. However, no serious adverse events were reported in any of the studies (one reported event was due to an unrelated cause[19]).

The absence of serious adverse events in clinical trials is in contrast to the several serious adverse events reported to the FDA. This suggests that the safeguards used in a clinical trial setting may have resulted in elimination of subjects with pre-existing diseases or on specific medications, and a consequent reduction in the probability of a serious adverse event. Second, the source of the herbal product and the dosage regimen are well defined in the trial setting. Thus, ephedra use under medical supervision appears to be safer compared to the self-administration of ephedra-containing dietary supplements. From a different perspective, however, since ephedra has been tested only in a few controlled studies and since adverse events in clinical trials are underreported overall[31,32], it is possible that more serious adverse events may be encountered when ephedra is used by the population at large, in spite of medical supervision. Irrespective of the argument, the probability of an adverse event appears to increase if ephedra is used as a dietary supplement.

PROBABLE CAUSES OF INCREASED ADVERSE EVENTS WITH EPHEDRA USE

The interpretation of the adverse event reports due to dietary supplements should be based on the considerations that they are probably underreported and those that are reported cannot always be verified for accuracy or causality[33]. Both these factors make it difficult to enforce regulations within the DSHEA that allows the FDA to ban a dietary supplement only if it can prove the hazards of using the supplement. Given these constraints, any reported adverse events should signal a safety issue and should be investigated.

Several factors could have been responsible for the increase in the adverse events with ephedra use and have been summarized here.

Lack of standardization of extract

Ephedra extract contains multiple alkaloids and possibly several other undefined ingredients[34]. Lack of consistency of extract composition with variations in the herb source and inadequate chemical analysis of the herbal extracts[35] could significantly affect the active ingredient concentrations in the recommended extract doses. In one study, 11 of 20 ephedra-containing dietary supplements tested either failed to list the ephedrine content on the label or varied in excess of 20% from the actual content and the label claims[36]. Lot-to-lot variability for one product exceeded 1000% for a constituent alkaloid, (-)-methylephedrine. These differences in the active constituent content and other contaminants are likely to increase the toxic effects of ephedra extract. Since the recommended ephedra dose is based only on ephedrine content, other undefined potent or toxic ingredients could be responsible for idiosyncratic reactions[34].

Combination with other herbs

Commercial ephedra products also contain additives such as caffeine containing stimulants and other herbal products[37]. The pharmacologic effects of ephedra are potentiated by these herbal stimulants, leading to an increase in the adverse events related to ephedra use[38]. According to the principles of traditional Chinese medicine, inappropriate combination of herbs can induce harmful adverse effects[21,39]. In traditional Chinese medicine, ephedra is typically combined with other herbs such as licorice, ginger, honey, cinnamon, and mulberry root[21,39,40] that improve therapeutic efficacy via synergistic action while reducing adverse effects. This could be one of the reasons that ephedra use in traditional medicine is not associated with significant adverse events[41].

Indications for ephedra use

Use of ephedra extract in traditional medicinal systems for respiratory ailments is prescribed only for acute situations and is contraindicated for long-term use[40]. Ephedra use as a dietary supplement in the USA, on the other hand, was self-administered by consumers as a treatment for obesity and for enhancing physical performance. Lack of any medical supervision may have resulted in the use of the supplement by patients with medical contraindications and in non-detection of early adverse drug reactions. Also, recommendations on the duration of ephedra use as a dietary supplement were not typically provided.

Myth of safety in natural products

A common myth is that dietary supplements are safe even at high doses because they are derived from natural sources. Thus, although the DSHEA requires manufacturers to provide recommended dosages on the product label, consumers may use higher doses than those recommended with the hope of achieving a greater effect.

POSSIBLE SOLUTIONS TO LIMIT RISKS RELATED TO DIETARY SUPPLEMENTS

Improve government oversight of herbal dietary supplements

Certain clauses within the DSHEA should be considered for amendment to protect consumers from the potential hazards of herbal dietary supplements.

- *Definition of dietary supplement*　The premise for classifying a substance as a dietary supplement must be redefined to exclude herbal extracts that contain constituents which are independently regulated by the FDA. Ephedra supplements contained FDA-regulated chemicals such as ephedrine (over-the-counter medication or OTC), norpseudoephedrine (a controlled substance), phenylpropanolamine, an ephedrine metabolite that has been withdrawn from the market[26], and a combination of stimulant 'amphetamine look-alike' alkaloids (that were banned)[36]

- *Safety standards and quality control*   Mandating good manufacturing practices and organizing expert panels to review the safety of dietary supplements are important amendments required for ensuring safety[33,42]. The FDA recently initiated the good manufacturing practice proposition for dietary supplements[23]

- *Manufacturer accountability*   Manufacturers should be required to obtain an approval from the FDA, based on the safety data, prior to marketing a supplement; to maintain records of consumer-reported adverse events; and to inform the FDA of serious adverse events within a stipulated time interval[33]

- *Burden of proof of safety*   The burden of proof should not be placed solely on the FDA. In accordance with the DSHEA, the FDA can ban or restrict use of a dietary supplement only if it can prove that the product is unsafe. An amendment to the Act should also require manufacturers to demonstrate reasonable safety of the dietary supplement to be marketed[33,42]. The guidelines for what the manufacturers should provide as a proof of safety and what the FDA needs to restrict marketing of a supplement deemed unsafe should be clearly defined. For example, in the case of ephedra, providing safety data on the basis of centuries of ephedra use in traditional medicinal systems is irrelevant when the extract preparation, combination with other herbs, duration of use, and the reasons for use of ephedra as a dietary supplement were distinctly disparate from ephedra use in traditional medicine.

Increase awareness among physicians

Organizations like the AMA and academic medical institutions should encourage education on complementary and alternative medicine to help future physicians understand the benefits and risks of herbal medications[43]. Obtaining a history of alternative medicinal modalities used by patients should be an integral part of a routine medical visit[44,45]. Additionally, physicians should report to the FDA any adverse reactions suspected to be caused by a dietary supplement.

Consumer education

Individuals should be advised to consume supplements made only by nationally known food and drug manufacturers, and should be able to obtain information on the safety and use of specific dietary supplements from government Internet sites[46,47]. Directing consumers to choose supplements that have undergone an independent, third-party verification is another means of helping ensure that only quality products are chosen[48]. Consumers need to be educated so that, in the event of an adverse reaction to a dietary supplement, they can report it directly to the FDA[46,47].

Conclusion

In comparison to the stringent control of the FDA over the quality and safety of prescription and OTC drugs, dietary supplements are regulated minimally. In the case of ephedra, this led to exposing consumers to significant health risks. Although it may not be practical to enforce on dietary supplements all the requirements that are enforced for drugs, certain basic requirements of safety and quality need to be clearly defined and mandated. Ephedra-containing dietary supplements have served as a model highlighting several regulatory deficiencies. Re-evaluation of these issues is of great importance for ensuring availability of safer dietary supplements.

References

1. United States Congress, 103rd Congress. Dietary Supplement Health and Education Act of 1994

2. Ephedra Education Council. The facts about ephedra (media center). Available at: www.ephedrafacts.com/thefacts.html, accessed 18 November 2002

3. Greenway FL. The safety and efficacy of pharmaceutical and herbal caffeine and ephedrine use as a weight loss agent. Obes Rev 2001; 2: 199–211

4. Bell DG, Jacobs I, Zamecnik J. Effects of caffeine, ephedrine and their combination on time to exhaustion during

high-intensity exercise. Eur J Appl Physiol Occup Physiol 1998; 77: 427–33

5. Food and Drug Administration. FDA announces rule prohibiting sale of dietary supplements containing ephedrine alkaloids effective April 12 (12 April 2004). Available at: www.fda.gov/bbs/topics/news/2004/NEW01050.html, accessed 8 August 2005

6. Boozer CN, Nasser JA, Heymsfield SB, et al. An herbal supplement containing Ma Huang-Guarana for weight loss: a randomized, double-blind trial. Int J Obes Relat Metab Disord 2001; 25: 316–24

7. Boozer CN, Daly PA, Homel P, et al. Herbal ephedra/caffeine for weight loss: a 6-month randomized safety and efficacy trial. Int J Obes Relat Metab Disord 2002; 26: 593–604

8. Aung HH, Dey L, Yuan CS. Warning: adverse effects of ephedra-containing dietary supplements. In Yuan CS, Bieber EJ, eds. Textbook of Complementary and Alternative Medicine. London: Parthenon Publishing, 2003: 289–98

9. Wolfe SM, Ardati AK, Woosley R. Petition to the Food and Drug Administration (FDA) requesting a ban on production and sale of dietary supplements containing ephedrine alkaloids. HRG publication 1590 (5 September 2001). Available at: www.citizen.org/publications/ release.cfm?ID=7053#_ednref19, accessed 19 December 2002

10. United States House of Representatives. Adverse Events on Metabolife (October, 2002). A report prepared by the US House of Representatives. Available at: http://reform. house.gov/min/ pdfs/pdf_inves/pdf_dietary_ephedra_metabolife_rep.pdf, accessed 19 December 2002

11. Haller CA, Jacob P, Benowitz NL. Short-term metabolic and hemodynamic effects of ephedra and guarana combinations. Clin Pharmacol Ther 2005; 77: 560–71

12. Vukovich MD, Schoorman R, Heilman C, et al. Caffeine–herbal ephedra combination increases resting energy expenditure, heart rate and blood pressure. Clin Exp Pharmacol Physiol 2005; 32: 47–53

13. Greenway FL, De Jonge L, Blanchard D, et al. Effect of a dietary herbal supplement containing caffeine and ephedra on weight, metabolic rate, and body composition. Obes Res 2004; 12: 1152–7

14. McBride BF, Karapanos AK, Krudysz A, et al. Electrocardiographic and hemodynamic effects of a multicomponent dietary supplement containing ephedra and caffeine: a randomized controlled trial. J Am Med Assoc 2004; 291: 216–21

15. Gardner SF, Franks AM, Gurley BJ, et al. Effect of a multicomponent, ephedra-containing dietary supplement (Metabolife 356) on Holter monitoring and hemostatic parameters in healthy volunteers. Am J Cardiol 2003; 91: 1510–13, A9

16. Haller CA, Jacob P, III, Benowitz NL. Pharmacology of ephedra alkaloids and caffeine after single-dose dietary supplement use. Clin Pharmacol Ther 2002; 71: 421–32

17. Gurley BJ, Gardner SF, White LM, Wang PL. Ephedrine pharmacokinetics after the ingestion of nutritional supplements containing Ephedra sinica (ma huang). Ther Drug Monit 1998; 20: 439–45

18. White LM, Gardner SF, Gurley BJ, et al. Pharmacokinetics and cardiovascular effects of ma-huang (Ephedra sinica) in normotensive adults. J Clin Pharmacol 1997; 37: 116–22

19. Coffey CS, Steiner D, Baker BA, Allison DB. A randomized double-blind placebo-controlled clinical trial of a product containing ephedrine, caffeine, and other ingredients from herbal sources for treatment of overweight and obesity in the absence of lifestyle treatment. Int J Obes Relat Metab Disord 2004; 28: 1411–19

20. Kalman D, Incledon T, Gaunaurd I, et al. An acute clinical trial evaluating the cardiovascular effects of an herbal ephedra–caffeine weight loss product in healthy overweight adults. Int J Obes Relat Metab Disord 2002; 26: 1363–6

21. Krapp K, Longe JL. The Gale Encyclopedia of Alternative Medicine. Detroit: Gale Group, 2001

22. Shekelle P, Morton S, Maglione M. Ephedra and ephedrine for weight loss and athletic performance enhancement: clinical efficacy and side effects. Evidence Report/Technology Assessment No 76, 2003. (Prepared by Southern California Evidence-based Practice Center, RAND Corporation.) Agency for Healthcare Research and Quality. Rockville, MD. Available at: www.fda.gov/OHRMS/DOCKETS/98fr/95n-0304-bkg0003-ref-07-01-index.htm, accessed 8 August 2005

23. Food and Drug Administration. Statement of Lester M. Crawford, DVM, PhD Deputy Commissioner, Food And Drug Administration before the Subcommittee on Oversight of Government Management, Restructuring and The District of Columbia Committee on Governmental Affairs, United States Senate, 8 October 2002. The Regulatory Framework Under The Dietary Supplement Health And Education Act (DSHEA) of 1994. Available at: www.fda.gov/ola/2002/ephedra1008.html, accessed 19 December 2002

24. Food and Drug Administration. FDA statement on street drugs containing botanical ephedrine (HHS News, 10 April 1996). Available at: www.cfsan.fda.gov/~lrd/ hhsephe1.html, accessed 19 December 2002

25. CBS Evening News. DOJ eyes ephedra product (16 August 2000). Available at: www.cbsnews.com/stories/2002/08/15/eveningnews/main518873.shtml, accessed 19 December 2002

26. Food and Drug Administration. Center for Drug Evaluation and Research (CDER). Food and Drug Administration Public Health Advisory. Subject: safety of phenylpropanolamine (6 November 2000). Available at: www.fda.gov/cder/drug/info page/ ppa/ advisory.htm, accessed 7 January 2003

27. United States House of Representatives. Minority Staff Report, Special Investigations Division, Committee on Government Reform, United States House of Representatives. Adverse event reports from Metabolife. Available at: http://reform.house.gov/min/pdfs/pdf_inves/pdf_dietary_ephedra_metabolife_rep.pdf, accessed 19 December 2002

28. Food and Drug Administration. FDA News. Secretary Thompson urges strong warning labels for ephedra (8 October 2002). Available at: www.fda.gov/bbs/topics/ NEWS/2002/NEW00844.html, accessed 19 December 2002

29. American Medical Association. AMA testifies before Congress in effort to ban ephedra (8 October 2002, news from the American Medical Association). Available at: www.ama-assn.org/ama/pub/article/2403-6837.html, accessed 7 January 2003

30. Food and Drug Administration. Consumer alert: FDA plans regulation prohibiting sale of ephedra-containing dietary supplements and advises consumers to stop using these products. Available at: www.fda.gov/oc/initiatives/ ephedra/december2003/advisory.html, accessed 12 August 2005

31. Ioannidis JP, Lau J. Completeness of safety reporting in randomized trials: an evaluation of 7 medical areas. J Am Med Assoc 2001; 285: 437–43

32. Corrigan OP. A risky business: the detection of adverse drug reactions in clinical trials and post-marketing exercises. Soc Sci Med 2002; 55: 497–507

33. Marcus DM, Grollman AP. Botanical medicines – the need for new regulations. N Engl J Med 2002; 347: 2073–6

34. Lee MK, Cheng BW, Che CT, Hsieh DP. Cytotoxicity assessment of ma-huang (ephedra) under different conditions of preparation. Toxicol Sci 2000; 56: 424–30

35. Straus SE. Herbal medicines – what's in the bottle? N Engl J Med 2002; 347: 1997–8

36. Gurley BJ, Gardner SF, Hubbard MA. Content versus label claims in ephedra-containing dietary supplements. Am J Health Syst Pharm 2000; 57: 963–9

37. Soni MG, Carabin IG, Griffiths JC, Burdock GA. Safety of ephedra: lessons learned. Toxicol Lett 2004; 150: 97–110

38. Young R, Gabryszuk M, Glennon RA. (-)Ephedrine and caffeine mutually potentiate one another's amphetamine-like stimulus effects. Pharmacol Biochem Behav 1998; 61: 169–73

39. Xu B. Chinese herbal medicine and formulation. In Yuan CS, Bieber EJ, eds. Textbook of Complementary and Alternative Medicine. London: Parthenon Publishing, 2002: 155–63

40. Bensky D, Gamble A. Warm, acrid herbs that release the exterior. In Bensky D, Gamble A, eds. Chinese Herbal Medicine: Materia Medica. Seattle: Eastland Press Inc, 1993: 28–9

41. Zhonghua Bencao Editorial Group. Zhonghua Bencao Editorial Group, Zhonghua Bencao (Chinese Herbal Medicine). Shanghai: Shanghai Science and Technology Publishing House, 1996

42. Burdock GA. Dietary supplements and lessons to be learned from GRAS. Regul Toxicol Pharmacol 2000; 31: 68–76

43. Greene J. Growing public interest in alternative medicine has led to a dramatic increase in the number of courses offered through medical schools, residency programs and CME (17 January 2002, from the American Medical News). Available at: www.ama-assn.org/sci- pubs/amnews/ pick_00/prsa0117.htm, accessed 7 January 2003

44. De Smet PA. Herbal remedies. N Engl J Med 2002; 347: 2046–56

45. Bauer BA. Herbal therapy: what a clinician needs to know to counsel patients effectively. Mayo Clin Proc 2000; 75: 835–41

46. Food and Drug Administration. FDA Consumer (September–October, 1998). Kurtzweil P. An FDA guide to dietary supplements. Available at: www.cfsan.fda.gov/~ dms/fdsupp.html, accessed 24 August 2005

47. Food and Drug Administration. Center for Food Safety and Applied Nutrition. Dietary Supplements. Consumer Education and General Information. Available at: www.cfsan.fda.gov/ ~dms/ds-info.html, accessed 8 August 2005

48. American Botanical Council. Herbalgram 2004; 64: 30–3. Whybark M. Third-party evaluation programs for the quality of dietary supplements. Available at: www.herbalgram.org/herbalgram/articleview.asp?a=2752, accessed 24 August 2005

Traditional Chinese Medicine: an overview 9

W. Xuan

INTRODUCTION

Traditional Chinese Medicine (TCM) is an ancient medical science in China. TCM is based on the collected and valuable experiences gained from the battle of the Chinese people against disease over thousands of years, and has become an important component in Chinese culture. TCM is a science of the physiology and pathology of the human body as well as the prevention, diagnosis, and treatment of diseases under the guidance of its unique theory – a theory that is deeply influenced by both ancient philosophy and accumulated clinical experience. It originated thousands of years ago and came to maturity a few hundred years before Christ. The earliest classical book on TCM, *Huang Di Nei Jing*, was written during The Period of Spring–Autumn War State 475–221 BC. *Huang Di Nei Jing* set up the underlying theory of TCM, and laid the foundation for its contemporary practice.

TCM is mainly composed of the theory and the therapeutic methods. Among these are Chinese materia medica (including Chinese herbal medicine, animal medicine and mineral medicine), acupuncture, moxibustion, and naprapathy (*Tui Na*).

THE FUNDAMENTAL THEORY OF TRADITIONAL CHINESE MEDICINE

The Fundamental Theory of TCM explains the physiology and pathology of the human body, as well as the etiology, prevention, and treatment of diseases. TCM can be divided into eight theories:

(1)   The theory of the *Yin* and *Yang*;

(2)   The theory of the movement/changes among five elements;

(3)   The theory of the *Zang-Xiang*;

(4)   The theory of the *Qi*, *Xie* and *Jin Ye*;

(5)   The theory of the channels and collaterals;

(6)   The theory of the causes and occurrence of diseases;

(7)   The theory of pathogenesis; and

(8)   The theory of the principles of prevention and treatment of diseases.

The theory of *Yin* and *Yang*

This theory is employed to interpret the structure and physiologic functions of the human body and the models of occurrence or development of diseases so as to guide the clinical diagnosis and its treatment.

Yin/Yang, dating back to the Zhou Dynasty (approximately 1000–770 BC), was a symbolic representation of the universe that embodied the concept of patterns, process, change, and relationships that can be seen graphically in the *Yin/Yang* symbol (Figure 9.1). The concept of *Yin/Yang* is the most important and distinctive theory in TCM. All Chinese medical physiology, pathology, diagnosis, and treatment can eventually be reduced to the fundamental theory of *Yin/Yang*. *Yin/Yang* represents the opposite but also interdependence. Each could consume, but also support its opposite. *Yin and Yang* can be inter-transformed because *Yin* contains the seed of *Yang* and vice versa. Moreover, *Yin/Yang* can be further subdivided into another level of *Yin/Yang* and so on until infinity. From Table 9.1, it can be seen that *Yin* and *Yang* are essentially an expression of a duality and an alternation of two opposite stages in time.

Yin and *Yang* are related in that they are in opposite stages of a cycle, which constitutes the motive force of all the changes, development, and decay of things. *Yin* and *Yang* are interdependent, although they are opposite, one cannot exist without the other. *Yin* and *Yang* are in a constant state of dynamic balance, which is maintained by a continuous adjustment of their relative levels. *Yin*

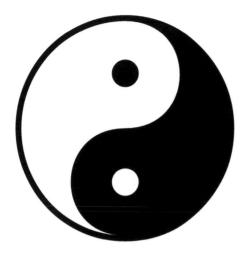

Figure 9.1   The symbol of *Yin* and *Yang*

and *Yang* transform into each other; *Yin* can change into *Yang* and vice versa. *Yin* and *Yang* within a human's body structure are shown in Table 9.2.

The theory of Wu-Xing

Wu-Xing is often translated into 'five elements' in English TCM books or articles, which is not quite right. This is because the five elements only refer to five different materials, such as wood, fire, earth, gold, and water, which were originally considered to be the most basic substances in people's daily life in ancient China. However, Xing implied the movement and changes, and Wu-Xing actually indicated movement and changes among the five elements as the Chinese ancient philosophers deeply believed that everything in the physical universe was formed on the basis of movement and changes among the five elements mentioned above, and so did the TCM practitioners. Therefore, the English translation for Wu-Xing in the fundamental theory of TCM should be written as the movement and changes among five elements.

The theory of the movement and changes among five elements, together with the theory of *Yin* and *Yang*, constitutes the basics of TCM theory. As explained above, the five elements refer to wood, fire, earth, gold, and water. Among them, each one has its own characteristic properties. The theory originally explained the composition and phenomena of the physical universe by applying concepts of 'inter-generating, inter-controlling, over-controlling, and inter-insulting' relationships

Table 9.1   Indications for general identification of *Yin* and *Yang*

Yin	Yang
Darkness	Light
Moon	Sun
Shade	Brightness
Rest	Activity
Earth	Heaven
Flat	Round
Space	Time
West	East
North	South
Right	Left
Water	Fire
Cold	Hot
Quiet	Restless
Wet	Dry
Soft	Hard
Inhibition	Excitement
Slowness	Rapidity
Substantial	Non-substantial
Storage	Transformation
Sustaining	Change

Table 9.2   *Yin* and *Yang* within the structure of the human body

Yin	Yang
Inferior	Superior
Interior	Exterior
Anterior–medial surface	Posterior–lateral surface
Front	Back
Structure	Function
Body	Head
Organs	Skin/muscles
Below the waist	Above the waist
Blood and body fluids	*Qi*

among the five elements. It was later used in TCM to expound the unity of the human body and the natural world. Clinically, this theory helps practitioners to identify the root causes of health problems.

Figure 9.2 illustrates different relationships among the five elements and those among internal organs. Interrelationships between the five elements and natural phenomena are shown in Table 9.3. In the inter-generating sequence, each element generates

Table 9.3   Introduction of natural phenomena to the five elements

	Wood (expansive/outward)	*Fire (upward)*	*Earth (neutrality)*	*Gold (contractive/inward)*	*Water (downward)*
Direction	east	south	center	west	north
Season	spring	summer	late summer	autumn	winter
Colors	green	red	yellow	white	black
Climate	wind	heat	dampness	dryness	cold
Tastes	sour	bitter	sweet	pungent	salty
Organs	Liver/GB	Heart/SI	Spleen/Stomach	Lungs/LI	Kidney/Bladder
Sense	Eyes	tongue	Mouth	Nose	Ears
Tissues	Sinews	vessel	Muscles	Skin	Bones
Grains	wheat	beans	rice	hemp	millet
Stage	birth	growth	transformation	harvest	storage

GB, gallbladder; SI, small intestine; LI, large intestine

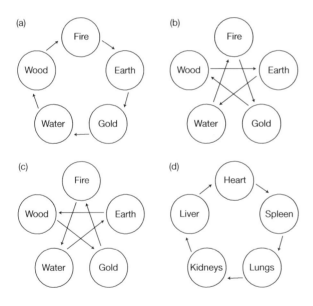

Figure 9.2   The inter-generating sequence (a); the inter-controlling and over-controlling sequence (b); the inter-insulting sequence (c); the inter-generating sequence among internal organs (d)

another and is generated by an element. In the inter-controlling sequence, each element controls another and is controlled by an element. In the over-controlling sequence, the same sequence is followed as the controlling one, but each element 'over-controls' another, so that it causes the other to decrease. In the inter-insulting

sequence, the sequence takes place in the reverse order from the controlling sequence.

The theory of movement and changes among five elements can be applied to TCM physiology and pathology. The inter-generating and the inter-controlling sequences provide the basic model of physiologic relationship among the internal organs. The over-controlling and the inter-insulting sequences provide a clinically useful pattern of pathologic relationship among the internal organs. The inter-generating sequence can also give rise to pathologic conditions when it is out of balance. The essence of the five element relationship is 'balance'. The inter-generating and the inter-controlling sequences keep a dynamic balance among the elements. When this balance is out of control for a prolonged period of time, disease occurs.

The theory of movement and changes among five elements can also be employed in TCM diagnosis. For example, a green color of the face indicates stagnation of the Liver-*Qi*; a red color of the face means excess/fullness of the heart-fire; a yellow or sallow complexion suggests deficiency/emptiness of the Spleen-*Qi*; a white color of the face implies deficiency/emptiness of the Lung-*Qi*; and a gray or black color recommends deficiency/emptiness of the Kidney-*Yang*.

The theory of movement and changes among five elements can be utilized to guide TCM treatment. For instance, whenever the empty Liver-Blood is noted, the following (based on the relationships among the five elements) should always be considered: the mother element (water/Kidney) fails to nourish the son element (wood/Liver); gold/Lung overcontrols wood/Liver; the son element (fire/Heart) is drawing too much from the mother element (wood/Liver); earth/Spleen is insulting the wood/Liver. It is necessary to keep all these relationships among the five elements in mind when determining treatment in TCM.

The theory of movement and changes among five elements is also used in determination of herbal or diet therapy. Diet therapy is partially based on the five-element model, and the principles underlying diet therapy are mostly the same as those in herbal therapy. Each food or herb has a certain flavor that is related to one of the elements, and is classified as having one of these flavors. The 'flavor' of a food or herb is not always related to its actual taste, although in most cases the two will coincide. For instance, lamb is classified as 'bitter' as is apple, which indicates that insomnia patients should avoid eating lamb and apple.

In addition, each of the flavors has a certain effect on the body. The sour flavor can generate body fluids and *Yin*, and control perspiration as well as diarrhea. The bitter flavor can clear away heat, tranquilize and harden, and calm down restlessness and subdue rebellious *Qi*. The sweet flavor tones, balances, and moderates. It is used to tone emptiness/deficiency, and to stop pain caused by emptiness. The pungent flavor scatters, and is used to expel pathogenic factors. The salty flavor flows downwards and softens hardness, and is applied to treat constipation and swelling.

It is important to know that particular organs and systems might be affected by different flavors. For example, the sour always goes to the nerves and can upset the Liver, and it should be avoided for Spleen disease. The bitter goes to the bones, and it should be avoided for Lung disease. The sweet goes to the muscles, and it should be avoided for Kidney disease. The pungent scatters the *Qi*, and should be avoided for Liver disease. The salty dries the Blood, and should be avoided for Heart disease.

Qi, *Xie*, and *JinYe*

TCM holds that *Qi*, *Xie*, and *JinYe* (also known as body fluid) are fundamental substances in the human body to sustain its normal vital activities. Together with the theory of *Zang-Xiang* and that of the channels and collaterals, they constitute the theoretical basis of TCM human physiology.

The concept of Qi in TCM

The ancient Chinese scholars believed that *Qi* was the most basic substance of which the universe was composed, and everything in the universe resulted from the movement and changes of *Qi*. It was then introduced into the TCM field, and was gradually used to form the theory of TCM. Since TCM practitioners emphasize the interrelationship between the universe and human beings, they consider the human being's *Qi* as a result of the interaction of the heaven-*Qi* and the earth-*Qi*. There is an old Chinese saying: '*Qi* is the root of a human being'. Generally speaking, the word *Qi* in TCM covers both substance and function. There are many different 'names' for *Qi*, which we can find from TCM books. However, all the various *Qi* are ultimately one *Qi*, merely manifesting in different forms. *Qi* varies by its names according to its source, location and function.

The substantial *Qi*:

- Source *Qi* (*Yuan Qi*): also known as congenital *Qi* as it is derived from the congenital essence of the parents

- Pectoral *Qi* (*Zong Qi*): a combined *Qi* from the *Qi* essence of food and drink and the air inhaled, which serves as the dynamic force of respiration and blood circulation

- Nutritive *Qi* (*Ying Qi*): transformed from the essence of food and drink, and flows with the blood in all 14 channels and collaterals

- Defensive *Qi* (*Wei Qi*): also transformed from the essence of food and drink, but moves outside the channels and collaterals

- Clean *Qi* (*Qing Qi*): the air inspired in the lung

- Waste *Qi* (*Zhuo Qi*): the air expired and the dense part of food.

The functional *Qi*:

- Heart-*Qi*

- Liver-*Qi*

- Spleen-*Qi*

- Lung-*Qi*

- Kidney-*Qi*

- Stomach-*Qi*.

The functions of *Qi* vary. First, *Qi* is of promoting action to activate the growth and development of the human body, and to speed up the formation and the circulation of the Blood. Second, *Qi* has a warming action as the main source to keep the body warm. Third, *Qi* guards the body surface against invasion of exogenous pathogenic factors, with a defending action. Fourth, *Qi* has a holding action, to hold, control, and govern the secretion and excretion of liquid materials, such as sweat, urine, and saliva, and to hold the internal organs in the abdominal cavity. Fifth, with a transforming action, *Qi* can metabolize fundamental substances, vital energy, *Xie*/Blood, and *JinYe*.

The concept of Xie in TCM

'*Xie*' here is always translated into 'blood' in English TCM books. However, *Xie* in TCM has a different meaning from blood in Western medicine. Therefore, in order to help verbally recognize them, *Xie*/Blood should be employed instead. According to TCM, *Xie*/Blood itself is a form of *Qi*, and is inseparable from *Qi*; *Qi* infuses liveliness into *Xie*/Blood, and without it, *Xie*/Blood would only be an inert fluid; *Xie*/Blood is derived mostly from the food-*Qi* produced by the Spleen. The Spleen then sends food-*Qi* upward to the Lungs, and, through the pushing action of Lung-*Qi*, the food-*Qi* is sent to the Heart, where it is transformed into *Xie*/Blood. As for *Xie*/Blood's function, it is to nourish and moisten the whole human body, and it is considered to play an important role in sustaining mental activity as *Xie*/Blood establishes the material foundation for the mind (Figure 9.3).

The concept of JinYe in TCM

JinYe is usually translated as body fluid in English. '*JinYe*' in TCM refers to the intracellular and the extracellular fluid in Western medicine. '*Jin*' indicates liquid that is diluted and moisturized, which is distributed under the skin and in muscles as well as pores/orifices of the body, while '*Ye*' means fluid that is sticky and hard to move, which infuses the joints, *Zang-Fu* organs, and brain and marrow of the body. *JinYe* originates from food and drink, which is transformed by the Stomach and transported by the Spleen. In addition, both the

Small Intestine separating the clarity from the turbidity and the Large Intestine absorbing fluid from the waste are closely related to the transformation of *JinYe*. As for the distribution of *JinYe*, it is mainly completed by the Spleen's transmission and transportation, by the Lung's dispersing and descending, and by the Kidney's vaporization (Figure 9.4).

The functions of *JinYe* are first, to moisturize and nourish the body; and second, to transform the *Xie*/Blood. *Jin* moisturizes the skin and hair, the muscles, the eyes, the nose, and the mouth, etc., while *Ye* nourishes the *Zang-Fu* organs, the brain, and the marrow. In addition, *JinYe* joins the *Xie*/Blood through the small collaterals (*Sun Mai*) and becomes a component part of the *Xie*/Blood.

All *Qi*, *Xie*/Blood, and *JinYe* derive from the essence of food and drink, but their properties and functions are different. Physiologically, they depend on each other, and they restrain and utilize each other. Pathologically, they also influence each other, and can cause imbalance of the other.

The relationship between Qi and Xie/Blood

Theoretically, TCM holds that 'The *Qi* is the commander of the *Xie*/Blood while the *Xie*/Blood is the mother of the *Qi*'. To explain this, we must look at how *Qi* acts on the *Xie*/Blood. First, *Qi* helps to transform *Xie*/Blood, and in fact is the primary power for transformation of *Xie*/Blood. Therefore, insufficient *Qi* may lead to *Xie*/Blood deficiency. Second, *Qi* drives the force to move the *Xie*/Blood, and is the driving power for circulation of the *Xie*/Blood, not only through its direct action, but also by means of relevant organs, such as the Heart-*Qi*'s pushing, the Lung-*Qi*'s dispersing or descending, and the Liver-*Qi*'s unrestrained flow/movement. Consequently, *Qi*'s stagnation or deficiency often causes poor *Xie*/Blood circulation or even *Xie*/Blood stasis. Third, *Qi* controls the movement of the *Xie*/Blood, and is able to keep the *Xie*/Blood circulated within the vessels, mainly through the Spleen-*Qi*. Whenever *Qi* becomes insufficient, various types of hemorrhage soon occur. Fourth, *Xie*/Blood carries the *Qi*, and *Qi* exists in the *Xie*/Blood. Last, *Xie*/Blood provides *Qi* with nutrients, and *Qi*, therefore, constantly receives nutrients from the *Xie*/Blood.

The relationship between Qi and JinYe

Qi transforms *JinYe*. *Qi* is the primary power for transformation of *JinYe*, although *JinYe* is mainly transformed

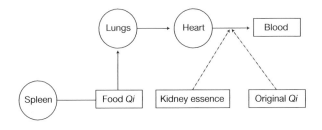

Figure 9.3   The origin of the *Xie*/Blood

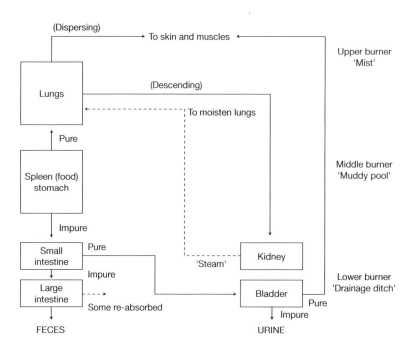

Figure 9.4   The origin, transformation, and excretion of *JinYe*

through the function of the Spleen and the Stomach. *Qi* promotes transportation of *JinYe*. *Qi* is the basic power for normal transportation and distribution of *JinYe*. *Qi* arrests excretion of *JinYe*. *Qi* is able to adjust and control excretion of *JinYe* so as to keep the balance between *JinYe*'s transformation and its excretion. *JinYe* is the carrier of *Qi* as *Qi* is always with *JinYe*. Therefore, loss of *JinYe*, such as profuse perspiring, frequent vomiting, or diarrhea, often results in deficiency of *Qi*.

The relationship between the *Xie*/Blood and *JinYe*

Both the *Xie*/Blood and *JinYe* derive from the essence of food and drink, and are substances of the liquid state. Their main function is to nourish and moisturize the body. Since the *Xie*/Blood becomes *JinYe* when it extravasates the collaterals and *JinYe* becomes a component of the *Xie*/Blood when it seeps into the small collaterals, both *JinYe* and *Xie*/Blood are believed to be from the same source. Therefore, insufficient *Xie*/Blood usually results in deficiency of *JinYe* and vice versa. In addition, the *Xie*/Blood and perspiration are also considered to come from the same source. Hence, TCM holds that 'Those who lose *Xie*/Blood cannot get themselves perspired, while those who perspire profusely will not have the same sufficiency of *Xie*/Blood as usual'.

The theory of *Zang-Xiang*

Zang-Xiang is usually translated into *Zang-Fu* organs in English TCM books, and is equivalent to internal organs in Western medicine. The theory of *Zang-Xiang* is on the basis of *Zang-Fu* organs, and explains the physiologic function and pathologic changes of each *Zang-Fu* organ and the mutual relationships among the organs. The theory also explains functional relationships that provide total integration of bodily functions, emotions, mental activities, tissues, and sense organs, as well as environmental influences. Although the name of each *Zang-Fu* used in TCM is basically the same as that of each internal organ used in Western medicine, their fundamental meanings are different, because the names of *Zang-Fu* not only indicate anatomic units, but also cover the physiologic and pathologic aspects of *Zang-Fu*. On the other hand, the names of internal organs used in Western medicine only point out the entities by means of anatomy.

In TCM, all *Zang-Fu* organs of the human body are classified into three groups. They refer to: five *Zangs*, including the Heart (and the Pericardium), the Liver, the Spleen, the Lungs and the Kidney; six *Fus*, involving the Gallbladder, the Stomach, the Large Intestine, the Small Intestine, the Urinary Bladder and the *SanJiao* (triple *Jiao*); *QiHengZhiFu*, also known as Extraordinary

Table 9.4   The 12 *Zang-Fu* organs in TCM

Zang (Yin)	Fu (Yang)	Tissues	Sense organs
Heart	Small Intestine	Channels and Collaterals	Complexion
Liver	Gallbladder	Sinews/Tendons	Nails
Spleen	Stomach	Muscles	Lips
Lung	Large Intestine	Skin and pores	Body hair
Kidney	Urinary Bladder	Bones	Hair
Pericardium	Triple *Jiao*		

Organs, referring to the Brain, the Marrow, the Bone, the channels and collaterals, the Gallbladder and the Uterus. The difference between *Zang* and *Fu* is that all *Zangs* functionally store vital substances, such as *Qi*, *Xie*/Blood, and *JinYe*, while all of the *Fus* digests food and drink and transmits the essence.

There are 12 *Zang-Fu* organs in TCM. Among them, six are *Yin* and six are *Yang* (Table 9.4). The functions of each of the *Zang-Fu* organs follow.

Five Zangs

(1) The Heart includes the Pericardium, and is considered the most important organ in the human body. It controls all the other organs' functions, and is therefore called the 'king of all the organs'. The Heart has three major functions. First, the Heart controls *Xie*/Blood circulation, and connects its channels. It is believed that the Heart is connected with the channels and collaterals to form a closed system, where the *Xie*/Blood is circulated by the Heart-*Qi*, which is considered as the motive power. Second, the heart houses the mind. 'Mind' in TCM indicates the mental activities of the human body. TCM holds that the Heart controls mental/thinking activities as well as consciousness by way of 'housing the mind'. Third, the Heart links the Tongue and manifests in the complexion because the collateral (*luo mai*) of the Heart channel ascends to connect the Tongue and the Heart has its outward manifestation in the face. The Pericardium is the peripheral tissue of the Heart. It prevents the Heart from being directly invaded by exterior pathogenic factors.

(2) The Liver is divided into the Liver-*Yin* (Liver itself and the *Xie*/Blood stored in it) and the Liver-*Yang*, including the Liver-*Qi*. The Liver has four major functions. First, the Liver promotes the unrestrained and smooth flow of *Qi*. Ancient Chinese medical scholars believed that wood or a tree tended to spread out freely, as did the Liver. To correspond to this character, the Liver is classified as 'wood' in the theory of the movement/changes among five elements of TCM. This is strongly associated with the Heart's function to sustain the normal mental activities of human beings with the Spleen/Stomach's function to keep normal digestion and absorption, and with keeping harmonious movement of both *Qi* and the *Xie*/Blood or removing any stagnated *Qi* within *SanJiao* so as to dredge or adjust the water passage. Second, the Liver stores the *Xie*/Blood and regulates the volume of the *Xie*/Blood according to physical activities at any time, which is a self-regulating process. Third, the Liver controls the sinews/tendons and manifests in the nails. The contraction and relaxation of the sinews/tendons depend on the nourishment of the *Xie*/Blood from the Liver, as do the nails. Finally, the Liver relates to the eyes. The eye is a sensory organ, but connected to the collateral of the Liver. It is the nourishment and moistening of the Liver-*Xie*/Blood that gives the eyes the capacity to see.

(3) The Spleen in TCM is believed to be located in the middle *Jiao*. As a major organ in the digestive system, the Spleen has five main functions. First, the Spleen dominates the transformation and transportation of food-*Qi*. The Spleen transforms food-*Qi* from ingested food and drink, which have been digested by the Spleen and Stomach, and transports this food-*Qi* and other refined parts of food and drink ('food essence') to the various organs and parts of the body to nourish them. In addition, the Spleen absorbs and transports water. Second, through its *Qi*, the Spleen keeps the *Xie*/Blood circulated within the channels and collaterals. Third, the Spleen controls the muscles and the four limbs because the muscles, the major components of the four limbs, are mainly nourished by the food-*Qi*,

which is transformed and transported by the Spleen. Fourth, the Spleen chains the mouth and manifests on the Lips. When the Spleen's function is normal, the sense of taste is good, the lips are moist and rosy, and the action of chewing that prepares food for the Spleen to transform and transport its food essence is proper. Fifth, the Spleen raises the 'clear *Qi*' and keeps all the *Zang-Fu* organs at their locations. This means that the Spleen has an ability to send the food essence (food-*Qi*) upward to the Lung, where the essence is distributed, and to keep all internal organs at their original locations.

(4) The Lung, believed in TCM to consist of the Lung-*Yin* and the Lung-*Qi*, has four main functions. First, the Lung governs *Qi*, which covers two aspects. The Lung controls respiration because the Lung is the main organ where the 'clean *Qi*' from the environment and the 'waste *Qi*' from the human body are exchanged. The Lung combines food-*Qi* with inhaled clean *Qi* to form Pectoral *Qi* (*ZongQi*), which is further spread all over the body to nourish tissues and to promote physiologic processes. Second, the Lung controls the dispersion/descent and maintenance of water metabolism. The Lung can disperse or spread defensive *Qi* and the essence of food and drink all over the body warmly to moisturize skin and muscles and to nourish the whole body. In addition, since the Lung is the uppermost organ in the body, the Lung-*Qi* must descend to communicate with the Kidney-*Qi*, and to push the water in upper *Jiao* downward to the Kidney and the Urinary Bladder. Third, the Lung connects the skin, perspiration glands, pores, and hair, and is capable of spreading *JinYe* and Defensive *Qi* to the skin, perspiration glands, pores, and hair to nourish and moisturize them so as to strengthen the body to fight against invasion of external pathogenic factors. Finally, the Lung relates to the nose, the gate of the lung through which the fresh air enters and the 'waste *Qi*' exhales. The major functions of the nose, ventilation and smelling, mainly depend on the Lung-*Qi*.

(5) The Kidney is often referred to as the Kidney essence (Kidney-*Yin*) and the Kidney-*Qi* (Kidney-*Yang*). The former is derived from the parents and established at conception, while the latter is transformed from the former after birth. Since Kidney-*Yin* and Kidney-*Yang* are the foundation of the *Yin*

and *Yang* for all the other *Zang-Fu* organs, they are also called 'original *Yin*' and 'original *Yang*', respectively. Kidney-*Yin* is the fundamental substance for birth, growth, and reproduction, while Kidney-*Yang* is the motive force of all physiologic processes. The Kidney has various functions. A primary function of the Kidney is to store the essence. The Kidney stores both 'inherited essence' and 'acquired essence', which are, respectively, obtained from the parents at conception and from refined essence extracted from food and drink through the transforming power of the other *Zang-Fu* organs. The inherited essence determines the basic constitution, growth, sexual maturation, fertility, development, strength, and vitality of the human body. The acquired essence is also known as 'essence of five *Zangs* and six *Fus*', part of which is stored in the Kidney in preparation for future needs. The second function of the Kidney is to dominate the regulation of water metabolism, which is to spread *JinYe* all over the body and to discharge the waste fluid produced by all the *Zang-Fu* organs inside the human body. The Kidney is like a gate that has the function of opening and closing. Under physiologic conditions, a balance between Kidney-*Yin* and Kidney-*Yang* exists, resulting in the normal regulation of the opening and closing of the 'gate'. Opening the gate eliminates the water (urine), while closing the gate helps retain the water (*JinYe*) needed by the organs. The third function of the Kidney is to control the reception of *Qi* (air). TCM holds that, to make use of the 'clear *Qi*' from the air, the Lung and the Kidney must work together. The Lung has a 'descending action' on *Qi*, which is directed down to the Kidney that responds by 'holding' this *Qi* down. The fourth function of the Kidney is to produce the Marrow to nourish the bones and fill up the Brain. Kidney-essence is the organic foundation for the production of the Marrow, which is stored in the bone cavity to supply the nourishment to bones. 'Marrow' in TCM means a substance that is the common matrix of bones, bone marrow, and Brain and Spinal cord. Thus, the Kidney-essence produces the Marrow, which generates the Spinal cord and 'fills up' the Brain. For this reason, the Brain has a physiologic relationship with the Kidney in TCM. The fifth function of the Kidney is to manifest on the hair. The hair is nourished by the *Xie*/Blood, but originates from the Kidney-essence, as it can transform the *Xie*/Blood. Therefore, the quality and color of the hair are related to the state of the Kidney-essence. The final primary function of the Kidney is to unite the ears and control the two lower orifices (Ear-*Yin*). The ears rely on nourishment from the essence for their proper function and are therefore physiologically related to the Kidney. The two lower orifices mean the front and the rear private parts, which include the urethra, the genitalia, and the anus. These orifices are functionally related to the Kidney.

Ming Men

Ming Men is often translated as 'The Gate of Vitality' in English. It first appeared in the classical TCM book *Huang Di Nei Jing* (475–221 BC), and many different explanations have been given since then. However, it is commonly believed that the real meaning of the term '*Ming Men*' is basically the same as that of the Kidney-*Yang*, and the term is only used to emphasize the importance of the Kidney-*Yang*.

Six Fus

Six Fus is a collective term for the Small Intestine, the Gallbladder, the Stomach, the Large Intestine, the Urinary Bladder, and the *SanJiao*.

(1)   The Small Intestine dominates the reception of food content from the Stomach, absorbs and digests the food content, and separates the useful/clarity from the waste/turbidity.

(2)   The Gallbladder stores and excretes bile, and dominates decision-making and judgment.

(3)   The Stomach receives food and drink, dominates the digestion of food, governs the transportation of the content of food/drink and directs Stomach-*Qi* downward.

(4)   The Large Intestine dominates transportation of waste.

(5)   The Urinary Bladder stores and eliminates urine.

(6)   The triple *Jiao* (*SanJiao*) has three components. The upper *Jiao* (*ShangJiao*) controls respiration and dominates the Lung's dispersing function. It spreads nutrients and vital energy throughout the whole body, which is why the upper *Jiao* is referred to as a 'sprayer'. The middle *Jiao* (*ZhongJiao*), also referred to as a 'fermentation tank', dominates the digestion of food and the transformation of the 'essence of food and drink'. The lower *Jiao* (*XiaJiao*) controls the separation of the useful (clarity) from the waste (turbidity), and eliminates (to filter and drain off) the waste. It is often described as a 'drainage ditch'.

Extraordinary organs

In addition to the regular *Yin* and *Yang* organs, there are also six extraordinary organs functioning like *Yin* organs (i.e. storing the essence but not excreting anything), and having the shape of *Yang* organs (i.e. hollow inside the organs). Functionally, all the six extraordinary organs are directly or indirectly related to the Kidney. The names of these organs are as follows: Brain, Marrow, Bones, channels and collaterals, Gallbladder, and Uterus.

Since the Brain and the Uterus were not mentioned in the previous paragraphs, they are introduced here. The Brain is formed by the Marrow and is contained in the cranial cavity. As predicted by TCM, 'the Brain is a sea of the Marrow'. The Brain controls thinking activity of the human body and dominates the audio and visual senses. TCM also believes that the Uterus' functions in producing menses and conceiving pregnancy are mainly related to the functions of the Heart (controlling the Blood circulation), the Liver (storing the Blood), the Spleen (keeping the Blood flow within the vessels), the Kidney (retaining the reproductive essence), and the *Ren* channel as well as the *Chong* channel (both supplying the Blood to the Uterus). Therefore, the Uterus in TCM refers not only to the organ itself but also to the different internal systems.

The theory of the channels and collaterals

This theory describes the mutual relationship between the physiology and pathology of the channels and collaterals. It forms the basis for acupuncture and naprapathy practitioners.

Channel means 'route' in Chinese, and is the main trunk distributed vertically in the whole system of channels and collaterals. The collateral implies 'net', and is the branch of a channel in the system. Different channels and collaterals are linked with each other and distributed to cover the whole human body so that the superficial, interior, upper, and lower portions of the body are connected into an organic whole.

The system of the channels and collaterals mainly consists of 20 channels, their branches, and their subsidiary parts. The channels are divided into 12 regular and eight extra ones. The collaterals, of which there are

15, are referred to as connective. Others may be superficial or small.

THE CAUSES OF DISEASE IN TCM

Identifying the root cause of the disease is a very important part in TCM practise. TCM stresses that balance is the key to a healthy body. Any long-term imbalance such as extreme climate change, overdue physical exercise, heavy workload, excessive rest, too frequent (or rare) sexual activity, unbalanced diet, sudden emotional changes, etc. can all be attributed to the cause of a disease. Therefore, the various causes of disease in TCM mainly include six exogenous factors, epidemic pathogenic factors, parasites, internal imbalance caused by seven emotional changes, improper diet, maladjustment between work/exercise and rest, trauma and the phlegm/fluid retention, and Blood stasis.

In recognizing the cause of a disease, TCM practitioners focus on analyzing signs as well as symptoms, and identifying different patterns, in addition to understanding the objective conditions that might be possible factors in a disease, called 'identifying the pattern to work out the causes'. The causes of disease are discussed below.

Six exogenous factors

'Six exogenous factors' is a general term for the six climatic conditions in excess: pathogenic wind, pathogenic cold, pathogenic summer heat, pathogenic dampness, pathogenic dryness, and pathogenic fire.

Pathogenic wind prevails in the spring, but occurs in all the seasons. It has the characteristics of being apt to move; tending to rise, disperse, and move upward and outward; being apt to migrate and change, leading to mobility; and causing all other diseases.

Pathogenic cold prevails in winter, but also exists in other seasons. Its characteristics are quickly consuming the *Yang* of the human body; coagulating *Qi* and the Blood in channels and collaterals or even blocking circulation of both *Qi* and the Blood; and causing contraction of the skin, muscles, channels and collaterals, tendons and ligaments.

Pathogenic summer heat prevails in summer, with characteristics of a hot nature; quickly exhausting *Qi* and consuming *JinYe*; and often accompanying pathogenic dampness.

Pathogenic dampness often occurs in late summer, a period of transition from summer to autumn. It always has characteristics of a heavy and turbid nature, of

viscousness, lingering in nature, of going downward, and of easily consuming the *Yang* of the human body.

Pathogenic dryness prevails in autumn. It quickly consumes the *JinYe* of the human body, and easily impairs the Lung.

Pathogenic fire is divided into external fire and endogenous fire. It is hot in nature; capable of flaring up; quickly consuming *JinYe* and exhausting *Qi*; able to produce endogenous wind, resulting from overconsuming the Liver-*Yin*; it causes various bleedings; easily causes carbuncles and sores; and frequently irritates the Heart and the mind.

Epidemic pathogenic factor

Epidemic pathogenic factor is a kind of pathogen with very strong infectivity, and also a minute pathogenic substance, such as a pathogenic micro-organism, which usually invades the human body through the mouth and nose, and cannot be directly observed by the human sensory organs. Sudden onset, similar manifestations, strong infectivity, and quick epidemicity are characteristics in common for all diseases caused by epidemic pathogenic factor.

Parasites

It was a long time ago when TCM started to demonstrate that parasites could cause diseases. The first discussion on treatment of ascariasis of the biliary tract can be traced back to the book *On Treatment of Diseases Caused by Pathogenic Wind and Cold* (Shang Han Lun), written in the third century AD. In the Sui dynasty, recognition of oxyuriasis and taeniasis was recorded in detail. Since then, it has been proved that Chinese herbs are safe and reliable in the treatment of parasitoses.

Internal imbalance caused by seven emotional changes

Seven emotional changes in TCM refer to seven different kinds of emotional reactions, such as joy, anger, melancholy, over-thinking, grief, fright, and shock. They are natural responses of the human body to environmental changes, and belong to the normal range of mental activities. However, seven emotional changes become pathogenic factors when sudden/violent or persistent changes of the environment occur, and when it is beyond the human body's endurance.

If joy becomes excessive excitement, the Heart has the potential to be harmed. Anger includes irritability, frustration and indignation, which affect the Liver. Melancholy/over-thinking indicates excessive mental work that weakens the Spleen. Grief includes sadness, which affects the Lung. Fright harms the Kidney and shock affects both the Kidney and the Heart.

Improper diet

Improper diet includes abnormal ingestion, contaminated food, and food preference. Any of these gives rise to diseases, such as acid regurgitation, anorexia, vomiting, and diarrhea.

Maladjustment between work/exercise and rest

Maladjustment includes physical over-strain, mental over-strain, sexual over-strain, and excessive rest. Any of the above over-strains would result in a different type of disease due to 'Qi exhaustion', 'over-consumption of the Heart–Blood/the Spleen-Qi' and 'over-consumption of the Kidney-essence'. Excessive rest could give rise to poor circulation of Qi and the Blood, and thus cause further diseases.

Traumas

Traumas include gunshot or incised wounds; traumatic injuries (injuries by knife or spear, fall or stumble, contusion, stabbing and abrasion, and by sports); injuries by heavy load, twist, sprain or wrench; burns or scalds; and bites by insects or beasts. Any of the above would cause at least bleeding, swelling and pain, fractures or joint dislocation, internal bleeding and, at most, even death.

Phlegm/fluid retention and blood stasis

Both phlegm/fluid retention and Blood stasis derive from the pathologic changes of the human body. When they are formed, they might, in turn, act directly or indirectly on some tissues or organs of the body to cause new diseases or different syndromes, in which phlegm/fluid retention and Blood stasis become another group of pathogenic factors.

Pathogenesis

Pathogenesis is the mechanism of the occurrence and the development of a disease. TCM believes that there are two major factors causing the occurrence of disease: the deficiency of the vital-Qi, which refers to the physiologic functions of the body, and the pathogenic-Qi, which

extensively covers any kind of pathogenic factor causing damage to the body. Basic pathogenesis includes vital-Qi fighting against pathogenic-Qi, an imbalance between *Yin* and *Yang* and lack of control of Qi's ascending or its descending.

METHODS OF DIAGNOSIS IN TCM

TCM diagnosis is intimately related to 'identification of disease patterns' as this provides the diagnostic tools necessary to identify the patterns, and is based on the fundamental principle that signs and symptoms reflect the condition of the internal organs. TCM uses not only symptoms and signs, but many other manifestations to form a picture of the disease pattern present in a particular person. Many of the so-called symptoms and signs would not be considered as such in Western medicine.

Over the centuries, TCM diagnosis has developed an extremely sophisticated system of correspondences between outward signs and internal organs. It includes four methods traditionally described with four words: observation, listening/smelling, inquiring, and palpation.

Observation

Expression

This is the outward manifestation of the vital activities.

Body

The body consists of five different constitutional body shapes. The 'wood type' is tall and slender. The 'fire type' has a small pointed head and small hands. The 'earth type' has a slightly fat body with a large head and belly, and wide jaw. The 'gold type' has broad and square shoulders, a strongly built body, and a triangular face. The 'water type' has a round face and body with a long spine.

Hair

The state of the hair is related to the condition of the Blood/Kidney essence.

Face color

Face color reflects the state of Qi/Blood and condition of the mind.

Eyes

The eyes reflect the state of the mind and the essence.

Nose

If the tip of the nose is green/blue, abdominal pain is indicated. If the tip of the nose is yellow, dampness is present. If the tip of the nose is white, Blood deficiency is a concern. If the tip of the nose is red, heat is present in the Lung and Spleen. If the tip of the nose is gray, an impairment of water movement is indicated.

Ears

If the color of the ears is white, a cold pattern exists. If they are black, pain is present. Dryness indicates extreme exhaustion of Kidney-*Qi*.

Mouth and lips

If the color of one's mouth and lips is very pale, emptiness of Blood or *Yang* is suggested. If the color is deep red, heat is present in the Spleen/Stomach. If the color is purple, Blood circulation is not functioning well. If the color is greenish, stasis of Liver-Blood and stagnation of Liver-*Qi* invading the Spleen could be problematic.

Teeth and gums

Teeth bright in color and dry like stone indicates heat. A dry and gray (like bones) presentation indicates empty-heat. Bleeding, painful or swollen gums suggests extreme heat in the Stomach. Swollen gums without pain indicate empty-heat. Very pale gums indicate deficiency of Blood.

Throat

Pain, redness, and swollen throat imply invasion of exterior wind-heat/fire in the Stomach. Sore and dry throat reveals a 'deficiency of Kidney-*Yin*' with empty-heat.

Limbs

If nails are pale, Blood deficiency may be suspected. Stasis of the Blood produces a bluish color.

Skin

Deficiency of Liver-Blood will cause the skin to dry. Itchy skin is caused by the wind. Edema produces swelling and is due to 'emptiness of Kidney-*Yang*'. Yellow skin indicates jaundice.

Tongue

A normal tongue is of proper size, light red in color, free in motion, and has a thin layer of white coating over the surface. It is neither dry nor over-moist. Tongue observation is based on the following:

(1) The tongue color indicates the conditions of Blood, nutritive *Qi* and *Yin* organs.

 (a) A pale tongue indicates patterns of empty-cold, caused by 'deficiency of *Yang-Qi*', 'insufficiency of both *Qi* and Blood', and invasion by exogenous pathogenic cold.

 (b) A red tongue indicates various patterns of excess-heat, due to invasion by pathogenic heat, and patterns of empty-heat resulting from over-consumption of *JinYe*.

 (c) A deep red tongue occurs in the severe stage of febrile disease in which the pathogenic heat has been transmitted to the inside body, and in patterns of empty-heat.

 (d) A purplish tongue indicates 'stagnation of both *Qi* and Blood' or 'preponderance of endogenous cold' due to 'deficiency of *Yang*'.

(2) A flabby tongue indicates deficiency of both *Qi* and *Yang* and 'retention of dampness' inside the body.

(3) A cracked tongue indicates over-consumption of *JinYe* by excess-heat, loss of kidney-essence and 'hyperactivity of empty-fire'.

(4) A thorny tongue indicates 'hyperactivity of pathogenic heat'.

(5) A rigid and tremulous tongue indicates invasion of exogenous heat and disturbance of the mind by damp-heat, or consumption of the Liver-*Yin* due to 'severe endogenous-heat stirring up the endogenous-wind', or 'obstruction of the collaterals due to the wind-phlegm'.

(6) A deviated tongue indicates a typical 'obstruction of the collaterals due to the wind-phlegm'.

The tongue coating indicates the state of the *Yang* organs. The moisture indicates the state of the *JinYe*.

Channels

In regard to channels, an observation of signs along the course of a channel including redness, white streaks, purple spots, and skin rashes is necessary.

Listening/smelling

Listening to speech:

- Speaking feebly and in low tones indicates patterns of emptiness

- Speaking lustily indicates patterns of excess/fullness

- Delirious speech indicates the heart collateral obstructed by phlegm-heat

- Muttering or extreme verbosity indicates disturbance of the mind

- Stuttering suggests collaterals obstructed by wind-phlegm.

Listening to breathing:

- A coarse and loud breathing sound indicates a full pattern

- A weak and thin breathing sound indicates an empty pattern.

Listening to the cough:

- A loud cough suggests a full pattern, such as the Lung invaded by wind-cold or obstructed by cold-phlegm

- A clear cough suggests a full pattern, but indicates the Lung invaded by wind-heat or obstructed by heat-phlegm

- A dry cough with little sputum indicates the Lung invaded by pathogenic dryness or 'deficiency of Lung-*Yin*' for a long time.

Smelling:

- A strong and foul scent is an indicator of heat

- An absence of scent indicates cold

- Foul breath indicates heat in the Stomach.

Inquiring

It is necessary to listen attentively to the complaints of the patient, inquire about the onset and duration of the illness, and record the medical history. To find out how the problem arose, TCM practitioners must inquire about the living conditions of the patient and his environment, both the emotional and familial environment. The most commonly used areas of questioning today are listed in Table 9.5.

Palpation

This mainly includes feeling the pulse and palpating channels and points (Figure 9.5). When feeling for a pulse, three fingers should be placed above the wrist joint where the radial artery throbs. The area for feeling the pulse is divided into three regions, named *Cun*, *Guan*,

Table 9.5   Areas of inquiry

Chills and fever
Perspiration
Head and body
Thorax and abdomen
Food and taste
Stools and urine
Sleep
Deafness and tinnitus
Thirst and drink
Pain

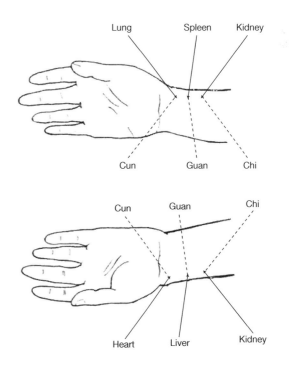

Figure 9.5   The three regions for feeling the pulse

Table 9.6   Relationship between regions of the pulse and internal organs

Pulse positions	Energy type	Triple Jiao	Organs (left/right)
Front/*Cun*	*Qi*	Upper	Heart/Lung
Middle/*Guan*	Blood	Middle	Liver/Spleen
Rear/*Chi*	*Yin*	Lower	Kidney/gate of vitality

and *Chi*. The region opposite to the styloid process of the radius is known as *Guan*, that distal to *Guan* is *Cun*, and that proximal to *Guan* is *Chi*. Finger force is exerted first lightly, then moderately, and finally heavily to get a general idea of the depth, frequency, rhythm, strength, and form of the pulse. The relationship between different regions of the pulse and internal organs is reflected in Table 9.6.

A normal pulse is of medium frequency (4–5 beats per breath) and regular rhythm. It must be even and forceful.

IDENTIFICATION OF DISEASE PATTERNS

TCM diagnoses diseases by using 'identification of disease patterns'. Identification of disease patterns is not made from a list of symptoms and signs, but from a reflection on the pathogenesis of the disease. Over centuries of accumulated clinical experience, TCM has developed a comprehensive and extremely effective diagnostic system and symptomatology to identify disease patterns. There are several methods in identifying disease patterns. These methods are based on the following.

Eight principles are based on the categories of exterior/interior, cold/hot, full/empty, and *Yin*/*Yang*, which are the foundation for all the other methods of disease pattern identification to identify the location and nature of the disease.

Qi, Xie/Blood, and *JinYe*, also known as vital substances in TCM, indicate the basic disharmonies such as deficiency, stagnation, and rebellion.

Zang-Fu is based on pathologic changes occurring in the internal organs.

Pathogenic factors are based on the pathologic changes occurring when the body is invaded by factors such as wind, cold, heat, dampness, dryness, and fire.

The five elements are based on the interpretation of clinical manifestations according to generating, over-controlling, and insulting sequences.

The channels and collaterals, based on the courses of different channels, is the oldest method that describes the symptoms and signs related to each channel or collateral rather than the organs.

The reflections on six channels is utilized mainly for the diagnosis and treatment of diseases caused by exterior-cold, which was formulated by *Zhang, ZhongJing*. It has been the bible for Chinese doctors, especially in northern China, for about 16 centuries. Reflections on:

(1) *Tai-Yang channel*: aversion to chills, headache, neck stiffness, superficial pulse, and fever;

(2) *Yang-Min channel*: aversion to heat, perspiring, thirst, restlessness, abdominal pain aggravated by pressure and constipation;

(3) *Shao-Yang channel*: alternate chills and fever, full sensation in the chest, bitter taste and thirst;

(4) *Tai-Yin channel*: full abdomen, vomiting, diarrhea, poor appetite, and weak and slow pulse;

(5) *Shao-Yin channel*: sleepiness, aversion to chills, cold limbs, diarrhea, and very weak pulse;

(6) *Ju-Yin channel*: delirium, loss of consciousness, extremely cold limbs, thirst, and poor appetite.

The four stages are the most important and most widely used method, devised by Ye, TianShi (1667–1746), for the treatment of febrile infectious diseases that start with invasion of the exterior wind-heat:

(1) *Stage I*: *Wei*/protective level;

(2) Fever, slight aversion to cold, headache, slight perspiring, slight thirst, superficial and fast pulse;

(3) *Stage II*: *Qi*/defensive level;

(4) Severe fever, aversion to heat, profuse perspiring, thirst, wheezing, scanty urine, constipation, and strong pulse;

(5) *Stage III*: *Yin* level;

(6) High fever (higher during nights), loss of consciousness, delirium, rashes, deep red tongue, yellow tongue coating, threadlike and rapid pulse;

(7) *Stage IV*: Blood level;

(8) Delirium, coma, convulsion, mania, bleeding, and extremely deep red tongue.

The triple Jiao is combined with the four stages to make 'identification of disease patterns' and to provide treatment principles for febrile infectious diseases starting with invasion of the wind-heat.

TRADITIONAL CHINESE MEDICINE TREATMENT AND TREATMENT PRINCIPLES

Treatment is only provided when 'treatment principles' are established. The treatment principles are usually set up right after the disease pattern is identified. Since disease patterns are different, treatment principles for each pattern should vary accordingly, and so does treatment.

For example, in the view of Western medicine, a cough is a symptom of many diseases, such as respiratory tract infection, bronchitis, bronchiectasis, pneumonia, and pulmonary tuberculosis. However, in TCM, it can be identified by the following patterns:

(1) *Pattern A*: wind-cold attacking the Lung (*Feng-HanSuoFei*);
Marked by cough with diluted sputum, profuse watery nasal discharge, chills, headache, stuffy nose, sneezing, thin and white tongue coating, and superficial pulse;

(2) *Pattern B*: wind-heat invading the Lung (*FengRe-FanFei*);
Manifested by cough with thick sputum, sore throat, thin and yellow tongue coating, and rapid as well as superficial pulse;

(3) *Pattern C*: phlegm-heat obstructing the Lung (*Tan-ReYongFei*);
Demonstrated by cough with thick and yellow or blood-stained sputum, chest pain, dyspnea, red tongue with yellowish greasy coating, and rapid rolling pulse;

(4) *Pattern D*: dryness-heat over-consuming the Lung-*Yin* (*ZaoReShangFei*),
Marked by cough without sputum or with very sticky sputum, chest pain with severe coughing, dry mouth, red tongue tip, thin and yellow tongue coating without moisture, and rapid but weak pulse;

(5) *Pattern E*: phlegm-dampness blocking the Lung (*TanShiZuFei*);
Indicated by cough with whitish sputum, stuffy sensation in the chest, white and greasy tongue coating, and rolling pulse;

(6) *Pattern F*: liver-fire attacking the Lung (*GanHuo-FanFei*);
Manifested by dry cough caused by upward adverse flow of the Lung-*Qi*, hypochondriac pain with severe coughing, red complexion, dry throat, thin and yellow tongue coating with little moisture, and wiry or rapid pulse;

(7) *Pattern G*: deficiency of the Lung-*Yin* (*FeiYinKuiXu*);
Indicated by dry cough or cough with little or blood-stained sputum, afternoon hot flush, night sweats, red tongue with little coating, and rapid but weak pulse.

Therefore, the treatment principles for each pattern mentioned above must be established and points selected as below:

(1) *Pattern A*: to expel the wind (*QuFeng*), disperse the cold (*SanHan*) and transform the phlegm (*HuaTan*) to stop coughing (*ZhiKe*);
Points: LI 4 (*HeGu*), L 7 (*LieQue*), B 13 (*FeiShu*), G 20 (*FengChi*), S 40 (*FengLong*);

(2) *Pattern B*: to expel the wind, clear away the heat (*QingRe*) and resolve the phlegm (*HuaTan*) to stop coughing;
Points: L 10 (*YuJi*), L 5 (*Chi Ze*), *TaiYang*, B 13 (*FeiShu*), G 20 (*FengChi*), S 40 (*FengLong*);

(3) *Pattern C*: to clear away the heat and resolve the phlegm to stop coughing;
Points: L 5 (*Chi Ze*), S 40 (*FengLong*), L 10 (*YuJi*), LI 11 (*QuChi*);

(4) *Pattern D*: to clear away the heat from the Lung and moisten the dryness (*RunZao*) to stop coughing;
Points: B 13 (*FeiShu*), L 5 (*Chi Ze*), CV 22 (*TianTu*), K 3 (*TaiXi*);

(5) *Pattern E*: to strengthen the Spleen (*JianPi*) to dispel the dampness (*Huashi*), and to transform the phlegm to stop coughing;

Points: B 13 (*FeiShu*), L 9 (*TaiYuan*), B 20 (*PiShu*), Sp 9 (*YinLingQuan*), S 40 (*FengLong*);

(6)   *Pattern F*: to reduce the fire from the Liver (*QingxieGanHuo*) and moisten the Lung (*RunFei*) to stop coughing;
Points: B 13 (*FeiShu*), L 5 (*Chi Ze*), G 34 (*YangLingQuan*), LR 3 (*TaiChong*);

(7)   *Pattern G*: to tonify *Yin* (*YangYin*) to distinguish the empty-fire in the Lung (*QingRe*) to stop coughing;
Points: B 13 (*FeiShu*), L 5 (*Chi Ze*), L 7 (*LieQue*), K 7 (*FuLiu*), H 6 (*YinXi*), Sp 6 (*SanYinJiao*).

Bibliography

Beijing College of Traditional Medicine. Essentials of Chinese Acupuncture. Beijing: Foreign Language Press, 1985

Maciocia G. The Foundations of Chinese Medicine, A Comprehensive Text for Acupuncturists and Herbalists. Singapore: Churchill Livingstone, 1995

TCM Group. The Foundation of Traditional Chinese Medicine. Shanghai: Science-Technology Press, 1996

Wang Z. New Edition on Selection of Acupuncture Points in TCM Internal Medicine. Beijing: Document Press of Science and Technology, 1995

Yang Z. Handbook of Practical Selection of Acupuncture Points. Beijing: Jin Dun Press, 1990

Chinese herbal medicine and formulations   10

B. Xu

CHINESE HERBS

Chinese herbal medicine, as the major component of the Chinese Medicine (CM) or Traditional Chinese Medicine (TCM), has played a very important role in the promotion of health, prevention of disease, and treatment of illnesses for Chinese people for several thousand years.

Nomenclature of Chinese herbs

China spans cold, warm, and hot zones, and has a very rich variety of medicinally used plants, animals, and minerals which all fall into the umbrella of Chinese herbal medicine. Different Chinese herbs usually have different names. The herbal names may appear confusing sometimes. However, there are some rules to follow in the nomenclature of Chinese herbs.

Most Chinese herbs are named by one of the following rules:

(1) *Named after growth place:* to stress the genuine medicinal materials, many Chinese herbs are named after the place where they are grown.

(2) *Named after growth property:* different herbs have different growth properties. Therefore, some Chinese herbs are named after their corresponding growth properties.

(3) *Named after appearance, color, or odor:* for intuitive reasons, some Chinese herbs are named after their appearance. Some are named after their colors. Others are named after their characteristic odor.

(4) *Named after functions:* to stress the medicinal functions of herbs, some Chinese herbs are named after their chief therapeutic functions.

(5) *Named after the medicinal parts:* most Chinese herbs use only a part of the original herb for medicinal use. To stress the part that is used, some herbs are named after the corresponding medicinal part.

(6) *Named after the discoverer:* to commemorate the discoverer of herbs, some Chinese herbs are named after the person who discovered the herb's medicinal function.

(7) *Named after translated name:* some herbs were originally grown in other nations. To emphasize the original place where the herb came from, some herbs are named by translated names.

Properties of Chinese herbs

The properties of Chinese herbs are governed by the theory of the nature of CM herbs. Based on the theory, all Chinese herbs can be characterized by *Qi*, flavor, channel tropism, and tendency.

Qi

The *Qi* is used to describe the cold, hot, warm, and cool properties of herbs. They differ only by degree. Cold and cool herbs have the function of heat-clearing, fire-purging, detoxicating, and removing heat from blood. Warm and hot herbs have the function of warming the middle-*Jiao* to dispel cold, restoring yang, and invigorating pulse beat.

Flavor

The flavor is used to describe the sour, bitter, sweet, acrid, salty, and bland properties of herbs.

(1) *Sour:* sour herbs have the property of astringency and astriction. They are used to treat sweating due to debility, diarrhea, seminal emission, and leucorrhea, etc.

(2) *Bitter:*   bitter herbs have the property of purging, drying, and consolidating the *Yin*. Bitter herbs are used to purge heat, relax the bowels, eliminate dampness, and keep *Yin*, etc.

(3) *Sweet:*   sweet herbs have the property of invigorating, regulating the stomach, and providing respite. Sweet herbs are used to strengthen the body by means of tonics, etc.

(4) *Acrid:*   acrid herbs have the property of dispersing and moving. They are used to disperse exterior syndrome, promote blood circulation, and stop pain, etc.

(5) *Salty:*   salty herbs have the property of softening a hard mass and purging. They are used to resolve hard lumps and relieve constipation, etc.

(6) *Bland:*   bland herbs have the property of excreting dampness and diuresis. They are used to treat difficulty in micturition and edema, etc.

The *Qi* and flavor of a herb are correlated with each other and act together to represent the property of the herb.

Channel tropism

Channel tropism represents the ability of an herb to act selectively on a specific part of the body. It is employed to match the herbs selected and the organ affected.

Based on channel tropism, some herbs may act as a 'medicinal guide'. A medicinal guide is a class of herbs meeting the following two criteria:

• Acting on a specific organ

• Leading other herbs to act on this organ.

Tendency

Tendency represents the acting direction of an herb. It includes ascending, descending, floating, and sinking. The ascending and floating herbs act upward and outward. The descending and sinking herbs act downward and inward.

Generally speaking, if the diseased location is up and exterior, ascending and floating herbs are needed. If the diseased location is low and interior, descending and sinking herbs are needed. If the disease trend is upward, descending herbs are needed. If the disease trend is downward, ascending herbs are needed. Tendency is correlated to herbal *Qi*, flavor, weight, processing, and compatibility.

Compatibility of herbs

An herbal formula or prescription usually contains different herbs. The herbs in a formula are not randomly selected. There are close relationships between these herbs. These relationships are summarized as compatibility of herbs.

Generally speaking, there are seven types of compatibility in a formula:

(1) *Using a single herb:*   this is the simplest case in which only one herb is used.

(2) *Mutual reinforcement:*   in this case, two herbs reinforce each other's functions.

(3) *Mutual assistance:*   in this case, an herb (ministerial herb) can promote the function of another herb (monarch herb).

(4) *Mutual restraint:*   in this case, one herb's side-effects and toxicity are reduced or eliminated by another herb.

(5) *Mutual detoxification:*   in this case, one herb can reduce or eliminate another herb's toxicity or side-effects. This is in fact another expression of mutual restraint.

(6) *Mutual inhibition:*   in this case, one herb reduces or nullifies another herb's function.

(7) *Antagonism:*   in this case, the combination of two herbs causes adverse side-effects and toxicity. This is where the herbs can be toxic or dangerous if applied inappropriately.

Due to current confusion and misunderstanding about herbs and herbal products, it is necessary to address the herbal safety issue further here.

There are significant differences between the adverse side-effects of chemical drugs and the adverse side-effects of herbs. The adverse side-effects of a chemical drug exist no matter whether the drug is applied appropriately or not. The side-effects of a chemical drug will exist even if the physician and the patient are following the correct directions. In other words, the adverse side-effects of the chemical drug are unconditional: they exist no matter whether the chemical drug is applied appropriately or not.

However, most adverse side-effects in Chinese herbal medicine arise from the inappropriate application of herbs. If the herbs are applied appropriately, the herbal side-effects can be reduced or even eliminated. In this case, it is appropriate to say that the herbal treatment has few or no side-effects. In other words, the adverse side-effects of Chinese herbs are conditional: they generally arise only when the herbs are applied inappropriately.

The inappropriate applications of Chinese herbal medicine include:

(1) Wrong diagnosis;

(2) Inappropriate selection of herbs;

(3) Inappropriate combination of herbs;

(4) Inappropriate processing of herbs;

(5) Inappropriate methods of administering herbs;

(6) Inappropriately high dosage;

(7) Inappropriately long application;

(8) Inappropriate administration of herbs with other drugs, etc.

Any one or more of the above inappropriate applications will lead to adverse herbal side-effects. Because only qualified CM doctors are capable of avoiding the above situations, it is recommended that the public does not take Chinese herbs without appropriate supervision. Otherwise, adverse herbal side-effects are unavoidable.

Therefore, there are many contraindications in Chinese herbal medicine. If a doctor of Chinese Medicine fails to observe these precautions, or if the public takes herbs by their own choice, serious side-effects or even fatal accidents may occur. There have been numerous lessons on the danger of herbs in Chinese Medicine history.

Currently in the United States, herbs are classified as food dietary supplements. This classification is inappropriate and even misleading. It has sent a wrong message to the public that herbs are as safe as other dietary supplements. As a result, many people take herbs of their own volition, and this leads to an increasing number of adverse side-effects.

In fact, herbs are very different from other dietary supplements. Herbs can be very dangerous or even fatal if they are administered inappropriately. Because of this safety consideration, we strongly recommend that herbs be taken out of the food dietary supplement category, and be classified into a new category.

Commonly used Chinese herbs

There are over 5000 documented Chinese herbs. It is beyond this book's scope to cover these. As examples, we will introduce a few commonly used Chinese herbs in the following sections.

Dan Shen (radix Salviae miltiorrhizae)

Properties   Bitter and mild cold. Belonging to the heart, pericardium, and liver channels.

Functions and indications

(1) Promoting blood circulation by removing blood stasis. *Dan Shen* is used to treat stasis due to blood heat.

(2) Promoting blood circulation to subdue swelling. *Dan Shen* is used to treat carbuncles and boils.

(3) Nourishing the blood and tranquilizing. *Dan Shen* is used to treat insomnia, headache, dizziness, and palpitations.

Dosage and directions   Approximately 3–15 g per day. Used in decoction.

Dang Gui (radix Angelicae sinensis)

Properties   Sweet, acrid, and warm. Belonging to the liver, heart, and spleen channels.

Functions and indications

(1) Enriching the blood and regulating menstruation. *Dang Gui* is used to treat blood deficiency.

(2) Promoting blood circulation to stop pain. *Dang Gui* is used to treat traumatic injury, carbuncles, boils, and arthralgia due to wind-dampness.

(3) Loosening the bowel to relieve constipation. *Dang Gui* is used to treat constipation of blood deficiency type.

Dosage and directions   Approximately 6–15 g per day. Used in decoction. The body of the herb is used to enrich blood. The tail is used to promote blood circulation.

Du Huo (radix Angelicae pubescentis)

Properties   Acrid, bitter, and mild warm. Belonging to kidney and urinary bladder channels.

Functions and indications

(1) Expelling wind, removing dampness, and alleviating pain. *Du Huo* is used to treat arthralgia due to wind-cold-dampness.

(2) Dispelling cold and relieving exterior syndrome. *Du Huo* is used to treat the effect of an exopathogen with wind-cold-dampness.

Dosage and directions Approximately 3–9 g per day. Used in decoction.

Attention and contraindications *Du Huo* should not be applied in arthralgia with deficiency of *Qi* and blood.

Ma Huang (herba Ephedrae)

Properties Acrid, mild bitter, and warm. Belonging to lung and urinary bladder channels.

Functions and indications

(1) Relieving superficies syndrome by means of diaphoresis. *Ma Huang* is used to treat the effect of wind-cold with aversion to cold, fever, headache, stuffy nose, anhidrosis, and floating and tense pulse.

(2) Facilitating the flow of Lung-*Qi* to relieve asthma. *Ma Huang* is used to treat dyspnea of excess type due to attack of pathogenic wind-cold and obstruction of the Lung-*Qi*.

(3) Inducing diuresis to alleviate edema. *Ma Huang* is used to treat edema of excess type with exterior syndrome, aversion to wind, and general edema with fever.

Dosage and directions Approximately 3–10 g per day. Used in decoction. Raw *Ma Huang* is usually used for (1) and (3), and honey-fried *Ma Huang* is usually used for (2).

Attention and contraindications The dosage of *Ma Huang* should not be too large. Patients with lung deficiency, hyperhidrosis, and cough with dyspnea should not take *Ma Huang*.

Mai Dong (radix Ophiopogonis)

Properties Sweet, mild bitter, and mild cold. Belonging to the heart, lung, and stomach channels.

Functions and indications

(1) Nourishing *Yin* and reinforcing the stomach. *Mai Dong* is used to treat consumption of body fluid caused by heat.

(2) Moistening the lung and clearing away the heart-fire. *Mai Dong* is used to treat *Yin* deficiency and dryness of the lung.

Dosage and directions Approximately 6–15 g per day. Used in decoction.

Attention and contraindications *Mai Dong* should not be applied to diarrhea with cold of insufficiency type and cough affected by wind-cold.

Ren Shen (radix Ginseng)

Properties Sweet, mild bitter, and mild warm. Belonging to the spleen and lung channels.

Functions and indications

(1) Invigorating *Qi* for emergency treatment of collapse. *Ren Shen* is used to treat collapse due to *Qi* deficiency.

(2) Invigorating *Qi* to strengthen the spleen. *Ren Shen* is used to treat lung, kidney, and spleen deficiency.

(3) Promoting the production of body fluid to quench thirst. *Ren Shen* is used to treat febrile disease with thirst and sweating.

(4) Tranquilizing the mind and promoting mentality.

Dosage and directions Approximately 3–9 g per day (maximum 30 g per day). Used in decoction.

Attention and contraindications *Ren Shen* cannot be used for heat of excess type, hyperactivity of the Liver-*Yang*, and retention of dampness with overabundance of heat. Incompatible with *Li Lu* (*Veratrum nigrum* L.). Antagonistic with *Wu Ling Zhi* (feces *Trogopterorum*).

Sheng Di (radix Rehmanniae)

Properties Sweet, bitter, and cold. Belonging to the heart, liver, and kidney channels.

Functions and indications

(1) Removing pathogenic heat from blood. *Sheng Di* is used to treat epidemic febrile disease.

(2) Removing heat from the blood to stop bleeding. *Sheng Di* is used to treat various types of bleeding due to blood-heat.

(3) Nourishing *Yin* and promoting production of body fluid. *Sheng Di* is used to treat consumption of body fluid caused by febrile disease.

Dosage and directions Approximately 6–15 g per day. Used in decoction. *Sheng Di* is used unprepared for (1) and is parched into charcoal for (2).

Attention and contraindications Patients with water retention due to hypofunction of the spleen, abdominal distension, and diarrhea should not use *Sheng Di*.

Yin Chen (herba Artemisiae capillaris)

Properties   Bitter and mild cold. Belonging to spleen, stomach, liver, and gallbladder channel.

Functions and indications

(1)   Clearing away heat, promoting diuresis, and treating jaundice. *Yin Chen* is usually used to treat jaundice due to damp-heat pathogen. It can also be applied to treat jaundice due to cold-dampness.

(2)   Expelling ascaris and relieving itching. *Yin Chen* is used to treat biliary ascariasis.

Dosage and directions   Approximately 9–15 g per day (maximum 30 g per day). Used in decoction. Avoid boiling for too long.

CHINESE HERBAL FORMULATION

A formula, or a prescription in Chinese herbal medicine is composed of a number of herbs. It is formed through careful selection of herbs based on diagnosis, differentiation of symptoms and signs, and treatment plan.

Principles of formulating a prescription

Generally speaking, a formula is composed of four kinds of herbs: monarch herb, ministerial herb, adjuvant herb, and conductant herb.

Monarch herb

The monarch herb is also called the principal herb. It is the herb in a formula that plays the major role in treating the chief complaint.

Ministerial herb

The ministerial herb is also called subsidiary herb. It has two functions in a formula:

(1)   Assisting the monarch herb to strengthen the treatment for the chief complaint.

(2)   Playing a major role in treating accompanying diseases and symptoms.

Adjuvant herb

An adjuvant herb has three functions in a formula:

(1)   *Assisting:*   to assist the monarch and ministerial herbs to strengthen the treatment function.

(2)   *Balancing:*   to eliminate or restrain the toxicity or drastic action of monarch or ministerial herbs.

(3)   *Corrigent:*   in some serious conditions, it is necessary to use a small dosage of corrigent herbs with a property opposite to that of the principal herbs in order to favorably modify the action of the principal herb.

Conductant herb

A conductant herb has two functions in a formula:

(1)   *Guiding:*   to lead other herbs in the formula to reach the diseased location.

(2)   *Mediating:*   to mediate between various herbs in the formula.

In a formula, there is no specific requirement for the number of monarch and ministerial herbs. The rule is to be concise. In addition, not all formulae contain complete monarch, ministerial, adjuvant, and conductant herbs. It all depends on the disease condition.

Variations of formulae

In addition to the principle of formulating a prescription, some changes of the formula might be needed in application. There are four types of changes to a formula:

(1)   *Changing medicinal ingredients:*   in this situation, the ministerial herbs are changed and the monarch herb remains. So the formula can be applied to treat different accompanying symptoms.

(2)   *Changing the compatibility:*   in this situation, the monarch herb is changed, and the formula's functions and indications are changed.

(3)   *Modifying the dosage:*   in this situation, no herbal component is changed. Only the dosage of each component herb is changed. This may also lead to change in the formula's functions and indications.

(4)   *Changing the dosage form:*   in this situation, only the dosage form is changed. For example, the decoction form is changed to pill or tablet form, etc. This change will affect the formula's function and indications too.

Dosage forms of formulae

There are many dosage forms in Chinese Medicine formulae. In the following we will introduce some of the commonly used dosage forms.

Decoction

A decoction is made by decocting prepared herbs in water or another solvent for a certain time. Then the soup is kept as a decoction. A decoction takes effect quickly and can be modified easily. It is the most widely used dosage form in CM.

Pill

A pill is prepared by blending the powdered herbs with honey, water, or other excipient to make into a bolus. A pill takes effect slowly but lasts longer, and is applicable to chronic disease. It is convenient to administer, store, and carry.

Powder

A powder is a preparation of herbs ground into granules for oral administration or external application. It can be easily absorbed, and is convenient to carry.

Medicinal extract

A medicinal extract is prepared by boiling the herbs with water or vegetable oil to a concentrated state. It can be used for both oral administration and external application.

Pellet

A pellet is made of melted or sublimated minerals. It can be used for both oral administration and external application.

Tincture

A tincture is prepared by soaking the herbs in alcohol for days. It is used for deficiency conditions, pain due to wind-damp, or traumatic injury.

Medicinal tea

Medicinal tea is a brick tea-like preparation made of coarse powdered herbs (with or without tea leaves) and adhesive excipient. It is convenient to carry and administer.

Herbal distillate

An herbal distillate is a preparation obtained through the distillation process via an herb and water.

There are other dosage forms that are beyond the scope of this book.

Commonly used Chinese Medicine formulae

There are thousands of documented Chinese formulae. It is impossible to cover them in detail here. In the following, I will discuss a few formulae as examples of how Chinese formulae work.

An Shen Wan (sedative bolus)

Composition   *Huang Lian* (rhizoma *Coptidis*) 4.5 g, *Zhu Sha* (*Cinnabaris*) 3 g, *Sheng Di* (radix *Rehmanniae*) 1.5 g, *Dang Gui Shen* (radix *Angelicae sinensis* body) 1.5 g, *Zhi Gan Cao* (radix *Glycyrrhizae preparata*) 1.5 g.

Directions   Prepared as pills. Administered before sleep every night. Take 9 g each time. It also can be prepared as a decoction.

Functions   Relieves palpitations and tranquilizes; replenishes *Yin* and removes heat.

Indications   Heart-*Yin* deficiency and flaring-up of the heart-fire with palpitations and insomnia.

Bai Tou Weng Tang (radix Pulsatillae decoction)

Composition   *Bai Tou Weng* (radix *Pulsatillae*) 15 g, *Huang Bai* (cortex *Phellodendri*) 12 g, *Huang Lian* (rhizoma *Coptidis*) 6 g, *Qin Pi* (cortex *Fraxini*) 9 g.

Directions   Prepared as decoction.

Functions   Clears away heat and toxic materials, eliminates pathogenic heat from blood and treats diarrhea.

Indications   Dysentery due to damp-heat pathogen with diarrhea, abdominal pain, tenesmus, bloody mucous stool, burning sensation of the anus, yellowish and greasy tai, slippery and rapid pulse.

Gui Zhi Tang (ramulus Cinnamomi decoction)

Composition   Gui Zhi (ramulus *Cinnamomi*) 4.5–9 g, Bai Shao (radix *Paeoniae alba*) 4.5–9 g, Gan Cao (radix *Glycyrrhizae*) 3–6 g, Sheng Jiang (rhizoma *Zingiberis recens*) 2–4 g, Da Zao (fructus *Jujubae*) four pieces.

Directions   Prepared as a decoction. Administer twice a day, and finish one unit per day. After administering the decoction, the patient should take a little warm gruel to obtain mild sweating.

Functions   Expels pathogenic factors from muscles and skin, and regulates *Ying* and *Wei*.

Indications   Wind-cold exterior syndrome of deficiency with headache, fever, sweating, aversion to wind, arthralgia, myalgia, thin and white tai, and floating and moderate pulse.

Liu Wei Di Huang Wan (bolus of six drugs including Rehmannia)

Composition   Shu Di (radix *Rehmanniae Preparata*) 24 g, Shan Zhu Yu (fructus *Corni*) 12 g, Shan Yao (rhizoma *Dioscoreae*) 12 g, Ze Xie (rhizoma *Alismatis*) 9 g, Fu Ling (*Poria*) 9 g, Mu Dan Pi (cortex *Moutan*) 9 g.

Directions   Prepared as pills. Take 6–9 g each time. Administer 1–2 times a day. It also can be prepared as a decoction.

Functions   Nourishing Kidney-*Yin*.

Indications   Kidney-*Yin* deficiency with lassitude in loin and leg, dizziness, tinnitus and deafness, night sweat, seminal emission, hectic fever, diabetes, red tongue, scanty tai, thin and rapid pulse.

Ma Huang Tang (Ephedra decoction)

Composition   Ma Huang (*Ephedra*) 4.5–9 g, Gui Zhi (ramulus *Cinnamomi*) 6 g, Xin Ren (bitter apricot seed) 9 g, Gan Cao (radix *Glycyrrhizae*) 3 g.

Directions   Prepared as a decoction. After administering the decoction, cover the patient with a quilt to produce mild sweating.

Functions   Relieves superficies syndrome by means of diaphoresis and facilitates the flow of the Lung-*Qi* to relieve asthma.

Indications   Wind-cold exterior syndrome of excess type with aversion to cold, fever, headache, aching pain, anhidrosis, asthma, thin and white tai, and floating and tense pulse.

Si Wu Tang (decoction of four ingredients)

Composition   Shu Di (radix *Rehmanniae Preparata*) 12 g, Dang Gui (radix *Angelicae Sinensis*) 9 g, Bai Shao (radix *Paeoniae alba*) 9 g, Chuan Xiong (rhizoma *Chuanxiong*) 6 g.

Directions   Prepared as a decoction.

Functions   Enriches the blood and regulates menstruation.

Indications   Blood deficiency and stagnation with irregular menstruation, dysmenorrhea, scanty menstruation, blood stasis, metrorrhagia and metrostaxis, dizziness, palpitations, pale tongue, thin and small pulse.

Xiao Chai Hu Tang (minor decoction of Bupleurum)

Composition   Chai Hu (radix *Bupleuri*) 9 g, Huang Qin (radix *Scutellariae*) 6 g, Ban Xia (rhizoma *Pinelliae*) 6 g, Ren Shen (radix *Ginseng*) 6 g, Zhi Gan Cao (radix *Glycyrrhizae Preparata*) 3 g, Sheng Jiang (rhizoma *Zingiberis recens*) 6 g, Da Zao (fructus *Jujubae*) four pieces.

Directions   Prepared as a decoction.

Functions   Treats Shaoyang diseases.

Indications   Shaoyang disease with alternate attacks of chills and fever, feeling of fullness and discomfort in chest and hypochondrium, bitter taste and dry throat, vexation and nausea, thin and white tai, and string pulse.

Yin Chen Hao Tang (Oriental wormwood decoction)

Composition   Yin Chen Hao (herba *Artemisiae capillaris*) 18 g, Zhi Zi (fructus *Gardeniae*) 9 g, Da Huang (radix et rhizoma *Rhei*) 9 g.

Directions   Prepared as a decoction. Finish one unit per day. Continue taking several units.

Functions   Clears away heat, promotes diuresis, and treats jaundice.

Indications   Jaundice due to damp-heat pathogen with skin and sclera yellow or orange color, yellow and reddish urine, constipation, oppressed feeling in chest, thirst, greasy tai, and slippery and rapid pulse.

CLINICAL APPLICATIONS

After learning the basic knowledge of Chinese herbal medicine, readers might be interested to know how Chinese herbs are applied in clinical settings.

The major diagnostic methods used in Chinese herbal medicine are called the Four Diagnostic Methods, and the major treatment methodologies used in Chinese herbal medicine are called Bian Zheng Lun Zhi, which is the summary of the complete process of diagnosing, analyzing, understanding, and treating a disease in Chinese medicine. These are very different from the counterparts in Western medicine. In the following we will use two examples to demonstrate how Chinese herbal medicine works in clinical practice.

Chronic gastritis

Chronic gastritis is an inflammatory disease affecting the gastric mucosa. In Chinese herbal medicine, it is further classified into the following *Zheng* types.

Stagnation of liver and stomach Qi

Zheng   Stomach distension and moving pain triggered by anxiety and anger and reduced by belching and flatus, hypochondrium distension, nausea, vomiting, gastric discomfort, acid regurgitation, pink tongue, thin and white tai, and string pulse.

Treatment method   Soothe the liver and regulate the circulation of *Qi*; regulate the stomach and stop the pain.

Formula   *Chai hu shu gan san.*

Insufficiency of stomach Yin

Zheng   Burning pain in stomach, poor appetite, stomach distension after meal, fondness for sour and sweet foods, thirst, constipation, red tongue, thin and dry tai, thin and fast pulse.

Treatment method   Nourish the *Yin* to strengthen the stomach.

Formula   *Yi wei tang.*

Spleen–stomach deficiency of cold type

Zheng   Continuous dull pain in stomach, fondness for warmth and pressure, poor appetite, stomach distension after meal, spitting clear saliva, dim complexion, fatigue, cold hands and feet, diarrhea, pale tongue, white tai, and deep thin weak pulse.

Treatment method   Strengthen the spleen and replenish the *Qi*; warm the middle *Jiao* and soothe the stomach.

Formula   *Huang qi jian zhong tang.*

Channel blockage by blood stasis

Zheng   Long-lasting, fixed, needle-like pain in the stomach, refusing pressure, hematemesis, black stools, dim purple tongue with ecchymosis, and uneven pulse.

Treatment method   Promote the blood circulation to remove obstruction in the meridian channels.

Formula   *Ge xia zhu yu tang.*

Hypertension

Hypertension is a group of diseases characterized by increased blood pressure. In Chinese herbal medicine, it is further classified into the following *Zheng* types.

Flaming-up of the liver-fire

Zheng   Dizziness, headache, tinnitus, bitter taste, flushed face, redness of eyes, anxiety, constipation, dark yellow urine, red tongue, yellow and dry tai, and string pulse.

Treatment method   Clear away the liver-fire.

Formula   *Long dan xie gan tang.*

Hyperactivity of Yang due to Yin deficiency

Zheng   Dizziness, headache, heaviness in the head and lightness in the feet, fast temper, vexation, insomnia, sore waist, tinnitus, warm centers of the hands and feet, red tongue, yellow tai, string thin fast pulse.

Treatment method   Nourish the *Yin* and suppress the excessive *Yang.*

Formula   *Tian ma gou teng yin.*

Liver and kidney Yin deficiency

Zheng   Dizziness, dry eyes, tinnitus, headache, waist and knee sores, warm centers of the hands and feet, seminal emission, red dry tongue, thin tai, and string thin pulse.

Treatment method   Nourish the liver and kidney.

Formula   *Qi ju di huang wan.*

Yin and Yang deficiency

Zheng   Dizziness, headache, tinnitus, palpitations, shortness of breath, intolerance of cold, cold extremities, waist soreness, weak legs, polyuria in night, pale tongue, white tai, deep thin pulse.

Treatment method   Nourish the *Yin* and restore the *Yang*.

Formula   *Shen qi wan.*

Stagnation of phlegm in the interior

Zheng   Fullness of head, dizziness, headache, chest and diaphragm distension, spitting and vomiting phlegm, vexation, insomnia, pale tongue, greasy tai, string and slippery pulse.

Treatment method   Clear the phlegm.

Formula   *Ban xia bai zhu tian ma tang.*

Comments

In Western medicine practice, the burden of designing protocols and procedures rests upon the Western medical profession as a whole. The physicians need to follow and implement the protocols and procedures. In this sense, Western medicine is a standardized medicine.

In contrast to Western medicine, Chinese Medicine is an individualized, tailored medicine. The burden of designing protocols and procedures in Chinese Medicine practice rests upon the doctors of Chinese Medicine. Thus, it usually takes greater clinical practice and experience to become a qualified doctor of Chinese Medicine (CMD) than to qualify as a physician of Western medicine.

RESEARCH METHODOLOGIES AND APPROACHES IN CHINESE HERBAL MEDICINE

As Chinese herbal medicine has become more and more popular around the world, research into Chinese herbal medicine has increased as well. This is a good trend that will help to elucidate the underlying processes and mechanisms of Chinese herbal medicine. However, the global increase in Chinese herbal medicine research has brought some problems to light. These problems have drawn increasing attention and concern to the profession of Chinese Medicine.

Some new researchers of Chinese herbal medicine have not received adequate education and training in Chinese Medicine. They applied the methods and techniques of Western medicine directly to Chinese herbal medicine research, and have reached some inappropriate conclusions, which have caused some adverse effects among patients and the public. For example, the ephedra event has not only hurt patients and the public, but also damaged the reputation and image of Chinese herbal medicine. To prevent similar incidents from happening again, it is necessary to elucidate the differences between Chinese herbal medicine research and Western medicine research[1].

System differences

The root cause of the above situation lies in the fact that Western medicine and Chinese herbal medicine involve two different systems, as will be discussed.

Western medicine

A chemical drug usually contains one or a few active ingredients. Models studying chemical drugs belong to a multi-body, linear system or a single-body, non-linear system.

Chinese herbal medicine

Generally speaking, a single Chinese herb contains many ingredients. A formula consisting of many herbs contains many more ingredients. During decoction (a process of boiling the herbs together in a liquid such as water) there are cross-reactions between these ingredients, which make the decoction even more complicated. *In vivo*, the pharmacokinetics of herbal medicine usually involves many ingredients, some of them may act together, 'couple and interact with each other'. As a result, models for the study of Chinese herbal medicine fall into multi-body, non-linear systems.

Theoretical differences

Differential equations for the pharmacokinetics of the Western medicine system are solvable. Therefore, it is possible to control and analyze the chemical drug's process analytically and accurately in Western medicine's pharmaceutical research. The Western medicine pharmaceutical system can be reduced to a mathematically solvable system. This is the mathematical basis on which the randomized, double-blind, control study method can be applied to Western medicine research.

Currently, differential equations for multi-body, non-linear systems cannot be solved accurately. Approximations are necessary in Chinese herbal medicine study. Therefore, there is no mathematical tool with which to study Chinese herbal medicine pharmacokinetic processes *in vivo* analytically and accurately. The Chinese herbal medicine system cannot be reduced to a mathematically solvable system. This is the rationale by which the randomized double-blind control study method cannot be directly applied to Chinese herbal medicine research.

Methodology differences

Because the differential equations for the Western medicine systems are solvable, it is possible to apply the randomized, double-blind, control study method to the pharmaceutical research. However, the differential equations for multi-body, non-linear systems cannot be solved accurately. Therefore, it is impossible to apply the randomized, double-blind, control study method directly to Chinese herbal medicine research.

When applying modeling and other pharmaceutical study methods to Chinese herbal medicine, some studies make assumptions and approximate the Chinese herbal medicine system into a linear system or single-body, non-linear system. These assumptions may not reflect the true process involved in the Chinese herbal medicine pharmacokinetics. If the multi-body, non-linear property is not essential to the normal function of the system, a linear approximation is acceptable. However, if this multi-body, non-linear property is essential to the normal function of the system, the approximation should not violate the nature of the multi-body, non-linear system.

When the non-linear property is essential to the normal function of the multi-body system, linear approximation is inappropriate. Without linear approximation, it is very difficult to solve the differential equations of multi-body, non-linear systems. This is the theoretic difficulty underlying modern scientific studies on Chinese herbal medicine.

Experimental differences

Experimentally, Chinese herbal medicine is very different from Western medicine research. Generally speaking, there are two types of Chinese herbal medicine research.

It is important to study each individual ingredient of an herb. However, due to the system difference, it is inappropriate to apply the conclusion of the study of an individual ingredient (a single body, linear system) to a formula (a multi-body, non-linear system). Therefore, for the efficacy and safety of an herbal formula, it is necessary to study the original herbal formula in its formula state directly.

The experimental difficulty in conducting systematic and rigorous research into Chinese herbal medicine is the control of variable settings. Because conclusions from an isolated ingredient study may be different from those in a formula study, it is inappropriate to draw a conclusion based on the former. Thus, it may be inappropriate to conclude which ingredient is active, and which is not, simply based on the study of isolated ingredients. A complete, rigorous research on a formula demands a full study of all variable settings in the formula state.

Because the ingredient variable is more accurate than the herb variable, the study should concentrate on the variable of ingredient. However, this is sometimes very difficult to implement. For example, if a formula consists of 50 ingredients (this is a conservative estimate), and each variable (ingredient) takes on 10 different values (e.g. 10 different 'strengths') during the control study, there will be an astronomical number of variable settings to study. There is neither sufficient time nor funds to support these studies. Thus, simply applying pharmaceutical study methods to Chinese herbal medicine study will not work. This is why it is very rare (if it even exists) to see a complete, systematic, and rigorous study (controlling and comparing all variable settings) on a Chinese herbal formula.

To simplify the situation, some studies simply assume many ingredients to be inactive based on conclusions of studies on their isolated states. This leads to the control study on a few assumed 'active' ingredients. However, it runs the risk of making inappropriate and subjective assumptions.

Many other studies concentrate on the control of single component herbs rather than on ingredients in an herbal formula. This greatly reduces the number of variables, but it actually goes back to the traditional way of Chinese herbal medicine study. Even for the control of component herbal variables, there are still many variable settings for a complete, systematic, and rigorous study. Most studies simply choose one or a few variable settings (based on researchers' experience or literature) to conduct studies. These fixed-setting studies provide conclusions for these settings only. They do not provide information on the optimum setting. Neither do they provide information on the 'dangerous' settings.

For the above reasons, Chinese herbal medicine studies are very complicated, difficult, costly, and time-consuming. There are thousands of formulae in Chinese herbal medicine. However, up to today, there is still no medical school, university, company, science foundation, or even country that can afford a systematic, complete, and rigorous study and research into one of the formulae in Chinese herbal medicine. This fact indicates the challenges that lie ahead in the field of research and study on Chinese herbal medicine.

However, these only reflect the defects and inadequacies in Chinese herbal medicine's study and research methodologies and approaches. As for the Chinese herbal medicine itself, it is a complete, systematic, and rigorous medicinal system.

CONCLUSION

Western medicine and Chinese Medicine differ in culture, origins, history, philosophy, theory, principles, approaches, diagnosis, treatment, therapeutic outcomes, etc. Despite all of the differences, however, one thing is common to them – they are both medicines. Chinese Medicine, as an integral part of Chinese culture, is relatively new to most people who have grown up in Western culture. To them, the major component of Chinese Medicine – Chinese herbal medicine – is still a mystery, and there are many puzzling questions regarding Chinese Medicine and Chinese herbal medicine.

Because Chinese Medicine and Chinese herbal medicine are new to many countries, many governments do not have adequate information or preparation on how to regulate them. Thus, they decide not to regulate them. The decision not to regulate Chinese Medicine is based on a misunderstanding about Chinese Medicine and Chinese herbal medicine, and has played an important role in increasing the occurrence of Chinese Medicine side-effects. In the best interest of patients, and to protect the integrity of the Chinese Medicine profession, we recommend that regulations on the profession of Chinese Medicine should be installed, either through the government or from the Chinese Medicine profession itself.

Reference

1. Xu B. Mathematical Herbal Medicine. Acupuncture Today 2005; 6 June

Bibliography

FDA Overview of Dietary Supplements, US Food and Drug Administration, Center for Food Safety and Applied Nutrition, 3 January 2001. Available at: www.fda.gov

He ZG. Chinese Medicine. Beijing: The People's Medical Publishing House, 1989

Molony D, Molony MP. The American Association of Oriental Medicine's Complete Guide to Chinese Herbal Medicine. New York: Berkley Books, 1998

Wang XH. Fundamentals of Chinese Medicine. Shanghai: Shanghai Science and Technology Publishing House, 1995

Wang YY. Chinese Medicine Internal Medicine. Shanghai: Shanghai Science and Technology Publishing House, 1997

Xu B. Recommendation on Chinese Medicine in the United States of America to White House Commission on Complementary and Alternative Medicine Policy, December 2001. ACMA Publication Issue December 2001. Available at: www.AmericanChineseMedicineAssociation.org

Xu B. Letter to the Congress. ACMA Publication Issue August 2002. Available at: www.AmericanChineseMedicineAssociation.org

Xu B. Fundamental Characteristics of Chinese Medicine: Holism and Bian Zheng Lun Zhi. ACMA Publication Issue February 2003. Available at: www.AmericanChineseMedicineAssociation.org

Acupuncture

11

Y. G. Wang

INTRODUCTION

Acupuncture is a medical therapy that uses the insertion of an acupuncture needle into the skin of certain points of the body, called acupuncture points, at different depths to treat a patient's syndrome or disease. Acupuncture dates back 4000 years in China since the Stone Age. It was adopted worldwide over the centuries: by Korea in AD 541, by Japan in AD 562 and by Europe in the sixteenth century[1]. The first person who introduced acupuncture into the USA is believed to be Dr Franklin Bache, grandson of Benjamin Franklin, in 1825[1]. However, acupuncture was not acknowledged by the USA until 1971, when, following China's ping-pong diplomacy, Henry A. Kissinger made his historical visit to Beijing. This not only resulted in President Nixon's visit to China the following year, but also introduced acupuncture to the USA through popular media and the medical profession. The story tells of Kissinger's visit, during which a staff member was treated with acupuncture when he suffered from post-surgical complications. When he returned from his trip, he wrote of his experience in the *New York Times*[2]. As a result, more and more doctors visited China to see it with their own eyes. Dr Rosenfield was one of them.

Parade Magazine carried Rosenfield's article 'Acupuncture goes mainstream (almost)' in 1998[3]. Accompanying the article was a color photograph taken on one of his hospital visits during the tour, which showed a wide-awake young woman in the middle of open-heart surgery under acupuncture anesthesia, smiling at the camera! Dr Rosenfield wrote:

> *'I first witnessed acupuncture at the University of Shanghai about 20 years ago. The patient was a 28-year-old woman about to have open-heart surgery. She was placed on the operation table, wide awake and smiling. Then to my astonishment, the surgeon proceeded to open her chest. Her only 'anesthetic' was*

> *an acupuncture needle in her right earlobe that was connected to an electrical source. She never flinched. There was no mask on her face, no intravenous needle in her arm. This account is not hearsay. I was there and took the photo on this page.'*

Acupuncture has been accepted as conventional medical practice in most countries in the world for many years. The World Health Organization (WHO) listed more than 40 conditions for which acupuncture may be effective[4].

This chapter focuses on fundamental acupuncture issues. It covers the following topics:

- Acupuncture needles

- Common meridians and most common acupuncture points

- Auricular and scalp acupuncture

- Acupuncture for common syndromes (including migraine headache, low back pain, and insomnia) and indication of acupuncture therapy

- Cautions in using acupuncture therapy

- Who visits an acupuncturist

- Physiologic bases of acupuncture analgesia.

THE ACUPUNCTURE NEEDLE

Acupuncture involves a thin needle inserted into specific points of the body to stimulate its own natural system to treat the disease. The needle is called an acupuncture needle and the point is called an acupuncture point, or simply an acupoint.

Figure 11.1a shows the acupuncture needle, which mainly consists of two parts: the handle and the stem or needle body. Figure 11.1b shows the Chinese character

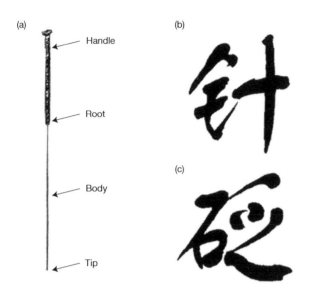

Figure 11.1   The acupuncture needle (a), the Chinese character for needle (b), and the Chinese character for stone puncture (c)

for needle. The left side of the character means metal and the right side represents a sharp instrument. Therefore, an acupuncture needle is a sharp instrument made of metal, mostly stainless steel today. In the Stone Age, the acupuncture needle was made of stone. Figure 11.1c shows the Chinese character for stone puncture. The left part of the character means stone and the right side is the sound of the word, pronounced as '*bian*'.

In the USA, most acupuncturists use disposable needles, for a single acupuncture point only. The needle has a guide tube. The acupuncturist places it on a selected acupuncture point and taps the needle tail with the index finger to insert the needle. Acupuncture needles are not treated with any drug, which is why they are sometimes referred to as 'dry needles'.

Unlike a regular needle, in which there is a hollow channel for injecting drugs or withdrawing fluids, an acupuncture needle is solid and very fine. Most needles used in clinics measure 30 or 32 gauge in diameter. The length of the needle varies from half an inch (13 mm) to 5 inches (125 mm). Shorter needles are used in superficial areas, such as the head and face, and longer ones in fleshy regions. The required depth of insertion is given with each formula point, but variations occur in different body types and the acupuncturist's own judgment should be used. Normally, when a needle reaches the desired depth, the patient will feel a sensation of fullness or radiating warmth (*De Qi* sensation). Because the tip

of acupuncture needles is sharp and round, acupuncture needles do not normally cut or damage skin and muscles as regular needles do when they penetrate through them; therefore, they cause only slight bleeding and leave almost no needle holes afterwards.

MERIDIANS AND ACUPUNCTURE POINTS

The theoretic basis of acupuncture is the theory of the meridians, in which the *Qi* and blood of the human body are circulated. Meridians pertain to the *Zang-Fu* organs interiorly and extend over the body exteriorly, forming a network and linking the tissues and organs into an organic whole. Meridians are divided into regular meridians and extra meridians. The 12 pairs of regular meridians constitute most of the meridian system. There are eight extra meridians. Twelve regular meridians plus two of the eight extra meridians, one running along the midline of the abdomen and chest and the other along the midline of the back, are the 14 meridians that fall into four groups.

The three *Yin* meridians of the hand

The lung meridian (LU), pericardium meridian (PC), and heart meridian (HT) run through the anterior aspect, midline, and posterior aspect of the anterior side of the upper part of the body from the chest to the hands. They are collectively called the three *Yin* meridians of the hand (Figure 11.2).

The three *Yang* meridians of the hand

The large intestine meridian (LI), triple energizer meridian (TE), and small intestine meridian (SI) run through the anterior aspect, midline, and posterior aspect of the medial side of the upper body from the hands to the head. They are collectively called the three *Yang* meridians of the hand (Figure 11.3).

The three *Yin* meridians of the foot

The spleen meridian (SP), liver meridian (LR), and kidney meridian (KI) run respectively through the anterior aspect, midline, and posterior aspect of the medial side of the lower limbs from the feet to the abdomen and the chest. They are collectively called the three *Yin* meridians of the foot (Figure 11.4).

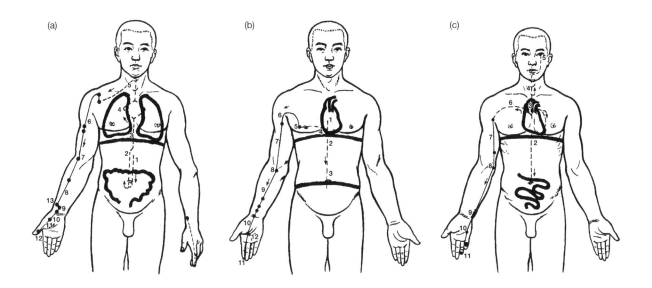

Figure 11.2 Three *Yin* meridians of the hand: the lung meridian (LU (a)), pericardium meridian (PC (b)), and heart meridian (HT (c))

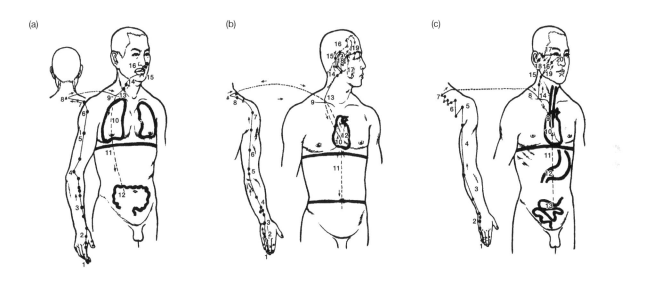

Figure 11.3 The three *Yang* meridians of the hand: the large intestine meridian (LI (a)), triple energizer meridian (TE (b)), and the small intestine meridian (SI (c))

The three *Yang* meridians of the foot

The stomach meridian (ST), gallbladder meridian (GB), and bladder meridian (BL) run from the head through the trunk to the feet along the anterior aspect, midline, and posterior aspect of the lateral side of the lower limbs. They are collectively called the three *Yang* meridians of the foot (Figure 11.5).

Conception vessel and governor vessel

The extra meridian running along the meridian system of the abdomen and chest upward to the lower lip is called the conception vessel (CV). The extra meridian running along the meridian system of the back upward to the top of the head and then downward to the middle of the face is called the governor vessel (GV) (Figure 11.6).

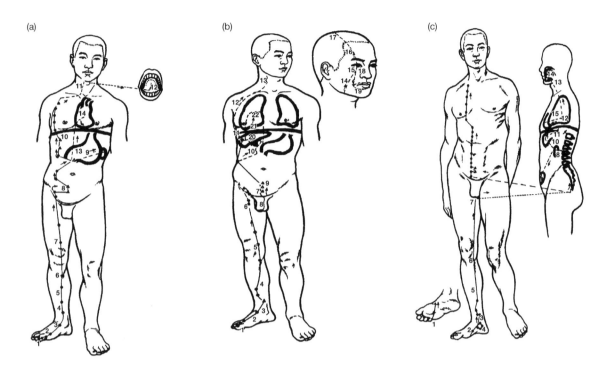

Figure 11.4   The three *Yin* meridians of the foot: the spleen meridian (SP (a)), liver meridian (LR (b)), and kidney meridian (KI (c))

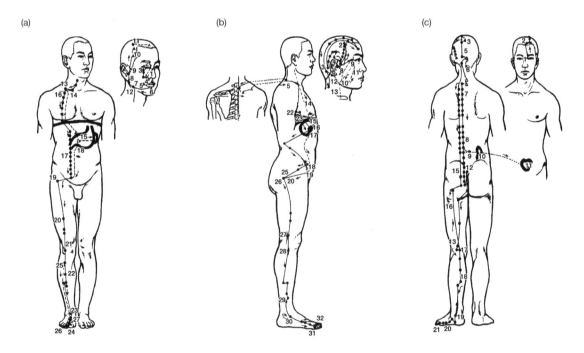

Figure 11.5   The three *Yang* meridians of the foot: the stomach meridian (ST (a)), gallbladder meridian (GB (b)), and bladder meridian (BL (c))

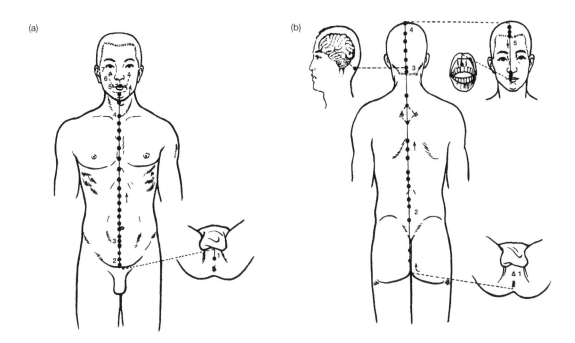

Figure 11.6 Conception vessel and governor vessel. The extra meridian running along the meridian system of the abdomen and chest upward to the lower lip is called the conception vessel (CV (a)). The extra meridian running along the meridian system of the back upward to the top of the head and then downward to the middle of the face is called the governor vessel (GV (b))

A total of 361 acupuncture points have been identified along the 14 meridians. The standard nomenclature of these points consists of the Chinese phonetic (*pinyin*) name followed by the alphanumeric code in parentheses. Apart from these, there are a number of acupuncture points with specific therapeutic properties not on the 14 meridians. They are called extraordinary points.

The acupuncture point and its action

Each acupuncture point has its own therapeutic action. For example, the point *Hegu* (LI 4), located between the first and second metacarpal bones, can sedate pain in the head and mouth, indicated for headache, toothache, and sore throat (Figure 11.7). The point *Shenmen* (HT 7), located on the medial end of the transverse crease of the wrist, can induce tranquilization and remedy insomnia (Figure 11.8). *Yanglingquan* (GB 34) is located at the lateral aspect of the knee joint, in the depression anterior and inferior to the head of the fibula. It is indicated in the treatment of gallbladder diseases, shoulder pain, and stiff neck (Figure 11.9). *Yinlingquan* (SP 9), located in the depression on the lower border of the medial condole of the tibia (Figure 11.10), is indicated in the treatment of retention or incontinence of urine and seminal emission.

The *Ashi* point is any point where, when the doctor presses it, the patient groans with pain. 'A' is pronounced 'Ah' in Chinese and '*Shi*' means yes. It is the same as a trigger or tender point. Inserting an acupuncture needle directly into an *Ashi* point is recommended to treat pain. An *Ashi* point (trigger point) may be found outside abdominal muscles and in skin, scars, tendons, joint capsules, ligaments and periosteum. The cause of tenderness at trigger points may be poor inactivation of calcium by muscle sarcoplasmic reticulum, which causes calcium to cross-link the actin and myosin, with ensuing permanent contraction[5]. How needling rectifies this problem, however, is unclear.

Anatomy of acupuncture points

Dung[6] listed ten structures in his review, which are found in the vicinity of acupoints. In decreasing order of importance they are listed as follows:

(1) Large peripheral nerves;

(2) Nerves emerging from a deep to a more superficial location;

(3) Cutaneous nerves emerging from deep fascia;

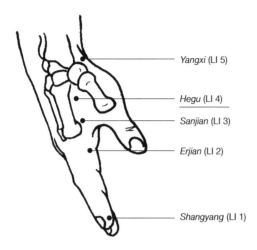

Figure 11.7   The location of the *Hegu* (LI 4) acupoint

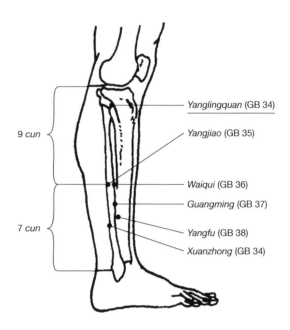

Figure 11.9   The location of the *Yanglingquan* (GB 34) point

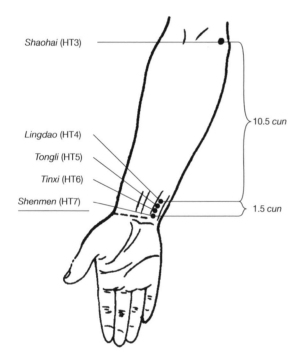

Figure 11.8   The location of acupoint *Shenmen* (HT 7)

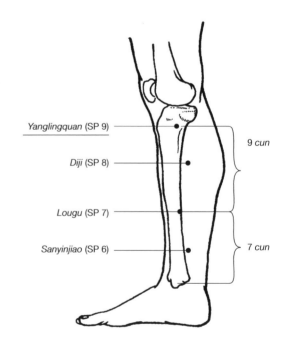

Figure 11.10   The location of the *Yinlingquan* (SP 9) point

(4)   Nerves emerging from bone foramina;

(5)   Motor points of neuromuscular attachments (a neuromuscular attachment is the area where a nerve enters the muscle mass);

(6)   Blood vessels in the vicinity of neuromuscular attachments;

(7)   Nerves composed of fibers of varying sizes (diameters), more likely on muscular nerves than on cutaneous nerves;

(8)   Bifurcation points of peripheral nerves;

(9)   Ligaments (muscle tendons, joint capsule, fascial sheets, collateral ligaments), rich in nerve endings;

(10) Suture lines of the skull.

Heine[7] revealed that 80% of acupoints correlate with perforations in the superficia of cadavers. Through these holes, a cutanous nerve vessel bundle penetrates the skin. If replicated, this finding could be the morphologic basis for acupoints.

Location of acupuncture points

Several experiments have shown that acupuncture needling of true acupoints produces marked analgesia for acute laboratory-induced pain in human subjects, while needling of sham points produces very weak effects[8–10]. Cho and *et al.*[11,12] used acupuncture needling on *Zhiyin* (UB 67), *Guangmin* (GB 37), and *Xiaxi* (GB 43), all located on the legs and toes, to treat eye disease. They are related to the eyes according to traditional meridian theory. Stimulating these points by acupuncture needles can, surprisingly, activate the visual cortex, which is detected by functional magnetic resonance imaging (fMRI). In contrast, stimulating the sham points on the same leg cannot activate the visual cortex. The results provided the first scientific evidence that acupuncture 'signals' are projected to neocortical areas of the brain for central processing. The data also demonstrated that accurately locating the true acupoints to treat disease could be important clinically, because sham points are not able to achieve effective results.

In order to locate acupoints accurately, the descriptions of the exact anatomic position must be followed, obviously the simplest method. Unfortunately, there are many acupoints that do not fall into an exact location. Their individual locations depend upon the dimensions of the patient. In order to account for variations in body size, the Chinese developed the 'human inch' called '*cun*' as an acupuncture measuring unit (AMU). The AMU uses either the finger length of the patient as a unit (finger equivalent unit) or the bone length between joints of the patient as unit (bone equivalent unit).

Finger equivalent unit

As a variation of this finger equivalent unit, the width of the patient's thumb (not the medical provider's!) may be regarded as one *cun*. The combined breadth of index, middle, ring, and little fingers of the hand at the level of the second metacarpophalangeal joints may be considered three *cun*. The distance between the two creases of the interphalangeal joints of the patient's middle finger, when flexed, represents one *cun*. Figure 11.11 is an illustration of a modern version of the finger equivalent units.

Bone equivalent unit

A list of the proportional measurement is as follows:

- The bone equivalent unit of the head is calculated by one of the following measurements: midline of the anterior hairline to midline of the posterior hairline equals 12 *cun*; the distance between the anterior hairline and the glabella is 3 *cun*; the distance between the posterior hairline and the seventh cervical spinous process is 3 *cun* (Figure 11.12).

- The bone equivalent unit of the back is calculated by measuring the distance from the midline to the medial border of the scapula, which is 3 *cun*. The distance between the nipples is 8 *cun*, as is the lower end of the sternum to the umbilicus. The distance between the umbilicus and the upper border of the symphysis pubis is 5 *cun* (Figure 11.13).

- The bone equivalent unit of the upper arm is calculated by measuring from the axillary fold to the cubital elbow crease, which is 9 *cun* (Figures 11.12 and 11.13).

- The bone equivalent unit for the upper leg is calculated by measuring from the proximal point of the greater trochanter to the lower aspect of the patella, a

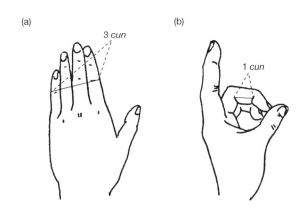

Figure 11.11   Finger equivalent units

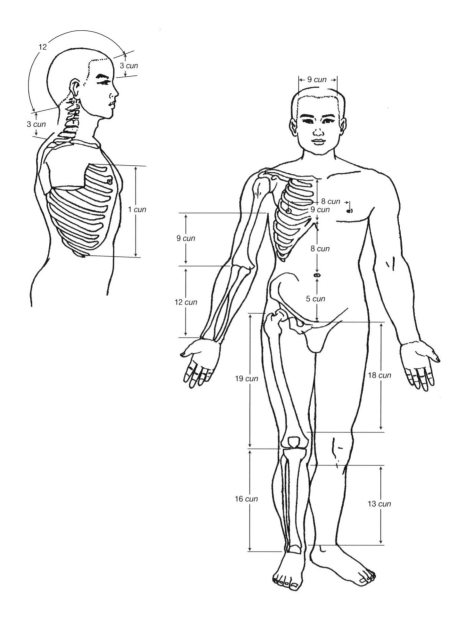

Figure 11.12 Bone equivalent units of the front and right side of the body

distance of 19 *cun*. The lower leg is calculated by measuring either the distance from the middle of the patella to the prominence of the lateral melleolus, which is 16 *cun*, or the distance from the medial condyle of the tibia to the prominence of the medial malleolus, which is 13 *cun* (Figures 11.12 and 11.13).

De Qi sensation

The results of acupuncture treatment eventually depend upon the response of the body to acupuncture stimula-

tion. In a clinical setting, the efficacy of acupuncture therapy may rely on receiving *De Qi* sensation created by acupuncture needling, choosing acupoints, and accurately locating them. *De Qi* is a kind of sensation to which the patient responds. In the process of acupuncture needling, the patient feels numbness, fullness, and sometimes soreness around the acupoint, or feels an electric sensation traveling to a certain area of the body. Similarly, the acupuncture provider feels the acupuncture needle to be heavy, or as if 'a fish is biting the bait'. Chiang and Chang[13] showed that the essential correlate of acupuncture analgesia was a *De Qi* sensation. By injecting procaine (2%) into the acupoints LI 4 and

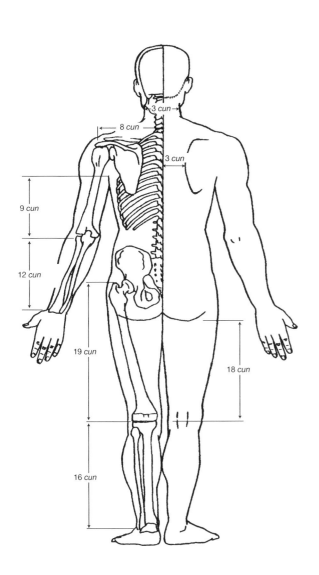

Figure 11.13   Bone equivalent units of the back of the body

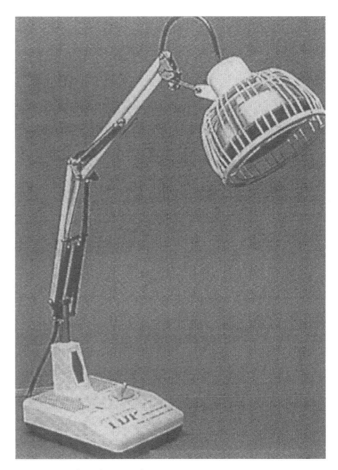

Figure 11.14   The DTP lamp

MOXIBUSTION

In the clinic, an acupuncturist may use heat by burning a moxa made of an herb called *Ai* (dried leaves of *Artemesia vulgaris*), over the acupuncture point and the surrounding tissues, a technique called moxibustion, rather than inserting acupuncture needles. Some moxa are smokeless. Some clinics now use a heat source called a DTP light (Figure 11.14) to replace moxa. Moxibustion is usually used for the conditions caused by deficiency, weakness, or 'cold'.

ELECTROACUPUNCTURE

In most circumstances, acupuncturists also connect the acupuncture needle to a mild electrical stimulator, a technique called electroacupuncture. The electrical pulses administered via the acupuncture needle stimulate the deep tissues. The intensity (1–3 mA), pulse width (0.2–1.0 ms), and frequency (1–500 Hz) can thus be precisely determined. Generally, low-frequency,

LI 10 in humans, he determined that the subcutaneous injection did not block *De Qi* sensations, while intramuscular procaine abolished them. Moreover, whenever *De Qi* sensations were blocked, so was acupuncture analgesia. Perhaps the best experiment of all was performed on humans with direct microelectrode recordings from single fibers in the median nerve while acupuncture was performed distally[14]. They showed that when the *De Qi* sensation was achieved, type II muscle afferents produced numbness; type III gave sensations of heaviness, distension, and aching; and type IV (unmyelinated fibers) produced soreness. As soreness is uncommon in *De Qi*, the main components of *De Qi* are carried by types II and III afferents (small myelinated afferents from muscles).

high-intensity stimulation pulses of needling work through the endorphin system and acts in all three centers (spinal cord, midbrain, and hypothalamus–pituitary), as mentioned below. The method produces analgesia of slower onset, but the analgesia lasts longer than fast-frequency stimulation and its effects are cumulative, continuing to improve after several treatments. In contrast, the high-frequency, low-intensity analgesia is rapid in onset, but of very short duration and without cumulative effects.

Because low-frequency, high-intensity analgesia produces a cumulative effect, repeated treatment produces more and more benefit for the patient[15,16] or laboratory animal[17].

AURICULAR ACUPUNCTURE

Ear acupuncture or auricular acupuncture is stimulation achieved by inserting acupuncture needles into the acupoints located on the auricle.

The ear has the highest density of acupoints, comprising 10% of the acupoints of the whole body. There are more than 43 auricular points that have proven therapeutic values. The acupuncture points in the ear represent different body parts, including inner organs (Figure 11.15). Methods of ear acupuncture include needling, blooding the acupoint on the ear, and massaging the ear[18].

Because every part of the external ear is reflected through a microsystem to remote reflexes of every part of

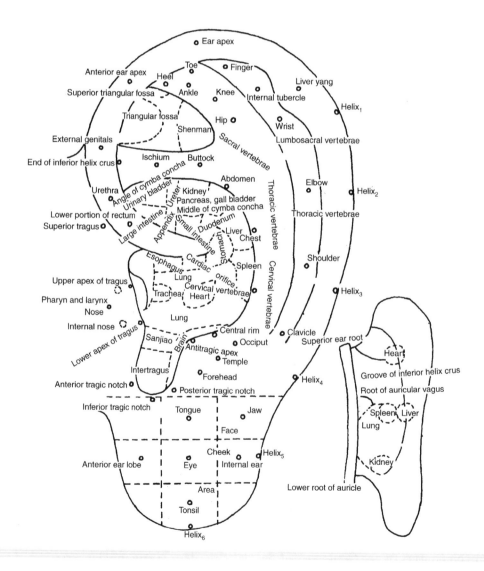

Figure 11.15   Ear acupoints

the body, a wide variety of health problems are relieved by auricular acupuncture therapy. Almost all health conditions can be affected to some degree by stimulating reactive ear points. The most commonly reported uses of auricular acupuncture therapy have been for the control of chronic pain, detoxification from addictive drugs, relief of nausea, and reduction of hypertension.

SCALP ACUPUNCTURE

Scalp acupuncture is acupuncture needling of the acupoints on the scalp, mainly over the cortical area, to treat diseases, for example, hemiplegia. The acupuncture needle is inserted at the area of the scalp over the motor cortex of the brain. Its efficacy needs further investigation, particularly for such self-limiting diseases as cerebral vascular accidents.

INDICATIONS FOR ACUPUNCTURE

List of the World Health Organization

In 1979, the WHO listed more than 40 conditions for which acupuncture may be effective. Based on this list, conditions that we treat with acupuncture alone and which respond well include the following but are not limited to:

(1) *Neurologic*: headache, migraine, neuralgia, postoperative pain, stroke residuals, Parkinson's disease, and facial pain;

(2) *Emotional*: trauma, hypertension, insomnia, depression, anxiety, nervousness, and neurosis;

(3) *Digestive*: abdominal pain, hyperacidity, chronic diarrhea, indigestion, and constipation;

(4) *Musculoskeletal*: backache or pain, muscles cramping, localized traumatic injuries, sprains, strains, sports injuries, arthritis disc problems, sciatica, pain and weakness in the neck, shoulders, arms, hands, fingers, knees, legs, and feet;

(5) *Ear, eye, nose, dental*: poor vision, tired eyes, tinnitus, nervous deafness, toothache, post-extraction pain and gum problems;

(6) *Respiratory*: sinusitis, common cold, tonsillitis, bronchitis, allergy, and asthma;

(7) *Gynecologic*: impotence, premenstrual syndrome, cramps, menopause syndrome, and obstetrics;

(8) *Other benefits*: vitality and energy increase, stress reduction, deep relaxation, skin rejuvenation, weight control, smoking cessation, and other addiction problems.

When to use acupuncture?

As an alternative medicine in the USA, the indication for acupuncture therapy could also be summarized as follows:

(1) Any properly diagnosed patient when conventional treatments have not worked, or conventional medicine is less effective or with more side-effects;

(2) Any patient feeling sick or abnormal when conventional diagnostic techniques show normal and/ or when no conventional treatment is available;

(3) To increase the benefits of other medical care; for example, acupuncture for pain caused by cancer or for the side-effects of chemotherapy.

Principle of prescription and selection of acupoints

Before acupuncture treatment, the medical provider needs to decide how many acupoints to select and how to combine them for individual patients. Selection of acupoints and prescription of the combination of acupoints are based on the theory of meridians, the actions of acupoints, and the patient's symptoms or disease and their causes. The following is a brief introduction to the methods for selection of points and prescription.

Selection of acupoints on the diseased meridian

Acupoints are selected directly from the affected meridian. For example, *Zhonfu* (LU 1), *Chize* (LU 5), and other acupoints of the lung meridian are selected to treat a cough due to disease of the lung.

The combination of the exterior–interior acupoints

When a disease is on the *Yin* meridian, the prescription of acupoints could be selected from this *Yin* meridian itself. A *Yang* meridian is exteriorly–interiorly related to the *Yin* meridian, according to the theory of meridians.

For example, the kidney meridian is a *Yin* meridian and is related to the *Yang* bladder meridian in the leg. Thus, if the kidney meridian is affected, *Hunlun* (BL 60) and *Jinggu* (BL 64) of the bladder meridian are also selected to treat the kidney disease.

The combination of the anterior–posterior acupoints

Anterior is defined as the thoracic–abdominal region, belonging to *Yin*. Posterior is the lumbodorsal region, belonging to *Yang*. This method is also known as the combination of abdomen-*Yin* acupoints and back-*Yang* acupoints. Both acupoints on the anterior and posterior regions are selected to make up a prescription. For instance, select *Zhongwan* (Ren 12) on the abdomen and *Weishu* (BL 21) on the back to treat epigastric pain.

The combination of the distant–local acupoints

The selection of the acupoints on the diseased area and corresponding acupoints distant to the area simultaneously make up a prescription. For example, selecting *Jinming* (BL 1) near the eye and *Xingjian* (LR 2) distantly treats eye disease.

The combination of the left–right acupoints

According to the theory, the courses of the meridian cross each other. For example, select *Hegu* (LI 4) on the right side to treat facial paralysis on the left side, and vice versa. Because of the symmetric distribution of the meridian, acupoints on both sides are selected in the treatment of diseases of the internal organs, in order to strengthen the co-ordinating effects. However, it has been found that acupoints on the healthy side and no acupoints on the diseased side are selected in practice, such as in the treatment of hemiparalysis, arthralgic pain, etc. with a certain therapeutic result.

TREATMENT OF COMMON DISEASES WITH ACUPUNCTURE

Acupuncture for lower back pain

In the USA, lower back pain was among the top five primary reasons adult patients visit office-based physicians, according to a National Ambulatory Medical Care Survey[19] during 1980–90. Data show that 60–80% of adults have experience of lower back pain. Patients disabled from lower back pain increased by 168% from 1971 to 1986 and cost \$14 to \$20 billion annually in treatment, according to the 1986 report of the National Center for Health Statistics[19]. Surgery rates for lower back pain are five times higher in the USA than in England. Although operative procedures are frequently performed, 50–75% of the patients, unfortunately, continue to have disabling pain after the operation. Other conventional treatments are not very effective either. However, according to Liao *et al.*[19], acupuncture treatment could relieve the disabling lower back pain of 85% of the patients for the first time in many years.

Causative factors

Causative factors are the retention of pathogenic wind, cold, and damp in channels and collaterals; lumbar muscular strain, which is stagnation of *Qi* and blood in the lumbar region due to sprain or contusion; deficiency of *Qi* of the kidney due to excessive work; occupational sitting or standing for long periods of time; or excessive sexual activity causing loss of the essence of the kidney.

Select points

Select points are *Shenshu* (BL 23), *Weizhong* (BL 40), and a painful spot (i.e. *Ashi* point).

Acupuncture for headache

Headache is pain in the upper half of the head, excepting pain in the face. It is caused by many factors. Generally, it is divided into two main types: the diseases of inside the skull and outside the skull.

Causative factors

Factors causing pain are mainly cerebritis, meningitis and tumor. The disorders of the outside skull are mainly frontal sinusitis, tooth disease, ear disease, throat and pharyngitis, eye disease, as well as emotional stress and hypertension.

Select points

(1) *Migraine* (one-side headache): *Taiyang* (Extra 1), *Fengchi* (GB 20);

(2) *Forehead*: *Touwei* (ST 8), *Taiyang* (Extra 1);

(3) *Occipital region: Fengchi* (GB 20), *Dazhui* (DU 14), *Yintang* (Extra 2);

(4) *Whole potions: Yintang* (Extra 2), *Fengchi* (GB 20).

Acupuncture for stomachache

Stomachache is a symptom resulting from acute and chronic gastritis or peptic ulcer. Acute gastritis is expressed mainly as epigastric pain or upset, nausea, and vomiting, and it is accompanied by diarrhea and fever. Chronic gastritis is mainly indicated as epigastric upset or dull pain, anorexia, and postprandial distension. The peptic ulcer is rhythmic pain. The characteristic of pain includes anguish, distension, burning pain, and hungry sensations.

Causative factors

The causative factors of this disease include irregular meals, overindulgence, a fatty diet, and long-term alcohol intake, or it may arise from other *Zang-Fu* organ diseases. Some features of this disease are insidious onset, long incubation period, or following an acute attack of chronic pathogenic changes. Long-term treatment and watching one's diet are necessary.

Select points

These are *Zusanli* (ST 36), *Zhongwan* (Ren 12), *Qimen* (LR 14, right), *Weishu* (BL 21, cupping) and *Liangqiu* (ST 34).

Acupuncture for arthritis

Arthritis is inflammation in the joints, as a result of various causes. The main clinical manifestation is arthralgia and a functional disturbance to different degrees. There are three main clinical types of arthritis: rheumatic arthritis, rheumatoid arthritis, and osteoarthritis.

(1) *Rheumatic arthritis* occurs chiefly in adolescents. Before onset, it is commonly characterized by an upper respiratory infection. The acute stage is manifested as fever and profuse sweating. Characteristics are multiple with movement in large joints accompanied by acute inflammatory symptoms, such as redness, swelling, fever and pain, as well as functional disturbance. It often recurs.

(2) *Rheumatoid arthritis* occurs chiefly in the young and middle aged. The small joints of the hands and feet are the most commonly affected, usually symmetrically, but other large synovial joints (hip, knee, and elbow) are often also involved. Onset is insidious and mainly chronic. Acute onset is uncommon. At onset, the syndromes of pathogenic joint changes are similar to rheumatic arthritis, and they may be accompanied by fever.

(3) *Osteoarthritis* is also named hypertrophied or denatured arthritis. The disease usually presents in middle-aged persons (over 40 years of age). The joint lesions are chiefly at joints at dominant extremities, such as the lumbar vertebra, hip, knee, and finger. It is usually insidious in onset. Swelling is not present in the pathogenic joints.

Select points

(1) *Temporomandibular joint: Xiaguan* (ST 7), *Hegu* (LI 4);

(2) *Interspinal vertebrae joints:* correspond with *Jiaji* points;

(3) *Shoulder joints: Jianyu* (LI 15), *Jianliao* (SJ 14);

(4) *Elbow joints: Quchi* (LI 11), *Shaohai* (HT 3);

(5) *Wrist, metacarpophalangeal, digital joints: Waiguan* (SJ 5);

(6) *Lumbosacral joints: Yaoyangguan* (DU 3), *Ciliao* (BL 32);

(7) *Hip joints: Huantiao* (GB 30), *Fenshi* (GB 31);

(8) *Knee joints: Xiyan* (Extra 36), *Yanglingquan* (GB 34);

(9) *Ankle joints: Jiexi* (ST 41), *Kunlun* (BL 60).

Acupuncture for insomnia

Insomnia is difficulty in falling asleep, dream-disturbed sleep, sleeplessness in the whole night, and disturbed sleep accompanied by palpitations, dizziness, poor memory, lassitude, and listlessness.

Select points

Select points are *Shenmen* (HT 7), *Sanyinjiao* (SP 6), *Fengchi* (GB 20), and *Neiguan* (PC 6).

Acupuncture for constipation

Symptoms are dry stool, dysphasia, and 3–5 days or more required to relieve the bowels.

Select points

Select points are *Zhigou* (SJ 6), *Tianshu* (ST 25) and *Zusanli* (ST 36).

SIDE-EFFECTS

One of the great advantages of acupuncture is the infrequent occurrence of serious side-effects. Needles are either single-use disposable or sterilized, like any other medical instrument, under meticulous conditions. The acupuncturist can adjust treatment at any time to react to changes in an individual's condition.

Most people do not experience unpleasant side-effects. However, any time a needle is placed in the body, there is a risk of bleeding or infection. With the use of disposable needles, the risk of infection is remote and, in the hands of a competent acupuncturist, the risk of bleeding is minimal. Occasionally, a small vessel under the skin may be pricked, resulting in a bruise. Occasionally, people may feel dizzy, especially at the start of the first treatment and, more commonly, when acupuncture has not yet been experienced.

Occasionally the original symptoms worsen for a few days and other symptoms, that include changes in appetite, sleep, bowel or urination patterns, or emotional state, may be triggered. These should not cause concern, as they are simply indications that the acupuncture is starting to work. It is quite common for the first one or two treatments to induce a sensation of deep relaxation or even mild disorientation immediately following the treatment. These pass within a short time and never require anything more than a slight rest to overcome.

Cautions

(1) *San Yin Chiao* (SP 6) in conjunction with *He Gu* (LI 4) is forbidden for pregnant women, to avoid miscarriage. Stimulating certain acupuncture points, particularly those on or near the abdomen, can trigger uterine contractions and induce premature labor and possibly miscarriage. The acupuncturist should be informed of pregnancy if possible. Acupuncture can be implemented to treat morning sickness, but a physician should be consulted first.

(2) People on anticoagulant drugs may bleed easily, even when thin acupuncture needles are inserted. They should consult their physician before having acupuncture if such medication has been prescribed.

(3) Electroacupuncture can cause problems for people with pacemakers, because the stimulation pulses can interfere with the pacemaker-generated pulses. In addition, magnets, which are sometimes used to stimulate acupuncture points, may interfere with pacemakers.

(4) Anyone with a compromised immune system needs to be especially careful that the acupuncturist is using disposable needles.

(5) The acupuncturist should proceed with extreme caution when inserting needles into the limbs of diabetic patients. Even a small cut in a person with diabetic neuropathy can turn into a severe infection.

Risks

Improperly performed acupuncture can cause fainting, local hematoma (due to bleeding from a punctured blood vessel), pneumothorax (punctured lung), convulsions, local infections, hepatitis B (from non-sterile needles), bacterial endocarditis, contact dermatitis, and nerve damage.

WHO VISITS AN ACUPUNCTURIST?

Complementary and alternative medicine (CAM) therapies have increasingly attracted national attention from the media, the medical community, governmental agencies, and the public. Two national random-household telephone surveys[20,21] have indicated that the use of CAM therapies and the expenditures on them increased substantially in the USA between 1990 and 1997. Overall, prevalence of use increased by 25%; total visits by an estimated 47%, from 427 to 629 million; and expenditures on CAM services by an estimated 45%, totaling $21 billion.

Generally, most of the surveys, including the aforesaid, on CAM therapies covered all kinds of CAM treatments (more than 20 different CAM treatment types). Very few studies on a single type of CAM have been conducted.

The author has practiced acupuncture and traditional Chinese medicine in the Chicago area for 10 years. Based on the data from a total of 160 cases (40 cases per year) randomly selected from 4 consecutive years (1998–2001), our statistical analysis may be focused on the following areas to expose who visits an acupuncturist and how much they pay for each visit.

(1)   Patient's general information;

(2)   What kind of syndrome(s) the patient had;

(3)   Before visiting an acupuncturist, for how long the patient suffered from the syndrome(s) and for how long they utilized conventional medical treatment;

(4)   How the acupuncturist was found (by referral and from whom, through the Yellow Pages or the Internet); linear relationship and regression analysis tools will analyze the results;

(5)   The cost of the average visit.

Results

In the total of 160 cases, 41% were male and 59% female. The average age was 44.94 years (range 13–71 years) with a standard deviation of 25.57 and a 95% confidence interval of 44.94 ± 3.96. Of the patients, 63% were white, 10% black, 6% Asian–American, and 21% Hispanic and other races.

Of the patients, 86.25% had a college education or higher (11.25% had a doctorate degree). Similarly, the majority of the patients' occupations (91.25%) were professional, including a physician, psychologist, dentist, pharmacist, attorney, professor, trader, controller, musician, and company administrator. The number of disease(s) or syndrome(s) the patients suffered from when they visited the acupuncturist were 2.23 ± 2.16 (range 1–7, 95% confidence interval 2.23 ± 0.33).

Overall, a patient visited an acupuncturist because of pain (27.53%), fatigue (12.36%), cardiovascular disease (8.99%), weight problems (8.43%), mental disorder (4.49%), allergy (4.49%), migraine headache (3.93%), digestive system problems (3.37%), insomnia (3.37%), skin disease (2.81%), upper respiratory disease (2.25%), and other causes (17.98%). Figure 11.16 shows the top ten diseases and syndromes causing a patient to visit an acupuncturist. The patients had been treated by conventional medicine for 4.96 ± 7.16 years (range 0.5–25 years, 95% confidence interval 4.96 ± 1.11).

As indicated in Table 11.1, some patients heard about acupuncture from a relative or friend; they varied between 75% and 85% (correlation coefficient, $r = -0.849$). Fewer patients used the Yellow Pages, and

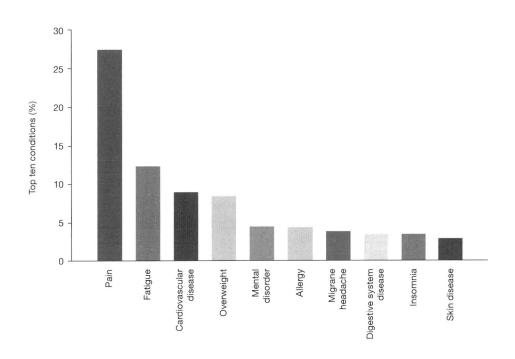

Figure 11.16   Top ten reasons why patients visit an acupuncturist

Table 11.1   How some patients found an acupuncturist

Year	Relative or friend		Website		Yellow pages		Doctor's referral	
	n	*%*	*n*	*%*	*n*	*%*	*n*	*%*
1998 (*n* = 40)	34	85	0	0	6	15	0	0
1999 (*n* = 40)	33	82.5	1	2.5	5	12.5	1	2.5
2000 (*n* = 40)	30	75	2	5	6	15	2	5
2001 (*n* = 40)	31	77.5	3	7.5	2	5	4	10

this number decreased each year from 15 to 5% (correlation coefficient, $r = -0.7502$). The number of patients learning from a website or following another medical practitioner's referral rose every year from 0 to 7.5% (correlation coefficient, $r = 1$) and from 0 to 10% (correlation coefficient, $r = 0.9827$), respectively. We calculated the equation of the regression line of website information to be $y = 2.5x - 4995$ and a physician's referral is $y = 3.25x - 6494$. Based on these equations, we predicted that patients' visits to an acupuncturist through a physician's referral would increase to 12.5%, and through a website would increase to 10% in 2002. Figure 11.17 demonstrates how the patients obtained information about an acupuncturist in the consecutive 4 years, and the regression lines.

Before 2001, payment for acupuncture treatment was out of a patient's own pocket. The average cost for each visit was $68 ± 27.16 (range $20–80, 95% confidence interval $68 ± 8.42) in 1998; $71 ± 23.43 (range $25–85, 95% confidence interval $71 ± 7.27) in 1999; $76 ± 18.80 (range $20–90, 95% confidence interval $76 ± 5.83) in 2000; and $82.75 ± 16.09 (range $30–120, 95% confidence interval $82.75 ± 4.99) in 2001. In 2001, 12.5% of patients treated by acupuncture were covered by insurance fully or partially.

PHYSIOLOGIC BASES OF ACUPUNCTURE ANALGESIA

Although acupuncture has been used in China for more than 4000 years and its efficacy has been proved by ample clinic experiences, its mechanisms of action are a recent focus of study. The facts of acupuncture anesthesia and its cures have astonished the modern medical field. The anesthesia produced by acupuncture is very different from that produced by drugs. First of all, consciousness is maintained, allowing the patient to eat, talk, and co-operate with doctors during surgery.

Second, stimulation of specific acupuncture points is essential to maintain analgesia. Third, analgesia persists long after stimulation has been terminated, allowing the patient to move immediately or much earlier without pain postoperatively. Thus, the patient recovers from surgery sooner.

How can an acupuncture needle inserted in the hand possibly relieve toothache? Because such phenomena do not conform to accepted physiologic concepts, scientists are puzzled and skeptical. They were confused by the way traditional Chinese medicine explained *Yin–Yang*, the five elements, the eight principles of diagnosis and the functioning of organs by *Zang-Fu*. In 1973, Chinese scientists published the model of a cross-circulation experiment. The effect of acupuncture analgesia was transmitted from a donor rabbit, which received acupuncture, to a normal recipient. The pain threshold of both rabbits significantly increased. The experiment offered for the first time some evidence that acupuncture must have produced in the animals some kind of chemical substance or substances that potentially suppresses pain. It is now known that acupuncture may activate the endogenous systems of analgesia to be able to alleviate pain in the clinic.

According to Pomeranz[22], the mechanism of acupuncture analgesia is as follows: when an acupuncture needle penetrates an acupuncture point, the needle and electrical impulses stimulate nerve fibers in the muscle, which send impulses to the spinal cord and activate three centers (spinal cord, midbrain, and hypothalamus/pituitary) to cause analgesia. The spinal site uses enkephalin and dynorphin to block incoming messages with low-frequency stimulation and other transmitters (perhaps γ-aminobutyric acid) at high-frequency stimulation. The midbrain uses enkephalin to activate the raphe-descending system, which inhibits spinal cord pain transmission by a synergistic effect of the monoamines serotonin and norepinephrine (noradrenaline). The midbrain also has a circuit, which

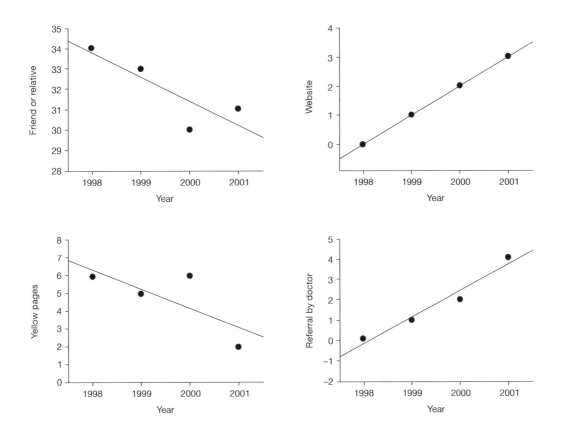

Figure 11.17 How patients learned about acupuncture in the years 1998–2001 in the author's experience

bypasses endorphinergic links at high-frequency stimulation. Finally, at the third (hypothalamus/pituitary) center, the pituitary releases β-endorphin into the blood and cerebrospinal fluid to cause analgesia at a distance. The hypothalamus also sends long axons to the midbrain and activates the descending analgesia system via β-endorphin. This third center is not activated at high-frequency stimulation, but only at low frequencies.

The endorphin–acupuncture analgesia hypothesis is supported by the following:

(1) Naloxone, an endorphin antagonist, can antagonize acupuncture analgesia[23,24] and increasing the doses of naloxone produces increasing blockade, showing a dose–response curve[25].

(2) Acupuncture analgesia is enhanced by protecting endorphins from enzyme degradation[26–31].

(3) Lesions of the periaqueductal gray matter (site of endorphins) or the arcuate nucleus of the hypothalamus (the site of β-endorphins) abolish acupuncture analgesia[32,33].

(4) The level of *c-Fos* gene protein, which measures increased neural activity, is elevated in endorphin-related areas of the brain during acupuncture analgesia[34–36].

(5) Rats deficient in endorphin show poor acupuncture analgesia[31,37].

(6) Mice genetically deficient in opiate receptors show poor acupuncture analgesia[38].

SUMMARY AND FUTURE PROSPECT

Patients who visit acupuncturists in the Chicago Metropolitan Area are similar to those who utilize other alternative medicines. The majority of patients are female, educated, white, and middle aged. The top ten reasons for visiting an acupuncturist are pain, fatigue, cardiovascular disease, weight problems, mental disorder, allergy, migraine headache, digestive system disease, insomnia, and skin disease. Our data indicate that more and more patients will find acupuncturists from websites and from their regular physician's referral, and that full and partial insurance coverage for acupuncture treatment is to be executed.

To enhance the acceptance of acupuncture in the USA, the panel convened by the National Institutes of Health in 1997[39] suggested six points for the future: first, improvement in understanding between acupuncturists and the conventional health-care community; second, improvement in training and more uniform licensing, certification, and accreditation of acupuncturists; third, full information for patients about their treatment options, prognosis, relative risks, and safety practices; fourth, strengthened communication between health-care provider groups; fifth, coverage of acupuncture treatment by insurance; and sixth, identification of important areas for future acupuncture research.

References

1. Liao SJ, Lee MH, Ng LK. The historic background. In Principles and Practice of Contemporary Acupuncture. New York, NY: Marcel Dekker, 1994: 8–41

2. Reston J. News about my operation in Peking. New York Times, 26 July 1971

3. Rosenfeld I. Acupuncture goes mainstream (almost). Parade Magazine, 16 August 1998: 10

4. Bannerman RH. Acupuncture: the WHO view. World Health 1979; (December): 27–8

5. Travell J, Sommons D. Myofascial Pain and Dysfunction. The Trigger Point Manual. Baltimore, MD: Williams and Wilkins, 1983

6. Dung HC. Anatomical features contributing to the formation of acupuncture points. Am J Acupunct 1984; 12: 139–43

7. Heine H. Akupunkturtherapie – Perforationen der oberflächlichen Körperfaszie durch hutane Gefäß-Nervenbndel. Therapeutikon 1988; 4: 238–44

8. Stacher G, Wancura I, Bauer P, et al. Effect of acupuncture on pain threshold and pain tolerance determined by electrical stimulation of the skin: a controlled study. Am J Chin Med 1975; 3: 143–6

9. Chapman CR, Chen AC, Bonica JJ. Effects of intrasegmental electrical acupuncture on dental pain: evaluation by threshold estimation and sensory decision theory. Pain 1977; 3: 213–27

10. Brockhaus A, Elger CE. Hypalgesic efficacy of acupuncture on experimental pain in men. Comparison of laser acupuncture and needle acupuncture. Pain 1990; 43: 181–5

11. Cho ZH, Chung SC, Jones JP, et al. New findings of the correlation between acupoints and corresponding brain cortices using functional MRI. Proc Natl Acad Sci 1998; 95: 2670–3

12. Cho ZH, Na CS, Wang EK, et al. Functional magnetic resonance imaging of the brain in the investigation of acupuncture. In Stux G, Hammerschlag R, eds. Clinical Acupuncture, Scientific Basis. Berlin: Springer, 2001: 83–95

13. Chiang CY, Chang CT. Peripheral afferent pathway for acupuncture analgesia. Sci Sin 1973; 16: 210–17

14. Wang K, Yao S, Xian Y, Hou Z. A study on the receptive field of acupoints and the relationship between characteristics of needle sensation and groups of afferent fibres. Sci Sin 1985; 28: 963–71

15. Martelete M, Fiori AM. Comparative study of the analgesic effect of transcutaneous nerve stimulation (TNS), electroacupuncture (EA), and meperidine in the treatment of postoperative pain. Acupunct Electrother Res 1985; 10: 183–93

16. Walker JB, Katz RL. Nonopioid pathways suppress pain in humans. Pain 1981; 11: 347–54

17. Pomeranz B, Warma N. Potentiation of analgesia by two repeated electroacupuncture treatments: the first opioid analgesia potentiates a second, nonopioid analgesia response. Brain Res 1988; 452: 232–6

18. Lichun H, Williams H. Methods of ear acupuncture. In Introduction to Auricular Medicine. Fern Park, Florida: Auricular Medicine International Research & Training Center, Inc., 2004: 5–6

19. Liao SJ, Lee MH, Ng LK. Acupuncture for chronic pain and surgical analgesia. In Principles and Practice of Contemporary Acupuncture. New York, NY: Marcel Dekker, 1994: 290–326

20. Eisenbarg DM, Kessler RC, Foster C. Unconventional medicine in the United States – prevalence, costs and patterns of use. N Engl J Med 1993; 328: 246–52

21. Eisenberg DM, Davis RD, Ettner SL, et al. Trends in alternative medicine use in the United States, 1990–1997: results of a follow-up national survey. J Am Med Assoc 1998; 280: 1569–75

22. Pomeranz B. Acupuncture analgesia – basic research, In Stux G, Hammerschlag R, eds. Clinical Acupuncture, Scientific Basis. Berlin: Springer, 2001: 1–28

23. Pomeranz B, Chiu D. Naloxone blocks acupuncture analgesia and causes hyperalgesia: endorphin is implicated. Life Sci 1976; 19: 1757–62

24. Mayer DJ, Price DD, Raffii A. Antagonism of acupuncture analgesia in man by the narcotic antagonist naloxone. Brain Res 1977; 121: 368–72

25. Cheng R, Pomeranz B. Electroacupuncture analgesia is mediated by stereospecific opiate receptors and is reversed by antagonists of type 1 receptors. Life Sci 1979; 26: 631–9

26. Zou K, Yi QC, Wu SX, et al. Enkephalin involvement in acupuncture analgesia. Sci Sin 1980; 23: 1197–207

27. Cheng R, Pomeranz B. Monoaminergic mechanisms of electroacupuncture analgesia. Brain Res 1981; 215: 77–92

28. Chou J, Tang J, Yang HY, Costa E. Action of peptidase inhibitors on methionine 5-enkephalin-arginine 6-phenylalanine 7 (YGGFMRF) and methionine 5-enkephalin (YGGFM)

metabolism and on electroacupuncture antinociception. J Pharmacol Exp Ther 1984; 230: 349–52

29. Ehrenpreis S. Analgesic properties of encephalinese inhibitors: animal and human studies. Prog Clin Biol Res 1985; 192: 363–70

30. Hishida F, Takeshige C. Effects of d-phenylalanine on individual variation of analgesia and on analgesia inhibitory system in their separated experimental procedures [Japanese with English abstract]. In Takeshige C, ed. Studies on the Mechanism of Acupuncture Analgesia Based on Animal Experiments. Tokyo: Showa University Press, 1986: 51

31. Murai M, Takeshige C, Hishida F, et al. Correlation between individual variations in effectiveness of acupuncture analgesia and those in contents of brain endogenous morphine-like factors. [Japanese with English summary]. In Takeshige C, ed. Studies on the Mechanism of Acupuncture Analgesia Based on Animal Experiments. Tokyo: Showa University Press, 1986: 542

32. Wang Q, Mao L, Han J. The arcuate nucleus of hypothalamus mediates low but not high frequency electroacupuncture in rats. Brain Res 1990; 513: 60–6

33. Takeshige C, Zhao WH, Guo SY. Convergence from the preoptic area and arcuate nucleus to the median eminence in acupuncture and nonacupuncture stimulation analgesia. Brain Res Bull 1991; 26: 771–8

34. Guo HF, Cui X. C-Fos proteins are not involved in the activation of preproenkephalin gene expression in rat brain by peripheral electric stimulation (electroacupuncture). Neurosci Lett 1996; 207: 163–6

35. Lee JH, Beitz AJ. The distribution of brainstem and spinal nuclei associated with different frequencies of electroacupuncture analgesia. Pain 1993; 52: 11–28

36. Pan B, Castro-Lopes JM, Coimbra A, et al. C-fos expression in the hypothalamic pituitary system induced by electroacupuncture or noxious stimulation. Neuroreport 1994; 5: 1649–52

37. Takahashi G, Mera H, Kobori M. Inhibitory action on analgesic inhibitory system and augmenting action on naloxone reversal analgesia of d-phenylalanine. [Japanese with English summary]. In Takeshige C, ed. Studies on the Mechanism of Acupuncture Analgesia Based on Animal Experiments. Tokyo: Showa University Press, 1986: 608

38. Peets J, Pomeranz B. Studies of suppression of nocisensor reflexes using tail flick electromyograms and intrathecal drugs in barbiturate-anaesthetized rats. Brain Res 1987; 416: 301–7

39. National Institutes of Health. Acupuncture, NIH Consensus Statement, Vol. 15, Number 5. Bethesda, MD: NIH, 1997

Tai Chi

12

S. Xutian, F. Sun and S. Tai

INTRODUCTION

Tai Chi or Taiji is short for Taijichuan, which is very popular all over the world[1]. It is a combination of Chinese martial arts with Chinese breath training (Tu Na – a special breath training program for health cultivation), energy flowing guidance (Dao Yin – guiding the *Qi*-vital bio-energy circulation of the body by mind for health purposes), and meditation progress. Indeed, Taiji is a kind of traditional Chinese Yanshenshu (a mind–body harmonizing technique for health improvement and longevity), an important part of Traditional Chinese Medicine (TCM).

Originally used for the purposes of martial arts, the slow and graceful movements of Taiji, however, also reflect the natural movements of animals and birds, as symbols or 'pictures', which were designed to focus on the mind and breathing through a complex series of execution of forms. As the forms are practiced in slow but continual and fluidic movements, the breathing is regulated as an integral part of this flowing meditation. The effect of mind regulation produces a sedative state directly on the central nervous system, which in turn helps to stimulate and improve other systems of the body. The calm and graceful movements of Taiji themselves are like physical poetry and meditative dance as well.

When practiced properly, *Qi* energy is increased, and one often feels a 'tingling' of fingers and toes, and a warming up of the body. The mind becomes clear and relaxed. The movements help loosen tight muscles, make the joints flexible, increase the posture, stability, and balance the whole body.

There are various schools or styles of Taiji: Chen, Yang, Wu, Sun, and Hao styles[2]. In 1956, the Simplified Taiji was compiled to address the above problems, which is also known as the Beijing Style. It comprises 24 forms (movements), mostly from the traditional Yang Style 108 forms. The Simplified Taiji was the result of many Taiji masters working towards standardizing and simplifying Taiji, and focusing on the purpose of promoting health. One of the most important characteristics of the Simplified Taiji is that even though the 24 forms of Taiji constitute a simplified version, it is still a 'traditional' sequence, with the original martial art applications in every movement. In 1979, the Chinese State Physical Education and Sports Committee again commissioned another change[2]. The current Taiji version is composed of 48 forms (movements) which inherited the best and strongest points from the Chen, Yang, and Wu styles.

Taiji was popular from the nineteenth century in China as a kind of martial art and slowly transferred to Western countries. In the modern world, the main purpose is no longer for fighting but just for health, fitness, disease prevention, and therapy. During the past 30 years, Taiji has spread throughout the world, propagated by immigrant populations and the opening of China from the mid 1970s. The traditional disciplines of acupuncture, herbal remedies, and Qigong therapies are now regaining public interest and respect as they gradually become supported by modern scientific research evidence.

It is estimated that there are 12 million people of all ages who practice Taiji in China[2]. It is regulated and organized by the Chinese National Sports Association. There are national 'instructor' exams and coaching seminars as well as organized competitions within individual family styles. Taiji is also one of the official competition events in the larger national and international martial arts competitions and has been proposed to the International Olympic Committee as a competition event in the 2008 Olympic games.

HISTORY AND PHILOSOPHY

There are some legends about the early history of Taiji. It is difficult to make a completely unified history story about the origin of Taiji, because the secret of Taiji was kept within individual families for many generations before it was taught to the public. Written records are missing. The origin of Taiji was argued about for hundreds of years. Most people believed that Taiji was developed to the present style by some martial art masters during the late Ming and early Qing dynasties.

The most recent research shows solid evidence that the earliest 'Taiji 13 Forms for Health Cultivation' was created in Qianzai Temple in Tang village by Chen Yu-Ting (1600~) from Chen Jiagou village, Wen County, and Li Yan (1606~1643) from Tang village, Beai County, Henan Province of China[3]. Wang Zong-Yue (1750~) learned Taiji from Li He-Lin in Tang village and wrote a text entitled *Taijiquan Lun*, which is the most important part of a collection of classical writings that form the guidelines for all styles of Taiji[3].

Another legend says that the credit for formalizing the soft-style series of exercises into a unified whole belongs to a Taoist Priest, Zhang (or Chang) San-Feng (1270–1364). He lived as a recluse on Mount Wu-Tang in the Hebei Province of China. As the legend goes, Mr Zhang happened to be walking in the woods when he encountered a crane fighting with a snake. The crane was jabbing at the snake with its long beak in straight angular strikes. The snake was able to avoid the crane by changing its shape and position (staying very soft and resilient), slithering away, and quickly counterattacking while the bird was still committed to its original thrust. Mr Zhang gleaned from this that it would be possible for a weaker opponent to overcome a stronger one if he became soft and elusive. He incorporated this lesson into a new, softer version of a martial art and at the same time a health-promoting program. He reworked the original forms of Shao Lin with a new emphasis on breathing and inner energy balance. It is reputed that he learnt and created the so-called 'internal' boxing method. He then started a school which was known as the Wu-Tang School of Internal Boxing.

However, Taiji's essential principle, no doubt, has its roots in ancient Chinese philosophy, which inherited Daoism, Buddhism, and Confucianism. Some postures of style were inherited from Dao Yin's *Yellow Emperor's Classic of Internal Medicine*[4], the first important book for TCM (about 206 BC–AD 220), and *Frolics of the Five Animals* (tiger, deer, bear, monkey, and bird), created by the ancient famous Chinese doctor Hua Tuo (about AD 220–265)[5]. Serious students of Taiji understand many of the terms and concepts used in TCM[5], such as *Yin Yang*, Five Elements, Meridians, as well as the circulation of *Qi*, in addition to the historic martial arts roots.

The theory is that Zhang San-Feng originated a soft style that combined both existing combat techniques and other movements, primarily designed to increase the flow of *Qi* energy through the body, thus creating a form that was a physical manifestation of Taoist thinking.

Going back even further, we can see the ancestors of Taiji. In the third century, Hua Tuo created a system of exercise to improve the digestion and circulation of the human body, based on the movements of animals and birds. The essence of this system was to move every part of the body. In the sixth century, Buddha Dharma visited the Shao Lin monastery and developed a system of exercise for the monks, who were in poor physical condition because of too much meditation. This was known as the Eighteen Form Lohan Exercise. Later, in the eighth century, this was developed into the 37-form Long Kung-Fu, which, unlike other styles of Kung-Fu, was based upon a 'soft' or internal approach, rather than a 'hard' external one.

Modern, non-violent Taiji as a form on its own, rather than being a part of martial art, was developed much later, as the need for combat gradually decreased, although the Taiji practitioner is always aware that the forms that he is using are the same as those of combat, but slower. The Chen style contained jumps, leaps, and explosions of strength all within a circular path. The Yang style, formulated in the mid-nineteenth century, is softer, and is the most popular system[2].

Taijichuan, the original combat form of Taiji, translated by words means Supreme Ultimate Fist, but the word Taiji was in fact one of the various changeable energy states or modes of description of the universe, such as Huang Ji, Yuan Ji, Wu Ji, etc. The word Taiji was born from Wu Ji, in the moment between motion and still transforming, or starting polarization or separating to, *Yin* and *Yang*[1]. Now we use the word Taiji as the name of a combat form or a fitness exercise. Unlike many other martial arts, which were aggressive or outward, the main principle of Taiji was that of a soft combat – absorbing the opponent's aggressive energy and using it against him. This is a principle of *Yin* and *Yang*, a balance of opposites where the soft is used to overcome the hard, as described in the maxim 'using a force of four ounces to defeat that of a thousand pounds' or 'overcome a weight of a thousand carries by a force of four ounces'. Imagine an opponent twice your weight throwing a powerful punch – the Taiji adept would step back and absorb the punch by grasping the fist and pulling it past him, using his opponent's own forward energy and motion to overbalance the attacker. Or he might respond in any number of ways, always using the same principles.

So, if we want to understand more about Taiji, we should know the essence of Chinese philosophy and culture, as illustrated in the following key points of view.

Tao is action – only vague and intangible. Yet, in the vague and void, there is image, there is substance; within the intangible there is essence, there is marrow; this essence is real. Within this real being, there is validity, trust and information[6].

There is something evolved from void and born before the making of heaven and earth. It is inaudible and invisible. It is independent and immutable. It is forever orbiting. It is the parents of all things of heaven and earth[6].

The Chinese ancient philosophy considers that there is intangible energy called *Qi* (or *Chi*) full of the universe, no matter whether the object is large or small, *Qui* is in anything anywhere. This is an important aspect of Chinese culture. It suggests that *Qi*, a concept that is sometimes referred to as special energy, has features of energy, image, material, essence, information, and consciousness. *Qi* exists in the entire universe and is considered to be the basic unit of everything in the universe. *Qi* is the most essential substance making up the world and *Qi* generated everything in the universe. Therefore, *Qi* is the root of a myriad things and everything has the spirit *Qi*. It seems like the astronomic theory: before anything was created, the universe was in a state of chaos at first, called *Wu Ji*; when it separated to *Yin* and *Yang* it became the *Taiji* state, like the fog and dew, then created all things. That is 'Tao engenders One, One engenders Two, Two engenders Three, and Three engenders ten thousand things'[6]. As a part of the universe, the human body is related to the universe as a single union. It is believed that, through systematic discipline (mental, moral, and physical), human beings can accumulate *Qi* and cultivate the potential to achieve health, intelligence, and longevity[5].

Under this philosophy, Taiji was created and developed; it incorporates therapy and fitness, but always involves the *Qi* principle. It maintains that a person not only has a physical body, but also has an intangible energy body – *Qi* system (meridian system, aura, etc.) – enclosed with the human spirit.

Based on this background, Taiji practitioners should understand this philosophy first, then learn physical postures combining with mind and breath training, called *Xin Fa* (the main principle of the mind–body harmonious practice technique). Most people find it hard to understand how the invisible *Qi* circulates in the body and how energy and messages are exchanged between the human body and the universe.

PUBLIC SIMPLIFIED PRACTICE PROGRAM

Principles for Taiji practice

The main principle of Taiji, originating from traditional Chinese philosophy, is the holistic harmony and the balance of *Yin* and *Yang*. The main purpose of Taiji practice in modern society is to achieve health benefits and longevity by balancing *Yin* and *Yang* in order to reach holistic harmony. There are variations in the principles of Taiji practice, but the following principles are central to gaining more benefits, above and beyond the health-related ones.

'Stand like a balance and move like a wheel' (Wang Zong-Yue)[7]

When you are standing you should be very stable, like a balance; when you are moving you should be very flexible, like a wheel. In this way of Taiji training, you can gradually get rid of rigidity and obtain flexibility in body, mind, and personality. Each body part moves like a wheel turning smoothly and stably and any individual movement of a body part is accompanied and counterbalanced by the rest of the movements of the other parts. In each movement, every part of the body should be light, agile, and strung together, and each movement is slow but continually fluidic, endless but independent, and effortless but powerful.

'Suspend head, relax shoulder, and sink elbow, and concentrate on Dantian' (Qi sinks in Dantian, which is located just below the navel in the lower abdomen) (Wu Yu-Nang)[7]

Suspend the head to keep it straight and upward as if there is an invisible thread fixed at Baihui (meridian point GV20 on the top of the head)[5], lightly lifting the head up throughout the neck and trunk. Only when you relax the shoulders and sink the elbows, can you sink *Qi* in Dantian. This is the ideal way to harmonize the upper with the lower part of the body, and void and soft with hard and solid. In this way, you can naturally relax the whole body and mind, and facilitate both the energy circulation inside the body and the energy exchange between the body and the universe.

The waist is the commander of body movements[7]

Subtle attention should always be paid to the waist to achieve a real relaxation with extremely stable and flexible movements of the whole body, because the energy center (Dantian) is in the waist area of the body, and the whole body movements are initiated from the waist area. The waist movement directs the movement of other parts of the body like a commander, and also leads the energy flowing to the whole body. It can make a real combination of movement and tranquility; movement and tranquility always accompany each other. 'It represents a balance, in which movement is characterized by tranquility and tranquility is represented by movement'(Wu Yu-Nang)[7].

'Keep mind calm when body moving' (Wu Yu-Nang)[7]

During Taiji practice, the body is moving, but the mind is always calm. The mind is the general commander. Only when the mind is calm, can it intelligently command the movement of the body. One draws the energy up from the earth through the *Yongquan* (meridian point K1 on the bottom of the foot)[5], and the waist directs the flow of energy to the head and limbs, like water flowing through a garden hose. In addition, a powerful mind may ensure a stable and peaceful body movement. On the other hand, skillful and natural body movements may improve mind power.

Taiji is also a special moving meditation

Taiji is considered a form of meditation with slow body movements, deep breathing exercises, energy guidance, and mind adjustment. Taiji is sometimes called a moving meditation or Chinese moving yoga because it integrates and coordinates the body, mind, energy or potent force and conscious or subconscious function into a single whole, mind body as one. In particular, natural, deep, and even breathing is required, and the conscious and subconscious function is trained to be coordinated. The mind is the director and energy is the guide, so the mind governs energy and energy leads the body movement (Wu Yu-Nang)[7].

In summary, 'by applying the inside energy and power to the whole body, all the movements of bending or pulling and stretching or pushing of Taiji actually lead to continuous collecting and releasing of energy. This is only a cultivation of energy through a closing or filling/opening or emptying activity to achieve health and longevity' (Chen Xin)[7].

Twenty-four forms[8]

Figure 12.1 shows 24 form styles. It should be noted that:

(1) In the illustrations of Figure 12.1, the paths of the movements to be executed are indicated by arrows drawn in solid lines for the right hand and left foot, and dotted lines for the left hand and the right foot.

(2) Movement directions are given in terms of the 12 hours of the clock. Begin by facing 12 o'clock, with 6 o'clock behind you, 9 o'clock at your left and 3 o'clock at your right. Thus a turn to one o'clock is one of 30° to the right, and a turn to 1.30 is one of 45°.

(3) The requirements of the standing posture are: head erect, torso straight, waist and hips relaxed, legs extended naturally, knee in line with toes.

Form 1: commencing form

(1) Stand upright with feet shoulder-width apart, toes pointing forward, and arms hanging naturally at sides. Look straight ahead (Figure 12.1,1).

Points to remember: hold head and neck erect, with chin drawn slightly inward. Do not protrude chest or draw abdomen in.

(2) Float arms slowly forward to shoulder level, palms down (Figure 12.1, 1–2).

(3) Bend knees as you press palms down gently, with elbows dropping towards knees. Look straight ahead.

Points to remember: keep torso erect and hold shoulders and elbows down. Fingers are slightly curved. Body weight is equally distributed between legs. While bending knees, keep waist relaxed and buttocks slightly pulled in. The lower arms should be coordinated with the bending knees.

Form 2: part wild horse's mane on both sides

(1) With torso turning slightly to the right (1 o'clock) and weight shifted onto right leg, raise right hand until forearm lies horizontally in front of right part of chest, while left hand moves in a downward curve until it comes under the right hand, palms facing each other as if holding an energy ball

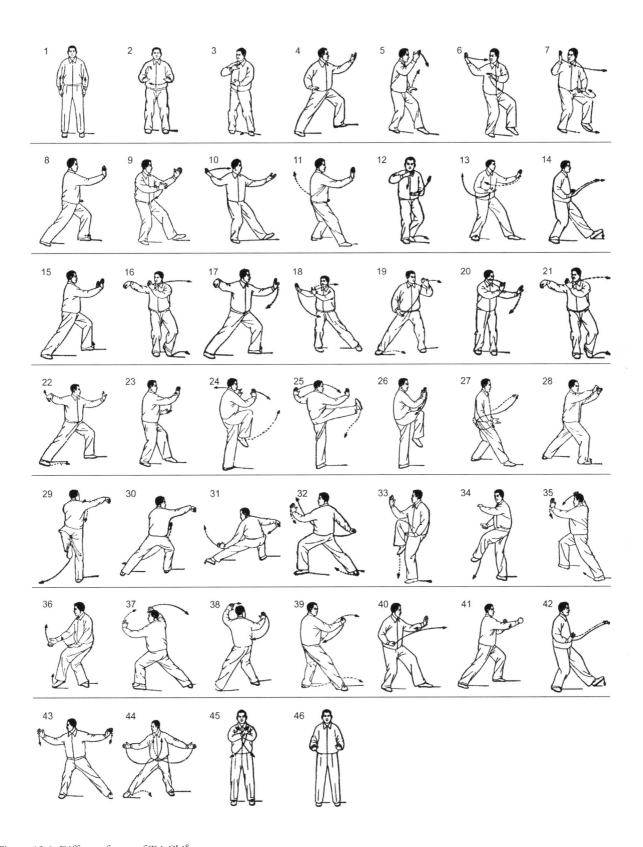

Figure 12.1 Different forms of Tai Chi[8]

(henceforth referred to as 'hold-ball gesture'). Move left foot to the side of right foot, toes on floor. Look at right hand (Figure 12.1, 3).

(2) Turn body to the left (10 o'clock) as left foot takes a step towards 8–9 o'clock, bending knee and shifting weight onto left leg, while right leg straightens with whole foot on the floor for a left 'bow stance'. As you turn body, raise left hand to eye level with palm facing obliquely up and elbow slightly bent, and lower right hand to the side of right hip with palm facing down and fingers pointing forward. Look at left hand (Figure 12.1, 4).

(3) Repeat movements in (1)–(2), reversing 'right' and 'left' (Figure 12.1, 3–4).

Points to remember: hold torso erect and keep chest relaxed. Move arms in a curve without stretching them when you separate hands. Use waist as the axis in body turns. The movements in making a bow stance and separating hands must be smooth and synchronized in tempo. When taking a bow stance, place front foot slowly in position, with heel coming down first. The knee of the front leg should not go beyond the toes, while the rear leg should be straightened, forming an angle of 45° with the ground. There should be a transverse distance of 10–30 cm between heels. Face 9 o'clock in final position.

Form 3: white crane flashes its wings

(1) With torso turning slightly to the left (8 o'clock), make a hold-ball gesture in front of the left part of the chest, left hand on top. Look at left hand.

(2) Draw right foot half a step towards left foot and then sit back. Turn torso slightly to the right (10 o'clock), with weight shifted onto right leg and eyes looking at right hand. Move left foot forward a bit, toes on floor for a left 'empty stance', with both legs slightly bent at knee. At the same time, with torso turning slightly to the left (9 o'clock), raise right hand to the front of right temple, palm turning inward, while left hand moves down to the front of left hip, palm down. Look straight ahead (Figure 12.1, 5).

Points to remember: do not thrust chest forward. Arms should be rounded when they move up or down. Weight transfer should be coordinated with the raising of the right hand. Face 9 o'clock in the final position.

Form 4: brush knee on both sides

(1) Turn torso slightly to the left (8 o'clock) as right hand moves down while left hand moves up. Then turn torso to the right (11 o'clock) as right hand circles past abdomen and up to ear level with arm slightly bent and palm facing obliquely upward, while left hand moves in an upward–rightward–downward curve to the front of right part of chest, palm facing obliquely downward. Look at right hand (Figure 12.1, 6).

(2) Turn torso to the left (9 o'clock) as left foot takes a step in that direction for a left bow stance. At the same time, right hand draws leftward past right ear and, following body turn, pushes forward at nose level with palm facing forward, while left hand circles around left knee to stop beside left hip, palm down. Look at fingers of right hand (Figure 12.1, 7–8).

(3) Repeat movements in (1)–(2), reversing 'right' and 'left' (Figure 12.1, 6–8).

Form 5: strum the lute

Move right foot half a step towards left heel. Sit back and turn torso slightly to the right (10–11 o'clock), shifting weight onto right leg. Raise left foot and place it slightly forward, heel coming down on floor and knee bent a little for a left empty stance. At the same time, raise left hand in a curve to nose level, with palm facing rightward and elbow slightly bent, while right hand moves to the inside of the left elbow, palm facing leftward. Look at forefingers of left hand (Figure 12.1, 9).

Points to remember: body position should remain steady and natural, chest relaxed and shoulders and elbows held down. Movement in raising left hand should be more or less circular. In moving right foot half a step forward, place it slowly in position, toes coming down first. Weight transfer must be coordinated with the raising of the left hand. Face 9 o'clock in the final position.

Form 6: curve back arms on both sides

(1) Turn torso slightly to the right, moving right hand down in a curve past abdomen and then upward to shoulder level, palm up and arm slightly bent. Turn left palm up and place toes of left foot on floor. Eyes first look to the right as body turns in that

direction, and then turn to look at left hand (Figure 12.1, 10).

(2) Bend right arm and draw hand past right ear before pushing it out with palm facing forward, while left hand moves to waist side, palm up. At the same time, raise left foot slightly and take curved step backward, placing down toes first and then the whole foot slowly on floor with toes turned outward. Turn body slightly to the left and shift weight onto left leg for a right empty stance, with right foot pivoting on toes until it points directly ahead. Look at right hand.

(3) Repeat movements in (1)–(2), reverse 'right' and 'left' (Figure 12.1, 10–11).

(4) Repeat movements in (1)–(2) and (3).

Points to remember: hands should move in curves when they are being pushed out or drawn back. While pushing out hands, keep waist and hips relaxed. The turning of the waist should be coordinated with hand movements. When stepping back, place toes down first and then slowly set the whole foot on the floor. Simultaneously with the body turn, point front foot directly ahead, pivoting on toes. When stepping back, the foot should move a bit sideways so that there will be a transverse distance between the heels. First look in the direction of the body turn and then turn to look at the hand in front. Face 9 o'clock in final position.

Form 7: grasp the bird's tail – left style

(1) Turn torso slightly to the right (11–12 o'clock), carrying right hand sideways up to shoulder level, palm, while left palm is turned downward. Look at left hand.

(2) Turn body slightly to the right (12 o'clock) and make a hold-ball gesture in front of right part of chest, right hand on top. At the same time, shift weight onto right leg and draw left foot to the side of right foot, toes on floor. Look at right hand (Figure 12.1, 12).

(3) Turn body slightly to the left, taking a step forward with left foot towards 9 o'clock for a left bow stance. Meanwhile, push out left forearm and back of hand up to shoulder level as if to fend off a blow, while right hand drops slowly to the side of right hip, palm down. Look at left forearm (Figure 12.1, 13).

Points to remember: keep both arms rounded while pushing out one of them. The separation of hands, turning of waist, and bending of leg should be coordinated.

(4) Turn torso slightly to the left (9 o'clock) while extending left hand forward, palm down. Bring up right hand until it is below left forearm, palm up. Then turn torso slightly to the right while pulling both hands down in a curve past abdomen – as if you were taking hold of an imaginary foe's elbow and wrist in order to pull back his body – until right hand is extended sideways at shoulder level, palm up, and left forearm lies across chest, palm turned inward. At the same time, shift weight onto right leg. Look at right hand (Figure 12.1, 13).

Points to remember: while pulling down hands, do not lean forward or protrude buttocks. Arms should follow the turning of the waist and move in a circular path.

(5) Turn torso slightly to the left as you bend right arm and place right hand inside left wrist; turn torso further to 9 o'clock as you press both hands slowly forward, palms facing each other and keeping a distance of about 5 cm between them, with left arm remaining rounded. Meanwhile, shift weight slowly onto left leg for a left bow stance. Look at left wrist.

Points to remember: keep torso erect when pressing hands forward. The movement of hands must be coordinated with the turning of waist and bending of front leg.

(6) Turn both palms downward as right hand passes over left wrist and moves forward and then to the right, until it is on the same level as the left hand. Separate hands shoulder-width apart and draw them back to the front of abdomen, palms facing obliquely downward. At the same time, sit back and shift weight onto right leg, which is slightly bent, raising toes of left foot. Look straight ahead (Figure 12.1, 14).

(7) Transfer weight slowly onto left leg while pushing palms in an upward-forward curve until wrists are shoulder high. At the same time, bend left leg for a left bow stance. Look straight ahead. Face 9 o'clock in the final position (Figure 12.1, 15).

Form 8: grasp the bird's tail – right style

Repeat movements (1)–(7), reversing 'left' and 'right' (Figure 12.1, 12–15).

Form 9: single whip

(1) Sit back and shift weight gradually onto left leg, turning toes of right foot inward. Meanwhile, turn body to the left (11 o'clock), carrying both hands leftward, with left hand on top, until left arm is extended sideways at shoulder level, palm facing outward, and right hand is in front of left ribs, palm facing obliquely inward. Look at left hand.

(2) Turn body to the right (1 o'clock), shifting weight gradually onto right leg and drawing left foot to the side of right foot, toes on floor. At the same time, move right hand up to the right until arm is at shoulder level. With right palm now turned outward, bunch fingertips and turn them downward from wrist for a 'hook hand', while left hand moves in a curve past abdomen up to the front of right shoulder, palm facing inward. Look at left hand (Figure 12.1, 16).

(3) Turn body to the left (10 o'clock) while left foot takes a step towards 8–9 o'clock for a left bow stance. While shifting weight onto left leg, turn left palm slowly outward as you push it forward with fingertips at eye level and elbow slightly bent. Look at left hand (Figure 12.1, 17).

Points to remember: keep torso erect, waist relaxed, and shoulders lowered. Left palm is turned outward slowly, not abruptly, as hand pushes forward. All transitional movements must be well coordinated. Face 9 o'clock in the final position, with right elbow slightly bent downward and left elbow directly above knee.

Form 10: wave hands like clouds – left style

(1) Shift weight onto right leg and turn body gradually to the right (1–2 o'clock), turning toes of left foot inward. At the same time, move left hand in a curve past abdomen to the front of right shoulder, palm turned obliquely inward, while right hand is opened, palm facing outward. Look at left hand (Figure 12.1, 18).

(2) Turn torso gradually to the left (10–11 o'clock), shifting weight onto left leg. At the same time, move left hand in a curve past face with palm turned slowly leftward, while right hand moves in a curve past abdomen up to the front of left shoulder, with palm slowly turning obliquely inward. As right hand moves upward bring right foot to the side of left foot so that they are parallel and

10–20 cm apart. Look at right hand (Figure 12.1, 19–20).

(3) Repeat movements in (1) and (2) (Figure 12.1, 18–20), reversing 'left' and 'right'.

(4) Repeat movements in (1)–(2) and (3) twice.

Points to remember: use your lumbar spine as the axis for body turns. Keep waist and hips relaxed. Do not let your body rise and fall abruptly. Arm movements should be natural and circular and follow waist movements. Pace must be slow and even. Maintain a good balance when moving lower limbs. Eyes should follow the hand that is moving past face. Body in final position faces 10–11 o'clock.

Form 11: single whip

(1) Turn torso to the right (1 o'clock), moving right hand to right side for a hook hand, while left hand moves in a curve past abdomen to the front of right shoulder, with palm turned inward. Shift weight onto right leg, toes of left foot on floor. Look at left hand (Figure 12.1, 21–22).

(2) Repeat movements in (3) under Form 9 (Figure 12.1, 16–17).

Points to remember: the same as those for Form 9.

Form 12: high pat on horse

(1) Draw right foot half a step forward and shift weight gradually onto right leg. Open right hand and turn up both palms, elbows slightly bent, while body turns slightly to the right (10–11 o'clock), and raising left heel gradually for a left empty stance. Look at left hand.

(2) Turn body slightly to the left (9 o'clock), pushing right palm forward past right ear, fingertips at eye level, while left hand moves to the front of left hip, palm up. At the same time, move left foot a bit forward, toes on floor. Look at right hand (Figure 12.1, 23).

Points to remember: keep torso erect, shoulders lowered and right elbow slightly downward. Face 9 o'clock in the final position.

Form 13: kick with right heel

(1) Turn torso slightly to the right (10 o'clock) and move left hand, palm up, to cross right hand at

wrist as you pull left foot a bit backward, toes on floor. Then separate hands, moving both in a downward curve with palms turned obliquely downward. Meanwhile, raise left foot to take a step towards 8 o'clock for a left bow stance, toes turned slightly outward. Look straight ahead.

(2) Continue to move hands in a downward–inward–upward curve until wrists cross in front of chest, with right hand in front and both palms turned inward. At the same time, draw right foot to the side of left foot, toes on floor. Look forward to the right.

(3) Separate hands, turning torso slightly to 8 o'clock and extending both arms sideways at shoulder level, with elbows slightly bent and palms turned outward. At the same time, raise right knee and thrust foot gradually towards 10 o'clock. Look at right hand (Figure 12.1, 24–25).

Points to remember: keep your balance. Wrists are at shoulder level when hands are separated. When kicking right foot, left leg is slightly bent and the kicking force should be focused on heel, with ankle dorsiflexed. The separation of hands should be coordinated with the kick. Right arm is parallel with right leg. Face 9 o'clock in the final position.

Form 14: strike opponent's ears with both fists

(1) Pull back right foot and keep thigh level. Move left hand in a curve to the side of right hand in front of chest, both palms turned inward. Bring both hands to either side of right knee, palm up. Look straight ahead (Figure 12.1, 26).

(2) Set right foot slowly on floor towards 10 o'clock, shifting weight onto right leg for a right bow stance. At the same time, lower hands to both sides and gradually clench fists; then move them backward with an inward rotation of arms before moving them upward and forward for a pincer movement that ends at eye level, with fists about 10–20 cm apart, knuckles pointing upward to the back. Look at right fist (Figure 12.1, 27–28).

Points to remember: hold head and neck erect. Keep waist and hips relaxed and fists loosely clenched. Keep shoulders and elbows lowered and arms rounded. Face 10 o'clock in the final position.

Form 15: turn and kick with left heel

Repeat movements in Form 13, but reversing 'right' and 'left'.

Form 16: push down and stand on one leg – left style

(1) Pull back left foot and keep thigh level. Turn torso to the right (7 o'clock). Hook right hand as you turn up left palm and move it in a curve past face to the front of right shoulder, turning it inward in the process. Look at right hand (Figure 12.1, 29).

(2) Turn torso to the left (4 o'clock), and crouch down slowly on right leg, stretching left leg sideways towards 2–3 o'clock. Move left hand down and to the left along the inner side of the left leg, turning palm outward. Look at left hand (Figure 12.1, 30–31).

Points to remember: when crouching down, turn toes of right foot slightly outward and straighten left leg with toes turned slightly inward, both soles flat on floor. Keep toes of left foot in line with right heel. Do not lean torso too much forward.

(3) Turn toes of left foot outward and those of right foot inward; straighten right leg and bend left leg onto which weight is shifted. Turn torso slightly to the left (3 o'clock) as you rise up slowly in a forward movement. At the same time, move left arm continuously to the front, palm facing right, while right hand drops behind the back, still in the form of a hook, with bunched fingertips pointing backward. Look at left hand (Figure 12.1, 32).

(4) Raise right knee slowly as right hand opens into palm and swings to the front past outside of right leg, elbow bent just above right knee, fingers pointing up and palm facing left. Move left hand down to the side of left hip, palm down. Look at right hand (Figure 12.1, 33).

Points to remember: keep torso upright. Bend the supporting leg slightly. Toes of the raised leg should point naturally downward. Face 3 o'clock in the final position.

Form 17: push down and stand on one leg – right style

Repeat Form 16 movements, but reversing 'left' and 'right'.

Form 18: work at shuttles on both sides

(1) Turn body to the left (1 o'clock) as you set left foot on floor in front of right foot, toes turned outward. With right heel slightly raised, bend both knees for a half 'cross-legged seat'. At the same time, make a hold-ball gesture in front of left part of chest, left hand on top. Then move right foot to the side of the foot, toes on floor. Look at left forearm (Figure 12.1, 34).

(2) Turn body to the right as right foot takes a step forward to the right for a right bow stance. At the same time, move right hand up to the front of right temple, palm turned obliquely upward, while left palm moves in a small leftward–downward curve before pushing it out forward and upward to nose level. Look at left hand (Figure 12.1, 35)

(3) Repeat (1)–(2), reversing 'right' and 'left'.

Points to remember: do not lean forward when pushing hands forward, nor raise shoulders when moving hands upward. Movements of hands should be coordinated with those of waist and legs. Keep a transverse distance of about 30 cm between heels in bow stance. Face 2 o'clock in the final position.

Form 19: needle at sea bottom

Draw right foot half a step forward, shift weight onto right leg, and move left foot a bit forward, toes on floor for a left empty stance. At the same time, with body turning slightly to the right (4 o'clock) and then to the left (3 o'clock), move right hand down in front of body, up to the side of right ear, and then obliquely downward in front of body, palm facing left and fingers pointing obliquely downward, while left hand moves in a forward–downward curve to the side of left hip, palm down. Look at floor ahead (Figure 12.1, 36).

Points to remember: do not lean too much forward. Keep head erect and buttocks in. Left leg is slightly bent. Face 3 o'clock in the final position.

Form 20: flash arm

Turn body slightly to the right (4 o'clock) and take a step forward with left foot for a left bow stance. At the same time, raise right hand with elbow bent to stop above and in front of right temple, palm turned obliquely upward with thumb pointing down, while left palm moves a bit upward and then pushes forward at nose level. Look at left hand (Figure 12.1, 37).

Points to remember: keep torso erect and waist and hips relaxed. Do not straighten arm when you push left palm forward. The movement should be synchronized with the taking of the bow stance, with your back muscles stretched. Keep a transverse distance of less than 10 cm between heels. Face 3 o'clock in the final position.

Form 21: turn to deflect downward, parry and punch

(1) Sit back and shift weight onto right leg. Turn body to the right (6 o'clock), with toes of left foot turned inward. Then shift weight again onto left leg. Simultaneously with body turn, move right hand in a rightward–downward curve and, with fingers clenched into fist, past abdomen to the side of left ribs with palm turned down, while left hand moves up to the front of forehead, with palm turned obliquely upward. Look straight ahead (Figure 12.1, 38).

(2) Turn body to the right (8 o'clock), bringing right fist up and then forward and downward for a back-hand punch, while left hand lowers to the side of left hip with palm turned down. At the same time, right foot draws towards left foot and, without stopping or touching floor, takes a step forward, toes turned outward. Look at right fist (Figure 12.1, 39).

(3) Shift weight onto right leg and take a step forward with left foot. At the same time, parry with left hand by moving it sideways and up to the front, palm turned slightly downward, while right fist withdraws to the side of right hip with forearm rotating internally and then externally, so that the fist is turned down and then up again. Look at left hand (Figure 12.1, 40).

(4) Bend left leg for a left bow stance as you strike out right fist forward at chest level, turning palm left-ward, while left hand withdraws to the side of right forearm. Look at right fist (Figure 12.1, 41).

Points to remember: clench right fist loosely. Follow the punch with right shoulder by extending it a bit forward. Keep shoulders and elbows lowered and right arm slightly bent. Face 9 o'clock in the final position.

Form 22: apparent close-up

(1) Move left hand forward from under right wrist and open right fist. Separate hands and pull them back

slowly, palms up, as you sit back with toes of left foot raised and weight shifted onto right leg. Look straight ahead.

(2) Turn palms down in front of chest as you pull both hands back to the front of abdomen and then push them forward and upward until wrists are at shoulder level, palms facing forward. At the same time, bend left leg for a left bow stance. Look straight ahead (Figure 12.1, 42).

Points to remember: do not lean backward or protrude buttocks when sitting back. Do not pull arms back straight. Relax your shoulders and turn elbows a bit outward. Hands should be no further than shoulder-width apart when you push them forward. Face 9 o'clock in the final position.

Form 23: cross hands

(1) Bend right knee, sit back, and shift weight onto right leg, which is bent at knee. Turn body to the right (1 o'clock) with toes of left foot turned inward. Following body turn move both hands sideways in a horizontal curve at shoulder level, palms facing forward and elbows slightly bent. Meanwhile, turn toes of right foot slightly outward and shift weight onto right leg. Look at right hand (Figure 12.1, 43).

(2) Shift weight slowly onto left leg with toes of right foot turned inward. Then bring right foot towards left foot so that they are parallel to each other and shoulder-width apart; straighten legs gradually. At the same time, move both hands down in a vertical curve to cross them at wrist, first in front of abdomen and then in front of chest, left hand nearer to body and both palms facing inward. Look straight ahead (Figure 12.1, 44–45).

Points to remember: do not lean forward when separating or crossing hands. When taking the parallel stance, keep body and head erect with chin tucked slightly inward. Keep arms rounded in a comfortable position, with shoulders and elbows held down. Face 12 o'clock in the final position.

Form 24: closing form

Turn palms forward and downward while lowering both hands gradually to the side of hips. Look straight ahead (Figure 12.1, 46).

Points to remember: keep whole body relaxed and draw a deep breath (exhalation to be somewhat prolonged) when you lower the hands. Bring left foot close to right foot after your breath is even. Walk about for complete recovery.

THE REAL FITNESS AND THERAPY PRINCIPLE

Based upon the Western view of human anatomy and biology, a practitioner may only accept a human being as a solid body, which contains many systems and organs made by different cells. However, according to the exploration of the human being's potential ability, TCM philosophy recognizes that a human being not only has a solid body, but also has an intangible energy body (meridian system, aura and energy system, etc.)[4].

We will now use an example to illustrate the way TCM philosophy looks at the body, and how it is different from the Western view. From Western understanding, according to the laws of dynamics and mechanical analysis, the organs inside the human body could not maintain their regular positions suspended in the cavity space of the body like blooming flowers or satellites in the universe, and would collapse if they only relied on the integrity of muscles and tendons. So the question is: what force holds these organs in place all the time with their active functions? TCM philosophy said that it is the bio-energy field that holds everything together in the proper place. Without the support of the energy field in cavity space, organs will collapse, and eventually wither and die. To TCM practitioners, the force of the energy field is as inherent as the cosmic force that holds the stars suspended in the universe.

Everyone knows that all plants on earth rely not only on water and nutrition from earth, but also on the products of photosynthesis, from chlorophyll in leaves reacting with sunlight, the energy from the universe. TCM philosophy believes that, like plants, human beings have a similar ability to exchange energy with the universe for life vitality, governed by the subconscious mind.

This basic principle of Taiji is greatly influenced by the *Yellow Emperor's Classic of Internal Medicine*, which says: 'Keep your mind in a quiet, calm and void state, guide your conscious deep inside, how could you get an illness?'[4], which means that human beings could prevent all diseases and achieve self-healing by balancing *Yin* and *Yang*, and improving the energy circulation of our bodies.

Within our solid body there are many spaces. TCM named four big spaces:

(1) The chest space between the spine and chest ribs (called upper *Jiao*);

(2) The upper abdomen space between the diaphragm and navel (called middle *Jiao*);

(3) The lower abdomen space between the navel and pubis (called lower *Jiao*);

(4) The back space between the spinal column and organs, from the top of the head to the coccyx (called back *Jiao*).

These spaces seem empty and void, but are actually full of invisible energy fields, like the universe space[9,10].

Both Western and Eastern medicine philosophies share the cell theory. The cells open to emit the energy out to the surrounding space and close to absorb the energy from the space. The human body is like a universe, called a 'small universe'. The cavity space is full of various kinds of energy, which congregates, collides, emerges, activates, circulates, and reacts to generate even newer energy. This is the human being's intangible body, including the aura light, meridian system, inside-organ light, etc. The energy in the space forms an energy field like magnetic or gravity fields. The density and characteristics of the energy field influence the activities of cells and finally the health condition[9,10].

TCM has recognized that the energy field in the body space greatly influences the health condition of human beings. The influence is very simple and strictly follows the law of physics, diffusion theory: whatever is in a higher concentration gradient will eventually diffuse into an area of lower concentration.

If the density of the energy field in the space outside the organ is too high, the energy existing inside cells cannot be emitted to the space, because the law of physics would not allow that to happen. If the energy cannot be emitted, the cells will not open properly, which in turn will cause the stagnation of the energy and retention of damp and heat inside the cells or organs. Further, this may cause inflammation and/or even mutation of the cells, eventually developing into cancers. If the density of the energy field in the space outside the organ is too low, it is easy for the cells to emit the energy from inside to the space, but difficult to absorb the energy from the space to inside. This will result in a lack of energy in the organ, showing weakness and low function of the organ. This theory is a new development in TCM, which can be called 'body space

medicine', and greatly promotes the further development of TCM[10].

The therapeutic techniques of TCM, such as some Chinese herb prescriptions, can change the energy pressure of the body space to promote lucidity ascending and turbidity descending, and can use the energy radiation of cell colonies as a dynamic force to improve human function and health condition. By the method of TCM treatment, the pressure difference and consistency difference of body space energy are increased to form a sharp contrast between void and solid, which will reach an 'extreme solid and extreme void' state, so establishing high pressure between them to induce energy movement with high-speed, powerful collisions among the cells and a great change in the energy field. As a result, the energy circulation becomes smooth and the human body returns to its normal condition[10]. With its similar underlying principles, Taiji practice can also help people in this way.

As an example, we will consider how to help patients with liver problems. According to the theory and healing methodology of TCM[10], if something is wrong (usually caused by energy stagnation) in the liver, the liver will not be treated directly. Instead, the stagnating energy in the space (the high-energy zone) around the liver will not only be cleaned, but also utilized at the same time. TCM recognizes that the stagnating energy around the liver is a potential dynamic energy, which, during its movement, might be able to generate a kind of promoting force to exert the following beneficial effects:

(1) Promoting and activating the cells around the heart, called 'wood can produce fire';

(2) Promoting the movement of the diaphragm, which plays an important role in the adjustment of lucidity ascending and turbidity descending;

(3) Enhancing liver function, which further promotes the returning circulation of hepatic portal veins.

Therefore, TCM can intelligently and fully utilize the dynamic energy produced by adjusting the energy stagnation[10]. With a similar therapeutic strategy, Taiji also can play an important role in health improvement.

The function of cell energy follows the 'entropy' principle of thermodynamics. The energy stagnation inside the cells is called 'positive entropy', which cannot be utilized. The cells can only emit this energy to other organs, benefiting them, and then the cells will be empty themselves, which state is called 'negative entropy'. Only in this situation can the cells absorb energy from outside and utilize it. This natural principle is entirely analogous to the Christian philosophy: to give and to receive. The more you give, the more you will get[9,10].

Therefore, life is simply the activation, circulation, and exchange of energy. If the movement of energy stops, life will end. If the movement of energy is stagnating in some parts, those parts of the body will become diseased. The original reason for illness is not infection by micro-organisms such as bacteria and viruses, but energy stagnation. The infection by viruses is the result of energy stagnation for a period of time. For example, in the early stage of lung infection there is no micro-organism in the lung, but the density of energy in the chest space is abnormally high and the energy inside the lung cells is stagnating. Once this condition has prevailed for a while, micro-organisms will appear. Thus TCM treats the patient holistically, with the emphasis on prevention and self-healing strategy. In most cases, TCM does not directly attack the abnormal organs or parts, like the allopathic approach, but adjusts the whole body to reinforce the energy circulation in the abnormal area[10].

From the point of view of the martial arts, every posture of original Taiji probably has some special meaning about fighting. However, in modern society, we are more concerned with the health purpose of Taiji. So the following discussion emphasizes on *Xin Fa* (the main principle of the mind–body practice technique for mind training) of *Dao Yin* (use the mind to guide the *Qi* movement) related to fitness and therapy beyond the original meaning.

For example, the commencing form requires you to relax the whole body, breathing evenly, slowly, deeply, and smoothly, calming the mind, imagining your body empty, loose, and melted with the universe; while waiting for the energy, push your hands up and exchange the energy with the outside by your skin pores. It is important to rid yourself of everyday burdens and enter the special Taiji training state at the beginning.

The hold-ball gesture is one of the most basic gestures and appears many times in the whole Taiji routine. Holding a concentrated *Qi* ball between two hands in front of abdomen (lower *Jiao*) or chest (upper or middle *Jiao*) can strengthen the energy in the Dantian area, which is the vital sea of human energy, or strengthen the energy in the chest by utilizing the outside energy field.

According to experiment and research, there are six meridian channels starting or ending on each hand, which are connected to the whole body. There is a strong energy field around the hands. When the hands are moving through or staying beside some part of the body,

they will influence the energy field of the body space, which will be stroked and changed.

During the Taiji movement, following the hand posture change, the energy function of corresponding organs will be adjusted. For instance:

- The *brush knee on both sides* (Form 4) will adjust the *Qi* circulation on the shoulders, neck, head, ears, and knees;

- The *grasp the bird's tail* (Form 7) will adjust the *Qi* circulation of three *Jiaos* (triple energizer) in the chest, and upper and lower abdomen, especially benefitting heart and kidneys;

- The *single whip* (Form 9) could open the *Bai Hui* to exchange the energy with the universe and help the energy circulation of the liver;

- *Wave hands like clouds* (Form 10) is mostly beneficial for the head, face, and all organs on the face;

- *Push down and stand on one leg* (Form 16) may let the energy of the universe connect and go through the body, especially benefitting the kidneys;

- *Cross hands* (Form 23) and *closing form* (Form 24) keep the energy stored in the body.

Of course, the Taiji program has a holistic function for fitness and therapy and is not separated for special parts or organs, but we can select some individual postures for at-a-standstill training.

SUGGESTIONS FOR TAIJI PRACTITIONERS

For health purposes, we pay more attention to the fitness and therapy functions of Taiji; the methods and requirements of Taiji practice are somewhat different from those of the martial arts.

(1) After practicing for a while and becoming familiar with the routine of physical movements, you should gradually slow down the movements. For instance the 'simplified Taiji (24 forms)'[8] usually needs only 5 minutes, but now you should practice it for half an hour or even longer. Only in this way can you have time to adjust your breath and put the *Xin Fa* in it to train your mind. It looks very simple but it is not easy, and needs time and effort to practice and train.

(2) Read some books about Chinese culture and philosophy, especially TCM, which will help you to understand the essence of Taiji *Xin Fa* and yourself.

(3) According to your individual situation, you may select one or more postures as the still style of training or meditation, as well as the regular Taiji practice.

(4) The last but not the least requirement is: cultivate your high moral standard of being responsible for society, and loving people and life. Only in this way can you keep your mind peaceful, and continue for your lifetime so as to improve your practice gradually and obtain benefits continuously.

SCIENTIFIC RESEARCH EVIDENCE

Taiji, although practiced for balancing mind and body to cultivate physical and psychologic health benefits in China for hundreds of years, has only recently gained the interest of researchers in Western countries as an alternative form of exercise. There is a steady increase in scientific research documenting the benefits of Taiji[11].

Literature reviews published between 1999 and 2001 began to offer conclusions based on reviews of clinical studies from a discipline or a focused clinical area perspective. Chen and Snyder[12] reviewed the growing evidence for Taiji as a potential nursing intervention, and concluded that Taiji practice had demonstrated benefits of balance improvement, falls prevention, cardiovascular enhancement, and stress reduction.

In a 2001 publication, Li *et al.*[13] reviewed 31 topic-related articles, including both controlled experimental clinical trials and descriptive or case–control studies, designed to assess either physiologic response or the general health and fitness effect of Taiji practice. These authors concluded that Taiji is 'a moderate intensity exercise that is beneficial to cardiopulmonary function, immune capacity, mental control, flexibility, and balance control; it improves muscle strength and reduces risk of falls in the elderly'[13]. Fascko and Grueninger[14] confirmed the conclusions of Li *et al.*[13] after an extensive review of the relevant literature assessing the effects of Taiji on physical and psychologic health that included over 30 relevant articles published before 2001.

In March 2004, Wang *et al.*[15] published a systematic review of Taiji as a therapeutic intervention for chronic conditions. They reviewed 9 randomized critical trials, 23 non-randomized controlled studies, and 15 observational studies. The authors concluded that Taiji has physiologic and psychosocial benefits and is also safe and effective in promoting balance control, flexibility, and cardiovascular and respiratory function in older patients with chronic conditions.

Most recently, a critical review by Klein and Adams[11] has offered an update on the current breadth and strength of research evidence regarding comprehensive therapeutic benefits of Taiji practice. Controlled research evidence was found to confirm the therapeutic benefits of Taiji practice with regard to improving quality of life, physical function including activity tolerance and cardiovascular function, pain management, balance and risk of falls reduction, enhancing immune response, and improving flexibility, strength, and kinesthetic sense. Figure 12.2 illustrates the distribution of therapeutic effect revealed in the 17 studies included in this critical analysis[11]. Of the dependent variables examined in controlled research, improved indicators of quality of life were most often assessed and validated. Quality of life is a complex construct encompassing multiple and overlapping domains of life function. The effects related to general health and well-being, psychologic, social, cognitive, and behavioral foci were grouped together under the collective subheading of quality of life. The second most frequently studied beneficial effect was improved physical function.

According to the critical analysis by Klein and Adams[11], of the > 300 topic-related articles identified through electronic search of the literature, > 200 of those titles were judged to be original, topic-relevant, scholarly or scientific reports. Of > 200 published reports examined, 17 controlled clinical trials[16–31] were judged to meet a high standard of methodologic rigor. Evidence from chronologic descriptive analysis of date of publications, number, and design rigor categorized as levels I–IV (controlled clinical trials; randomized clinical trials; observational case studies, pilot studies; and one group trial) reveals that the amount and strength of research evidence has exponentially increased in the past 5 years. Topic-related output within that time period has more than doubled the output for the previous 20 years (Figure 12.3)[11]. Geographic distribution of publications examined includes scientific studies conducted in the United Kingdom, United States, Canada, Australia, Israel, China, and South Korea, etc., showing the global clinical and research interest evident within this body of published literature.

Within the larger body of scientific reports and clinical studies including levels I–IV, a variety of clinical populations were studied. These included children with

Outcome effect

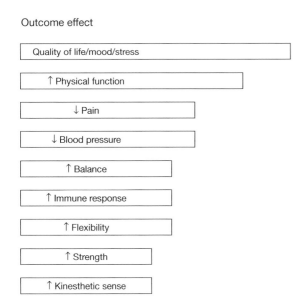

Figure 12.2 Summary of frequency of outcome benefits of Taiji practice from 17 clinical trials[11]. Physical function includes measures of improved aerobic conditioning

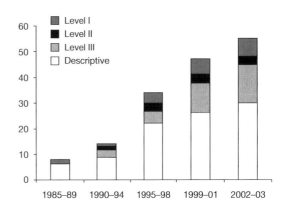

Figure 12.3 Pattern of proliferation of reports related to Taiji[11]. Sources: medical and health-related English language publications from the past two decades, subcategorized by level of evidence ($n = 154$ clinically based articles). Level I: randomized clinical trials (randomized group assignment); level II: controlled clinical trials (non-randomized group assignment); level III: correlational and observational, including one group or case study with pre-testing/post-testing; descriptive: scholarly discussions and literature reviews

attention deficit[32], adults with cardiac dysfunction [17,33,34], and individuals with rheumatoid arthritis[35–37], fibromyalgia[38], chronic back pain[18], osteoporosis[39,40], hemophilia[41], osteoarthritis[19,42], ankylosing spondylitis[43], Alzheimer's disease[44], multiple sclerosis[45,46], head trauma[47], Parkinson's disease[48], acquired immunodeficiency syndrome[44], and immune vulnerability[20].

A total of 1035 subjects participated in the 17 research studies included in the critical review by Klein and Adams[11]. Demographic distributions showed that at least 70% of the subjects were older adults, 60% or more were women, and >80% of subjects represented non-clinical populations. Taiji intervention most often conformed to characteristics of *Yang* style[49] and most often included simplified forms modified from the traditional *Yang* style 108 (movements) forms[50]. The lengths of Taiji intervention training ranged from 6 weeks to 12 months. Frequencies of supervised intervention ranged from once to three times weekly. Activity duration ranged from <15 minutes to >1 hour per session.

The Taiji groups did so well in all these clinical trials that an article in the *Journal of the American Geriatrics Society* recommended Taiji as a low-technology approach to conditioning that can be implemented at relatively low cost in widely distributed facilities throughout the community[51].

Beneficial effects on the cardiovascular and pulmonary system

Taiji exercise has recently gained the attention of Western researchers as a potential form of aerobic exercise[52]. The aerobic capacity provides important information about cardiopulmonary function. It is important to know the effect of Taiji exercise on aerobic capacity if clinicians want to recommend Taiji as an alternative form of aerobic exercise.

A study by Lai *et al.*[53] found that elderly Taiji exercisers showed a significant improvement in oxygen uptake compared to an age-matched control group of sedentary elders. The authors concluded that the data validated the practice of Taiji as a means of delaying the decline in cardiopulmonary function commonly considered 'normal' for aging individuals. In addition, Taiji was shown to be a suitable aerobic exercise for older adults[53]. Another study by Lai *et al.*[54] showed that Taiji is an aerobic exercise of moderate intensity. The other cardiovascular study comparing elderly Taiji practitioners with a sedentary group also found that the Taiji group showed a 19% higher peak oxygen uptake in comparison with their sedentary counterparts'[55].

In a year-long clinical trial[34], individuals who had recently undergone coronary bypass graft surgery ($n = 20$) were non-randomly assigned to either a Taiji practice group or a home-based exercise group after completion of an aerobic cycling cardiac phase II exercise program. The Taiji group members were found to exercise at an intensity of 48–57% of the maximum heart rate range. Graded exercise tests performed before and after 1 year of intervention found that those in the Taiji group showed a significant increase in the oxygen peak (10% increase) and peak work (12% increase) as compared with the control group.

One intriguing finding of the current research concerns evidence for a conditioning effect at low training heart rates. Young *et al.*[22] reported that, in a randomized control study, individuals regularly performing Taiji with a mean exercising heart rate of 75 beats/min had a similar beneficial cardiovascular response related to a decreased resting systolic blood pressure (mean change 7.0 mmHg) as compared to a group who participated in a walking program at a mean exercising heart rate of 112 beats/min (mean change in resting systolic blood pressure 8.4 mmHg).

In another cardiac-related study[17], an 8-week randomized clinical trial (*n* = 126) was conducted to evaluate the effect of Taiji practice for individuals with recent myocardial infarct. Results revealed that both the aerobic exercise group and the Taiji group showed a trend to reduced systolic blood pressure, but only the Taiji group showed a trend to reduced diastolic blood pressure, suggesting that Taiji practice outcome may be mildly superior to aerobic exercise programs for this clinical population.

The beneficial effects of Taiji on blood pressure, lipid profile, and anxiety status have been shown in a randomized controlled trial using a Taiji group and a group of sedentary lifestyle controls (in total 76 healthy subjects with blood pressure at high normal or stage I hypertension)[56]. After 12 weeks of Taiji training, at a frequency of three times per week, compared with controls, the treatment group showed a significant decrease in systolic blood pressure of 15.6 mmHg and in diastolic blood pressure of 8.8 mmHg. The serum total cholesterol level decreased by 15.2 mg/dl and high-density lipoprotein cholesterol increased by 4.7 mg/dl. Both trait anxiety and state anxiety were decreased. This study shows that, under well-designed conditions, Taiji exercise training could decrease blood pressure, result in favorable lipid profile changes, and improve subjects' anxiety status, suggesting that Taiji could be used as an alternative modality in treating patients with mild hypertension, with a promising economic benefit[56].

The collective research data, with respect to cardiovascular rehabilitation applications, provide evidence that Taiji practice is a safe, effective, low-intensity exercise regimen suitable for use as an exercise option with this vulnerable clinical population. Although the mechanism of effect is not fully understood, the possibility of increasing aerobic capacity without stressing a compromised cardiac system is desirable. Although collaborating clinical research is needed, there is theory-based rationale to generalize these conclusions to pulmonary rehabilitation as well.

Balance improvement and falls prevention

One of the challenges faced by people of advancing age is decreased postural stability and an increased risk for falls. There has been an increased interest and research over the past decade in using Taiji as an intervention exercise for improving postural balance and preventing falls in older people[57–61].

Improved balance is one of the most commonly attributed benefits of Taiji practice. One of the earliest well-known studies addressing this effect comes from a correlation study[15]. In the article published in 1992, Tse and Bailey[62] reported that balance abilities among experienced Taiji practitioners were observed to be superior to balance abilities among sedentary subjects. This early work became part of the justification for the belief that Taiji practice had a potential use in falls reduction programs. The findings in a controlled clinical study by Tsang and Hui-Chan[63] indicated that even 4 weeks of intensive Taiji training are sufficient to improve balance control in the elderly subjects. These improvements were maintained even at follow-up 4 weeks afterwards. Furthermore, the improved balance performance from week 4 onwards was comparable to that of experienced Taiji practitioners. A randomized controlled study by Jacobson *et al.*[30] observed improved lateral balance stability in healthy volunteer adults (*n* = 24) after just 12 weeks of Taiji practice.

In a prospective controlled clinical study (*n* = 38), Lan *et al.*[28] observed improved time on balance in the Taiji group as compared with controls. Subjects were older adults, and the study was conducted over a 12-month period. The mean frequency of practice was 4.6 times per week. The style of Taiji practiced in both studies was the 108 *Yang* form. Another randomized controlled trial showed that 6 months of low-intensity Taiji training could maintain the beneficial effects on balance and strength of 3 months of intensive balance and/or weight training[64]. Subjects were 110 healthy community dwellers (mean age 80). Significant gains persisted after 6 months of Taiji training. Most recently, in a 2005 publication by Tsang and Hui-Chan[65], the results demonstrate that long-term Taiji practitioners have better knee muscle strength, less body sway in perturbed single-leg stance, and greater balance confidence. Significant correlations among these three measures uncover the importance of knee muscle strength and balance control during perturbed single-leg stance in older adults' balance confidence in their daily activities.

Research evidence supporting the clinical use of Taiji in the area of falls prevention comes in major part from the well-known multiple-center FICSIT (Frailty and Injuries: Cooperative Studies on Intervention Techniques) studies[23,24]. The Atlanta group of the federally-funded, prospective FICSIT study randomly assigned community-dwelling older adults ($n = 200$) to one of three groups: a 15-week course of Taiji exercises, computerized balance training, or education (control). Subjects were grouped in cohorts of 10–12. The Taiji groups met twice weekly, and the balance training and control groups met once weekly. Biomedical, functional, and psychosocial outcome variables were measured immediately and 4 months post-intervention. Although improvements in physiologic response to exercise were found in the Taiji group, the most cited finding of the follow-up study report[24] is a 47% reduction in falls risk or delay of next fall in the Taiji group.

Whereas the FICSIT studies suggested a reduction in the number of falls, a more recent randomized clinical trial ($n = 163$) conducted in Australia provides primary evidence. Barnett *et al.*[66] randomly assigned community-dwelling elders known to have a risk of falling to either a control or a Taiji exercise group. The Taiji intervention consisted of weekly group instruction in Taiji combined with daily home practice. Physical performance and general health measures were assessed through repeated measures. After 1 year of Taiji practice, the experimental group was found to have a 40% reduction in falls. Furthermore, in a 6-month, randomized controlled trial ($n = 256$), Li *et al.*[67] concluded that improved functional balance through Taiji training is associated with subsequent reductions in fall frequency in older persons.

Recently, the potential benefits in healthy younger age cohorts and for wider aspects of health have also received attention. The study by Thornton *et al.*[68] documented prospective changes in balance and vascular responses for a community sample of middle-aged (33–55 years) women ($n = 34$). Dynamic balance measured by the Functional Reach Test was significantly improved following a 12-week Taiji exercise program (three times per week), with significant decreases in both mean systolic (9.71 mmHg) and diastolic (7.53 mmHg)

blood pressure, compared with sedentary controls. The data confirm that Taiji can be a good choice of exercise for middle-aged adults, with potential benefits for the aging as well as the aged.

Pain management in chronic back pain and osteoarthritis

Taiji practice has been shown to be effective in pain management. Bhatti *et al.*[18] reported preliminary findings of a randomized clinical trial ($n = 51$) investigating the efficacy of Taiji practice as a strategy to manage chronic pain. Adult subjects with a long-standing diagnosis of chronic back pain were assigned to either a control group or a Taiji exercise group. Study results after 6 weeks of Taiji practice revealed significant reductions in average, lowest, and worst pain experienced in the last week, measured on a visual analog scale, and self-reported improvements in mood.

Osteoarthritis (OA) is the most common form of arthritis in the United States and causes functional limitations and pain that worsen an individual's quality of life. Reducing the pain associated with OA is an important consideration in managing OA. In a randomized clinical trial of adults with lower limb OA ($n = 33$), Hartman *et al.*[19] found that, after 12 weeks of twice-weekly supervised exercise sessions, subjects in the Taiji group reported significant increases in self-efficacy for arthritis symptoms and improved satisfaction with general health as compared with controls. Similarly, Adler *et al.*[21] demonstrated, in a pilot study, that pain intensity scores for individuals ($n = 16$) with chronic arthritis pain decreased as compared with controls. The experimental intervention employed was a 10-week program of once-weekly supervised Taiji exercise.

The safety of Taiji for rheumatoid arthritis (RA) patients was evaluated in a study ($n = 55$) by Kirsteins *et al.*[36] RA patients, who received 1 hour of Taiji instruction once and twice a week for 10 weeks in two separate studies, showed no deterioration in their clinical disease activities compared with the corresponding controls. No significant exacerbation of joint symptoms using this weight-bearing form of exercise was observed. Taiji exercise appears to be safe for RA patients and may serve as an alternative for their exercise therapy and part of their rehabilitation program.

Improved flexibility, strength, and kinesthetic sense

In physical rehabilitation, there is agreement that a relationship can exist between a reduction in impairment and an improvement in function. Variables such as flexibility, strength, and kinesthetic sense are impairments that are associated with the complex construct of physical function. Evidence, generated through controlled clinical research, has demonstrated the beneficial effects of Taiji practice on these three variables. In addition to improvements in lateral body stability related to balance, Jacobson *et al.*[30] found significant improvements in leg extensor strength and kinesthetic sense in healthy subjects after 12 weeks of Taiji. Sun *et al.*[25] observed lower resting systolic and diastolic blood pressure and an increase in shoulder and knee flexibility in older adults who participated in a 12-week program of Taiji exercises as compared with randomly assigned controls. In a prospective controlled trial ($n = 36$), Chen and Sun[29] observed increased flexibility measured using a sit-n-reach box. The Taiji intervention employed in the latter study consisted of the *Yang*-style 24-movement form and was conducted over 16 weeks at a frequency of twice-weekly classes. Such demonstrations of beneficial changes in physical variables, often addressed as goals of physical rehabilitation, make Taiji practice an exercise intervention option with potential to achieve improved flexibility, strength, and kinesthetic sense.

Potential immune response effects

A potential immune response effect of Taiji practice is a frequent claim of Taiji enthusiasts. Preliminary evidence of this phenomenon was provided in a two-group study of Taiji practitioners who reported 6 years or more of regular Taiji practice. Xusheng *et al.*[31] found positive changes in humoral activity attributed to a single episode of practice and indications of humoral immunity associated with long-term Taiji practice.

Clinical evidence to assess the effect of Taiji practice on immune response within novice Taiji practitioners is just emerging. Both the incidence and severity of herpes zoster (shingles) increase markedly with increasing age in association with a decline in varicella-zoster virus (VZV)-specific cell-mediated immunity. In a randomized clinical trial ($n = 36$), Irwin *et al.*[20] exposed older adults with no previous Taiji experience to 15 weeks of practice at a frequency of three times a week. Results revealed a nearly 50% increase in VZV-specific, cell-mediated immunity in the Taiji group as compared with demographically similar, wait-list controls. In addition, Taiji was associated with improvements in physical health functioning, with the greatest effects in those older adults who had impairments of physical status at entry into the study. Evidence of this enhanced immune effect suggests clinical applications for the elderly who naturally experience some decline in immune response and for immune-suppressed individuals. This is an under-researched area with great potential.

Psychologic benefits

Taiji augments the exercise effects through the use of both mental concentration and relaxation of tension, which are thought to benefit emotional states. The psychologic benefits of Taiji practice have been shown in a number of studies[26,27,69,70] and reviews[15,71].

The stress reduction effects of Taiji exercise, as measured by heart rate, blood pressure, urinary catecholamine, and salivary cortisol level, were compared with groups of brisk walking, meditation, and quiet reading in a randomized controlled trial ($n = 96$) by Jin[27]. In general, it was found that the stress-reduction effect of Taiji characterized those physiologic changes produced by moderate exercise. Heart rate, blood pressure, and urinary catecholamine changes for the Taiji exercise group were similar to those changes occurring in the walking group. Additionally, the Taiji group expressed enhancement of 'vigor' and a reduction in anxiety states.

In a randomized controlled trial ($n = 118$), Li *et al.*[72] reported significant improvement in self-rated sleep quality in older adults with moderate sleep complaints who participated in a 24-week program of Taiji exercises (a 60-minute session, three times per week) as compared with low-impact exercise controls. Taiji appears to be effective as a non-pharmacologic approach to sleep enhancement for sleep-disturbed elderly individuals.

In summary, the scientific literature validating the physical and physiologic therapeutic effects of regular Taiji practice has grown exponentially over the past 5 years. The documented range of benefits validates the attribute of comprehensiveness of effect. The research evidence supports benefits of improved quality of life; physical function including cardiovascular, pain management, balance, and risk of falls reduction; enhanced immune response; and improved flexibility, strength, and kinesthetic sense attributed to Taiji practice. Based on evidence generated from controlled clinical trials, Taiji program exploration is justified in the areas of cardiac rehabilitation, chronic pain management, falls prevention programs, and health and wellness intervention for individuals who are immune suppressed and for fitness exercise programs for the elderly and individuals with exercise precautions due to arthritis-related conditions. Applied theory and preliminary research serve as justification for future controlled clinical study of the benefits of Taiji intervention with individuals with neurologic disease, particularly multiple sclerosis, parkinsonism, neurodevelopmental motor performance dysfunction, pulmonary insufficiency, and systemic musculoskeletal disorders. It is anticipated from existing research and the mind/body theoretic model that potential benefits from Taiji practice could be expanded to include both physical and behavioral applications.

CONCLUSIONS

Although most Western people know Taiji as a traditional Chinese physical exercise, it is in fact a kind of traditional Chinese Yanshenshu (a mind–body harmony technique for health improvement and longevity), an important part of TCM, when it is practiced with Taiji principles (the natural principles for harmonizing body and mind). The scientific literature validating the physical and physiologic therapeutic effects of regular Taiji practice has increased exponentially.

After practicing Taiji, most people realize that Taiji is not a regular physical exercise but a special body–mind training technique, which is closely related to traditional Chinese philosophy, culture, and medicine. The relationship between the human body and mind, as well as between human beings and the natural environment is greatly emphasized in Taiji. According to TCM literature, 'the advanced doctors would like to treat patients before their symptoms become detectable'[4]. Taiji, as a part of TCM, has been effectively applied in most of the Oriental countries for hundreds of years. It is a wiser, easier, more economic, convenient, and effective medicine.

How much benefit a practitioner obtains from Taiji practice depends on how much he understands the Taiji philosophy and whether he practices it correctly. Since the former is much more important than the latter, more details on Taiji *Xin Fa* (the main principle of the mind–body practice technique for mind training) have been introduced in this chapter. It is hoped that readers will be able to achieve greater benefit from Taiji practice after reading this chapter.

Following the Taiji principle, human beings could self-cultivate and reinforce the defensive system to prevent diseases and improve health through adjusting their inner bio-energy circulation, and harmonizing the body and mind with the universe. According to official statistics, China, where more people follow the Oriental health principle and utilize TCM including Taiji, used only about 1–2% of the health-care expense of the world to manage about 22% of the population of the world at the end of the 1970s and the beginning of the 1980s[73]. In contrast, a great part of the GDP is used for health care in most Western countries. According to one report[74], about 6–7% of that GDP (about 1.3 trillion USD/year) was used for health care in the United States in recent years. If more Western people were to apply Taiji as a complementary and alternative health-care technique, significant benefits would be achieved.

References

1. Delza S. Taiji Chuan. New York: State University of New York Press, 1985
2. Gu L. Taijiquan Technique. Shanghai: Shanghai Educational Publishing House, 1982
3. Yuan F. The historical origin of Taijiquan has been discovered after misunderstood for hundreds of years. Da He News, China, 26 March 2005
4. Veith I. The Yellow Emperor's Classic of Internal Medicine [translation]. Berkeley and Los Angeles: University of California Press, 2002
5. Cheng X. Chinese Acupuncture and Moxibustion. Beijing: Foreign Languages Press, 1987
6. Watson B. Lao-Tzu Tao Te Ching. Indianapolis: Hackett Publishing Company, 1984
7. Yu J. Taiji Healthy Express. Beijing: Chinese Tourism Publishing House, 2005
8. China Sports Magazine. Simplified Taijiquan. Beijing: People's Spots Publishing House of China, 1999
9. Guo Z. Chinese Intelligent Medicine. Shijiazhuang: Hua-Shen Publishing House, China, 1992
10. Guo Z. The Introduction of Body Space Medicine. 4th Annual CAMera Research Sysposium – Building CAM Research: Case by Case, Edmonton, Canada, June, 2005
11. Klein PJ, Adams WD. Comprehensive therapeutic benefits of Taiji: a critical review. Am J Phys Med Rehabil 2004; 83: 735–45
12. Chen K, Snyder M. A research-based use of Tai Chi/movement therapy as a nursing intervention. J Holistic Nurs 1999; 17: 267–79
13. Li F, Harmer P, McAuley E, et al. An evaluation of the effects of tai chi exercise on physical functioning among older persons: a randomized clinical trial. Anal Behav Med 2001; 23: 139–46

14. Fascko D, Grueninger W. T'ai Chi Ch'uan and physical and psychological health: a review. Clin Kinesiol 2001; 55: 4–12

15. Wang C, Collet JP, Lau J. The effect of Tai Chi on health outcomes in patients with chronic conditions: a systematic review. Arch Intern Med 2004; 164: 493–501

16. Lumsden DB, Baccala A, Martire J. T'ai chi for osteoarthritis: an introduction for primary care physicians. Geriatrics 1998; 53: 84–8

17. Channer K, Barrow D, Barrow R, et al. Changes in hemodynamic parameters following Tai Chi Chuan and aerobic exercise in patients recovering from acute myocardial infarction. Postgrad Med J 1996; 72: 349–51

18. Bhatti TI, Gillin JC, Atkinson JH, et al. T'ai Chi Chih as a treatment for chronic low back pain: a randomized, controlled study. Proceedings of the Third Annual Alternative Therapies Symposium Creating Integrated Healthcare, San Diego, 1–4 April 1998. Am Assoc Crit Care Nurs 1998; 7: 216–18

19. Hartman CA, Manos TM, Winter C, et al. Effects of t'ai chi training on function and quality of life indicators in older adults with osteoarthritis. J Am Geriatr Soc 2000; 48: 1553–9

20. Irwin MR, Pike JL, Cole JC, et al. Effects of a behavioral intervention, Tai Chi Chih, on varicella-zoster virus specific immunity and health functioning in older adults. Psychosom Med 2003; 65: 824–30

21. Adler P, Good M, Roberts B, et al. The effects of Tai Chi on older adults with chronic arthritis pain. J Nurs Scholarship 2000; 32: 7

22. Young D, Appel L, Jee SH, et al. The effects of aerobic exercise and T'ai Chi on blood pressure in older people: Results of a randomized trial. J Am Geriatr Soc 1999; 47: 277–8

23. Wolf SL, Barnhart HX, Ellison GL, et al. The effect of Tai Chi Quan and computerized balance training on postural stability in older subjects: Atlanta FICSIT Group. Frailty and Injuries: Cooperative Studies on Intervention Techniques. Phys Ther 1997; 77: 371–81

24. Wolf SL, Barnhart HX, Kutner NG, et al. Reducing frailty and falls in older persons: an investigation of Tai Chi and computerized balance training. Atlanta FICSIT Group. Frailty and Injuries: Cooperative Studies of Intervention Techniques. J Am Geriatr Soc 1996; 44: 489–97

25. Sun WY, Dosch M, Gilmore GD, et al. Effects of Tai Chi Chuan program on Hmong American older adults. Educ Gerontol 1996; 22: 161–7

26. Brown DR, Wang Y, Ward A, et al. Chronic psychological effects of exercise and exercise plus cognitive strategies. Med Sci Sports Exerc 1995; 27: 765–75

27. Jin P. Efficacy of Tai Chi, brisk walking, meditation, and reading in reducing mental and emotional stress. J Psychosom Res 1992; 36: 361–70

28. Lan C, Lai J, Chen S, et al. 12-month Tai Chi training in the elderly: its effect on health fitness. Med Sci Sports Exerc 1998; 30: 345–51

29. Chen WW, Sun WY. Tai Chi Chuan, an alternative form of exercises for health promotion and disease prevention for older adults in the community. Int Q Comm Health Educ 1997; 16333–9

30. Jacobson B, Ho-Chen C, Cashel C, et al. The effect of T'ai Chi Chuan training on balance, kinesthetic sense, and strength. Percept Motor Skills 1997; 84: 27–33

31. Xusheng S, Yugi X, Zhu R. Detection of ZC rosette-forming lymphocytes in the healthy aged with Taichiquan (88 style) exercise. J Sports Med Phys Fitness 1990; 30: 401–5

32. Hernandez-Reif M, Field TM, Thimas E. Attention deficit hyperactivity disorder: benefits from Tai Chi. J Bodywork Mov Ther 2001; 5: 30–3

33. Fontana JA, Colella C, Baas LS, et al. T'ai Chi Chih as an intervention for heart failure. Nurs Clin North Am 2000; 35: 1031–47

34. Lan C, Chen S, Lai J, et al. The effect of Tai Chi on cardiorespiratory function in patients with coronary artery bypass surgery. Med Sci Sports Exerc 1999; 31: 634–8

35. van Deusen J, Harlowe D. The efficacy of the ROM dance program for adults with rheumatoid arthritis. Am J Occup Ther 1987; 41: 90–5

36. Kirsteins A, Dietz F, Hwang S. Evaluating the safety and potential use of a weight-bearing exercise, Tai Chi Chuan, for rheumatoid arthritis patients. Am J Phys Med Rehabil 1991; 70: 136–41

37. Ng G, Yeung D. Tai-Chi Chuan Training for Rehabilitation of Rheumatoid Arthritis. Poster presentation at the 14th International WCPT Congress 2003, Barcelona, 7–12 June 2003

38. Taggart HM, Arsianian CL, Bae S, et al. Effects of T'ai Chi exercise on fibromyalgia symptoms and health-related quality of life. Orthop Nurs 2003; 22: 353–60

39. Qin L, Au S, Choy W, et al. Regular Tai Chi Chuan exercise may retard bone loss in postmenopausal women: a case-control study. Arch Phys Med Rehabil 2002; 83: 1355–9

40. Prior JC, Barr SI, Chow R, et al. Physical activity as therapy for osteoporosis. CMAJ 1996; 155: 940–4

41. Danusantoso H, Heijnen L. Tai Chi Chuan for people with haemophilia. Haemophilia 2001; 7: 437–40

42. Song R, Lee EO, Lam P, et al. Effects of tai chi exercise on pain, balance, muscle strength, and perceived difficulties in physical function in older women with osteoarthritis: a randomized clinical trial. J Rheumatol 2003; 30: 2039–44

43. Koh TC. Tai chi and ankylosis spondylitis: a personal experience. Am J Chinese Med 1982; 10: 59–61

44. Briggs N. Teachers Exchange and Success Stories. Presented at Taijiquan Teachers Exchange Weekend, Douglassville, PA, 24–26 October 2003

45. Mills N, Allen J: Mindfulness of movement as a coping strategy in multiple sclerosis: a pilot study. Gen Hosp Psychiatry 2002; 22: 425–31

46. Husted C, Pham L, Hekking A, et al. Improving quality of life for people with chronic conditions: the example of T'ai Chi and multiple sclerosis. Altern Ther Health Med 1999; 5: 70–4

47. Shapira MY. Tai Chi Chuan practice as a tool for rehabilitation of severe head trauma: three case reports. Arch Phys Med Rehabil 2001; 82: 1283–5

48. Calkins J. Taiji and Parkinson's. Presented at Taijiquan Teachers Exchange Weekend, Douglassville, PA, 24–26 October 2003

49. Liang SY, Wu WC. Tai Chi Chuan, 2nd edn. Roslindale, MA: YMAA, 1996

50. Zhongwen F. Mastering Yang Style Tai Chi. Berkeley, CA: North Atlantic Books, 1999

51. Blair SN, Garcia ME. Get up and move: a call to action for older men and women. J Am Geriatr Soc. 1996; 44: 599–600

52. Taylor-Piliae RE, Froelicher ES. Effectiveness of Tai Chi exercise in improving aerobic capacity: a meta-analysis. J Cardiovasc Nurs 2004; 19: 48–57

53. Lai JS, Lan C, Wong MK. Two-year trends in cardiorespiratory function among older Tai Chi Chuan practitioners and sedentary subjects. J Am Geriatr Soc 1995; 43: 1222–7

54. Lai JS, Wong MK, Lan C, et al. Cardiorespiratory responses of Tai Chi Chuan practitioners and sedentary subjects during cycle ergometry. J Formos Med Assoc 1993; 92: 894–9

55. Lan C, Lai JS, Wong MK, et al. Cardiorespiratory function, flexibility, and body composition among geriatric Tai Chi Chuan practitioners. Arch Phys Med Rehabil 1996; 77: 612–16

56. Tsai JC, Wang WH, Chan P, et al. The beneficial effects of Tai Chi Chuan on blood pressure and lipid profile and anxiety status in a randomized controlled trial. J Altern Compl Med 2003; 9: 747–54

57. Gillespie LD, Gillespie WJ, Robertson MC, et al. Interventions for preventing falls in elderly people. Cochrane Database Syst Rev 2003; 4: CD000340

58. Wu GJ. Evaluation of the effectiveness of Tai chi for improving balance and preventing falls in the older populations: a review. J Am Geriatr Soc 2002; 50: 746–54

59. Gillespie LD, Gillespie WJ, Robertson MC, et al. Interventions for preventing falls in elderly people. Cochrane Database Syst Rev 2001; 3: CD000340

60. Wolf SL, Barnhart HX, Kutner, NG, et al. Selected as the best paper in the 1990s: reducing frailty and falls in older persons: an investigation of Tai Chi and computerized balance training. J Am Geriatr Soc 2003; 51: 1794–1803

61. Choi JH, Moon JS, Song R. Effects of Sun-style Tai Chi exercise on physical fitness and fall prevention in fall-prone older adults. J Advanced Nurs 2005; 51: 150–7

62. Tse SK, Bailey DM. T'ai Chi and postural control in the well elderly. Am J Occup Ther 1992; 6: 295–300

63. Tsang WW, Hui-Chan CW. Effect of 4- and 8-wk intensive Tai Chi training on balance control in the elderly. Med Sci Sports Exerc 2004; 36: 648–57

64. Wolfson L, Whipple R, Derby C, et al. Balance and strength training in older adults: intervention gains and Tai Chi maintenance. J Am Geriatr Soc 1996; 44: 498–506

65. Tsang WW, Hui-Chan CW. Comparison of muscle torque, balance, and confidence in older Tai Chi and healthy adults. Med Sci Sports Exerc 2005; 37: 280–9

66. Barnett A, Smith B, Lord SR, et al. Community-based group exercise improves balance and reduces falls in at-risk older people: a randomized controlled trial. Age Aging 2003; 32: 407–14

67. Li F, Harmer P, Fisher KJ, et al. Tai Chi: improving functional balance and predicting subsequent falls in older persons. Med Sci Sports Exerc 2004; 36: 2046–52

68. Thornton EW, Sykes KS, Tang WK. Health benefits of Tai Chi exercise: improved balance and blood pressure in middle-aged women. Health Prom Int 2004; 19: 33–8

69. Jin P. Changes in heart rate, noradrenaline, cortisol and mood during tai chi. J Psychosom Res 1989; 33: 197–206

70. Ross MC, Bohannon AS, Davis DC, et al. The effects of a short-term exercise program on movement, pain, and mood in the elderly. Results of a pilot study. J Holistic Nurs 1999; 17: 139–47

71. Sandlund ES, Norlander T. The effects of Tai Chi Chuan relaxation and exercise on stress and well-being. Int J Stress Manage 2000; 7: 139–49

72. Li F, Fisher KJ, Harmer P, et al. Tai Chi and self-rated quality of sleep and daytime sleepiness in older adults: a randomized controlled trial. J Am Geriatr Soc 2004; 52: 892–900

73. Chen Yongjie, Jia Qian. The diagnoses for Chinese medicine and herbology development. People's Daily, Beijing, China, 2003

74. Eisenberg DM, Davis RB, Ettner SL, et al. Trends in alternative medicine use in the United States, 1990–1997: results of a follow-up national survey. J Am Med Assoc 1998; 280: 1569–75

Qigong

13

N. J. Manek and C. Lin

A healer in every family and a world without pain

INTRODUCTION

Over the preceding decade, Western medical researchers have increasingly turned their gaze on traditional medical systems. Much of the interest and funding for such research has come on the heels of David Eisenberg's 1993 report that vast numbers of Americans were turning to a range of alternative health practices[1]. The phenomenon appears to be increasing, as shown by a replication in 1997 of a national survey carried out in 1990[2]. There is a growing acceptance of the principles of Traditional Chinese Medicine (TCM) in the Western world[3,4]. Anyone studying TCM will be introduced to the ancient Chinese notions of harmony and well-being that have been a sustaining theme of Chinese culture. These ancient notions not only survive until today but also remain viable approaches to both personal health care and medical intervention. Qigong, a key component of Chinese medical practice, contains a balance between body, mind, and spirit and works well with other healing modalities, complementing them. Qigong, like Western biofeedback therapy, is a systematic training in psychophysiologic self-regulation and helps develop skills that can have very broad applications. The central idea of Qigong is working with the life force or universal energy. This force, although invisible, has measurable effects, as the science of quantum physics is beginning to discover. Science and the venerable tradition of Qigong are joining hands, and helping usher in a new era of energy medicine[5,6].

A BRIEF HISTORY OF QIGONG

In the thousands of years of development of Qigong many texts have been written about the practice and philosophy of this ancient art. One of the key texts is *The Yellow Emperor's Classic of Internal Medicine*, dating back to the Han Dynasty (206 BC to AD 220)[7]. It is considered a medical bible in Chinese medicine. In this text there are explicit techniques for guiding the *Qi* and the importance of fundamental elements for modern day Qigong were clearly recognized then as they are today: breathing, body postures, and the mind. A set of fitness exercises called 'the five-animal play', which mimicked the movements and gestures of the tiger, deer, bear, monkey, and bird, were developed to improve circulation and prevent disease, and specific energy techniques were expounded for a variety of chronic illnesses. Thus, early Chinese medical practice propounded oneness with nature, i.e. the universe, and combined concepts of philosophy and religion. Three main features that recur with great frequency in Chinese religious philosophy are the concepts of:

(1) Tao;

(2) *Yin* and *Yang*; and

(3) The theory of the five elements: metal, water, wood, fire, and earth.

A further description of Qigong is contained in the Daoist philosophical works of the third and fourth centuries BC. In the classic *Tao Te Ching* (Dao De Jing; The Middle Way), Lao Tzu[8], the patriarch of Daoism, writes:

Can you coax your mind from its wandering and keep to the original oneness?

Can you let your body become supple as a newborn child's?

Daoism, China's original spiritual tradition, is pragmatic, emphasizing simplicity and harmony with nature. The references to Tao (Dao) are generally in conjunction with the two component parts of the universe, the *Yin* and the *Yang*, which come from 'emptiness' and thus eventually return to the 'emptiness'. In order to achieve a balance of *Yin* and *Yang* energy and keep the mind and body healthy, Daoists practiced and developed many styles of Qigong.

There are thousands of individual monastic or family styles of Qigong and many are steeped in mysticism. The term 'Qigong' is actually quite recent and has been used in its present specialized sense only since the twentieth century. The therapeutic (medical) use of the term dates from 1936, and since that time Qigong has come to represent most Chinese self-healing exercises and meditation disciplines[9]. The period of modern Qigong practice and research (from the 1980s to the present) has gradually emerged into a practice found in the public domain and scientific research. As Qigong has gained increasing popularity in therapeutic use in Western cultures, it has stimulated discussion, research, and clinical practice as a form of complementary therapy. There is also growing interest in its application in the community and social arena – for example, a recent pilot study reported on the feasibility of integrating Qigong into the daily school curriculum and school-children who were taught Qigong had improved social behavior and grades[10].

MODERN PERSPECTIVES IN ENERGY MEDICINE

Conventional or Western medicine considers that the cellular organisms operate largely via the following sequence of reactions:

$$\text{function} \Leftrightarrow \text{structure} \Leftrightarrow \text{chemistry}$$

When an organ is not functioning properly, the cause is often ascribed to structural defects in the cellular system arising out of chemical imbalances. However, the emerging mind–body field has gradually moved beyond the notion of segmented biologic systems, to one of inseparable components of a dynamic system. Although the immune system is clearly central to the healing endeavor, the healing system is larger than one subset of organs, tissue, and cells: it encompasses the integral activities of virtually all biologic subsystems, including those associated with 'mind' and 'emotion'[11]. However, to ask a deeper question: What is the immaterial substrate that animates and propels the entire healing system? Rachel Naomi Remen refers to it as the 'life force.' Levin hypothesizes the role of a 'superempirical force', an energetic phenomenon that is tapped or accessed through committed spiritual or religious practice[12]. Levin emphasizes that, in future, this force may no longer be considered superempirical, but empirical. The yogic, Qigong, and Sufi traditions, among others, have recognized this force from time immemorial.

In the West, some scientists in the field of quantum physics have been successful in measuring bioenergy fields[5]. It appears that from a deep meditative state, humans can, by specific intention, have a dramatic effect on the characteristics of physical reality[5]. It has been shown that a simple human intention can be embedded into an electronic device which can then statistically influence, to a significant degree, the results of either an *in vivo* or an *in vitro* biologic target, depending upon the nature of the intention[13]. Examples of target materials selected were the pH of water, a liver enzyme, alkaline phosphatase (ALP), and the major cell energy store, adenosine triphosphate (ATP)[14]. A new category of communicative channel, then, is available in nature that is able to drive an energetic process that alters properties of materials in line with the specific intention. These experimental data usher in a new era for quantum physics' scientific investigation of the mysteries of nature's life force, and a shift in the paradigm of the connection between matter and energy[5]. One must now deal with the following equation:

$$\text{mass} \Leftrightarrow \text{energy} \Leftrightarrow \text{consciousness}$$

Einstein quantified the connection between the first two terms of this equation. There is abundant evidence of a connection between the last two terms and, although at present physics cannot quantify it, consciousness must be included in any discussion of energy and conservation laws. While these studies in physics do not test Qigong directly, they examine correlates of healing energy and it is reasonable to infer that scientists are therefore also measuring correlates of *Qi*.

QIGONG DEFINED

The word 'Qigong' (pronounced chee gong) is a combination of two ideas: *Qi* is the fundamental 'vital energy' or 'dynamic force' of the entire manifest universe, the basic energy force that comprises all matter and animates all living beings. There is no English equivalent for *Qi*. It has also been referred to as Chi, *Ki* in Japan, and *Prana* in the Hindu tradition, which forms the basis of yoga and Ayurvedic medicine. 'Gong' means the skill of working with, or cultivating, self-discipline, perseverance, and achievement through which one is able to strengthen and direct this vital energy. The *Qi* tends to flow unobstructed through the body and thus promotes health and well-being. Alteration of this energy by blockage of flow can result in states of excess or deficient energy. This abnormal state of energy relates to subsequent disease or injury[15]. An improvement in *Qi* balance is the ultimate objective of Qigong practice. This skill, then, is acquired through regular practice of specific exercises which are based on three main principles:

(1)   Harmonizing or tuning the breath;

(2)   Harmonizing or tuning one's posture and body movements;

(3)   Harmonizing or tuning one's mind.

It should be noted that the practices described by the term Qigong are extraordinarily diverse: they include practices designed to aid in martial arts, practices working with sound and visualization, meditations to achieve spiritual purification, and practices designed to increase health and vitality.

THE MERIDIAN SYSTEM

It is believed that the *Qi* vital energy circulates throughout the human body in a system of channels and collaterals, smaller channels that branch off to reach all parts of the body, that are generally the same as the meridian system used in acupuncture. There are 12 main channels in the body (Table 13.1) and eight reservoir channels. The distribution of the meridian system is related to both internal and external structures and is not solely determined by nerves, muscles, or blood vessels. Most acupuncture points and meridians correspond to the high electrical conductance points on the body surface[16]. During Qigong the conductivity of acupuncture points – that is, the ability of these points to conduct an electric charge – changes dramatically. When a Qigong practitioner concentrates on a particular acupoint, the skin resistance at that point goes down relative to other acupoints on the body[9]. It has been shown that the application of polarized agents to both the acupuncture points

Table 13.1   The major energy channels (meridians) in Qigong

Organ system	Meridian
Lung	starts on chest in front of the shoulder, ends in thumb
Heart	starts under armpit, ends in little finger
Large intestine	starts in index finger, ends at side of nostril
Stomach	starts under the eye, ends in second toe
Spleen	starts in big toe, ends at side of chest
Small intestine	starts in little finger, ends in front of ear
Urinary bladder	starts at inside corner of the eye, ends in little toe
Kidney	starts on sole of foot, ends at top of the chest
Gallbladder	starts at outside corner of the eye, ends in fourth toe
Liver	starts in big toe, ends on front of chest or below nipple
Triple heater*	starts in the fourth finger, ends by outside corner of eyebrow
Heart constrictor**	starts beside the nipple, ends in middle finger

*An area described as between the diaphragm and lower abdomen and containing the pancreatic gland. It may also be described as a hollow organ that separates into upper, middle, and lower portions and functions to regulate the activities of other viscera and participates in the control of food metabolism. There is no real anatomic equivalent in the Western tradition

**Described by Master Lin (personal communication) as a meridian envelope or case akin to the pericardium serving as protection for the heart. Qigong meridian considers that the central nervous system function has some relation to the pericardium and to non-acupuncture points on a meridian illicits the pressure pain reaction. However, in the case of the acupuncture points the effect usually lasts considerably longer compared to non-acupuncture points[17]. Other electro-dermal techniques such as Electropuncture According to Voll (EAV) have provided information on the energy distribution of the meridians[18]. Using a low-voltage current, EAV measures the electric conductance of the skin above individual acupuncture points. Diagnosis depends on measuring the relative electric conductance and its time dependence. A diagnostic criterion of degeneration of an organ is an indicator drop when the conductance decreases from an apparent maximum value and levels off during measurement[18]. Qigong practice appears to decrease standard deviations of individual electro-dermal responses[19] which suggest *Qi* balance. Interestingly, a circadian rhythm can be observed in that larger average electro-dermal responses occur in the afternoons compared to the mornings[19].

Manipulation of the meridian system by acupuncture, mechanical pressure, and Qigong activates the self-organizing system of an organism. The major *Qi* meridian energy points are distributed on the body surface (Figures 13.1 to 13.3)[20]. A light stroking of the arms, legs, head, and torso along the meridians improves the circulation of the energy, and similarly a state of 'awakening of the body' may be achieved through light tapping of the body along the meridian lines[21].

Many factors either individually or in combination create energy blockages in the meridian system. These include emotions, poor or incorrect nutrition, environmental and weather changes, wrong medication, and injury[21]. The emotions, like *Qi,* must be fluid and changeable, not stuck in extreme positions. These factors contribute to energy blockages and imbalance in *Yin* and *Yang* energy (Table 13.2). *Yin* is earthy energy, female, passive, and spiritual. *Yang* energy is male, active, and physical. *Qi* is considered neutral, at the midpoint between the positive and negative pole. It is neither *Yin* nor *Yang* itself, yet is capable of functioning in either capacity.

THE ART OF PRACTICE

Cultivation of Qi energy

Qigong is called 'practice' or 'training' because, unlike medication, it is not 'prescribed' for a limited period of time, but, rather, practiced daily. This is easy to do

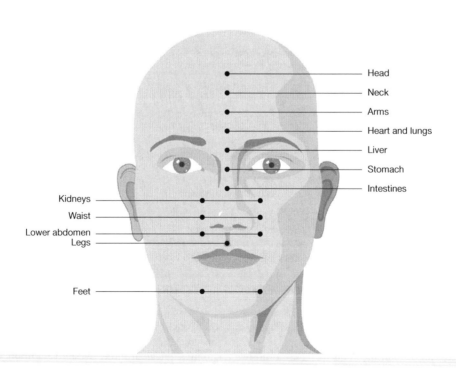

Figure 13.1 Energy points on head and face with corresponding organ systems

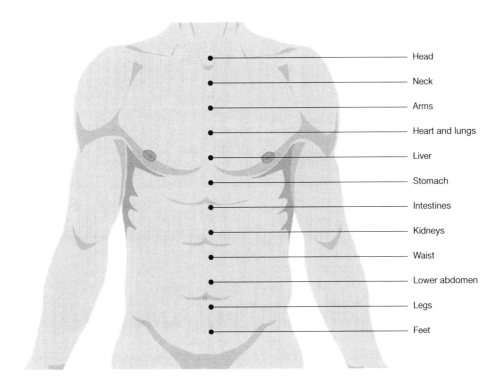

Figure 13.2 Energy points on chest and torso with corresponding organ systems

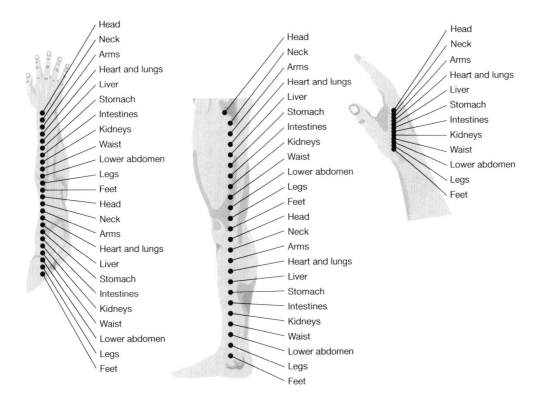

Figure 13.3 Energy points on the upper arm, lower extremity, and hand with corresponding organ systems

Table 13.2 Characteristics of *Yin* and *Yang* energy

Yin	Yang
Female	Male
Moon	Sun
Earth	Heaven
Night	Day
Water	Fire
Cold	Heat
Dampness	Dryness
Darkness	Light
Flows downwards	Flows upwards

because Qigong is as enjoyable as any exercise, yet does not require a great expenditure of time or money. Qigong incorporates both physical and meditative elements, which makes it distinctly different from conventional treadmill or bicycle workouts (Table 13.3). It is relatively non-strenuous and low-impact, and is characterized by postural alignment and relaxed movements coupled with diaphragmatic breathing, characteristics which in themselves are conducive to an enhanced feeling of well-being[21]. Students generally practice an average of 20 to 40 minutes each day. There is emphasis on a gradual progression of movement paced to suit each individual; inability to perform a movement is not regarded in any sense as failure. Movements are encouraged to be performed slowly, in a relaxed graceful fashion. The practice also involves bringing attention to areas of muscular tension. Qigong includes standing, seated, and supine methods. With only slight adjustments in technique, it is possible to practice most standing exercises from a seated or lying down position. This makes Qigong an ideal exercise for the disabled. Beyond these advantages, Qigong is easy to implement (e.g. indoors or outdoors) in clinical care or community settings[10] and promotes socialization. Other concepts of cultivating *Qi* involve eating nutritious food and achieving mental peace with meditation.

Mindful meditation

The goal of Qigong meditation is to cultivate a stable and non-reactive awareness of one's internal (e.g. cognitive–affective–sensory) and external (social–environmental) experiences as contrasted with the tendency humans have to react quite reflexively to the myriad situations (whether stressful or challenging, or not) encountered in daily life[22]. Meditative Qigong has

the goal of 'a sound mind in a sound body' and thus is always practiced as a complement to medical Qigong. Qigong meditation includes two types of practices. The first is 'entering tranquility', which means training the mind to be silently aware without any particular point of focus. It is 'emptiness'. The other kind of Qigong meditation consists of healing visualization and concentration techniques. The movement practice can assist in the experience of achieving stillness and achieving deeper states of meditation. Chants or sounds may also be used to aid in the meditation and guide the Qigong visualization. In the visualization, there is conscious production of mental images and the body is visualized as fully healed or nourished with healing energy.

THE SCIENTIFIC EVIDENCE TO DATE

Most of the clinical studies investigating the effects of Qigong are from China and evidence has been presented in journals inaccessible to the West. The Qigong database assembled by the Qigong Institute provides the only record in English of the vast amount of research on Qigong from China[23]. This database has collected over 1500 abstracts and publications from various conferences and journals. There remains, however, a relative lack of Western medical literature on this practice and research into the efficacy of Qigong clearly is in the beginning stages using Western academic standards.

A fundamental issue that frequently confronts Western trained medical investigators as they construct randomized clinical trials on a practice such as Qigong is that, in order to form a hypothesis, they first have to specify what properly belongs to the 'context' surrounding Qigong and what properly forms the 'active' part of the practice. The problems of practitioner motivation and experience often do not receive formal consideration in the planning of trials. Furthermore, it needs to be acknowledged that the Qigong practitioner and the biomedical researcher may possess two different explanatory models for understanding how a mind–body intervention such as Qigong might prove therapeutic[24,25]. The real 'payoff' of such studies may be a comparison of the different effects or qualitative measures felt by patients with different belief systems and coping strategies. Therefore, it is difficult to perform an 'efficacy' study of a complex intervention. Instead, it may be more relevant to perform an 'effectiveness' study. Such designs have been common in behavioral interventions and they examine how well an intervention works in a 'real-life' setting, usually examining the incremental effect of an

Table 13.3 Aspects of Qigong practice

(1) *Slow*: one should perform Qigong slowly. The slower one performs Qigong, the more effective the exercises.

(2) *Focus*: full concentration is required in Qigong practice. The practice may be performed with the eyes closed to avoid distraction. It is not advisable to carry out practice while watching television or listening to music as the distraction may reduce the effectiveness of the exercise. However, music that is calming and relaxing can enhance the practice and is recommended.

(3) *Breathing*: practitioners of Qigong learn to incorporate the physical movements and the breathing. One develops the imagery to direct the *Qi* flow during the breath from the nostril to the *Dan Tien*, a location 3 inches below the umbilicus and 2.5 inches deep from the surface. Initially, visualization of *Qi* flow is necessary. As the practice becomes more advanced, one may feel the *Qi* in the body and one may intentionally direct the *Qi* to different parts of the body to heal injury or to direct the *Qi* from the body.

(4) *Correct movement*: the Qigong movements themselves open up the major channels of the front and back, *Yang* and *Yin*, respectively. The open body posture can be carried out standing, sitting, or lying down, depending on the current ability of the person.

(5) *Relaxation*: relaxing is one of the most important aspects of practicing Qigong. One needs to be loose and relaxed and without tension. Tension results in muscle contraction, impairs the blood flow, and decreases the *Qi* flow.

(6) *Correct intention:* a sense of readiness and openness is conveyed. Some Masters may even give a 'pass word' to prepare for practice. This is a feature of the spiritual cultivation that often accompanies Qigong practice and acknowledges the field of immense energy or 'emptiness' from which *Qi* itself draws its energy. A sense of gratitude is also imparted in the intention.

Adapted from reference 21

intervention as compared to a group randomized to receive 'usual customary care'[26].

With these caveats in mind, the limited number of clinical research studies offer important preliminary evidence for Qigong as a complementary therapy.

Cardiovascular system

Very few controlled studies of the effects of Qigong regarding the cardiovascular system exist[27]. A review of 30 representative studies looking at Qigong and hypertension highlighted many areas of concern of the research methodology, including the lack of random assignment and selection biases[28] which limited interpretation. Nevertheless, the weight of evidence suggests that practicing Qigong may have a positive effect on hypertension by reducing the drug dosage requirement for blood pressure control, as well as the incidence and mortality of stroke[29]. Qigong practice appears to have beneficial physiologic effects that indicate stabilization of the cardiovascular system, including a decrease in the heart rate, respiratory rate, and systolic blood pressure[30] in healthy volunteers. It is recommended that persons wishing to practice Qigong undergo a general medical and blood pressure check before embarking on this form of isometric exercise[31].

Neurologic system

A pilot study suggested that training in mindfulness movement similar to Qigong practice may offer patients with multiple sclerosis a self-help method to increase physical and psychologic functioning[32]. Qigong may serve as an exercise alternative to enhance levels of physical activity in patients with muscular dystrophy and other forms of neuromuscular disease[33]. The same investigators report that Qigong may be a useful adjunct therapy regimen in patients with muscular dystrophy in that it can bring about a decreased rate of decline in general health using quantitative measures of health-related quality of life, depression, and coping levels[34].

Cancer

Integrative centers such as the Stanford Cancer Supportive Care Program (SCSCP) have been developed to provide support for patients with cancer undergoing traditional cancer therapies[35]. Qigong classes have been offered as part of the Stanford program and of the 334 patients who evaluated Qigong, 78% felt a reduction in their sense of stress, 74% noted an increased sense of well-being, 58% noted an increase in energy, 43% mentioned more restful sleep, and 22% achieved some pain reduction[35]. For the patients with cancer, the emotional effect of Qigong may be as important as the energetic effect. In China, Qigong is commonly prescribed as an adjunct to chemotherapy and radiation[9]. In a review of more than 50 studies of Qigong therapy for cancer in China, *in vitro* studies reported the inhibitory effect of *Qi* emission on tumor growth[36] and *in vivo* studies of cancer-infected animals reported longer survival times. Another study showed preliminary results which, although not conclusive, appear to suggest that Qigong treatment had a tumor-inhibitory effect in a mouse model of lymphoma[37]. Anecdotal reports have documented a reduction in tumor markers such as prostate-specific antigen (PSA) after Qigong in a patient with an elevation of this marker but without any other treatments[38].

Pulmonary system

Qigong practice incorporates diaphragmatic breathing exercises which could improve respiratory symptoms when used in combination with drug management[29]. A pilot study investigating Qigong as a complementary therapeutic measure in asthma patients found a decrease in peak flow variability, reduced hospitalization rate, less sickness leave, reduced antibiotic use, and fewer emergency consultations resulting in reduced treatment costs over a period of one year of self-conducted Qigong exercises[39]. In healthy volunteers who practiced Qigong, an overall improvement in ventilatory efficiency for oxygen uptake and carbon dioxide production was observed[40,41]. As yet, no medical evidence for Qigong and chronic obstructive pulmonary disease (COPD) has been reported. Anecdotal evidence for Qigong practice and substantial improvement in more serious pulmonary conditions such as alveolar proteinosis has been reported (see case report below)[20].

Endocrine system

Qigong movement may be beneficial in reducing plasma glucose after a meal without inducing a large increase in the heart rate in patients with diabetes[42]. *Qi* training has been shown to modulate secretion of growth hormone, insulin-like growth factor (IGF-1), and testosterone[43,44]; however, the applicability of Qigong in diseases such as osteoporosis remains unknown.

Psychiatry and depression

The meditative aspect of Qigong and, therefore, its link with the psychological state of the individual is also an important element of the Qigong practice. Qigong has been studied as a therapy for detoxification of heroin addicts compared to medical and non-medical treatments. Withdrawal symptoms were reduced more rapidly in the group practicing Qigong, with lower levels of anxiety compared to the group receiving the detoxification drug lofexidine-HCL[45]. Qigong is promising as an alternative intervention for the elderly with chronic physical illness[46] and has the effect of alleviating clinical depression in this group[47]. Other studies have also shown a beneficial effect in more serious psychiatric diseases such as bipolar disorder[48] and in suicide prevention[49].

Musculoskeletal system

Treatment recommendations for chronic pain syndromes such as fibromyalgia include non-pharmacologic modalities of physical and/or occupational therapy which set the groundwork for subsequent exercise programs. Individualized programs can be tailored to include Qigong[50]. It may be an effective adjunct to pharmacologic treatment, particularly in terms of helping foster a greater sense of control and self-efficacy to meet the challenges of a chronic and difficult to treat syndrome[51–53]. A pilot study confirmed that a package including education and Qigong movement therapy weekly for 8 weeks resulted in a significant improvement in symptoms and signs in subjects with fibromyalgia, with benefits sustained for at least 4 months[53].

Immune system

Preliminary evidence from a small, non-randomized, uncontrolled study has shown that short-term practice of Qigong lowers cortisol levels, with concomitant changes in numbers of cytokine-secreting cells in healthy subjects[54]. It is possible that the influence of Qigong on the immune system may be partially mediated by its psychologic effect. A mutual regulation exists between the neuroendocrine and immune systems; the neuroendocrine system influences immune function through hormonal and neural pathways, while the immune system affects neuroendocrine function by means of cytokines[55]. The psychologic state may be the main link between the immune and neuroendocrine systems[56]. After practicing Qigong for a period of one month, subjects have been shown to exhibit lower values than controls in innate immune response cells including monocytes and granulocytes, as well as lower levels of complement proteins[57]. The authors of this study suggested that Qigong practice may constitute an effective psycho-social method for immune modulation, which may be of clinical relevance[57]. Further studies are required to assess the functionality of these leukocyte subsets, including their cytotoxicity after Qigong training. In this regard, a recent study reported enhanced neutrophil bactericidal function in trained individuals[58]. The effects of Qigong practice may be at the gene expression level; there appears preliminary evidence for mind–body interaction and regulation of gene expression at the transcription level[59].

EXTERNAL QIGONG

Although Qigong is practiced mainly as a self-healing method, *Qi* emission, or external *Qi* therapy (EQT), has been a part of medical Qigong to assist others regain health. It is said that practitioners develop an awareness of *Qi* sensations in their bodies and can use their intentions to guide the *Qi*[60,61]. With enough practice and sufficient skill, the Qigong practitioner can direct his/her *Qi* energy to help others break *Qi* blockages and induce excess *Qi* out of the body, so as to bring about an energy balance, alleviate pain, or abate disease[38]. In an anecdotal pilot trial, a positive response with some effect on pain relief in 10 patients with chronic orofacial pain receiving EQT was demonstrated[62]. Similarly, EQT has been used successfully in managing symptoms of premenstrual syndrome[63].

Does EQT exert its effect (if any) through the power of suggestion, or does it have a direct effect on biological systems? This question has been addressed using laboratory sample targets of the practitioners' treatment[64]. Such *in vitro* models eliminate from experiments the factor of psychological cueing and can be subject to replication under strictly controlled conditions. These studies have investigated the ability of experienced Qigong practitioners to enhance the growth of healthy human cells by the application of EQT. The observed increase in cultured cells following EQT was not replicated in a subsequent experiment[64]. Another study of the possible healing effects of EQT found that external Qigong had an inhibitory effect on the withdrawal symptom in morphine-dependent mice and rats[65].

There has been speculation that the effectiveness of Qigong therapy may be related to Chinese culture and lifestyle. Examples of two successful case reports of patients from different ethnic backgrounds who had not been exposed to TCM follow.

Case report 1

A 51-year-old Hispanic lady presented to a tertiary medical center with progressive shortness of breath over a period of 1 year. She was a non-smoker. Physical examination revealed an obese patient who was tachypneic at rest and had crepitations throughout both lung fields.

Preliminary investigations revealed widespread infiltrates on chest radiography. Blood gas analysis demonstrated hypoxia with a pO_2 of 50% on room air, and she required chronic oxygen therapy. Lung function tests revealed a moderately severe restrictive lung defect, with a reduction in the diffusion factor. A CT scan of the chest demonstrated diffuse alveolar infiltrates. Open lung biopsy was obtained and pathology revealed amorphous eosinophilic proteinaceous material in the alveoli. The diagnosis was alveolar proteinosis. Over the next 6 years she underwent multiple therapeutic broncho-alveolar lavage (BAL), with only minor improvement after each procedure. As her clinical course deteriorated, she underwent a course of high-dose steroids again, with little change in her pulmonary status. It was finally recommended that she would need a lung transplant.

On the urging of her son, she presented to a Qigong Master who recommended a series of weekly sessions of Qigong practice with daily home practice[20]. The practice was coupled with Qigong meditation practice. She also underwent eight sessions of external Qi healing by the Master. Her clinical status rapidly improved over 8 weeks and she no longer required oxygen therapy. Her exercise tolerance improved and she was no longer housebound. Whereas alveolar proteinosis can spontaneously improve, this case is unusual in that over a period of 7 years since the diagnosis, her clinical status had been progressively deteriorating until she was on oxygen therapy 24 hours a day. After a period of just 8 weeks of Qigong intervention she no longer required oxygen for the first time in 7 years. She also described a change in her attitude which accompanied Qigong practice, from a depressed, hopeless chronically ill individual to one who could once again participate in life. She did not require lung transplantation and she remains well 9 years after the initial Qigong therapy. This patient, in fact, no longer follows up with her pulmonologist and did not get further chest or lung imaging.

Case report 2

A 47-year-old Caucasian female presented with a 2-week history of trouble refocusing her eyes after rapid head turning. She was a non-smoker with no past history of hypertension. Her gait seemed unsteady and she stopped driving. She had had one episode of nausea and vomiting around the time her symptoms started. She also noted that her speech was 'stuttering' at times. She had no extremity weakness or sensory loss, but did experience diplopia with gaze directed to the left. Neurologic examination showed nystagmus on gaze to the right, and some mild difficulty standing on the left foot alone.

A non-contrast CT scan of the head demonstrated a hemorrhagic 1.5-cm lesion at the ponto-medullary region. Magnetic resonance image studies as well as a cerebral angiogram showed the presence of a 1.5-cm, angiographically occult, vascular malformation at the ponto-medullary junction. These findings confirmed a cavernous hamangioma which had recently bled. The natural history of such lesions was a significant likelihood of recurrent bleeding, and the malformation was felt amenable to surgical removal. While awaiting a neurosurgical opinion at a tertiary center, she underwent four sessions of EQT and also started Qigong self-practice.

A repeat MRI of the head showed resolution of the bleed and surgery was no longer deemed necessary, to the astonishment of her neurologist. This patient remains well with no further cerebral bleeds 6 years after the Qigong intervention.

WHICH QIGONG HEALER TO PICK?

As Qigong gains popularity in the West, it is imperative to select a good teacher who has been trained and certified by a Master. The teacher can only assist individuals in their own development of health, well-being, healing, and spiritual cultivation. The Qigong practice technique should be clear, with adjustments if necessary, with an understanding of what is required in terms of practice times (active exercises and meditation) from the student. A good teacher relies on the invisible wisdom of the body and nature, instead of always trying to *make* things happen. In other words, there is no vested interest in the outcome, but rather one 'lets go' of expected results. There is

respect for the science in the Western tradition and Qigong practice is taught as a complementary therapy.

CONCLUSIONS

The Western medical tradition can gain much from the study of Qigong and learn from the Chinese concepts of what it means to be a healthy human being and how that health can be enhanced, protected, and preserved. Qigong clearly has wide application as a complementary therapy to patients of all backgrounds, but, even more importantly, serves as a preventative measure. The *Yellow Emperor's Classic of Internal Medicine* is the source of the often quoted teaching of Chinese medicine: the wise physician cures diseases before they develop, rather than after they manifest. The following passage from the *Classic* reads:

> *Tao was practiced by the sages and admired by the ignorant people. Obedience to the laws of Yin and Yang means life; disobedience means death. The obedient ones will rule while the rebels will be in disorder and confusion. Anything contrary to harmony (with nature) is disobedience and means rebellion to nature.*
>
> *Hence the sages did not treat those who were already ill; they instructed those who were not yet ill. They did not want to rule those who were already rebellious; they guided those who were not yet rebellious. This is the meaning of the entire preceding discussion. To administer medicines to diseases which have already developed is comparable to the behavior of those persons who begin to dig a well after they have become thirsty, and of those who begin to cast weapons after they have already engaged in battle. Would these actions not be too late?*

Cultivating *Qi* is an ideal way to maintain the body, mind, and spirit, and achieve optimal health.

References

1. Eisenberg DM, Kessler RC, Foster C, et al. Unconventional medicine in the United States. Prevalence, costs, and patterns of use. N Engl J Med 1993; 328: 246–52
2. Eisenberg DM, Davis RB, Ettner SL. Trends in alternative medicine use in the United States, 1990–1997: results of a follow-up national survey. J Am Med Assoc 1998; 280: 1569–75
3. Cassidy CM. Chinese medicine users in the United States. Part I: Utilization, satisfaction, medical plurality. J Altern Complement Med 1998; 4: 17–27
4. Cassidy CM. Chinese medicine users in the United States. Part II: Preferred aspects of care. J Altern Complement Med 1998; 4: 189–202

5. Tiller WA. A personal perspective on energies in future energy medicine. J Altern Complement Med 2004; 10: 867–77

6. Cassidy CM. What does it mean to practice an energy medicine? J Altern Complement Med 2004; 10: 79–81

7. Ilza V. The Yellow Emperor's Classic of Internal Medicine [translation]. Berkeley and Los Angeles, California: University of California Press, 2002

8. Mitchell S. Tao Te Ching. The Book of The Way [translation]. Harper and Row, Publishers, Inc., 2000

9. Cohen KS. The Way of Qigong. The Art and Science of Chinese Energy Healing. New York: Ballantine Books, 1997

10. Witt C, Becker M, Bandelin K, et al. Qigong for schoolchildren: a pilot study. J Altern Complement Med 2005; 11: 41–7

11. Pert CB, Dreher HE, Ruff MR. The psychosomatic network: foundations of mind–body medicine. Altern Ther Health Med 1998; 4: 30–41

12. Levin JS. Religion and health: is there an association, is it valid, and is it causal? Soc Sci Med 1994; 38: 1475–82

13. Kohane MJ, Tiller WA. Biological processes, quantum mechanics and electromagnetic fields: the possibility of device-encapsulated human intention in medical therapies. Med Hypotheses 2001; 56: 598–607

14. Tiller WA, Dibble WE Jr, Nunley R, Shealy CN. Toward general experimentation and discovery in conditioned laboratory spaces: Part I. Experimental pH change findings at some remote sites. J Altern Complement Med 2004; 10: 145–57

15. Dorcas A, Yung P. Qigong: harmonising the breath, the body and the mind. Complement Ther Nurs Midwifery 2003; 9: 198–202

16. Shang C. Emerging paradigms in mind–body medicine. J Altern Complement Med 2001; 7: 83–91

17. Friedman MJ, Birch S, Tiller WA. Towards the development of a mathematical model for acupuncture meridians. Acupunct Electrother Res 1989; 14: 217–26

18. Sancier KM. The effect of Qigong on therapeutic balancing measured by Electroacupuncture According to Voll (EAV): a preliminary study. Acupunct Electrother Res 1994; 19: 119–27

19. Sancier KM. Electrodermal measurements for monitoring the effects of a Qigong workshop. J Altern Complement Med 2003; 9: 235–41

20. Lin C. Born a Healer. Minneapolis: Spring Forest Publishers, 2002

21. Lin MC. Spring Forest Qigong. Level 1 for Health, 2nd edn. Minnesota: Learning Strategies Corporation, 2002

22. Ott MJ. Mindfulness meditation: a path of transformation and healing. J Psychosoc Nurs Ment Health Serv 2004; 42: 22–9

23. Sancier KM. Search for medical applications of Qigong with the Qigong Database. J Altern Complement Med 2001; 7: 93–5

24. Kerr C. Translating 'mind-in-body': two models of patient experience underlying a randomized controlled trial of qigong. Cult Med Psychiatry 2002; 26: 419–47

25. Chu DA. Tai Chi, Qi Gong and Reiki. Phys Med Rehabil Clin N Am 2004; 15: 773–81, vi

26. Clauw DJ. Clinical research into alternative and complementary therapies: how do we tell if the glass is half empty or half full? J Rheumatol 2003; 30: 2088–9

27. Luskin FM, Newell KA, Griffith M, et al. A review of mind–body therapies in the treatment of cardiovascular disease. Part 1: Implications for the elderly. Altern Ther Health Med 1998; 4: 46–61

28. Mayer M. Qigong and hypertension: a critique of research. J Altern Complement Med 1999; 5: 371–82

29. Sancier KM. Therapeutic benefits of Qigong exercises in combination with drugs. J Altern Complement Med 1999; 5: 383–9

30. Lee MS, Kim BG, Huh HJ, et al. Effect of Qi-training on blood pressure, heart rate and respiration rate. Clin Physiol 2000; 20: 173–6

31. Leung KP, Yan T, Li LS. Intracerebral haemorrhage and Qigong. Hong Kong Med J 2001; 7: 315–18

32. Mills N, Allen J. Mindfulness of movement as a coping strategy in multiple sclerosis. A pilot study. Gen Hosp Psychiatry 2000; 22: 425–31

33. Wenneberg S, Gunnarsson LG, Ahlstrom G. Using a novel exercise programme for patients with muscular dystrophy. Part I: a qualitative study. Disabil Rehabil 2004; 26: 586–94

34. Wenneberg S, Gunnarsson LG, Ahlstrom G. Using a novel exercise programme for patients with muscular dystrophy. Part II: a quantitative study. Disabil Rehabil 2004; 26: 595–602

35. Rosenbaum E, Gautier H, Fobair P, et al. Cancer supportive care, improving the quality of life for cancer patients. A program evaluation report. Support Care Cancer 2004; 12: 293–301

36. Chen K, Yeung R. Exploratory studies of Qigong therapy for cancer in China. Integr Cancer Ther 2002; 1: 345–70

37. Chen KW, Shiflett SC, Ponzio NM, et al. A preliminary study of the effect of external Qigong on lymphoma growth in mice. J Altern Complement Med 2002; 8: 615–21

38. Chen KW, Turner FD. A case study of simultaneous recovery from multiple physical symptoms with medical Qigong therapy. J Altern Complement Med 2004; 10: 159–62

39. Reuther I, Aldridge D. Qigong Yangsheng as a complementary therapy in the management of asthma: a single-case appraisal. J Altern Complement Med 1998; 4: 173–83

40. Lim YA, Boone T, Flarity JR, Thompson WR. Effects of qigong on cardiorespiratory changes: a preliminary study. Am J Chin Med 1993; 21: 1–6

41. Lan C, Chou SW, Chen SY, et al. The aerobic capacity and ventilatory efficiency during exercise in Qigong and Tai Chi Chuan practitioners. Am J Chin Med 2004; 32: 141–50

42. Iwao M, Kajiyama S, Mori H, Oogaki K. Effects of Qigong walking on diabetic patients: a pilot study. J Altern Complement Med 1999; 5: 353–8

43. Lee MS, Kang CW, Ryu H, et al. Effects of ChunDoSunBup Qi-training on growth hormone, insulin-like growth factor-I, and testosterone in young and elderly subjects. Am J Chin Med 1999; 27: 167–75

44. Lee MS, Kang CW, Ryu H, Moon SR. Endocrine and immune effects of Qi-training. Int J Neurosci 2004; 114: 529–37

45. Li M, Chen K, Mo Z. Use of Qigong therapy in the detoxification of heroin addicts. Altern Ther Health Med 2002; 8: 50–9

46. Tsang HW, Mok CK, Au Yeung YT, Chan SY. The effect of Qigong on general and psychosocial health of elderly with chronic physical illnesses: a randomized clinical trial. Int J Geriatr Psychiatry 2003; 18: 441–9

47. Tsang HW, Cheung L, Lak DC. Qigong as a psychosocial intervention for depressed elderly with chronic physical illnesses. Int J Geriatr Psychiatry 2002; 17: 1146–54

48. Gaik F. A Preliminary Study Applying Spring Forest Qigong to Depression as an Alternative and Complementary Treatment. Adler School of Professional Psychology, 2002

49. Ismail K, Tsang HW. Qigong and suicide prevention. Br J Psychiatry 2003; 182: 266–7

50. Morris CR, Bowen L, Morris AJ. Integrative therapy for fibromyalgia: possible strategies for an individualized treatment program. South Med J 2005; 98: 177–84

51. Astin JA, Berman BM, Bausell B, et al. The efficacy of mindfulness meditation plus Qigong movement therapy in the treatment of fibromyalgia: a randomized controlled trial. J Rheumatol 2003; 30: 2257–62

52. Hadhazy VA, Ezzo J, Creamer P, Berman BM. Mind–body therapies for the treatment of fibromyalgia. A systematic review. J Rheumatol 2000; 27: 2911–18

53. Creamer P, Singh BB, Hochberg MC, Berman BM. Sustained improvement produced by nonpharmacologic intervention in fibromyalgia: results of a pilot study. Arthritis Care Res 2000; 13: 198–204

54. Jones BM. Changes in cytokine production in healthy subjects practicing Guolin Qigong: a pilot study. BMC Complement Altern Med 2001; 1: 8

55. Webster JI, Tonelli L, Sternberg EM. Neuroendocrine regulation of immunity. Annu Rev Immunol 2002; 20: 125–63

56. Ryu H, Lee MS, Jeong SM, et al. Modulation of neuroendocrinological function by psychosomatic training: acute effect of ChunDoSunBup Qi-training on growth hormone, insulin-like growth factor (IGF)-I, and insulin-like growth factor binding protein (IGFBP)-3 in men. Psychoneuroendocrinology 2000; 25: 439–51

57. Manzaneque JM, Vera FM, Maldonado EF, et al. Assessment of immunological parameters following a Qigong training program. Med Sci Monit 2004; 10: CR264–CR270

58. Lee MS, Jeong SM, Kim YK, et al. Qi-training enhances respiratory burst function and adhesive capacity of neutrophils in young adults: a preliminary study. Am J Chin Med 2003; 31: 141–8

59. Li QZ, Li P, Garcia GE, et al. Genomic profiling of neutrophil transcripts in Asian qigong practitioners: a pilot study in gene regulation by mind–body interaction. J Altern Complement Med 2005; 11: 29–39

60. Lin MC. Spring Forest Qigong. Level 2 for healing. Minneapolis: 2002

61. Chen KW. An analytic review of studies on measuring effects of external QI in China. Altern Ther Health Med 2004; 10: 38–50

62. Chen KW, Marbach JJ. External Qigong therapy for chronic orofacial pain. J Altern Complement Med 2002; 8: 532–4

63. Jang HS, Lee MS. Effects of qi therapy (external Qigong) on premenstrual syndrome: a randomized placebo-controlled study. J Altern Complement Med 2004; 10: 456–62

64. Yount G, Solfvin J, Moore D, et al. In vitro test of external Qigong. BMC Complement Altern Med 2004; 4: 5

65. Mo Z, Chen KW, Ou W, Li M. Benefits of external Qigong therapy on morphine-abstinent mice and rats. J Altern Complement Med 2003; 9: 827–35

Diet and nutrition in Traditional Chinese Medicine

14

M. E. Jones

INTRODUCTION

The role of food in the prevention of disease and maintenance of health has been a major research focus of nutrition during the past two decades. Every 5 years the US Department of Health and Human Services (HHS) jointly publishes with the Department of Agriculture (USDA) a *Dietary Guidelines for Americans*. The *Guidelines* provide science-based advice to promote health and to reduce risk for major chronic diseases through diet and physical activity. Diet plays a key role in the prevention of at least six of the ten leading causes of death in the United States, for example, cardiovascular disease, type 2 diabetes, hypertension, and osteoporosis.

In the practice of Traditional Chinese Medicine (TCM), there is, and always has been, a strong emphasis on utilizing diet and nutrition for maintaining health, preventing illness, and supporting recovery from illness. TCM strongly emphasizes prevention of illness primary to the curing of illness and stresses the importance of lifestyle choices in maintaining health. This is exemplified by the public practice of Tai Qi, an ancient form of energy movement, throughout the country. It is part of the national culture to practice a physical activity that will benefit the health of the body.

Western Medicine, being a trauma/critical-care-based medicine, has been slow to understand the importance of nutrition in the care of patients. However, research has shown that including nutrition in the care and treatment of patients, especially chronically ill patients, is vital to improving their state of health. Nutrition is elemental in treating, preventing and curing many diseases, including heart disease, renal disease, hepatic disease, cancer, anemia, eating disorders, and infection[1]. It is also elemental to the human body's healing and recovery process. For example, specific studies show that vitamin D is essential in promoting calcium and phosphorus absorption and normal bone development, and in preventing osteomalacia and rickets[2]. A folic acid supplement given to a woman trying to get pregnant can help prevent neural tube defects[3]. Severe vitamin B1 (thiamine) deficiency can result in beri beri, neuritis, and cardiovascular dysfunction[4]. These and other clinical studies have helped to improve the quality of people's lives as well as prevent illness. They prove the necessity of a well-balanced nutritious diet.

THE ROLE OF THE DIGESTIVE SYSTEM IN HEALTH AND HEALING

In the practice of TCM, the importance of food, nutrition, and a strong digestive system has been primary in treatment for thousands of years. Before any discussion about diet and nutrition can be started, one needs to understand the workings of the digestive system in order to be able to recommend foods that will not only benefit the whole body and the body's health but also benefit the digestive system and maintain its strength. There is an extraordinary amount of clinical evidence pointing to the importance of a strong digestive system primary to a healthy, nutritious diet.

In China during the late 1100s, a distinguished scholar and renowned Chinese medical physician, Li Dong-yuan, published *The Treatise on Spleen/Stomach*. This is the seminal textbook substantiating the necessity of a strong and healthy digestive system, namely the spleen and stomach, in maintaining health as well as healing illness. According to Li, it is of paramount importance to protect the spleen/stomach if people want to stay healthy and to strengthen them once they have become diseased, no matter what other viscera or bowels are also affected[5]. In order to achieve and maintain health, it is vital to have a strong digestive system coupled with a balanced and nutritious diet. When one's digestive system is strong, vitamins and minerals can be absorbed and utilized. When one's digestive system is weak, even the most balanced and complete diet will not bring about health and well-being.

TCM understands the connection between the prognosis of an individual and the strength of their digestive system. If the digestive system is weak, it will be a slow and difficult process to affect a cure for illness or repair damage from injury. If digestion is strong, the prognosis is much better and healing will be faster.

Patients with weak digestion

Estimates show that 40 to 50% of hospitalized patients are malnourished[6]. As more research has been done in the area of nutrition, hospitals have improved the diet they feed their patients. Yet, still we see many malnourished patients. This is due in part to the fact that hospitals feed patients food that a normal healthy person would eat, without consideration to the strength or weakness of the patient's digestive system.

Most patients who are hospitalized will enter the hospital with a weak or compromised digestive system. This is simply because illness and disease weaken digestion as they weaken the entire body. If a person is ill or diseased, their digestive system is compromised. If a person has been injured they may not enter the hospital with a weak digestive system, but their digestive system can become taxed by the medication, surgery, and/or other treatment given to heal them.

In order to support the healing prescriptions given to an ill, injured, or hospitalized patient, attention needs to be given to the food that the patient eats, as well as how it is prepared. When a person is ill or injured, their digestive system is not strong enough to break down the food that a healthy person's digestive system can. If a person's digestive system is weak, then a highly nutritious diet cannot be absorbed, which will lead to malnourishment.

In general, Western medicine places preventive health care secondary to treatment and management of illness. This is antithetical to TCM, which places more importance on prevention than cure. In an ancient Chinese medical textbook it is written, 'A superior doctor will cure a disease before its onset'. Whereas preventive health care is only cursorily addressed in Western medical textbooks, virtually all Chinese medical textbooks discuss details outlining philosophical, lifestyle, dietary, and emotional recommendations on how to live a long, healthy, happy life. Since it is the understanding of Chinese medicine that digestion is the source of good health, these textbooks contain a great deal of information on diet and food preparation that will help keep digestion healthy and strong.

Food as the source of energy and nutrients

Chinese medicine has a concept that Western medicine had historically acknowledged, but over the past 40 years has disavowed[7]. This is the concept of *Qi* or 'vital energy force'. This vital energy force is what all living beings use throughout their lives to live, to grow, to function, and to heal. It is the fundamental material of human life. In fact, there are many nature-based medical constructs that accept and understand the concept of *Qi*, such as Ayurvedic medicine, Siberian shamanism, and Native American herbalism.

According to TCM, this essential energy, *Qi*, is required for every metabolic activity and every transformation. One TCM school of thought holds that *Qi* is produced in the body in three basic forms[8]:

(1) Blood essence, including all the elements that constitute and are carried by blood, i.e. red and white blood cells, water, and various nutrients assimilated from digested food;

(2) Hormone essence, consisting of two forms: life essence, essential hormones secreted by the endocrine system, neurochemicals, cerebrospinal fluids, and enzymes, and sexual essence, various hormones associated with sexual functions including sperm and ova; and

(3) Essential fluids, heavier fluids like lymph and mucus, synovial fluid, tears, perspiration, and urine.

These vital fluids are synthesized from essential nutrients extracted by digestion. Excellent digestive functioning is critical to *Qi* formation. After we are born, there are only three sources from which we are able to build *Qi* – food, drink, and air.

Food is the main source of *Qi*; it provides the largest amount of energy for us to live on. Food is full of nutrition, sugars, carbohydrates, and proteins, and provides the basics we need to grow, rebuild, repair, and heal. The quality of the body's fluids, bones, organs, muscles, tendons, and other body parts is directly dependent upon the quality of the nutrients in the diet and the efficiency of digestion and metabolism. This is why both a highly nutritious diet and a strong digestive system are so critical to people's health.

The human body as a cohesive functioning system

TCM views the human body, composed of a variety of tissues, organs, channels, and collaterals, each performing their particular function, as an integral whole. The various parts are intimately interconnected and maintain a close connection with the external environment[9]. Western medicine views the human body as separate and distinct parts, each working together, but not necessarily in need of each other. For example, Western medicine believes the tonsils, appendix, uterus, ovaries, and even the spleen are non-essential pieces of the whole human body. These organs can be taken out routinely when there is repeated illness, infection, or disease. TCM, on the other hand, does not have a history of performing surgery or removing organs. In TCM all the tissues, organs, and parts of the human body are essential. This is because TCM views each of the organs and tissues as inseparable in structure and function. They are a cohesive functioning system.

Western medicine believes that, although organs, tissues, and other parts of the human body clearly can work together, they are essentially separate and need to be studied and treated separately. It is interesting to note that as Western medicine has become more research based, it has left behind many parts of medicine that it used to believe and teach, such as the connection between a person's health and the environment they live in. Evidence of this can be found in Western medical textbooks written in the early 1900s.

Vitalism vs mechanism

There are many differences between Western and Chinese medicine. One of the most important to understand, for the purposes of this chapter, is how TCM envisions both the anatomy and physiology of the organs that make up the digestive system, as well as how the digestive system works as a whole. Up until the middle of the nineteenth century, Western medicine had a vitalistic approach to physiology. The primary thinking was that living beings must possess 'some mysterious vital life force' in order to fuel the amazing act of living. This way of thinking is called vitalism[10].

This vitalistic view of physiology began to change as more emphasis was placed on clinical research. Physiologists began to believe and teach that living organisms functioned more like machines, albeit ones remarkably complex in nature. This mechanistic approach to life has led to more and more clinical research in the belief that everything can be understood by studying the working parts of an organism. This explains why Western medicine separates each of the organs for diagnosis, study, and treatment, and why we have so many doctors who specialize in understanding different parts of the human body.

TCM has a vitalistic view of physiology. It believes that the body needs *Qi* in its many forms to fuel the body, mind, and spirit. Chinese medicine, like Western medicine, has a very complex understanding of anatomy and physiology. The difference is that medical doctors in China only recently (in the last 600 years) performed the first dissection of a human body. Six hundred years may seem like a long time, but consider that Chinese medicine has been practiced in a similar fashion to today for at least 5000 years. That means that the Chinese had a very sophisticated understanding of the human body and its processes without ever having access to the modern medical equipment we use today, nor having performed an autopsy or dissection.

DIGESTION AND TCM

Digestion is the process of extracting essential nutrients from food and synthesizing the various fluids that sustain life. Digestion is the process that food goes through as it is broken down into simpler compounds such as carbohydrates, fats, vitamins, minerals, and proteins. These are the essential substances the body needs to absorb and utilize in order to build bones, build the immune system, keep our organs healthy and strong, repair damage from injuries, and generally keep our body and mind developing, repairing, living, and functioning.

According to Western physiology, enzymes that catalyze hydrolytic reactions accomplish digestion of food macromolecules. For example, amylase begins carbohydrate digestion in the mouth, while pepsins begin protein digestion in the stomach, but most digestion is accomplished in the small intestine by enzymes from the pancreas or attached to the brush-border membranes of the intestine[11]. This is a simple description of some of the basic pieces of the process of digestion. Digestion is a far more complex process involving intricate cooperation between organs, enzymes, fluids, and catalytic reactions. Yet, Western science spends very little time researching and understanding this process. Although Western medicine understands the connection between proper nutritional intake and health, it does not recognize the connection between being able to absorb nutrients and a well functioning digestive system.

Anatomy of the digestive system in TCM

In a general sense, Western and Chinese medicine are remarkably similar in their understanding of the anatomy and physiology of the human digestive system. However, some of the details and the philosophical view are different. Keeping in mind that Chinese medicine views the human body as an integrated whole, the organs are seen as essential parts of a whole system rather than as separate organs.

From this point on in this chapter, I will capitalize the names of organs when I am referring to their anatomic and physiologic definitions from TCM in order to differentiate them from the Western anatomic and physiologic definitions.

In TCM, all the organs in the human body play roles in digestion alongside the two major players – the Spleen and the Stomach. The Spleen, along with the Stomach, is the source of digestion. The Spleen's main function is to assist the Stomach's digestion by transporting and transforming food essences, absorbing the nourishment from food, and separating the usable from the unusable part of food[12]. The Spleen is a very essential organ in TCM because, physiologically speaking, it 'governs' the digestive system. When translating Chinese anatomy into Western anatomy there are some discrepancies on the exact correlations. However, generally speaking, the Spleen in TCM refers to the spleen, the pancreas, and the lymphatic tissue and organs in the body, including the tonsils and lymph glands. The Stomach, in Chinese medicine, refers to the stomach, the duodenum, and the first 6 inches of the small intestine as referred to in Western medicine[13].

Physiology of the digestive system in TCM

Physiologically, one of the main functions of both the Spleen and the Stomach is to govern transportation and transformation of food and water[14]. An ancient Chinese medical textbook, the *Huang-Di Nei Jing*, describes the physiology of digestion as, 'Food enters the Stomach, the refined part goes to the Liver, the excess goes to the sinews. Food enters the Stomach, the unrefined part goes to the Heart, the excess goes to the blood vessels… fluids enter the Stomach… the upper part go to the Spleen, the Spleen transports the refined essence upwards to the Lungs'[15]. This very complex and intricate process requires each of the organs involved to be healthy and working in harmony.

The Spleen plays a key role in separating the usable from the unusable parts of food. It directs the *Qi*, in this case the food-*Qi*, to the Liver, to the Heart, and to the Lungs. When the Spleen's function is impaired this will lead to fatigue, gas, diarrhea, poor digestion, and bloating.

The Spleen also governs the transformation, separation, and movement of fluids. 'The Spleen separates a usable from an unusable part from the fluids ingested; the 'clear' part goes upwards to the Lungs to be distributed to the skin and the 'dirty' part goes downward to the Intestines where it is further separated. If the Spleen function is impaired, the fluids will not be transformed or transported properly and may accumulate to form Dampness or Phlegm or cause edema'[16]. When the Spleen's function is strong, the person will have a good appetite, good digestion, plenty of energy, and good muscle tone.

The Stomach is the other key player in digestion. The Stomach controls the process of digestion called 'rotting and ripening'. An ancient Chinese medical textbook, *Nan Jing Jiao Shi*, says, 'The Middle Burner is in the Stomach… And controls the rotting and ripening of food and drink'[17]. The Stomach transforms the food and drink, by a process analogous to fermentation, into something that the Spleen can then separate to extract the refined essence from food. After this fermentation and separation process, food then moves down to the Small Intestine for further separation and absorption.

The Spleen's function can be impaired by improper dietary habits and foods that tax the digestive system. The Stomach's function can also be impaired by improper dietary habits. It is said that the Spleen 'likes dryness'. In other words, the excessive consumption of cold foods, cold liquids, and icy drinks will overburden the Spleen's transporting and transforming function. In contrast, the Stomach 'likes moisture'. This means that the Stomach likes foods that are moist and not drying, such as oatmeal as opposed to dry toast. The Stomach does not like to be overburdened by overeating or overfilling the Stomach cavity.

Digestion is the root of good health in Chinese Medicine because the nutrients from food and drink are essential for the body to heal and repair itself. Digestion needs to be strong to be able to transform, transport, and absorb nutrients.

Analogies for digestion in TCM

In understanding the digestive process from the TCM perspective it is helpful to have a mental picture of what this process looks like. A very simple analogy to describe the digestive process is to equate digestion to the process of composting. Composting is similar to digestion in terms of the actual process of the breakdown of organic materials into simpler substances and nutrients. The process of digestion is the breakdown of foods and organic ingestible matter into simpler substances, such as nutrients, carbohydrates, and simple sugars that the body can absorb and utilize for building and repair. In order for the composting process to occur rapidly and completely, certain conditions are needed. Composting can occur under less desirable conditions, but there are definitely necessary conditions for any composting to occur. According to ancient Chinese Medical textbooks, the conditions for optimal digestion are the same as those needed for optimal composting. Again, digestion can occur under less desirable conditions, but for optimal digestion certain conditions are necessary.

The two most important conditions for both digestion and composting are warmth and moisture. Organic materials break down quickly and easily in the presence of moisture and warmth. Food substances also break down more quickly and easily in the presence of warmth and moisture.

Another analogy illuminating the details of this process is that of a pot of food cooking over a fire. Imagine the Stomach as the pot and the Spleen as both the fire below the pot and the distillation system that the pot is attached to. When a person eats food, the food enters the warm stomach and begins to be digested. Remember that the Stomach's function is that of 'rotting and ripening'. The Stomach is the first step in the digestive process; it creates a soup or mash. The Stomach 'likes wet'. This soup needs to be warm for the digestion process to occur just as compost needs to be warm in order for organic substances to break down. From this analogy, it is easy to see how taking in cold foods or cold beverages into the 'warm soup' in the Stomach impedes or impairs the function of the Stomach.

On the other hand, the Spleen 'likes dryness'. Using the current analogy of the Spleen as the fire, when fire gets wet or damp it goes out. If a person drinks a cold beverage or eats cold or raw foods, the body needs to generate more fire or energy to heat the food up in order to cook it or digest it. This is how the digestive system and whole body system is taxed over time.

Cold, at the least, slows the digestive process, and at its worst, stops the digestive process. It is analogous to throwing ice or cold water onto a compost heap. In that case, it would be the sun that would have to generate more warmth to melt the ice and re-warm the compost heap. In the case of digestion, it is the *Qi* of the Kidneys and the Spleen that generate the heat to re-warm the stomach and begin digestion again. I only mention the Kidneys here to be specific about their role in keeping the body warm and generating heat. As the Kidneys' role

in digestion is somewhat small in this context, I will not elaborate on it.

The most critical concept for Westerners to understand in the prevention of illness and the treatment of disease is that the excessive consumption of cold foods, cold beverages, and raw foods, which are considered cold in nature by Chinese nutrition, can tax the Spleen and Stomach so much so that it leads to weak digestion. This is to say that when a person is healthy they should consume minimal amounts of cold foods and beverages and when a person is ill they should only consume warm, cooked, and room temperature foods and beverages. Consuming only warm, cooked, and room temperature foods and beverages will allow the digestive system to work less hard, which will give it time to heal and recover.

Recalling our previous analogy, when excessive amounts of cold items are ingested, it dampens the fire of the Spleen and Kidneys. When the fire is dampened the cooking process slows down. If iced and frozen items are ingested it can stop the cooking process. Over time, digestion is weakened. If digestion is weak, people become easily fatigued, health will be poor, and recovery from illness will be slow.

In Western Medicine we look at countless clinical studies which prove the importance of proper and complete nutrition. Let us look to the thousands of years of clinical experience provided by Chinese Medicine for evidence proving the necessity of strong digestion in health and well-being. If digestion is weak, food cannot be broken down, nutrients cannot be absorbed, and the body cannot maintain health, repair damage, and recover from illness. It is easy to see how poor digestion can lead to poor absorption of the essential vitamins, minerals, and other substances the body needs.

DIETARY GUIDELINES BASED ON TCM

There are four categories of dietary guidelines:

(1) General dietary guidelines to benefit and maintain digestive health, including, environmental and psychologic conditions which favor digestion, cooking guidelines which benefit digestion, and the five flavors, i.e. energies and organic actions;

(2) Constitutional dietary guidelines;

(3) Dietary guidelines to adhere to when recovering from illness; and

(4) Dietary guidelines for health-specific issues.

Regardless of the disease, illness, or injury, the physiology of the digestive process remains the same, and, therefore, any treatment or food that benefits digestion will benefit health.

General dietary guidelines to maintain digestive health

Environmental and psychologic conditions which favor digestion

Historically, Western and Chinese Medicine had a similar understanding of the effect environmental and psychologic conditions can have on digestion. For example, in a Western Medical textbook for nurses written in 1937[18], four conditions that favor digestion and assimilation were listed:

(1) Freedom from painful emotions;

(2) Freedom from excessive mental or physical fatigue, strain, or other discomfort;

(3) Freedom from hurry, with regularity and punctuality in serving; and

(4) Attractive, pleasant surroundings and a cheerful atmosphere.

Whereas in the practice of TCM, those conditions are still recognized, currently in the practice of Western Medicine, there is little if any recognition of these effects on digestion. With regard to these and other circumstances that negatively or positively affect digestion, TCM has a list of general recommendations that will benefit digestion when followed:

(1) Eat only when truly hungry.

(2) Eat until satisfied. Overeating will tax your digestive system.

(3) Go to sleep hungry in order to give digestion a rest.

(4) Eat a variety of foods and not too much of one food.

(5) Do not eat too much at one sitting, it will injure the lung *Qi*.

(6) Do not wait too long before eating when hungry, it can injure the Stomach and Spleen *Qi*.

(7) Do not sleep or lay down immediately after eating, it causes the Stomach *Qi* to reverse.

(8) Do not eat too much food at night.

(9) Do not go out in the wind after eating spicy foods that causes sweating, this can cause a person to get sick.

(10) Eat and drink food and liquids that are warm or room temperature. Warmth favors digestion.

(11) Eat slowly and chew food well before swallowing.

(12) Use oils and fats sparingly.

(13) Do not eat greasy, fatty, fried foods. Greasy foods can clog the digestive system, causing one to feel fatigued, groggy, and cloudy headed.

(14) Eat regular meals at regular times. Skipping meals from day to day can weaken the Stomach.

(15) Eat consistent amounts of foods from day to day.

(16) Eat breakfast in the morning, and do not start your day with an empty stomach.

(17) Consume cold or raw foods sparingly.

Chinese Medicine maintains that the digestive system is the source of health and well-being. In order to maintain the health and strength of the digestive system, it is helpful to eat according to these recommendations. In order to rebuild or strengthen the digestive system when it has been damaged or weakened, it is critical to follow these recommendations.

Cooked food benefits digestion

Chinese nutrition favors cooked food over raw food even though, according to Western science, raw food has more nutritional value. This is because cooking food will begin the breakdown process, making digestion easier. Cooking can facilitate the Stomach's function of 'rottening and ripening'. Cold and raw foods require more energy to break down, digest, and absorb the nutrients.

Overcooking food can deplete it of its nutritional value. However, not cooking food at all or eating raw food makes digestion have to work hard to extract the nutrients and energy it needs for the body. It is recommended that all foods be at least lightly cooked. Cooking food helps to break down fibers, cellulose, and other materials that are hard to digest. Lightly cooking foods will not break down all the fiber in food, and fiber is good for the digestive system.

When a person is sick their energy needs to be used for healing, and it is important that they eat easily digestible foods. They should adhere more strictly to the rule of lightly cooking food before eating. If one's digestive system is weak, then food should be cooked more, such as in soups and stews. People recovering from illness, the elderly, and young children still developing their digestive systems should eat nourishing, easily digestible soups and stews. Soups and stews are rich in nutrients. These nutrients are also more readily available to the body.

It is important to use oils and fats sparingly when cooking. Oils and fats are hard to digest; they can clog the digestive system and overwork the Spleen function. This can lead to accumulation of damp and phlegm, causing a person to have diarrhea, a fuzzy head feeling, fatigue, headache, and/or lassitude.

Warm food and drink

According to the ancient Chinese medical text, *Ling Shu*, 'If food and drink are never burning hot nor chilling cold, but moderately cold or hot, *Qi* will be sustained and (the person will be) immune to the attack of pathogens'[19]. Using the analogy of the stomach being the pot of stew cooking over the Spleen's fire it is obvious why excessive consumption of cold, chilled, or frozen foods and drink can be damaging to the digestive system. Cold obviously negates heat, and water puts out fire. Cold foods and liquids impede the warm digestive function. If the Spleen and Stomach are impeded in their transforming and transporting function, accumulation begins to happen. This accumulation can be phlegm, toxins, dampness, or stagnant food.

A diet consisting mainly of raw fruits and vegetables is cooling, not necessarily because these foods are chilled, but because they promote the use of extra energy to break down the food to get the nutrients needed for health. In essence, they promote the loss of body heat and secretion of fluid. For example, if a person eats an ice cream, it requires more energy or expenditure of heat to warm the ice cream for digestion.

Balanced diet according to TCM

In the Western diet, foods are considered for their protein, calorie, carbohydrate, vitamin, and other nutrient content; while in the Chinese diet, foods are considered for their flavors, energies, organic actions, and their effect on individual constitution. A balanced diet in Chinese nutrition refers to a diet consisting of a variety of the five flavors, energies, and organic actions. A balanced diet can be individual, based on one's constitution, or general, based on simple principles that benefit, strengthen, or support digestive health.

THE FIVE FLAVORS

According to the *Nei Jing*, an ancient Chinese medical textbook, there are five flavors, each entering, strengthening, and nourishing a particular organ. The *Su Wen* specifically outlines the organs that each of the flavors travels to, 'Sour travels to the liver. Pungent travels to the lungs. Bitter travels to the heart. Salt travels to the kidneys. Sweet travels to the Spleen. And these are called the five entering routes'[20]. The *Ling Shu* goes further to describe this relationship between flavor and organ, 'Each of the five tastes moves to what it likes. Sour travels to the tendons. Pungent travels to the *Qi*. Bitter travels to the heart. Salt travels to the bones. Sweet travels to the flesh. Such are called the five travels'[21]. When seeking to recommend a balanced diet according to Chinese nutritional concepts, it is important to understand about balancing the flavors to affect healing and enhance health.

The five flavors are first determined by their taste. Second they are determined by their common use in the body. For example, if a food is used as a tonic or something that strengthens the body, then it is considered sweet in flavor. There are some foods that are said to be a certain flavor, but do not taste like that flavor. For example, a food is listed as a sour food, but it doesn't taste sour. In this example its effect determines its flavor.

When a person is ill, food therapy can be applied to bring about health. In general, it is important to eat a balanced diet of the five flavors. When the diet contains an excess of one or more of the five flavors, the body system can become imbalanced. The resulting symptoms can cause great suffering.

The five flavors and their application

Bitter travels to the Heart

Bitter clears heat, dries dampness, and has the ability to strengthen and build *Yin*. If a person has diarrhea and they eat a bitter food, it has the ability to strengthen the *Yin* to stop the diarrhea. In excess, bitter can dry the skin, cause problems with the bones, and can cause the stomach energy to become tight and stuck. Examples of bitter foods are: apricot seed, asparagus, bitter gourd, wild cucumber, celery, coffee, hops, lettuce, radish leaf, and vinegar.

Sweet travels to the Spleen

Sweet tonifies, harmonizes, and has the ability to moderate or slow down. In excess, sweet can cause achy bones, phlegm and damp to accumulate, and heaviness in the limbs. Examples of sweet foods are: honey, sugar, peach, apricot, cantaloupe, banana, cheese, nuts, pasta, beef, pork, bean curd, black sesame seeds, carrot, cherry, chicken, chicken egg, fresh water clam, walnut, corn, pumpkin, star fruit, and wheat.

Hot/pungent travels to the Lungs

Hot/pungent disperses, spreads, and has the ability to move horizontally. Some pungent foods are able to moisten. In excess, hot/pungent can cause withering of the fingernails and toenails, irritate the lungs, and cause muscles to become tight. Examples of hot/pungent foods are: pepper, cayenne, onion, garlic, hot sauce, ginger, radish, turmeric, clove, chive root, chive seed, cinnamon bark, clove, fennel, ginger, peppermint, rosemary, spearmint, sweet basil, tobacco, and white pepper.

Salty travels to the Kidneys

Salty purges, nourishes *Yin*, and softens what is hard, e.g. tumors or masses. In excess, salty can cause bone weakness, facial pallor, and edema and kidney problems. Examples of salty foods are: salt, miso, soy sauce, watermelon, green olives, pickles, cheddar cheese, chips, barley, pork, duck, ham, kelp, and crab.

Sour travels to the Liver

Sour contains, contracts, draws inwards, and has the ability to astringe. In excess, sour can cause lips to become dry and cracked, the liver to produce excess saliva, the muscles to contract, and the skin to become wrinkled and tough. Examples of sour foods are: lemon, grapefruit, apple, crab apple, pickles, sauerkraut, lecithin, mango, olive, pineapple, plum, orange, mandarin, raspberry, small red or adzuki bean, star fruit, strawberry, tomato, tangerine.

THE FIVE ENERGIES

The five energies of foods refer to their capacity to generate sensations – ranging from hot to cold – in the human body. It is important to know the energy of a food in order to understand how a certain food will act on the body. This especially comes into play when choosing foods for an individual constitutional body type. Even though a food may be cold when it comes out of the

refrigerator, it may still generate heat in the body. If a person with a hot constitution eats a hot natured food, they will become hotter. It is important to eat foods that will balance one's constitutional nature.

The five energies of food are:

(1)   Cold, e.g. bamboo shoot, licorice, peppermint, clam, crab, grapefruit, lettuce, kelp, persimmon, salt, sugar cane, water chestnut, sea grass, seaweed, watermelon;

(2)   Cool, e.g. apple, barley bean curd, chicken egg, common button mushroom, lily flower, peppermint, mango, pear, radish, sesame oil, strawberry, tangerine, wheat, wheat bran, mung bean;

(3)   Hot, e.g. black pepper, cinnamon bark, ginger, green pepper, red pepper, soybean oil, white pepper, anise;

(4)   Warm, e.g. sweet rice, chicken liver, butter; and

(5)   Neutral, e.g. apricot, beef, black fungus, black sesame seeds, carrot.

The common actions of foods refer to the general action that food has without referring to their action on a specific organ. There are actions that can be easily understood by a Western medical practitioner, such as 'strengthens the body' or 'promotes urination'. However, there are many actions that are not easily understood without some background in TCM. Table 14.1 is a brief summary of 24 specific foods alongside their organic actions. Every food has properties and functions. Some have more therapeutic properties than others.

THE EIGHT CONSTITUTIONAL BODY TYPES

Generally speaking, there are eight different constitutional body types. There are two considerations that make up a person's constitution. The first consideration is heredity or congenital factors. The second is the factors that contribute to the constitution after birth. The constitution is not easy to change or alter. The constitution a person comes into this world with is more or less the constitution they have for the duration of their lives.

It is very important to understand a person's constitution when treating, diagnosing, and making dietary and lifestyle recommendations. There are certain foods and certain exercise habits that are actually detrimental to certain constitutions. Certain constitutions are prone to

Table 14.1 Specific foods and their organic actions[22–24]

Food	Properties	Functions	Clinical/notes
Adzuki bean	sweet, sour and neutral	clears heat; lets out water; disperses blood; eliminates edema	treats edema; good for obesity; good for skin sores with redness and swelling
Beef	sweet and neutral	tonifies the spleen and stomach; benefits the *Qi* and blood; strengthens the tendons and the bones	good for those who are weak and fatigued, and those with joint or bone soreness and weakness
Black bean	acrid and cool	invigorates the blood; lets out the water; eliminates toxins; tonifies kidneys; moistens and clears the skin	good for treatment of edema of the head and face; treats weakness of the low back and knees; good for the skin
Brown sugar	sweet and warm	invigorates blood; transforms stasis; tonifies middle *Qi*; moderates or slows down the liver	treats dysmenorrhea (with ginger and hawthorn berry)
Carrot	sweet and neutral	strengthens the Spleen; transforms dampness; harmonizes the intestines and the stomach; aids digestion	
Celery	sweet and cool	clears heat; calms the liver; dispels the wind	treats high blood pressure; treats headache and dizziness due to liver *Yang* rising; treats high cholesterol
Chicken	sweet and warm	warms the middle; benefits the *Qi*; tonifies the essence; builds the bone marrow	the best chicken is black chicken with black bones
Chili pepper	acrid and hot	warms the middle; disperses cold; promotes/improves the appetite; dispels dampness	treats pain from cold in the stomach
Corn	sweet and neutral	improves the appetite; lets out dampness	treats high blood pressure; treats high cholesterol; the husk is most effective for letting out dampness
Eggplant	sweet and cool	clears heat; invigorates the blood; eliminates edema	good for those with habitual blood in the stool
Fish	sweet and neutral or sweet and warm	tonifies the *Yang*; tonifies the *Qi*	
Garlic	acrid and warm	kills parasites; eliminates toxins; strengthens the stomach; digests accumulated foods	very good for treating diarrhea; reduces cholesterol; anticancer effects; should be eaten raw
Ginger, fresh	acrid and warm	releases the exterior; dispels cold; strengthens the stomach; stops vomiting; eliminates toxin	treats vomiting, mild cold, and rheumatoid arthritis
Goat's milk	sweet and warm	nourishes the blood; moistens dryness; benefits the *Qi*; tonifies deficiency	good for those with mouth sores and/or chronic fatigue
Lamb	sweet and warm	tonifies deficiency; warms the middle; warms the lower *Jiao*; tonifies the kidney *Qi*	treats impotence; treats post-partum abdominal pain; treats poor digestion

Continued

Table 14.1 *Continued*

Food	Properties	Functions	Clinical/notes
Mustard greens	acrid and warm	disseminates the lung *Qi*; brings up the phlegm; warms the middle; opens the *Qi*	if overeaten can cause blurred vision
Onion	acrid and warm	harmonizes the stomach; brings down the *Qi*; transforms dampness; dispels phlegm	good for diabetes and/or high cholesterol
Oyster	sweet, salty, and neutral	harmonizes the middle; tonifies deficiency	treats night sweats; treats anemia; increases memory
Peanut	sweet and neutral	harmonizes the stomach; stops bleeding; promotes lactation; moistens the lungs	peanut skin stops bleeding and treats all kinds of blood loss
Pumpkin	sweet and warm	tonifies the middle; benefits the *Qi*; eliminates inflammation; stops pain; eliminates toxins; kills parasites	eating too much can lead to abdominal distension
Rice, brown or white	sweet and neutral	tonifies the five organs; builds or strengthens body strength; builds the flesh	when prepared as congee is very suitable for convalescing
Shrimp	sweet and salty	tonifies the kidneys; strengthens the *Yang*; strengthens the stomach	improves appetite; transforms phlegm
Snow pea	sweet and neutral	harmonizes the middle; brings down the *Qi*; promotes urination; eliminates skin sore toxins	snow peas are difficult to digest therefore should not be over eaten
Walnut	sweet and warm	tonifies the kidneys; strengthens the lower back; secures the essence; stops wheezing; moistens the intestines	treats impotence, seminal emission, constipation, and frequent urination

specific illnesses that others are not. For example, some people, when they develop a cold, will almost always immediately develop a fever. There are other people who, when they develop a cold, will almost always contract pneumonia. And still there are other people who, when they develop a cold, will almost always go on to develop a cough. This is mainly due to their constitution.

There are six factors that contribute to a person's constitution after birth. It is important to pay attention to these factors, especially when treating children. The six post-natal factors that contribute to constitution are environment, nutrition/diet, lifestyle, emotions, disease/illness, and exercise. If an extreme of any of these factors occurs early in life, it can affect the constitution.

It is important to understand the difference between being ill and being of a certain constitutional type. The constitution does not mean illness; it is just a tendency towards certain health problems. People with particular constitutions do better on specific diets and eating

specific foods. They also do better to avoid certain foods that will aggravate their condition.

Avoiding foods does not mean that these foods should never be eaten. It means that if they are eaten they should be balanced with other foods. It also means that those foods should not be consumed in large quantities.

Diagnosis and treatment according to the constitution is a complicated piece of TCM. It should be studied well, in order to use it effectively, yet a basic understanding is helpful in applying TCM dietary principles to a balanced diet.

Normal constitution

Average weight; fairly strong; generally healthy; hair is abundant, shiny, moist, and healthy; skin color is radiant; eyes have life in them, not droopy or too animated; not excessively thirsty; there is nothing excessive about this body type in general; the personality is open, positive, and even tempered; healthy appetite; normal digestion and elimination; when this person catches a cold, it may be sudden or just a common sequelae of symptoms.

Yin deficiency constitution

Usually thin or emaciated; often taller than average; often has malar flush; often feels hot or feverish; may have red eyes, dry eyes, blurred vision, and/or spots in front of their eyes; often will be thirsty and have a dry mouth; likes to drink cold fluids; often their lips will be red and dry; they tend not to like hot climates; may be easily angered or can feel anxious; they tend to have more energy at night; bowel movements will tend to be dry; urine will tend to be scanty and more yellow; this constitution is related more to heredity, unless there has been chronic illness or major blood loss.

Foods that benefit

Foods that enrich or nourish the *Yin*; often foods that are sweet and cool in nature; bananas; Chinese pear; strawberries; lemon; duck egg; chicken egg; duck meat; pork; ham; cucumber; salt; green tea; clams; watermelon; milk; wheat; barley; plums; sea cucumber.

Foods to avoid

Dry and hot foods; deep fried or oily foods; ginger; scallion; garlic; chili pepper; black pepper.

Yang deficiency constitution

Tendency to overweight; tendency to lose hair easily; their face will lack luster, can be shiny and white; their skin will be white, flabby, and flaccid; they may have a bland taste in their mouth; their lips will be pale; they tend to be cold and have cold extremities; they will dislike cold on their back and their stomach; they become easily fatigued; they may be more introverted and quiet; they will prefer to eat warm foods and drink; they may easily suffer with diarrhea; they may have clear and profuse urination; this type of constitution is determined by heredity, or that they did not have adequate food, shelter, or support, or were extremely sick.

Foods that benefit

Rice; peanuts; mustard greens; carrot; garlic; onions; walnuts; pine nut; pumpkin; black pepper; cocoa; goat's milk; chicken; beef; lamb; shrimp; mussels; fish.

Foods to avoid

Oily and rich foods; banana; milk; soft shell turtle; cold or uncooked foods; increased intake of meats; warm foods.

Qi deficiency constitution

These people can swing in either direction with their weight, but more commonly are thin; their hair will be dry and brittle; their facial coloring tends to be yellow or white/grey; their eyes lack vitality; their lips are pale; these people tend to become easily fatigued; these people tend to have an aversion to both hot and cold; their personality will be quiet and have little desire to speak; they like to eat sweet foods because they get quick energy; their stools will be normal but sometimes difficult to pass; they may pass a larger amount of urine than normal; this constitutional type is caused by heredity or may be caused by internal injury to the spleen and stomach.

Foods that benefit

Rice; radishes; pumpkin; cocoa; honey; fish; potato; cabbage; carrot; Chinese date; chicken; beef; shrimp; sweet potato; mustard greens; fennel; lamb; oyster.

Foods to avoid

Similar to *Yang* deficiency; banana; oily and rich foods; acrid foods.

Blood deficiency constitution

These people are generally thin; their eyes lack vitality; they may see black spots in front of their eyes; their lips are pale; their eyes will be dry and scratchy; these people can easily become dizzy; often when they become upset, they may get heart palpitations; they tend to be absent minded; they have a quiet disposition; they will be unable to tolerate cold; in women, their menses will be scanty; this constitution is hereditary or may be caused by a major injury with large blood loss.

Foods that benefit

Sweet potato; black sesame; carrot; goat's milk; quail; peanut; spinach; lotus root; grape; cocoa; pork; clam; chicken egg; beef; important to eat meats and foods high in iron.

Foods to avoid

Oily and rich foods; milk; banana; cold or uncooked foods.

Phlegm/dampness constitution

Tend to be obese; they tend to have puffiness around their eyes, specifically their eyelids and under their eyes; they tend to feel that their body is heavy; they may have a bland or sweet taste in their mouth; they may feel that their mouth is slightly sticky; their facial color will be either dark or pale yellow; they may not have any specific temperament; this person likes to drink tea; their stools with be either normal or slightly soft; they may have cloudy urine.

Foods that benefit

Corn; mung bean; adzuki bean; pea; black bean; celery; amaranth; bamboo shoot; mushroom; banana; pear; watermelon; cucumber; tea leaves; duck; quail.

Foods to avoid

Also similar to *Yang* deficiency constitution; cold or uncooked foods; banana; milk.

Damp heat constitution

There is no particular body weight for this person; their face will often be shiny and oily; they may easily develop skin sores or in youth they may develop acne; the skin will be slightly yellow; the blood vessels in the eyes will be reddish and yellow; the area around the nose will tend to be oily and mucous membranes in the nose dry; this person may have a dry mouth with a slightly bitter taste; this person may be easy to anger; they may be somewhat impatient and anxious; they may feel fatigued and have a lack of energy; they like to eat oily, sweet, and deep fried foods; their stools are usually dry; they may feel that their bowel movements are incomplete; they may have scanty urine with strong yellow color; if these people become sick, it is often associated with emotional upset or associated with the food that they have eaten.

Foods that benefit

Celery; black bean; cucumber; wax gourd; Chinese pear; bamboo shoot; mung bean; snow pea; lima bean; carrot; winter squash; potato with skin; asparagus; mushroom; lemon; cranberry; huckleberry.

Foods to avoid

Oily and deep fried foods; acrid and warm foods; reduce the intake of shrimp and chives; often people who have a damp heat constitution and who eat oily foods will develop skin allergies.

Blood stasis constitution

This person will tend to be of average weight or thin; their complexion will be dark or blackish; they may have broken blood vessels around the nose or on the cheek bones; they may have loss of hair; this person's skin may look dark; there may be red spots or darker red spots on the body; they may have scaly skin, often seen on the legs of elderly people or on the skin of those people with advanced diabetes; the area around the eyes is rather dark; this person may have a dry mouth; they do not have a desire to drink but want only to rinse their mouth out; these people can be irritable, anxious, and impatient; the stools and urine are normal; when this person becomes sick they can easily develop masses; this type of constitution can develop from external injury, blood loss, long-term depression, or frequent energy from the cold.

Foods that benefit

Peanut; lotus root; peach; vinegar; crab; adzuki bean; chive; black fungus; brown sugar; cuttlefish; spinach; eggplant; rose.

Foods to avoid

There are no particular foods to avoid for the blood stasis constitution.

GENERAL GUIDELINES FOR HEALTH

Diagnosis

TCM and Western medicine differ in the way they diagnose illness. When there is disease, illness, or suffering a TCM doctor will look at all the symptoms a patient exhibits. He will look at the whole body system, including the emotions, in order to diagnose and treat the individual. In fact, a TCM doctor will also look at external circumstances, including weather and predominant climate, as it concerns their patient. A diagnosis will be arrived at based on the entirety of symptoms, the constitution of an individual, and the environmental and emotional influences affecting the individual.

After a diagnosis is reached, the doctor will proceed to treat the whole person for the illness or disease as well as the internal imbalance that led to the illness or disease. Chinese medicine rarely treats only the symptom.

In contrast, a Western medical doctor will separate out individual symptoms in order to arrive at a diagnosis. He will look at each of the individual organs, perhaps doing multiple tests on each organ or referring a patient to multiple specialists in order to determine what the problem is. It is not unheard of for a patient to have many doctors, each specializing in different parts of the human body, and/or different illnesses. A Western medical doctor will treat and prescribe medicine for each of the symptoms and diagnoses he determines needs treatment.

Diet therapy

Diet therapy is a very important part of TCM. In a chapter on diet therapy in *Qian Jin Yao Fang (Prescriptions Worth a Thousand Gold Pieces for Emergencies)*, Sun Simiao stated: 'First, gain a thorough understanding of the cause of the disease; when this is known, the disease can be attacked. Treat first with diet, but if this does not work, then use medicines'[25]. This statement clearly describes how important the use of diet therapy in the treatment of disease was at that time.

Diet therapy is just as important today. However, as diseases have become more complicated, the integration of diet therapy along with herbs and acupuncture to make up a complete treatment strategy is most helpful. A complete treatment strategy will produce faster recovery. Diet therapy is a complicated process involving consideration of individual constitution, particular disease, the five flavors, and the energies and actions of food. Diet therapy can become all the more complicated when certain foods have more than one energy or flavor. In this case, you see a single food acting on not just one but perhaps two or three organs. However, this analysis is simplified when one understands the physiology of how the organs support and work together to maintain health.

There are general dietary recommendations that are made based on maintaining the health of the digestive system. In TCM, the Spleen and the Stomach are the source of digestion, therefore emphasis is placed on maintaining the health and strength of these two organs.

The foods, food preparation techniques, and recipes that are prescribed support the digestive function and can be prescribed remedially for specific illnesses, disease, stages of recovery, injuries, and surgeries. If one's digestive system is strong, then recovery from illness or injury can be quick. If one's digestive system is weak, recovery will be slow and perhaps not at all.

Dietary guidelines to adhere to when recovering from illness

When a person is ill their body needs to focus its energy on healing. Therefore it is important to consume easily digestible food that can fortify the body. There are five main dietary guidelines for people recovering from illness or injury. The more serious the illness, the more strictly these guidelines should be followed:

(1) Eat cooked food;

(2) Do not eat cold foods;

(3) Follow the recommendations to benefit digestion;

(4) Eat a diet balanced with foods of the five flavors, five energies, and five actions; and

(5) Eat a balanced diet of vegetables, fruits, whole grains, legumes, seed and nuts.

If these guidelines are followed, the person will recover more quickly and have fewer complications. If a person is very seriously ill, or has undergone any sort of surgery, it is imperative that they eat only cooked foods. It is preferable that they eat highly nutritious, and easily digestible soups and stews until fully recovered.

CONCLUSIONS

Traditional Chinese Medicine is nature-based medicine. It has been successfully practiced for over 2000 years. It places great importance on the prevention and treatment of illness through dietary habits, lifestyle choices, exercise, and psychological well-being. It utilizes natural substances to heal, cure, and repair damage to the human body. It places primary attention on the health of the digestive system in effecting healing and in stimulating a healing response in the body. It is important to have at least a basic understanding of the TCM perspective of physiology of the digestive system, in order to make dietary recommendations that will benefit, support, and effect healing in the body.

TCM utilizes a complex system of diagnostics to determine what is best suited for each individual person. When a person is healthy, there are general dietary and lifestyle guidelines that can be followed to maintain health. When a person is ill there are specific guidelines to follow based on the nature of the illness or injury as well as the constitution of the person and the energy and flavors of the food. When those guidelines are not enough, a TCM doctor will recommend herbs, acupuncture, Qigong and other TCM healing modalities.

References

1. Greene HL. Clinical Medicine. Chicago: Mosby, 1991: 10–18
2. MacBryde CM, Elman R. Nutritional Requirements in Acute and Chronic Disease: Advances in Internal Medicine. New York, NY: Interscience, 1946; 53–92
3. MRC Vitamin Study Research Group. Prevention of neural tube defects: results of the Medical Research Council Vitamin Study. Lancet 1991; 338: 131–7
4. McLester JS. Nutrition and Diet in Health and Disease. Philadelphia: Saunders, 1943: 43–5
5. Yang S, Li J. Li Dong-yuan's Treatise on the Spleen and Stomach. Boulder, CO: Blue Poppy Press, 1993: 24–38
6. Thomson C. Diet and Nutrition. Chicago: Hills Publishing, 1996: 10–23
7. Schauf C. Human Physiology. St Louis: Times Mirror/Mosby College Publishing, 1990: 3–4
8. Clavey S. Fluid Physiology and Pathology in Traditional Chinese Medicine. New York, NY: Churchill Livingston, 1995: 7–50
9. NIH Publication No. 03-4082, Facts about the DASH Eating Plan, United States Department of Health and Human Services, National Institutes of Health, National Heart, Lung, and Blood Institute. J Am Dietetic Assoc 1999; 8: S19–27
10. Xiangcai X. The English–Chinese Encyclopedia of Practical Traditional Chinese Medicine. Beijing: Higher Education Press, 1989: 30–8
11. Schauf C. Human Physiology. St Louis: Mosby College Publishing, 1990: 3–5
12. Maciocia G. The Foundations of Chinese Medicine. New York, NY: Churchill Livingston, 1989: 50–2
13. Eckert A. Chinese Medicine for Beginners. Rocklin, CA: Prima Publishing, 1996: 14–16
14. Xinnong C. Chinese Acupuncture and Moxibustion. Beijing: Foreign Languages Press, 1987: 26–45
15. The Yellow Emperor's Classic of Internal Medicine – Simple Questions (Huang Di Nei Jing). Beijing: People's Health Publishing House, 1979: 32–40
16. Maciocia G. The Foundations of Chinese Medicine. New York, NY: Churchill Livingston, 1989: 34–50
17. A Revised Explanation of the Classic of Difficulties (Nan Jing Jiao Shi). Beijing: Nanjing College of Traditional Chinese Medicine, People's Health Publishing House, 1979
18. Harmer, B. Textbook of the Principles and Practice of Nursing. Chicago: The Macmillan Company, 1937: 126–8
19. Jing-Nuan, Wu J-N. Ling Shu or Spiritual Pivot. Washington, DC: University of Hawaii Press, 1993; 6: 38–63
20. The Yellow Emperor's Classic of Internal Medicine – Simple Questions (Huang Ti Nei Jing Su Wen). Beijing: People's Health Publishing House, 1979: 103–20
21. Ling Shu (The Miraculous Pivot), part of Huang Di Nei Jing (The Yellow Emperor's Internal Classic), Warring States period. Washington, DC: The Taoist Center, 1993: 62–80
22. Lu HC. Chinese Natural Cures: Traditional Methods for Remedies and Preventions. New York, NY: Black Dog & Leventhal Publishers, 1994: 22–44
23. Le K. The Simple Path to Health; A Guide to Oriental Nutrition and Well-being. Portland, OR: Rudra Press, 1996: 5–48
24. Eckert A. Chinese Medicine for Beginners. Rocklin, CA, 1996: 20–32
25. Bei Ji Qian Jin Yao Fang (Prescriptions Worth a Thousand Gold Pieces for Emergencies). Sun Simiao, 625: 32–40

Massage

15

D. J. Engen

HISTORY

Massage has a history in many cultures dating back to ancient times, and is considered by many to be one of the oldest forms of medical care. Greek and Roman physicians used massage therapy to alleviate pain. Julius Caesar was said to have been given a daily massage to treat his neuralgia. People giving massages are depicted in Egyptian tomb paintings. Massage is so ancient that the derivation of the word is uncertain – it may have come from the ancient Greek word *massin* (to knead), or the Arabic *mass*, or the Hebrew *mashesh* (to press). In the East, massage has continued to be seen as a holistic and beneficial part of health care continuing throughout the ages. Many Eastern cultures today utilize massage therapy regularly for health and wellness, and as one of the first forms of treatment with illness and injury. Some massage therapists are known as healers as they have apprenticed to learn ancient techniques for manipulating soft tissue to heal body illnesses.

Hippocrates, considered by many to be the father of Western medicine, in the fifth century BC, wrote in his *Corpus Hippocraticum*, 'The Physician must be experienced in many things, but assuredly in rubbing... for rubbing can bind a joint that is too loose, and loosen a joint that is too rigid'. In the Western world, massage has faced many struggles to maintain its existence. At the founding of the United States, medical practice relied on the use of herbs and therapeutic massage to a large extent. During World War I, nurses provided massage therapy to the injured to reduce anxiety and pain. In the 1930s, massage therapy became a therapeutic technique utilized by physical therapists to reduce pain and to aid in the recovery of muscle function.

CURRENT STATUS

With breakthroughs of medical technology and pharmacology, Western medical culture gradually adjusted. The result has been a reduction in the role of manual manipulation therapies and a rapid increase in diagnostics and treatment approaches using electrical instruments, surgery, and medications.

Funding has also been a key driver in the creation of current Western medicine medical practice. The relative lack of formal/validating research proving the benefits of massage therapy or soft tissue manipulation has resulted in reduced reimbursement from third party payers for massage therapy. In addition, whereas nurses once frequently employed massage in the routine care of patients, the nurse's role has evolved to the point where there has been a significant reduction in hands-on practice.

The American Massage Therapy Association (AMTA) reports that there is a rapidly growing interest in the benefits of massage therapy in conjunction with conventional medical treatments and to prevent and avoid injury or illness. The AMTA reported that 21% (1 in 5) of adult Americans received a massage in 2003, a 3% increase from 2002. Among adult Americans, 22% reported the use of massage therapy from a professional massage therapist for relaxation. The use of massage to treat severe back, neck, or shoulder pain was 25%, and for stress relief was 29%. In addition, 19% of those polled reported that they had discussed obtaining a therapeutic massage with their primary physician or health-care provider (an increase of 14% from 2002). Among those who discussed their use of massage with their health-care provider, 62% of their primary care providers strongly recommended or encouraged their patients to pursue therapeutic massage as a form of treatment.

American consumers are increasingly seeking methods for prevention and wellness as well as alternatives to medications and surgery. With the evolution of today's technology has come the changes in the the physical and mental nature of most jobs. With these changes has come a dramatic increase in stress – mental stress and physical stress (such as exemplified by repetitive use syndromes). For example, a person driving a car and/or sitting at a computer for hours, repetitively works the same set of muscles. Over time, the constantly working muscles become fatigued, contracted, and may start to become painful. Then, in the next effortful motion requiring the fatigued, contracted muscles to work, a painful muscle spasm may occur.

Americans seek massage therapy for many reasons. Some of these reasons are to reduce muscle aches and pain, reduce stiffness, increase range of motion and joint flexibility, relax, sleep better, recover faster after excessive exercise, break up scar tissue, reduce fibrosis and adhesions, improve mental alertness, improve exercise potential, and stretch tensed muscles. With the growth of consumer use, massage therapy is becoming more commonly accepted as a technique to improve or reduce some of these symptoms. Massage therapy may increase range of motion, relax tensed muscles, loosen connective tissue, relieve muscle spasms and associated pain, reduce stress-related tension, improve bowel function, lower heart rate, and blood pressure, improve circulation, mobilize muscle toxins, speed the recovery of fatigued muscles, improve the energy flow (*Qi*), and aid the body to release healing hormones.

Gertrude Beard, RN, RPT, former Associate Professor of Physical Therapy at Northwestern University Medical School in Chicago, Illinois, summarizes the findings of numerous research studies on the therapeutic effects of massage. Studies indicate that massage:

- Has a sedative effect upon the nervous system and promotes voluntary muscle relaxation

- Is effective in promoting recovery from fatigue produced by excessive exercise

- Can help break up scar tissue and lessen fibrosis and adhesions, which develop as a result of injury and immobilization

- Can relieve certain types of pain

- Provides effective treatment of chronic inflammatory conditions by increasing lymphatic circulation

- Helps reduce swelling from fractures

- Affects circulation through the capillaries, veins, and arteries, and increases blood flow throughout the muscles

- Can loosen mucus and promote drainage of fluids from the lungs by using percussive and vibratory techniques

- Can increase peristaltic action in the intestines to promote fecal elimination.

There are a number of studies demonstrating the beneficial effects of massage therapy in relation to the physiologic and psychologic aspects of stress. In one study, chair massage was provided twice a week for 5 weeks to 26 adult subjects, while 24 control subjects were asked to relax in the massage chair for 15 minutes. On the first and last days of the study all of the participants underwent EEG monitoring, before, during, and after the sessions. In addition, before and after the sessions they performed math computations, completed POMS depression and state anxiety scales, and provided a saliva sample for cortisol measurement. This small-scale study had outcomes suggesting that massage therapy offers benefits in not just alleviating the physiologic effects of anxiety, but also in improving mental alertness.

Research to determine which non-analgesic methods of pain control are effective and under what conditions has been an area of active and growing interest. A study was completed to test the effectiveness of massage as an intervention for cancer pain. Twenty-eight patients were randomly assigned to a massage or control group. The patients in the massage group were given a 10 minute massage to the back; the patients in the control group were visited for 10 minutes. The results showed massage to be an effective short-term nursing intervention for pain in males in this sample. No reduction of pain was found in the female population participating in this study.

A growing number of acute and long-term care facilities are instituting massage therapy programs to support their patients' health, healing, and quality of life. A study was conducted at a large university hospital to evaluate patient outcomes from a therapeutic massage program within an acute care setting. One hundred and thirteen hospitalized patients received one to four massages during the course of their hospital stay; 70 patients, 14 health-care providers, and 4 massage therapists completed surveys and narrative reports. The most frequently identified outcomes were increased relaxation (98%), a sense of well-being (93%), and positive mood change (88%). More than two-thirds of patients attributed enhanced mobility, greater energy, increased participation in treatment, and faster recovery to massage therapy. Thirty-five percent stated that benefits lasted more than one day. The study supported the value of this hospital-based massage therapy program and uncovered a range of benefits of massage therapy for hospitalized patients that require further study.

Today's Western medicine and third-party payors rely on valid research to change standards of practice and funding. Valid research showing that massage therapy can have medical benefits is growing, but more is needed. The massage techniques used are often missing from the research and the number of participants in the study is often quite small.

PHYSIOLOGIC EFFECTS

Understanding the physiologic workings of the human body might assist in the understanding of the techniques and impact of massage. The following sections outline three conceptual categories:

(1) Relaxation;

(2) Soft tissue (therapeutic); and

(3) Bioenergetic, related to the effects of massage therapy.

This is a broad and by no means all-inclusive overview of some of the concepts regarding the physiologic effects massage can have on the human body.

Relaxation effects

The body consists of a close interaction of organs and systems. 'The close inter-relationship between the somatic, autonomic and endocrine systems makes it impossible for pathologic changes to take place in any one structure without causing adaptive changes in other structures' (by Edner quoted in Chaitow). Richard Van Why compiled an abstracted collection of world literature showing scientific evidence supporting the claim that massage therapy is beneficial. With the interconnection of the body's systems, the effects massage therapy can have are theoretically unlimited.

For example, long slow massage strokes to a person's arm or back will have a local affect on the soft tissue of that area. These slow, rhythmic massage strokes affect the proprioceptive nerve fibers of the skin and underlying tissues of that area, which alert the brain to signal the release of relaxation-inducing hormones such as endorphins from the endocrine system. Such a release of hormones could be expected to bring the body to a parasympathetic (relaxation) state, (e.g. slowing of heart rate and respiratory rate), the effects expected from a relaxation massage.

Soft tissue (therapeutic) effects

The body is largely made up of a skeletal system, that creates structure, and soft tissue, which includes the muscles and connective tissue that protect the organs, autonomic, and circulatory systems, and create motion. The body functions as one unit and relies on muscle balance to function properly. Fluid, coordinated motion is created through muscle pull (concentric contraction) on the skeletal system, with the opposing muscle slowly lengthening (eccentric contraction). As muscles contract and shorten, they pull the skeletal system into a different position. The opposing muscle slowly lengthens to create coordinated/smooth motions, similar to pulley systems. Good muscle balance allows fluid movements, proper joint alignment for a full range of motion, and shock absorption.

With misalignment, decreased joint mobility, nerve impingement, and wear and tear of the joints can occur. If the joint is not moving in good alignment due to poor muscle balance, assisting/smaller (synergistic) muscles must do the extra work. Gradually the synergists become contracted, constricted, and fatigued. They can become ischemic (anoxia resulting from reduced peripheral circulation). With the chronic contraction and resulting reduced blood flow, the muscle loses the ability to clear all its waste products, developing chronic painful trigger points. The muscle shortens, weakens, and the fascial/connective tissue constricts around the muscle fibers. In addition, muscles that are out of balance and no longer working with a coordinated movement because of shortened and fatigued fibers are prone to spasm, fatigue, and pain. The result over time might be joint wearing, muscle tears, reduction in activity, or injury due to reduced coordination.

Therapeutic massage techniques can break up muscular waste deposits, stimulate circulation, loosen constricting fascia, and lengthen muscle fibers. The results include pain reduction, increased range of motion, improved balance, and the opportunity to strengthen muscle.

For most of today's work force, repetitive motions and motions that use one side of the pulley system and not the opposing muscle are becoming more and more common. With a therapeutic massage, the therapist assesses body posture and looks for misalignment, muscle imbalance, tightness, and weakness, toxin build-up, trigger points, etc. Using a variety of techniques, muscle toxins and muscle contractions can be released, connective tissue can be loosened, muscles can be lengthened to regain balance, and joint alignment can be gained. Muscles needing to be lengthened and strengthened can be identified for an exercise program to regain optimal function.

Bioenergetic effects

Eastern massage follows a belief system that the body has energy channels (meridians) flowing vertically throughout the body. Blockages in these energy channels are what create illness. The use of massage techniques to work on the flow of energy (*Ki* or *Qi*) throughout the body can help a person heal or prevent an illness.

DIFFERENT TECHNIQUES

The terms massage, therapeutic massage, bodywork, etc. are all terms meaning to promote health and healing through the intentional and systematic manipulation of the body's connective and muscle tissue. Deepak Chopra MD defines the term 'massage' as a form of bodywork, and includes deep tissue manipulation, movement awareness, and bioenergetic therapies under the category of bodywork, which includes therapies employed to improve the structure and functioning of the body. As massage has been a technique used for many centuries, it is not surprising that there are many specialty forms and/or techniques of massage therapy.

The following is an outline of some of the massage therapy and bodywork techniques outlined by the National Certification Board for Therapeutic Massage and Bodywork. The list is not all-inclusive, but contains some of the most often applied techniques in massage therapy and bodywork today.

Acupressure

Acupressure is a form of bodywork based on traditional Chinese meridian theory in which acupuncture points are pressed to stimulate the flow of energy or *Qi*.

Bodywork

Bodywork is a general term for practices involving touch and movement in which the practitioner uses manual techniques to promote health and healing in the recipient.

Chair massage

Chair massage refers to massage given with the recipient seated in an ordinary or special massage chair. Recipients remain clothed in chair massage. It has been called on-site massage when the chair is taken to a public place, such as an office or commercial establishment.

Craniosacral

In the 1900s, Dr William Sutherland, an osteopathic physician, proposed the concept of cranial pulsations, rhythmic movements of the brain. In the 1970s, Dr John Upledger, an osteopathic doctor, furthered Sutherland's concept and suggested such pulsations could be detected and corrected using very light pressure. Craniosacral therapy is a light touch manipulation of the head and bottom of the spine to restore optimal cerebrospinal fluid movement. It is purported to be useful in treating headaches, eye and ear problems, jaw problems, whiplash, and back pain.

Deep tissue massage

Deep tissue massage is also called deep muscle therapy or deep tissue therapy. It is an umbrella term for bodywork systems that work deeply into the muscles and connective tissue to release chronic aches and pains. Rolfing® and Hellerwork are examples of deep tissue massage.

Esalen massage

Esalen massage was developed at the Esalen Institute in Big Sur, California. The emphasis is on slow, long, flowing, gliding movements done to provide deep relaxation.

Feldenkrais Method

The Feldenkrais Method® is an educational system which uses movement to bring about more effective ways to function. Moshe Feldenkrais, a Russian-born Israeli, was a physicist, and mechanical and electrical engineer before developing his movement theories. Feldenkrais is offered in two forms. One form is called Functional Integration®, which is a one-on-one session. The other form is called Awareness Through Movement®, which is provided via group lessons. The goal is to 'rewire' or re-educate the nervous system.

Hellerwork

Joseph Heller, originally trained in Rolfing, developed Hellerwork after he studied with Judith Aston. Hellerwork is a series of eleven 90-minute sessions of deep tissue bodywork, movement education, and dialog designed to realign the body and release chronic tension and stress.

Jin Shin Do®

Jin Shin Do® (JSD), the 'way of the compassionate spirit', is Iona Marsaa Teeguarden's synthesis of Eastern and Western theories and practices. It is a method of releasing muscle tension and stress by applying deepening finger pressure to combinations of specific points on the body. It combines classic Chinese acupuncture theory, Taoist yogic philosophy and breathing methods, and Japanese acupressure techniques.

Manual lymph drainage

Manual lymph drainage is a gentle method of promoting movement of lymph into and through the lymphatic vessels. It is primarily used to reduce edema.

Myofascial release

During myofascial release, restrictions (stuck areas) are located and gentle sliding pressure is applied in the direction of the restriction to stretch the tissues. The stretching of tissues and the heat imparted by the practitioner's hands are thought to help produce a softer consistency of fascial tissues.

Neuromuscular therapy

Neuromuscular therapy (NMT) is a generic designation for trigger point work (see Trigger point massage).

Pregnancy massage

Pregnancy massage is the massage of pregnant women (prenatal) and women who have given birth (postpartum). It addresses the special needs of pregnant women such as discomforts in the lower back, feet, and legs.

Reiki

Reiki is a Japanese word pronounced 'ray-kee' and means 'universal life energy'. It is a light touch or no-touch technique for channeling this omnipresent energy to promote healing.

Reflexology

Reflexology is a form of bodywork based on the theory of zone therapy, in which specific spots of the body are pressed to stimulate corresponding areas in other parts of the body. Foot reflexology, in which pressure techniques are applied only to the feet, is the most common form of reflexology.

Rolfing®

Rolfing® is also called structural integration and was developed by Ida Rolf. Rolfing seeks to re-establish proper vertical alignment in the body by manipulating the myofascial tissue so that the fascia elongates and glides rather than shortens and adheres. The 10-session series can cause deep changes in the body that are physical as well as emotional.

Rosen Method®

The Rosen Method®, developed by physical therapist Marion Rosen, is a system of bodywork and movement that helps the client experience themself in a more accepting and loving way through non-intrusive, subtle touch, awareness of breath, movement exercises, and gentle coaxing.

Shiatsu

Shiatsu (Japanese for 'finger pressure') is a system for healing and health maintenance that has evolved over thousands of years. Shiatsu derives both from the ancient healing art of acupuncture and from the traditional form of Japanese massage, amma. The goal of each of the different types of shiatsu being practiced (e.g. Zen shiatsu, tsubo point therapy, shiatsu massage, and water shiatsu) is balancing energy flow.

Sports massage

Sports massage is applied to athletes to help them train and perform free from pain and injuries. Massage therapists blend classic Swedish strokes with such methods as compression, pressure-point therapy, cross-fiber friction, joint mobilization, hydrotherapy, and cryotherapy (ice massage) to meet the special needs of high-level performers and fitness enthusiasts.

Swedish massage

Swedish massage is also known as the Western or classic style of massage. It is credited to the Swedish fencing master and gymnastics instructor, Per Henrik Ling. It is a scientific system of manipulations on the muscles and connective tissues of the body for the purpose of relaxation, rehabilitation, or health maintenance. Swedish massage therapy comprises five basic strokes and their variations: effleurage, petrissage, friction, tapotement (or percussion), and vibration.

Therapeutic touch

Therapeutic touch was developed by nurses Dolores Krieger and Dora Kunz in the early 1970s after studying the ancient practice of laying on of hands. It is based on the idea that human beings are energy in the form of a field. In health, the field flows freely, while it becomes out of balance when disease is present.

Trigger point massage

Trigger point massage utilizes ischemic compression of individual areas of hypersensitivity in muscles, ligaments, tendons, and fascia. These trigger points are defined by their referral of pain to distant locations in muscles, connective tissues, and organs. Janet Travell, MD pioneered trigger point therapy in the United States.

Watsu®

Watsu®, or water shiatsu, is a system that employs the stretches of Zen shiatsu in a pool of warm water. The pool provides a deeply relaxing environment where weight and pressures are removed from the body. The client is floated and rocked as the spine is gently pulled and stretched, following the precepts of Zen shiatsu. Harold Dull originated Watsu®.

FINDING A MASSAGE THERAPIST AND A TECHNIQUE THAT IS RIGHT FOR YOU

'Not all massage therapists are created equal.' Today's massage therapy schools vary in their programs. Some offer massage training for a spa setting and others for therapeutic settings. For spa settings, the massage therapy student is provided with training to provide a relaxing and pampering massage. Proper use of techniques to alleviate soft tissue problems requires additional training beyond that used for general relaxation.

Along with adequate training, the massage therapist needs to incorporate their knowledge of techniques with their knowledge of the human body. Then, from hands-on experience, they have to incorporate their ability to assess or identify issues with utilizing the appropriate pressure and technique for each specific body type and problem. Most professional massage therapists learn an array of techniques and often interweave them into a massage session. The goal is to fit the talents of a therapist to your needs.

A MASSAGE SESSION

The massage therapist should first seek to learn what you want to get out of your session and, in turn, verbally help you understand what to expect. Certain types of massage therapy are uncomfortable during their application due to the strength of pressure and application to sensitive acupoints, trigger points, muscle spasms, or adhesions from old injuries or chronic physical stress. A good rule of thumb is, if a pressure point is painful, the pain should subside as soon as the pressure is removed. As your body adjusts to the changes made during the massage session, 24–36 hours of discomfort may be experienced. More persistent discomfort may indicate the session was too aggressive for you or too much change at once, or had caused some of the body's tissue to become bruised. Always stop a session if you are not confident with any experience of discomfort.

Massage techniques can be applied with the client seated or lying down. Some include oils or lotions, some do not. You should feel comfortable in knowing what to expect from the session, the amount of clothing you are to wear, and the draping to be used during the session. Always speak up and stop a session if it is not what you expected or desired.

STANDARDS OF PRACTICE

Massage therapy is regulated differently in every state. Many states require massage therapists to be licensed in order to practice; others have hours of training requirements, and other states have no standard requirements. At the time of this writing, 24 states and the District of Columbia currently offer licensure, certification, or registration. Most states, cities and counties require completion of a massage therapy training program. In addition to class hours, clinical practice hours are important in this hands-on profession. The National Certification Board for Therapeutic Massage and Bodywork is an organization seeking to increase the standards of practice through a written exam. Even with advanced training, massage providers are never licensed to diagnose any medical conditions or prescribe medications.

If you are seeking a therapeutic massage or specific skills, especially if more than a relaxation massage is desired, ask the therapist what and where they acquired their training, and ask for references of clients with similar issues. Seeking the advice of your primary care physician is also advisable.

Massage may not be appropriate, or certain areas of your body should be avoided if you have certain medical conditions, such as phlebitis, infectious disease, inflamed or infected tissue, deep vein thrombosis, or open wounds. Currently in the United States, a physician's prescription is required if you have active cancer. You may want to consult your physician if you have any of these conditions or other medical conditions before seeking the services of a massage therapist.

CONCLUSIONS

Massage is growing in use by consumers. Athletes are using massage therapy to increase performance and decrease the aches, pains, and stiffness after physical exertion. Professionals are seeking massage as a means to promote their health and wellness in an increasingly technologic, high-stress, overuse-syndrome-promoting work environment. Employers are also discovering the benefits of providing onsite massage therapy for their employees to promote mental and physical health. Hospitals are beginning to incorporate massage therapy into their care and treatments, and a growing number of health-care and insurance companies are now covering massage therapy services.

Even though the use of massage is growing by consumers, more validating research continues to be needed. The small amount of empirical research that does exist, more often than not, does not define the kind of touch or massage methodology employed, and massage is often rolled in with a range of other therapeutic methods.

As we have moved into a technologically advanced culture, ways to stay mentally, physically, and emotionally in balance, and maintain optimal health, become more difficult. Soft tissue manipulation through massage therapy is one method to positively impact the body's systems to improve health and well-being. Along with the physiologic benefits, a massage therapy session can also help you pay attention to your body. Awareness of tension, posture difficulties, weak or tight muscles, or muscle imbalances can help you adjust the ergonomics of your work environment, or your work-out exercise program. Awareness can help you incorporate optimal stretching and strengthening into your exercise program to promote optimal health and wellness. Consider exploring the possible benefits of massage not only in your personal self-care but for your patients as well.

Bibliography

ALTERNATIVES in health™ Vol 1;2 and Vol 1;5

Chopra D. Alternative Medicine, The Definitive Guide, 2nd edn. Berkeley, CA: Celestial Arts, 2002

Knaster M. Discovering the Body's Wisdom. New York: Bantam, 1996

Polly M, Teri K. Hospital-Based Massage Programs in Review, 3rd edn. Hospital-Based Massage Network, 2004

Smith MC, Stallings MA, Mariner S, Burrall M. J Nurse Midwifery 1999; 44: 217–30

Stillerman E. The Encyclopedia of Bodywork from Acupressure to Zone Therapy. Facts on File, 1996

Tappan F. Tappan's Handbook of Healing Massage Techniques. Appleton and Lange, 1998

The Bodywork Knowledgebase; Practitioner's Desk Reference, Vol 1 (1959–1988). Compiled by Richard van Why, 1989

Weinrich SP, Weinrich MC. The effect of massage on pain in cancer patients. Appl Nurs Res 1990; 3: 140–5

www.massagemag.com/2004/issue112/history112.htm, accessed on 9 August 2005

www.amtamassage.org/infocenter/current.html, accessed on 9 August 2005

www.online-ambulance.com/altermed/grp/1/art_grp /Bodywork/art/therapeutic_massage.html, accessed on 9 August 2005

www.secretsofisis.com/faq/states.html, accessed on 9 August 2005

www.ncbtmb.com/standards_of_practice.htm, accessed on 9 August 2005

Herbal antioxidants: potential and pitfalls

16

T. L. Vanden Hoek and Z.-H. Shao

INTRODUCTION

One important reason why herbal medication use has increased dramatically in the USA is the promise of youth. Many herbs contain antioxidant compounds which have great potential to lower the oxidant stress associated with aging. For example, 'To promote cardiovascular health' is one of the benefits posted on the bottle of some grape seed extracts. However, while oxidants may be associated with a number of disease processes associated with aging, they are also potentially beneficial in low levels as signaling molecules. Such oxidants are the means by which communication between and within cells of the body can occur quickly, and they may help the body adapt to stress.

This dual role of oxidants, both as culprits of disease and messengers for healthy adaptation, may explain why so many clinical trials of antioxidants have had equivocal results on long-term cardiovascular health. Oxidants may also be useful in fighting infection and in preventing cancer by initiating apoptosis. Thus, although a number of medicinal herbs have antioxidative properties, like other antioxidants the long-term effect on health is unclear. Their effects in certain settings when the body is placed under greater stress becomes even more uncertain. For example, up to 32% of patients in the preoperative setting have been reported to use herbal medications[1]. In addition to potential adverse effects and drug interactions, possibly due to a number of these herbal medications[2,3], one could ask whether a potent antioxidant could interfere with useful oxidant signaling which probably occurs when the body undergoes the major stress of surgery. A more complete understanding of oxidant physiology and pathophysiology will be necessary to fully appreciate the best role for medicinal herbs in preventing cardiovascular disease without harmful side-effects.

In addition to the possible benefits of preventing long-term oxidant stress, the antioxidants found in herbal medications may have great potential benefit for a second reason. Oxidants probably contribute to the tissue damage associated with certain medical emergencies in which blood flow is suddenly stopped to either particular organs or the entire body. These emergencies include stroke, myocardial infarction, shock, and cardiac arrest. The use of medicinal herbs for treating such medical emergencies has been less studied, but their antioxidant properties may be extremely useful in these particular settings. Traditional antioxidants such as vitamin E may not act quickly enough to be effective, whereas some herbal compounds may act fast enough to prevent rapid oxidant damage. Few studies have explored the potential for such acute treatment.

The goal of this chapter is to highlight these potential antioxidant benefits of herbal medications, both chronic and acute, and the potential dangers of interfering with the beneficial consequences of oxidants.

CARDIOVASCULAR DISEASE AND OXIDANT STRESS

Cardiovascular disease remains the leading cause of death in the USA, with 300 000 of these per year occurring outside the hospital as sudden cardiac arrest. While improvements in mortality have occurred, the actual numbers of people dying from cardiovascular diseases, including heart disease and stroke, have risen by 37% since 1950 because of aging and population growth, while improvements in age-adjusted mortality have slowed to negligible levels in the 1990s. In addition, congestive heart failure affects almost 5 million people in the USA, with 400 000 new cases diagnosed per year, and the prevalence is projected to increase 2–3-fold by 2010. Increased oxidant stress, when levels of oxidants within cells overwhelm antioxidant defenses, undoubtedly plays an important role in cardiovascular disease. Although

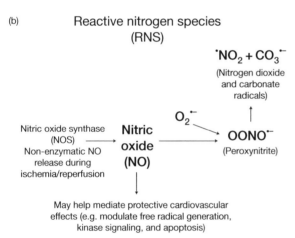

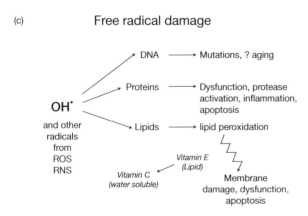

Figure 16.1 Overview of reactive oxygen (a), reactive nitrogen (b) oxidant species, and oxidant damage (c) that can occur both acutely and chronically in the cardiovascular system. Note that oxidants can play both damaging and protective roles depending upon species, amount, and conditions under which they are generated

critical for much life on our planet, oxygen has an important side-effect: it generates free radicals by interacting with sunlight, ionizing radiation, environmental chemicals, and our own intrinsic metabolic processes when we digest food (Figure 16.1).

These free radicals, highly reactive molecules with unpaired electrons usually containing oxygen or nitrogen, may lead to a number of degenerative diseases associated with aging and tissue oxidation. In particular, oxidative modification of low-density lipoproteins (LDLs) probably plays a major role in the progression of atherosclerosis, which in turn predisposes to diseases of heart attack and stroke – leading causes of death and disability, respectively, in the USA. What we eat can alter this outcome, in part by shielding us against this constant barrage of free radicals. A high intake of fresh fruits and vegetables rich in antioxidant flavonoids or nuts (rich in the antioxidant vitamin E) decreases cardiovascular risk of heart attack, stroke, and death[4–9].

CHRONIC EFFECTS OF ANTIOXIDANTS ON CARDIOVASCULAR DISEASE

Traditional antioxidants

Before discussing studies of the antioxidant cardiovascular effects of herbal medicines, much can be learned from research exploring the utility of traditional antioxidants, since this work has progressed further to multiple clinical trials. The use of antioxidant supplements to prevent cardiovascular disease has been an attempt to reproduce some of the benefits of a healthy diet. One of the most studied antioxidants is vitamin E, an antioxidant which affects smooth muscle proliferation and platelet adhesion, and in a number of smaller cohort studies appears to result in decreased risk of coronary artery disease[10,11]. However, a number of randomized clinical trials showed no benefit of vitamin E supplementation on coronary artery disease risk and high doses (≥ 400 IU/day) may increase all-cause mortality[12–14]. While one study suggested that vitamin E may decrease the risk of non-fatal myocardial infarctions, it did not decrease cardiovascular mortality[15].

Another antioxidant commonly studied in human clinical trials is β-carotene. Carotenoids represent over 500 different colored plant pigments, with β-carotene the most abundant in nature. β-Carotene, a highly effective free radical scavenger[16], has been associated with decreased LDL oxidation[17] and decreased risk of coronary artery disease[18]. However, prospective cohort studies have failed to show an association between carotenoid intake and coronary heart disease[19,20], and multiple primary prevention trials failed to show any reduction in coronary heart disease[21–24]. The potential dangers of antioxidants were highlighted in trials showing increased mortality among smokers taking β-carotene supplements[12,13].

In evaluating the potential benefits of herbal medications, the trials studying traditional antioxidants are very instructive. Although very promising as antioxidants in many models of free radical generation, antioxidants such as vitamin E and β-carotene have often failed to demonstrate a beneficial effect in human clinical trials. There may be many reasons for this failure, reasons which will need to be addressed in future evaluations of herbal medications. First, currently, there is no single good assay that can quickly and reliably measure changes in oxidant stress in the clinical setting. Thus, it is difficult to know if the dose of any antioxidant used is actually the most effective at reducing oxidants. Second, there are many types of species of oxidants generated in different compartments of the cell (e.g. mitochondrial vs cytosolic, lipid vs water-soluble phases) and body (e.g. organ-specific, liver vs brain vs heart). Since antioxidants have different mechanisms and sites of action, it is highly unlikely that any one antioxidant would be capable of attenuating oxidant stress in all cell compartments and organs of the body. Thus, a cocktail of antioxidants may be more beneficial than single agents. This is a potential advantage which herbal medicines possess. Many herbal formulations contain multiple phenolic compounds which may act in different ways to quench oxidant stress. They include flavonoids (over 5000 different compounds reported, including anthocyanidins, catechins, flavanones, flavones, flavonols, and isoflavones), tannins (ellagic acid, gallic acid), phenyl isopropenoids (e.g. caffeic acid, coumaric acids, ferulic acid), lignans, catechol, resveratrol (grape skins), rosmarinic acid (rosemary), and many others. (For a review of structures and antioxidant mechanisms see reference 25.)

Finally, the 'best' antioxidant(s) may not be the cocktail which quenches every trace of oxidants, including the beneficial effects of oxidants. Ideally, agents would augment oxidant defenses when needed but not decrease oxidant signaling, the use of oxidants to fight infections, or the role of oxidants in apoptosis and prevention of cancer. Toward this end, more sophisticated assays to evaluate such effects will be useful in the future to predict which formulations will be most effective.

Herbal antioxidants

Far fewer and smaller studies have examined the potential protective effects of antioxidant herbal preparations. There are some examples of herbal therapies which have been tested in small clinical trials. While the greatest use of herbal medications occurs in the East, controlled trials there are lacking because, in many instances, the use of placebo is considered unethical[26]. Experience with some of these compounds is also greater in Europe than in the USA. In Germany, Commission E of the Ministry of Health is a committee of physicians, pharmacists, scientists, and herbalists who evaluate the safety, quality, and efficacy of herbs. A significant portion of these herbs is prescribed for cardiovascular conditions and is evaluated in ongoing reports published by the Commission, and circulated by the American Botanical Council, and the reference text *PDR for Herbal Medicines*. Below is a highlight of some herbal remedies with potential cardiovascular benefits due to antioxidant activity. Unfortunately, a complete summary of potential antioxidant and pro-oxidant effects of each compound is not possible given the page limitations of this chapter. The level of detail in each section depends in part on the amount of human experience with the herb, as demonstrated by consumer interest and by clinical trials, and by work in our own laboratory with some of these compounds.

Danshen

Danshen (*Salvia miltiorrhiza*) has been used in Traditional Chinese Medicine for many years to promote blood flow and treat angina pectoris and acute myocardial infarction[27]. A constituent, terpene tanshinone, has been found to be a potent antioxidant against lipid peroxidation, including lipid peroxidation of LDLs[28] and myocardial mitochondrial membranes[29], without pro-oxidant effects[30]. Few placebo-controlled studies have been performed using danshen or its constituents. One double-blind study of 67 subjects reported symptomatic and electrocardiograph (ECG) improvement with tanshinone IIA. Adverse effects include acting as a vasoconstrictor of non-coronary arteries at higher doses[27], and a potentiation of warfarin when taken concurrently[31].

Garlic

Garlic (*Allium sativum*) is one of the over-the-counter preparations most widely used for medicinal reasons in the USA. The active substance in garlic is allicin, formed when alliin is broken down by alliinase as garlic is crushed[3]. Due to differences in bioavailability (in part due to preparation techniques and tablet composition) – with the additional difficulties of blinding studies and discontinuation by subjects due to odor – it has been difficult to perform randomized clinical trials to evaluate its possible effects on hyperlipidemia, hypertension, coagulation, and atherosclerosis. These effects are reviewed elsewhere within this book and by others[3]. Of note, the anti-atherosclerotic activity of garlic may be independent of its lipid-lowering effects and more due to its inhibition of lipid peroxidation[32]. Garlic used in patients with peripheral vascular disease increased their pain-free walking distance[33], and has been reported to decrease atherosclerotic plaque detected in the femoral artery or carotid bifurcation[34].

Ginkgo

Ginkgo (*Ginkgo biloba*) is one of the best-selling herbal preparations in the USA, derived from the leaves of the maidenhair tree. It has had mixed results in the few clinical trials designed to test whether it can improve measures of cognition in patients with vascular dementia, and has been reported to treat claudication and antagonize platelet-activating factor. Constituents of ginkgo, including the terpenoid compounds bilobalide and ginkgolides A and B, have antioxidant properties and are reported to attenuate reperfusion injury following ischemia[35–37]. A small, randomized, placebo-controlled trial of patients undergoing cardiopulmonary bypass or aortic valve replacement showed that high-dose pretreatment with *Ginkgo biloba* extract decreased indices of oxidant stress post-reperfusion (thiobarbituric acid-reactive species and electron spin resonance measures of the plasma ascorbate pool using dimethylsulfoxide/ ascorbyl free radical levels)[38]. However, the clinical outcomes in this small study were not significant. Of note, this is one of the few herbal studies which used both placebo controls and indices of oxidant stress.

Other benefits and possible adverse effects are important as this herbal medicine is used extensively. Of note, particularly in preoperative patients, are possible effects on bleeding and potentiation of warfarin.

American ginseng

American ginseng (*Panax quinquefolius*) is a perennial aromatic herb native to the northern region of the USA and Canada. It has a long, fleshy root, the shape of which somewhat resembles the human body. American ginseng extract is composed of a mixture of glycosides, essential oils, and a variety of complex carbohydrates and phytosterols as well as amino acids and trace minerals[39]. The bioactive constituents of American ginseng are dammarane saponins, commonly referred to as ginsenosides, which are present in root, leaf, stem, and berries[40]. American ginseng extract contains more than 30 ginsenosides such as Rg_1, Re, Ro, Rb_1, Rc, Rb_2, and Rd[41,42]. Among them, Rb_1 is a major bioactive component[43]. Based on high performance liquid chromatography/mass spectrometry (HPLC/MS) detection, ginsenoside 24(R)-pseudoginsenoside F_{11} is only present in American ginseng extract[44,45], while R_f is only present in Asian ginseng (*Panax ginseng* C.A. Meyer)[40,46]. This is an important parameter used to differentiate American ginseng from Asian ginseng.

Ginseng is one of the most valuable natural tonics in the East and West. Asian ginseng has been used in the Oriental East for over 4000 years. Many studies have shown that Asian ginseng affects various biologic processes and involves a wide range of pharmacologic actions, including antiaging, antitumor, and antistress effects[47]. Although many studies demonstrating beneficial effects of Asian ginseng can be found in the literature, relatively few studies have been performed with American ginseng. Until the past decade, researchers have found that American ginseng exerts beneficial effects on the cardiovascular system via its anti-ischemic, anti-arrhythmic and antihypertensive actions, and these actions have been attributed to its antioxidant activity. Ginsenosides extracted from American ginseng increase plasma high-density lipoprotein (HDL) content and decrease the lipid peroxide levels in hyperlipidemic rats[48]. At a high concentration (mg/ml range), ginsenosides directly reduce LDL oxidation[49]. At a low concentration (μg/ml range), ginsenosides significantly lessen LDL oxidation and reduce $CuSO_4$-induced oxidative changes in the presence of vitamin C (0.1–1 μmol/l), and significantly decrease the impairment of endothelium function induced by oxidized LDL in rat aorta[50]. American ginseng extract also protected cultured rat cardiac myocytes from oxidative damage[51]. Similarly, ginsenoside Rb_1 protected hippocampal neurons against ischemic injury[39]. It has been reported that Rb_1, Rd, Ra_1, and Ro inhibit protein tyrosine kinase activity induced by hypoxia/reoxygenation in cultured human umbilical vein endothelial cells, suggesting ginsenosides may play a pivotal role in preventing hypoxia/ reoxygenation injury[52]. In an *in vitro* study, American ginseng exhibited effective antioxidant activity in both lipid-soluble and water-soluble media by its chelating and scavenging activities. It is known that Fe^{2+} and Cu^{2+} ions catalyze hydroxyl ($OH^{.}$) radical formation, and thereby accelerate lipid peroxidation. American ginseng extract has a strong binding affinity to transition metal ions and inhibits the reduction of Fe^{3+} to Fe^{2+} and Cu^{3+} to Cu^{2+} to suppress the initiation of lipid peroxidation, and directly scavenges 1-diphenyl-2-picrylhydrazyl (DPPH) radicals and hydroperoxides (LOOH)[53].

Some work has been done in human trials to test whether the antioxidant effects of ginseng seen at the cellular level translate to the clinical setting. In a small randomized clinical trial of patients undergoing mitral valve replacement, the use of ginseng even more so than ginsenoside Rb in the cardioplegia improved post-bypass cardiac function (vs control patients), as measured by transesophageal echocardiography[54]. However, no index of oxidant stress was used in this study.

Hawthorn

Hawthorn (*Crataegus* species) is the subject of one of the largest herbal clinical trials initiated, approved by Commission E for use in treating New York Heart Association functional class II congestive heart failure. Hawthorn, a shrub native to both Europe and North America, contains a number of flavonoids and oligomeric procyanthin constituents within its leaves, flowers, and berries which have been formulated into a standard extract WS 1442. In addition to acting as an inotrope, vasodilator, and antihyperlipidemic agent, hawthorn also has potent antioxidant properties. It has been shown to decrease reperfusion injury in ischemic rat hearts[55]. Given its antioxidant properties, it may work in part via an attenuation of chronic reactive oxygen species released from nicotinamide adenine dinucleotide phosphate (NAD(P)H) oxidases and mitochondria – thought to be involved in the development and progression of heart failure[56]. Several clinical trials of hawthorn report improved symptoms and cardiac performance in patients with congestive heart failure[57,58]. These studies have culminated in the initiation of the Survival and Prognosis Investigation of Crataegus Extract (SPICE) trial, an international (120 centers, seven countries), randomized, placebo-controlled study of WS 1442 (450 mg/day for 24 months) in which it had hoped to enroll 2300 patients by the end of 2002 with New York Heart Association (NYHA) functional class II and III[59]. Study endpoints include mortality, cardiac events, and hospitalization. However, no results have been reported to date.

Scutellaria baicalensis

Scutellaria baicalensis, known as 'Huang-Qin' in China and as 'Hwang-Gum' in Korea, is a widely used herbal medicine. The major constituents of *Scutellaria baicalensis* extract are flavonoids, a group of polyhydroxy phenols[60], such as baicalein, baicalin, wogonin, and skullcapflavone I and II. These flavonoids have been shown to possess exceptional antioxidant activities[61–63]. Among the flavonoids, baicalein has attracted considerable attention, due to its phenolic hydrogens, and has been reported to exhibit anti-inflammatory, antihyperlipidemic and anti-arteriosclerotic effects.

Previous studies have shown that baicalein inhibits lipid peroxidation in rat liver homogenates[64], microsomes[65] and lecithin liposome membrane[66], and in brain cortex mitochondria[62]. It has been reported that baicalein prevents cell death induced by hydrogen peroxide in human neuroblastoma SH-SY5Y cells[63] and dermal fibroblasts[67], and protects against hippocampal neuronal death induced by 5 min of cerebral ischemia in gerbils[61].

In addition to preventing membrane and cell damage, *S. baicalensis* extract modulates nitric oxide (NO) production after concurrent treatment with interferon-γ (a NO inducer) in mouse peritoneal macrophages[68]. Baicalein has been shown to mediate the induction of quinone reductase and quinone reductase mRNA in the Hepa 1c1c7 marine hepatoma cell line[69]. A study has shown that *S. baicalensis* extract increases Bcl-2 protein, also known as antideath factor, while it decreases Bax protein level (a protein that induces apoptosis) in neuronal HT-22 cells during hydrogen peroxide exposure. Pretreatment with *S. baicalensis* extract increases cell viability and reduces oxidant stress-induced protein carbonyl formation. Two-dimensional electrophoresis showed that *S. baicalensis* extract decreases oxidized protein by 15%. It appears that *S. baicalensis* extract confers an anti-apoptotic effect through the interaction of *Bcl-2* and *Bax* genes[70].

It has been demonstrated that *S. baicalensis* extract and baicalein directly scavenge superoxide, hydroxyl radicals, DPPH radical, and alkyl radicals generated in chemical and enzyme systems[62,71]. Also, *S. baicalensis* extract inhibits xanthine oxidase, succinoxidase, and NADH-oxidase to suppress free radical formation[72,73].

Oxidants such as reactive oxygen species (ROS) have been shown to participate in myocardial ischemia/reperfusion injury. Antioxidants are known to protect against the ROS-mediated tissue injury, e.g. in cardiac ischemia/reperfusion. Recently, our studies have demonstrated that *S. baicalensis* extract and baicalein confer cardioprotection in a perfused, cultured cardiomyocyte during brief hypoxia, simulated ischemia/reperfusion, and mitochondria electron transport chain complex III inhibition with antimycin A. The results have showed that *S. baicalensis* extract and baicalein attenuate oxidant generation during all conditions studied and significantly decrease cell death at reperfusion after ischemia. Very interestingly, we found that *S. baicalensis* extract and baicalein, given only during the reperfusion phase, attenuate a ROS burst at 5 min after 1 h simulated ischemia in a dose-dependent fashion. Their protection may be related to the ability of the extracted chemicals to enter cells and orient in biomembranes. Baicalein, being free of sugar moieties, is more lipid soluble and may be able to penetrate the membrane with greater ease. An *in vitro* study revealed that *S. baicalensis* extract and baicalein possess potent ROS scavenging activity, using electron paramagnetic resonance spectroscopy with spin trap 5-methoxycarbonyl-5-methyl-1-pyrroline-*N*-oxide (MMPO) and a biochemical cell-free system[74,75]. These findings indicated that *S. baicalensis* extract and baicalein protect against oxidant-mediated cell injury in the ischemia/reperfusion model, presumably by virtue of its potent free radical scavenging ability and its ability to traverse cell membranes.

Possible pro-oxidant effects of herbal compounds

One important potential danger of herbal preparations is their ability to become pro-oxidants under certain conditions. For example, dietary polyphenols can be metabolized by peroxidases to form pro-oxidant phenoxyl radicals. Such radicals, particularly in the presence of Al, Zn, Ca, Mg, and Cd, can stimulate significant lipid peroxidation and have the potential to cause DNA damage[76,77]. Our own work has suggested that grape seed proanthocyanidin extract can, at higher doses, become a pro-oxidant, enough to activate apoptotic pathways leading to cell death[78]. Since there are few dosing guidelines followed by consumers of these products, the notion that 'more is better' could potentially lead to higher oxidant stress in the long term. This also points out the value of measuring oxidant stress levels in antioxidant trials. For example, the trials showing increased mortality among smokers taking β-carotene supplements[12] may have resulted in part from increased oxidant stress rather than decreased. Without measures of oxidant stress, it is difficult to know what higher doses,

or doses given in the context of other pro-oxidant agents, are doing to impact overall oxidant stress.

Why antioxidants may be detrimental: oxidants as helpful signaling molecules

The role of oxidants as potentially protective signaling molecules in the cardiovascular system was suggested by early preconditioning studies. Preconditioning was described in 1986 as a paradoxical protective effect on the heart in which brief episodes of ischemia increase the heart's tolerance to a subsequent sustained period of ischemia[79]. Originally, canine hearts were preconditioned with four 5 min occlusions of the coronary artery, each followed by 5 min of reperfusion[79]. When compared to controls, these hearts had 75% less infarcted myocardium after 40 min of occlusion. This early first window of preconditioning protection (within minutes to hours following the preconditioning stimulus) has been demonstrated in numerous *in vivo* models[80–86]. Since the work of Murry and colleagues, in which an antioxidant actually reversed the protective effects of preconditioning, it has become clear that oxidants may actually play an important role in the signaling induction of this protective adaptation[87]. Our own work shows that antioxidants attenuate oxidant signaling and abrogate preconditioning protection[88].

ACUTE EFFECTS OF HERBAL ANTIOXIDANTS ON CARDIOVASCULAR DISEASE

Herbal medications in treating acute cardiovascular disease

While much of the application of the antioxidant properties of herbal preparations has focused on chronic preventive effects, another important application is that of acute treatments, particularly for ischemic emergencies. Such diseases include myocardial infarction, stroke, cardiac arrest, and shock, and all involve ischemia and reperfusion – conditions which could quickly generate increased oxidant stress. The potential for impact by effective drugs which act quickly to attenuate oxidant stress is highlighted by cardiac arrest. Cardiac arrest affects 1000 women and men every day in the USA outside the hospital, occurring unexpectedly during their daily routines, with many under 50 years of age[89]. Survival is poor – usually less than 2–4%[90], most likely because irreversible injury to the brain and heart begins within minutes following global ischemia. This rapid rate of injury allows little time for all our modern efforts including mobile emergency medical services, cardio-pulmonary resuscitation, trauma centers, and over 5000 emergency rooms to make a difference. The survival rate is particularly dismal after failed defibrillation, and experts agree that a new approach is desperately needed[91].

Improving survival after cardiac arrest would have a significant impact on society and major causes of death, including treatment of other causes of arrest such as trauma and asphyxia, the leading causes of death in the young. In addition, any new therapy effective after such global ischemia would probably have a 'ripple' effect on the treatment of focal ischemic injuries to the heart and brain, i.e. myocardial infarction and stroke – leading causes of death and disability, respectively, in the USA[92]. The major barrier to treating all diseases of ischemia is time. During the global ischemia of cardiac arrest, cells within key organs such as the heart and brain begin to die within 10 min under normothermic conditions. Antioxidant agents which rapidly gain intracellular access have the potential to improve survival from cardiac arrest if oxidants are found to play an important role in post-resuscitation injury. For every 100 cardiac arrest patients treated outside the hospital, approximately 30 regain a pulse; yet ultimately only five or fewer leave the hospital alive, most dying due to heart and brain dysfunction. Thus, improvement in post-resuscitation care would have the potential to improve survival from cardiac arrest as much as six-fold. Efforts to improve post-resuscitation care are justified, since 75% of those discharged alive return to their communities with intact or only mildly impaired neurologic function. A signifi-cant cause of the subsequent heart and brain dysfunction that kills these patients likely includes oxidant injury and apoptosis. Recent evidence suggests that apoptosis occurs in the heart, not during ischemia, but during the early events of reperfusion, i.e. in the post-resuscitation phase, suggesting an association with the reintroduction of oxygen and, thus, oxidant generation.

Antioxidants and acute treatment of reperfusion injury at the cellular level

Much work supports the concept of free radical-mediated reperfusion injury following myocardial ischemia[93–95]. Antioxidants decrease injury in many studies, and measures of free radical production have detected surges of reactive oxygen species, particularly

the hydroxyl radical, during the first few seconds of reperfusion[95]. Controversy over the importance of reper-fusion oxidants is due in part to the failure of antioxidant therapy to provide protection in a number of studies[96]. However, work by us and others suggests two possible explanations for this failure:

(1) Many antioxidants will not gain intracellular access fast enough to prevent reperfusion injury[97–99];

(2) Antioxidants could actually worsen ischemia/reperfusion injury in tissue by blocking oxidant sig-naling, which can induce adaptive protection in surrounding cells[87,99,100].

Other investigators have found significant protection in ischemia/reperfusion injury when oxidant stress is atten-uated in ways which may not indiscriminately decrease signaling levels of oxidants. The work by Maulik *et al.* in a perfused mouse heart model of ischemia/reperfusion injury and apoptosis, showed significant protection in transgenic mouse hearts overexpressing glutathione per-oxidase, and worsened injury in knockout mice without this antioxidant enzyme[101]. Studies such as these support the notion that reperfusion ROS play a critical role in whether cells live or die after ischemia.

Herbal medicines with potential for treating acute oxidant injury

Grape seed proanthocyanidins

Proanthocyanidins, oligomers or polymers of polyhy-droxy flavan-3-ol units, are the major polyphenols in grape seeds and wine, particularly in red wine[102]. Over the past 10 years, increasing evidence has strongly sug-gested that moderate wine or alcohol consumption is associated with a reduced incidence of mortality and morbidity from coronary heart disease[103], possibly through the protective actions of polyphenolic com-pounds in grapes. The popular press carried stories on the beneficial constituents of red wine. People in south-ern France consume more fatty foods in comparison to those in North America, and yet, they suffer less from heart disease than people in North America or in the Northern regions of Europe. This incompatibility of a diet rich in fatty food with a decreased risk of heart dis-eases bears the name 'the French paradox'[104].

Grape seed proanthocyanidins have gained consider-able attention because of their wide range of biologic and pharmacologic properties, including the ability to scavenge free radicals[105,106]. Previous studies have demonstrated that grape seed proanthocyanidin extract (GSPE) inhibited TPA-induced lipid peroxidation and DNA fragmentation in mice brain homogenates and hepatic mitochondria. When compared with conventional antioxidants like vitamins C and E and β-carotene, GSPE proved to be a better antioxidant, as evidenced by decreased ROS formation in the peritoneal macrophages of mice[107]. GSPE pretreatment also showed a cytoprotective effect against hydrogen peroxide-induced oxidant stress in the cultured macrophage J774A.1, neuroactive adrenal pheochromocytoma PC-12 cells[107], and in rat primary glial cultures, murine macrophage-derived RAW264.7 cells[108].

In recent years, GSPE was found to function as an antioxidant and confer the cardioprotection in oxidant-mediated injury. There is ample evidence indicating the beneficial effects of GSPE in promoting recovery of post-ischemic myocardium, possibly through its antioxidant effect. When hearts obtained from GSPE-fed rats were exposed to ischemia/reperfusion, post-ischemic ventricular function was significantly improved and the extent of myocardial infarction was significantly reduced. The cardioprotective effect of GSPE was explained by its ability to scavenge peroxyl radicals directly and inhibit xanthine oxidase during ischemia/reperfusion and ischemic arrest[109–111]. A similar study further supported the cardioprotective effect of GSPE[112]. In addition, GSPE significantly reduced severe arteriosclerosis in the rabbit aorta and inhibited oxidation of LDL[113], and increased total antioxidant plasma capacity to make the perfused heart less susceptible to ischemia/reperfusion damage in the young and aged rats[114]. A study has recently been reported showing that GSPE protected cardiomyocytes from apoptotic cell death by reducing the expression of proapoptotic genes, *JNK-1*, and *c-Jun* during ischemia/reperfusion. The ischemia/reperfusion-mediated myocyte apoptosis is associated with enhanced expression of apoptotic factors, *JNK-1*, and *c-Jun* and resulted in ROS generation. Treatment with GSPE reduced the expression of both *JNK-1* and *c-Jun* in the reperfused myocardium and ameliorated free radical formation by almost 50–75%, and simultaneously reduced the appearance of the apoptotic cardiomyocytes in ischemia/reperfusion heart. These data indicate that the cardioprotective effect of GSPE may be attributed to its ability to block antideath signals by inhibiting pro-apoptotic factor and gene, *JNK-1*, and *c-Jun*[111].

It has been reported that low levels of nitric oxide (NO) can protect against ROS-mediated injury, whereas higher levels of NO may be toxic. GSPE treatment alone can cause a low level of NO production in rat primary glial cells and murine macrophage-derived RAW264.7 cells, but did not show any cytotoxicity. However, GSPE can protect cells from lipopolysaccharide/interferon-γ induced nitrosative stress by enhancing the endogenous glutathione (GSH) pool[108]. Recently, our own studies in a cardiomyocyte model of I/R have found that GSPE attenuates oxidant generation (Figure 16.2) and confers cardioprotection against this I/R injury (Figure 16.3) via increased NO generation at reperfusion (Figure 16.4).

Herbal medicines with potential for protecting against ischemia/reperfusion injury and inducing preconditioning cardioprotection

Resveratrol

Resveratrol (3,5,4′-trihydroxystilbene) is a naturally occurring polyphenolic antioxidant found abundantly in grape skins and seeds and in wines, especially in red wine[104]. It was found that resveratrol protects a variety of vital organs including kidney, heart, lung, and brain from I/R injury[115,116]. Resveratrol is a weak free radical scavenger *in vitro*, but possesses potent antioxidant capacity *in vivo*. It can directly scavenge peroxyl radicals which are formed as intermediate products of lipid peroxidation in membranes and lipoproteins and cause

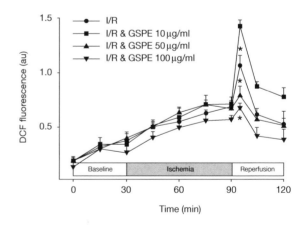

Figure 16.2 Effects of grape seed proanthocyanidin extract (GSPE) on 2′,7′-dichlorofluorescin (DCFH) oxidation (a marker of H_2O_2 and hydroxyl radical generation) during ischemia and reperfusion (I/R). A burst of DCF fluorescence was seen during 30 min of reperfusion following 1 h of simulated ischemia. When GSPE was administered at the start of reperfusion, DCF fluorescence was significantly attenuated. *$p < 0.01$ compared with untreated ischemic cardiomyocytes

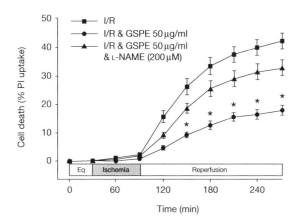

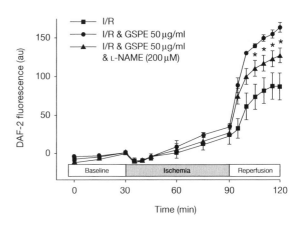

Figure 16.3 Effects of GSPE on cell death during I/R. Accelerated cell death occurred during 3 h of reperfusion following 1 h of simulated ischemia, as measured by propidium iodide uptake. When GSPE (50 µg/ml) was given at reperfusion, cell death was significantly reduced. Pretreatment with the NO synthase inhibitor, N_ω-nitro-L-arginine methyl ester (L-NAME, 200 µM) for 2 h and continuous perfusion during I/R partially reversed GSPE-conferred cardioprotection. *$p < 0.01$ compared with GSPE-treated ischemic cells vs untreated ischemic cells

Figure 16.4 Effects of GSPE on 4, 5-diaminofluorescein-2 (DAF-2) fluorescence (a marker of nitric oxide generation) during I/R. An increase in DAF-2 fluorescence was seen during the reperfusion. GSPE (50 µg/ml) given at reperfusion significantly increased DAF-2 fluorescence compared to untreated ischemic cells. Pretreated with L-NAME (200 µM) for 2 h and continuous perfusion during I/R abrogated the increase in DAF-2 fluorescence induced by GSPE. *$p < 0.01$ compared with L-NAME- and GSPE-treated ischemic cells vs GSPE-treated ischemic cells

tissue damage. The peroxyl radical scavenging activity of resveratrol may play a key role in reducing oxidative stress and lipid peroxidation during ischemia and reperfusion[117]. A number of studies have shown that resveratrol possesses potent cardioprotective properties. Acute treatment with resveratrol protects rat hearts from the damaging effects of ischemia and reperfusion injury, as evidenced by improved post-ischemic ventricular recovery and reduced myocardial infarction size[117,118]. Subsequent studies have shown that resveratrol exerts its cardioprotection against ischemia and reperfusion injury through NO-dependent and NO-independent pathways[119]. Short-term resveratrol treatment for 7 days renders the rat myocardium resistant to I/R injury. Resveratrol-fed hearts displayed improved cardiac functions and attenuated cardiomyocyte apoptosis. The mechanism by which resveratrol confers cardioprotection seems to be by a coordinated upregulation of iNOS (inducible nitric oxide synthase)-VEGF (vascular endothelial-derived growth factor)-KDR receptor-eNOS (endothelial nitric oxide synthase) pathway[120]. Resveratrol has been shown to provide cardioprotection through a mechanism involving pharmacologic preconditioning in a NO-dependent manner. Resveratrol-mediated cardioprotection was completely abolished by both N_ω-nitro-L-arginine methyl esterase (L-NAME), a

non-selective NOS inhibitor, and aminoguanidine (AG), an iNOS inhibitor. It was found that resveratrol at a low dose (10 µM) enhanced the induction of the iNOS expression and AG inhibited the iNOS expression, suggesting that resveratrol functioned through the induction of iNOS mRNA[121]. It was also demonstrated that resveratrol preconditions the rat hearts by activation of adenosine A_1 receptor via the PI3-kinase-Akt-Bcl-2 signaling pathway, and by activation of the adenosine A_3 receptor through a cAMP response element-binding protein (CREB)-dependent Bcl-2 pathway[122].

CONCLUSIONS

Given the importance of oxidants in both cardiovascular health and disease, it is likely that antioxidants will play important roles in both the chronic prevention and acute treatment of certain cardiovascular diseases. This chapter also highlighted recent thinking that some antioxidants at certain doses and under certain conditions can be harmful. Thus, it will be increasingly important to tailor our antioxidant therapies to attenuate harmful oxidants and not interfere with oxidants produced as part of healthy communication between cells and tissues. The promise of herbal medicines is great, as the numerous compounds they contain have the potential to treat quickly the oxidant stress of ischemic emergencies – an area not as extensively explored as chronic preventive

therapy. In addition, they have been time-tested, in some instances for centuries, and thus, may be safer as chronic therapies than even traditional antioxidants.

References

1. Kaye AD, Clarke RC, Sabar R, et al. Herbal medicines: current trends in anesthesiology practice – a hospital survey. J Clin Anesth 2000; 12: 468–71

2. Ang-Lee MK, Moss J, Yuan CS. Herbal medicines and perioperative care. J Am Med Assoc 2001; 286: 208–16

3. Valli G, Giardina EG. Benefits, adverse effects and drug interactions of herbal therapies with cardiovascular effects. J Am Coll Cardiol 2002; 39: 1083–95

4. Hertog MG, Feskens EJ, Hollman PC, et al. Dietary antioxidant flavonoids and risk of coronary heart disease: the Zutphen Elderly Study. Lancet 1993; 342: 1007–11

5. Gillman MW, Cupples LA, Gagnon D, et al. Protective effect of fruits and vegetables on development of stroke in men. J Am Med Assoc 1995; 273: 1113–17

6. Key TJ, Thorogood M, Appleby PN, Burr ML. Dietary habits and mortality in 11000 vegetarians and health conscious people: results of a 17 year follow up. Br Med J 1996; 313: 775–9

7. Hu FB, Stampfer MJ, Manson JE, et al. Frequent nut consumption and risk of coronary heart disease in women: prospective cohort study. Br Med J 1998; 317: 1341–5

8. Strandhagen E, Hansson PO, Bosaeus I, et al. High fruit intake may reduce mortality among middle-aged and elderly men. The Study of Men Born in 1913. Eur J Clin Nutr 2000; 54: 337–41

9. Bazzano LA, He J, Ogden LG, et al. Legume consumption and risk of coronary heart disease in US men and women: NHANES I Epidemiologic Follow-up Study. Arch Intern Med 2001; 161: 2573–8

10. Rimm EB, Stampfer MJ, Ascherio A, et al. Vitamin E consumption and the risk of coronary heart disease in men. N Engl J Med 1993; 328: 1450–6

11. Stampfer MJ, Hennekens CH, Manson JE, et al. Vitamin E consumption and the risk of coronary disease in women. N Engl J Med 1993; 328: 1444–9

12. Rapola JM, Virtamo J, Haukka JK, et al. Effect of vitamin E and beta carotene on the incidence of angina pectoris. A randomized, double-blind, controlled trial. J Am Med Assoc 1996; 275: 693–8

13. Miller ER, Postor-Barriuso R, Dalal D, et al. Meta-analysis: high-dosage vitamin E supplementation may increase all-cause mortality. Ann Intern Med 2005; 142: 37–46

14. Yusuf S, Dagenais G, Pogue J, et al. Vitamin E supplementation and cardiovascular events in high-risk patients. The Heart Outcomes Prevention Evaluation Study Investigators. N Engl J Med 2000; 342: 154–60

15. Stephens NG, Parsons A, Schofield PM, et al. Randomised controlled trial of vitamin E in patients with coronary disease: Cambridge Heart Antioxidant Study (CHAOS). Lancet 1996; 347: 781–6

16. Vile GF, Winterbourn CC. Inhibition of adriamycin-promoted microsomal lipid peroxidation by beta-carotene, alpha-tocopherol and retinol at high and low oxygen partial pressures. FEBS Lett 1988; 238: 353–6

17. Jialal I, Norkus EP, Cristol L, Grundy SM. beta-Carotene inhibits the oxidative modification of low-density lipoprotein. Biochim Biophys Acta 1991; 1086: 134–8

18. Morris DL, Kritchevsky SB, Davis CE. Serum carotenoids and coronary heart disease. The Lipid Research Clinics Coronary Primary Prevention Trial and Follow-up Study. J Am Med Assoc 1994; 272: 1439–41

19. Kushi LH, Folsom AR, Prineas RJ, et al. Dietary antioxidant vitamins and death from coronary heart disease in postmenopausal women. N Engl J Med 1996; 334: 1156–62

20. Evans RW, Shaten BJ, Day BW, Kuller LH. Prospective association between lipid soluble antioxidants and coronary heart disease in men. The Multiple Risk Factor Intervention Trial. Am J Epidemiol 1998; 147: 180–6

21. Blot WJ, Li JY, Taylor PR, et al. Nutrition intervention trials in Linxian, China: supplementation with specific vitamin/mineral combinations, cancer incidence, and disease-specific mortality in the general population. J Natl Cancer Inst 1993; 85: 1483–92

22. Greenberg ER, Baron JA, Karagas MR, et al. Mortality associated with low plasma concentration of beta carotene and the effect of oral supplementation. J Am Med Assoc 1996; 275: 699–703

23. Hennekens CH, Buring JE, Manson JE, et al. Lack of effect of long-term supplementation with beta carotene on the incidence of malignant neoplasms and cardiovascular disease. N Engl J Med 1996; 334: 1145–9

24. Omenn GS, Goodman GE, Thornquist MD, et al. Effects of a combination of beta carotene and vitamin A on lung cancer and cardiovascular disease. N Engl J Med 1996; 334: 1150–5

25. Rice-Evans CA, Miller NJ, Paganga G. Structure–antioxidant activity relationships of flavonoids and phenolic acids. Free Radic Biol Med 1996; 20: 933–56

26. Hesketh T, Zhu WX. Health in China. Traditional Chinese medicine: one country, two systems. Br Med J 1997; 315: 115–17

27. Lei XL, Chiou GC. Cardiovascular pharmacology of Panax notoginseng (Burk) F.H. Chen and Salvia miltiorrhiza. Am J Chin Med 1986; 14: 145–52

28. Niu XL, Ichimori K, Yang X, et al. Tanshinone II-A inhibits low density lipoprotein oxidation in vitro. Free Radic Res 2000; 33: 305–12

29. Zhao BL, Jiang W, Zhao Y, et al. Scavenging effects of Salvia miltiorrhiza on free radicals and its protection for myocardial

mitochondrial membranes from ischemia-reperfusion injury. Biochem Mol Biol Int 1996; 38: 1171–82

30. Ng TB, Liu F, Wang ZT. Antioxidative activity of natural products from plants. Life Sci 2000; 66: 709–23

31. Yu CM, Chan JC, Sanderson JE. Chinese herbs and warfarin potentiation by 'danshen'. J Intern Med 1997; 241: 337–9

32. Orekhov AN, Grunwald J. Effects of garlic on atherosclerosis. Nutrition 1997; 13: 656–63

33. Kiesewetter H, Jung F, Jung EM, et al. Effects of garlic coated tablets in peripheral arterial occlusive disease. Clin Invest 1993; 71: 383–6

34. Koscielny J, Klussendorf D, Latza R, et al. The antiatherosclerotic effect of Allium sativum. Atherosclerosis 1999; 144: 237–49

35. Janssens D, Remacle J, Drieu K, Michiels C. Protection of mitochondrial respiration activity by bilobalide. Biochem Pharmacol 1999; 58: 109–19

36. Liebgott T, Miollan M, Berchadsky Y, et al. Complementary cardioprotective effects of flavonoid metabolites and terpenoid constituents of Ginkgo biloba extract (EGb 761) during ischemia and reperfusion. Basic Res Cardiol 2000; 95: 368–77

37. Zhou LJ, Zhu XZ. Reactive oxygen species-induced apoptosis in PC12 cells and protective effect of bilobalide. J Pharmacol Exp Ther 2000; 293: 982–8

38. Pietri S, Seguin JR, d'Arbigny P, et al. Ginkgo biloba extract (EGb 761) pretreatment limits free radical-induced oxidative stress in patients undergoing coronary bypass surgery. Cardiovasc Drugs Ther 1997; 11: 121–31

39. Lim JH, Wen TC, Matsuda S, et al. Protection of ischemic hippocampal neurons by ginsenoside Rb1, a main ingredient of ginseng root. Neurosci Res 1997; 28: 191–200

40. Li T, Mazza, G, Cottrell, AC, Gao, L. Ginsenosides in root and leaves of American Ginseng. J Agric Food Chem 1996; 44: 717–20

41. Wang X, Sakuma T, Asafu-Adjaye E, Shiu GK. Determination of ginsenosides in plant extracts from Panax ginseng and Panax quinquefolius L. by LC/MS/MS. Anal Chem 1999; 71: 1579–84

42. Harkey MR, Henderson GL, Gershwin ME, et al. Variability in commercial ginseng products: an analysis of 25 preparations. Am J Clin Nutr 2001; 73: 1101–6

43. Li W, Gu C, Zhang H, et al. Use of high-performance liquid chromatography-tandem mass spectrometry to distinguish Panax ginseng C. A. Meyer (Asian ginseng) and Panax quinquefolius L. (North American ginseng). Anal Chem 2000; 72: 5417–22

44. Chan TW, But PP, Cheng SW, et al. Differentiation and authentication of Panax ginseng, Panax quinquefolius, and ginseng products by using HPLC/MS. Anal Chem 2000; 72: 1281–7

45. Li W, Fitzloff JF. Determination of 24(R)-pseudoginsenoside F(11) in North American ginseng using high performance liquid chromatography with evaporative light scattering detection. J Pharm Biomed Anal 2001; 25: 257–65

46. Smith RG, Caswell D, Carriere A, Zielke B. Variation in the ginsenoside content of American Ginseng, Panax quinquefolius L., roots. Can J Bot 1996; 74: 1616–20

47. Attele AS, Wu JA, Yuan CS. Ginseng pharmacology: multiple constituents and multiple actions. Biochem Pharmacol 1999; 58: 1685–93

48. Li JP, Lu ZZ, Lu YF. Lipoprotein-cholesterol metabolism and antioxidative effects of Panax quinquefolius saponins on experimental hyperlipidemic rat. Chung Kuo Yao Hsue Tsa Chi 1993; 28: 355–7

49. Li J, Huang M, Teoh H, Man RY. Panax quinquefolium saponins protects low density lipoproteins from oxidation. Life Sci 1999; 64: 53–62

50. Li JP, Huang M, Teoh H, Man RY. Interactions between Panax quinquefolium saponins and vitamin C are observed in vitro. Mol Cell Biochem 2000; 204: 77–82

51. Yang SJ, Qu JB, Zhang GG, Zhang WJ. Protective effects of Panax quinquefolius saponins on oxidative damage of cultured rat cardiac cells. Chung Kuo Yao Hsue Tsa Chi 1992; 17: 555–7

52. Dou DQ, Zhang YW, Zhang L, et al. The inhibitory effects of ginsenosides on protein tyrosine kinase activated by hypoxia/reoxygenation in cultured human umbilical vein endothelial cells. Planta Med 2001; 67: 19–23

53. Kitts DD, Wijewickreme AN, Hu C. Antioxidant properties of a North American ginseng extract. Mol Cell Biochem 2000; 203: 1–10

54. Zhan Y, Xu XH, Jiang YP. Protective effects of ginsenoside on myocardiac ischemic and reperfusion injuries. Zhonghua Yi Xue Za Zhi 1994; 74: 626–8, 648

55. Nasa Y, Hashizume H, Hoque AN, Abiko Y. Protective effect of crataegus extract on the cardiac mechanical dysfunction in isolated perfused working rat heart. Arzneimittelforschung 1993; 43: 945–9

56. Sorescu D, Griendling KK. Reactive oxygen species, mitochondria, and NAD(P)H oxidases in the development and progression of heart failure. Congest Heart Fail 2002; 8: 132–40

57. Leuchtgens H. Crataegus Special Extract WS 1442 in NYHA II heart failure. A placebo controlled randomized double-blind study. Fortschr Med 1993; 111: 352–4

58. Tauchert M, Gildor A, Lipinski J. High-dose Crataegus extract WS 1442 in the treatment of NYHA stage II heart failure. Herz 1999; 24: 465–74; discussion 475

59. Holubarsch CJ, Colucci WS, Meinertz T, et al. Survival and prognosis: investigation of Crataegus extract WS 1442 in congestive heart failure (SPICE) – rationale, study design and study protocol. Eur J Heart Fail 2000; 2: 431–7

60. Kimura Y, Okuda H, Tani T, Arichi S. Studies on Scutellariae radix. VI. Effects of flavanone compounds on lipid peroxidation in rat liver. Chem Pharm Bull 1982; 30: 1792–5

61. Hamada H, Hiramatsu M, Edamatsu R, Mori A. Free radical scavenging action of baicalein. Arch Biochem Biophys 1993; 306: 261–6

62. Gao Z, Huang K, Yang X, Xu H. Free radical scavenging and antioxidant activities of flavonoids extracted from the radix of Scutellaria baicalensis Georgi. Biochim Biophys Acta 1999; 1472: 643–50

63. Gao Z, Huang K, Xu H. Protective effects of flavonoids in the roots of Scutellaria baicalensis Georgi against hydrogen peroxide-induced oxidative stress in HS-SY5Y cells. Pharmacol Res 2001; 43: 173–8

64. Kimuya Y, Kubo M, Tani T, et al. Studies on Scutellariae radix. IV. Effects on lipid peroxidation in rat liver. Chem Pharm Bull (Tokyo) 1981; 29: 2610–17

65. Gao D, Sakurai K, Chen J, Ogiso T. Protection by baicalein against ascorbic acid-induced lipid peroxidation of rat liver

microsomes. Res Commun Mol Pathol Pharmacol 1995; 90: 103–14

66. Gabrielska J, Oszmianski J, Zylka R, Komorowska M. Antioxidant activity of flavones from Scutellaria baicalensis in lecithin liposomes. Z Naturforsch [C] 1997; 52: 817–23

67. Gao D, Tawa R, Masaki H, et al. Protective effects of baicalein against cell damage by reactive oxygen species. Chem Pharm Bull (Tokyo) 1998; 46: 1383–7

68. Kim HM, Moon EJ, Li E, et al. The nitric oxide-producing activities of Scutellaria baicalensis. Toxicology 1999; 135: 109–15

69. Park HJ, Lee YW, Park HH, et al. Induction of quinone reductase by a methanol extract of Scutellaria baicalensis and its flavonoids in murine Hepa 1c1c7 cells. Eur J Cancer Prev 1998; 7: 465–71

70. Choi J, Conrad CC, Malakowsky CA, et al. Flavones from Scutellaria baicalensis Georgi attenuate apoptosis and protein oxidation in neuronal cell lines. Biochim Biophys Acta 2002; 1571: 201–10

71. Shieh DE, Liu LT, Lin CC. Antioxidant and free radical scavenging effects of baicalein, baicalin and wogonin. Anticancer Res 2000; 20: 2861–5

72. Hanasaki Y, Ogawa S, Fukui S. The correlation between active oxygens scavenging and antioxidative effects of flavonoids. Free Radic Biol Med 1994; 16: 845–50

73. Hodnick WF, Duval DL, Pardini RS. Inhibition of mitochondrial respiration and cyanide-stimulated generation of reactive oxygen species by selected flavonoids. Biochem Pharm 1994; 47: 573–80

74. Shao ZH, Li CQ, Vanden Hoek TL, et al. Extract from Scutellaria baicalensis Georgi attenuates oxidant stress in cardiomyocytes. J Mol Cell Cardiol 1999; 31: 1885–95

75. Shao ZH, Vanden Hoek TL, Qin Y, et al. Baicalein attenuates oxidant stress in cardiomyocytes. Am J Physiol Heart Circ Physiol 2002; 282: H999–H1006

76. Galati G, Sabzevari O, Wilson JX, O'Brien PJ. Prooxidant activity and cellular effects of the phenoxyl radicals of dietary flavonoids and other polyphenolics. Toxicology 2002; 177: 91–104

77. Sakihama Y, Cohen MF, Grace SC, Yamasaki H. Plant phenolic antioxidant and prooxidant activities: phenolics-induced oxidative damage mediated by metals in plants. Toxicology 2002; 177: 67–80

78. Shao ZH, Vanden Hoek TL, Xie JT, et al. Grape seed proanthocyanidins induce pro-oxidant toxicity in cardiomyocytes. Cardiovasc Toxicol 2003; 03: 331–9

79. Murry CE, Jennings RB, Reimer KA. Preconditioning with ischemia: a delay of lethal cell injury in ischemic myocardium. Circulation 1986; 74: 1124–36

80. Li GC, Vasquez BS, Gallagher KP, Lucchesi BR. Myocardial protection with preconditioning. Circulation 1990; 82: 609–19

81. Schott RJ, Rohmann S, Braun ER, Schaper W. Ischemic preconditioning reduces infarct size in swine myocardium. Circ Res 1990; 66: 1133–42

82. Cohen MV, Liu GS, Downey JM. Preconditioning causes improved wall motion as well as smaller infarcts after transient coronary occlusion in rabbits. Circulation 1991; 84: 341–9

83. Asimakis GK, Inners-McBride K, Medellin G, Conti VR. Ischemic preconditioning attenuates acidosis in isolated rat heart. Am J Physiol 1992; 263: H887–94

84. Lawson CS, Downey JM. Preconditioning: state of the art myocardial protection. Cardiovasc Res 1993; 27: 542–50

85. Baxter GF, Yellon DM. Ischemic preconditioning of the myocardium: a new paradigm for clinical cardioprotection. Br J Clin Pharmacol 1994; 38: 381–7

86. Jenkins DP, Pugsley WB, Yellon DM. Ischaemic preconditioning in a model of global ischaemia: infarct size limitation, but no reduction of stunning. J Mol Cell Cardiol 1995; 27: 1623–32

87. Murry CE, Richard VJ, Jennings RB, Reimer KA. Preconditioning with ischemia: is the protective effect meditated by free radical induced myocardial stunning? Circulation 1988; 78 (Suppl II): 77

88. Vanden Hoek TL, Becker LB, Shao Z, et al. Reactive oxygen species released from mitochondria during brief hypoxia induce preconditioning in cardiomyocytes. J Biol Chem 1998; 273: 18092–8

89. Becker LB, Ostrander MP, Barrett J, Kondos GT. CPR Chicago: outcome of cardiopulmonary resuscitation in a large metropolitan area – where are the survivors? Ann Emerg Med 1991; 20: 355–61

90. Becker LB, Han BH, Meyer PM, et al. CPR Chicago: racial differences in the incidence of cardiac arrest and subsequent survival. N Engl J Med 1993; 329: 600–6

91. Weil MH, Becker LB, Budinger T, et al. Workshop executive summary report: post-resuscitative and initial utility in life saving efforts (PULSE). Circulation 2001; 103: 1182–4

92. National Heart, Lung and Blood Institute. Morbidity and Mortality: Chartbook on Cardiovascular, Lung, and Blood Diseases. Bethesda, MD: US Department of Health and Human Services, Public Health Service. National Institute of Health, Bethesda, Maryland, 1992

93. Zak R, Rabinowitz M. Metabolism of the ischemic heart. Med Clin N Am 1973; 57: 93–103

94. Hearse DJ. Stunning: a radical re-review. Cardiovasc Drug Ther 1991; 5: 853–67

95. Das DK. Cellular biochemical and molecular aspects of reperfusion injury. Ann NY Acad Sci 1994; 723: 116–27

96. Zweier JL, Flaherty JT, Weisfeldt ML. Direct measurement of free radical generation following reperfusion of ischemic myocardium. Proc Natl Acad Sci USA 1987; 84: 1404–7

97. Opie LH. Reperfusion injury and its pharmacologic modification. Circulation 1989; 80: 1049–62

98. Vanden Hoek TL, Shao Z, Li C, et al. Reperfusion injury in cardiac myocytes after simulated ischemia. Am J Phys 1996; 270: H1334–41

99. Vanden Hoek TL, Becker LB, Shao Z, et al. Preconditioning in cardiomyocytes protects by attenuating oxidant stress at reperfusion. Circ Res 2000; 86: 534–40

100. Das DK, Engelman RM, Maulik N. Oxygen free radical signaling in ischemic preconditioning. Ann NY Acad Sci 1999; 874: 49–65

101. Maulik N, Yoshida T, Das DK. Regulation of cardiomyocyte apoptosis in ischemic reperfused mouse heart by glutathione peroxidase. Mol Cell Biochem 2000; 196: 13–21

102. Ricardo da Silva JM, Darmon M, Fernandez Y, Mitjavila S. Oxygen free radical scavenger capacity in aqueous models of different procyanidins from grape seeds. J Agric Food Chem 1991; 39: 549–52

103. Rimm EB, Giovannucci EL, Willett WC, et al. Prospective study of alcohol consumption and risk of coronary disease in men. Lancet 1991; 338: 464–8

104. Renaud S, de Lorgeril M. Wine, alcohol, platelets, and the French paradox for coronary heart disease. Lancet 1992; 339: 1523–6

105. Bagchi D, Bagchi M, Stohs SJ, et al. Free radicals and grape seed proanthocyanidin extract: importance in human health and disease prevention. Toxicology 2000; 148: 187–97

106. Bagchi M, Kuszynski CA, Balmoori J, et al. Protective effects of antioxidants against smokeless tobacco-induced oxidative stress and modulation of Bcl-2 and p53 genes in human oral keratinocytes. Free Radic Res 2001; 35: 181–94

107. Bagchi D, Garg A, Krohn RL, et al. Protective effects of grape seed proanthocyanidins and selected antioxidants against TPA-induced hepatic and brain lipid peroxidation and DNA fragmentation, and peritoneal macrophage activation in mice. Gen Pharmacol 1998; 30: 771–6

108. Roychowdhury S, Wolf G, Keilhoff G, et al. Protection of primary glial cells by grape seed proanthocyanidin extract against nitrosative/oxidative stress. Nitric Oxide 2001; 5: 137–49

109. Facino RM, Carini M, Aldini G, et al. Procyanidins from vitis vinifera seeds protect rabbit heart from ischemia/reperfusion injury: antioxidant intervention and/ or iron and copper sequestering activity. Planta Med 1996; 62: 495–502

110. Sato M, Maulik G, Ray PS, et al. Cardioprotective effects of grape seed proanthocyanidin against ischemic reperfusion injury. J Mol Cell Cardiol 1999; 31: 1289–97

111. Sato M, Bagchi D, Tosaki A, Das DK. Grape seed proanthocyanidin reduces cardiomyocyte apoptosis by inhibiting ischemia/reperfusion-induced activation of JNK-1 and C-JUN. Free Radic Biol Med 2001; 31: 729–37

112. Pataki T, Bak I, Kovacs P, et al. Grape seed proanthocyanidins improved cardiac recovery during reperfusion after ischemia in isolated rat hearts. Am J Clin Nutr 2002; 75: 894–9

113. Yamakoshi J, Kataoka S, Koga T, Ariga T. Proanthocyanidin-rich extract from grape seeds attenuates the development of aortic atherosclerosis in cholesterol-fed rabbits. Atherosclerosis 1999; 142: 139–49

114. Facino RM, Carini M, Aldini G, et al. Diet enriched with procyanidins enhances antioxidant activity and reduces myocardial post-ischaemic damage in rats. Life Sci 1999; 64: 627–42

115. Constant J. Alcohol, ischemic heart disease, and the French paradox. Coron Artery Dis 1997; 8: 645–59

116. Giovannini L, Migliori M, Longoni BM, et al. Resveratrol, a polyphenol found in wine, reduces ischemia reperfusion injury in rat kidney. J Cardiovasc Pharmacol 2001; 37: 262–70

117. Ray PS, Maulik G, Cordis GA, et al. The red wine antioxidant resveratrol protects isolated rat hearts from ischemic reperfusion injury. Free Biol Med 1999; 27: 160–9

118. Hung LM, Chen JK, Huang SS, et al. Cardioprotective effect of resveratrol, a natural antioxidant derived from grape. Cardiovasc Res 2000; 47: 549–55

119. Hung LM, Su MJ, Chen JK. Resveratrol protects myocardial ischemia-reperfusion injury through NO-dependent and NO-independent mechanisms. Free Radic Biol Med 2004; 36: 774–81

120. Das S, Alagappan VKT, Bagchi D, et al. Coordinated induction of iNOS-VEGF-KDR-eNOS after resveratrol consumption A potential mechanism for resveratrol preconditioning of the heart. Vasc Pharmacol 2005; 42: 281–9

121. Hattori R, Otani H, Maulik N, Das DK. Pharmacological preconditioning with resveratrol: role of nitric oxide. Am J Physiol Heart Circ Physiol 2002; 282: H1988–95

122. Das S, Cordis GA, Maulik N, Das DK. Pharmacological preconditioning with resveratrol: role of CREB-dependent Bcl-2 signaling via adenosine A3 receptor activation. Am J Physiol Heart Circ Physiol 2005; 288: H328–35

Hawthorn

17

Z.-H. Shao and W.-T. Chang

INTRODUCTION

Herbal remedies were once popular methods for treating illness and diseases. Well before the advent of modern medicine, people relied on trial-and-error and inappropriate methods for the use of common plants, herbs, fruits, and other extracts found in nature to treat diseases. As science progressed, modern medicine became more common in the developed countries and soon replaced the role of herbal remedies. Herbal medicine, however, has started to regain people's attention as science looks towards more natural rather than molecularly engineered drugs to help ailing patients. A number of studies also show that herbal medicine exerts health protective effects[1–3]. With increasing popularity among the public, herbal therapy is currently estimated to be used by 12.1% to 14% of the population in the United States[4].

Hawthorn (*Crataegus*) has been used as food and medicine around the world for centuries. The Chinese used hawthorn for treating a variety of ailments including digestive problems, hyperlipidemia, poor circulation, and dyspnea[5]. In Europe, the hawthorn fruits, leaves and flowers were utilized as a cardiotonic, diuretic, and anti-atherosclerotic agent. It was not until the 1800s that hawthorn began to be used for the treatment of cardiovascular diseases[6]. Hawthorn's popularity in the United States did not occur until 1896 when it saw similar use as in Europe. Nowadays, it is gaining increasing attention for its potential cardiovascular enhancing and protective properties. Systematic evaluation has been done on its application in various heart diseases, especially congestive heart failure. In Germany, hawthorn extract has been approved and registered as a therapeutic agent for the treatment of minor forms of coronary heart disease and congestive heart failure[7]. Current claims suggest that hawthorn can be used as an alternative therapy for various cardiovascular diseases, such as angina, hypertension, hyperlipidemia, arrhythmia, and New York Heart

Association (NYHA) functional class II congestive heart failure[8]. Past and ongoing studies also suggest that its beneficial effect comes from the active component flavonoids, especially the oligomeric proanthocyanidins. With evidence from basic and clinical studies, hawthorn extract has been shown to exert the potential of being a viable, natural alternative treatment for heart diseases, as well as a promoter of general cardiovascular health.

PLANT AND CHEMICAL CONSTITUENTS

Hawthorn (*Crataegus*, more commonly known as haw, maybush, and whitethorn) belongs to the Rosaceae family. It is a bright red, fruit-bearing plant with bright green three- to five-lobed leaves and white flowers. Hawthorn can be found in Europe, East Asia, and eastern North America, and grows best in the northern temperate zones[5]. There are over 100 different kinds of hawthorn, among which *Crataegus oxyacantha*, *C. monogyna*, and *C. laevigata* are the forms most often used as medication.

There is currently intense interest in polyphenolic phytochemicals due to their antioxidant capacities and their great abundance in the diet and medicinal plants[9]. Polyphenols include the flavonoids, phenolic acids, stilbenes, and lignans. The flavonoids are naturally occurring antioxidants widely present in fruits, vegetables, and beverages (tea, wine, juice, etc.)[10]. They may be divided into several subclasses, such as flavanols (catechins and proanthocyanidins), flavanones (naringin, hesperidin), isoflavanones, flavonols (quercetin, myricetin), flavones (luteolin, apigenin), and anthocyanidins[11]. Epidemiologic studies have shown an association between the intake of flavonoids and reduced risks of cardiovascular diseases like myocardial infarction and stroke[12]. It appears to be attributed to their antioxidant properties. Hawthorn fruits, leaves, and flowers are considered the most potent parts of the plant. They contain a number of chemical components, such as flavonoids (quercetin, quercitrin, catechins, rutin, oligomeric proanthocyanidins), triterpene saponins (oleanolic acid, ursolic acid, crataegus acid), and amines (β-phenethylamine, tyramine, acetylcholine)[13–15]. Flavonoids, particularly oligomeric proanthocyanidins present in the hawthorn extract, are the major bioactive constituents that possess potent antioxidant activity. *In vitro* studies showed that hawthorn extract scavenges superoxide, hydrogen peroxide, and hypochlorous acid in the chemical cell-free system. It also decreases the malondialdehyde content in hepatic microsomal preparations[16]. In experimental atherosclerosis rats, it has also been demonstrated that hawthorn normalizes the levels of antioxidant enzymes in the hepatic, aortic, and cardiac tissues[17]. In hyperlipidemic mice, superoxide dismutase activity is increased by the hawthorn extract[18].

BASIC SCIENTIFIC STUDIES

Inotropic effect

Hawthorn extract may produce positive inotropic effects in the rat heart[19] and in patients with congestive heart failure[20]. Possible mechanisms include increase of the intracellular calcium concentration and inhibition of the cAMP phosphodiesterase activity[19]. Nevertheless, hawthorn extract LI132 was found to have no influence on the L-type calcium current in guinea pig ventricular cardiomyocyte, indicating that its positive inotropic effect may not be caused by cAMP phosphodiesterase inhibition[21]. Moreover, a common hydroalcoholic extract WS® 1442 from the hawthorn leaves and flowers was also found to significantly increase the contractile force of isolated papillary muscle strips via the cAMP-independent pathway[20]. However, the exact mechanisms underlying hawthorn's positive inotropic effect are still unclear.

Vasodilatory effect

Hawthorn extract has been shown to induce concentration-dependent relaxation in rat isolated mesenteric arteries, which, if the endothelium were denuded, would have a reduced effect[22]. The relaxation effect was also abolished by N_ω-nitro-L-arginine methyl ester (L-NAME), a nitric oxide (NO) synthase inhibitor, suggesting that the endothelium-derived relaxation factor NO may play a role in hawthorn-mediated vasodilatation. Similar results were also observed in the isolated rat aortic preparation, in which *Crataegus* extract caused endothelium-dependent vasodilatation by stimulating NO production and cGMP accumulation[23]. These results suggest that the active components of hawthorn extract may act on the endothelial cells, leading to release of NO and relaxation of the blood vessels. This may also explain the effects of blood pressure lowering and coronary blood flow enhancement mediated by hawthorn[7]. As to what constituent is responsible for the effect, crataegus acid (triterpene carboxylic acid) rich in hawthorn berry was considered the active component that mediates the coronary vasodilation[6].

Protective effect against ischemia/reperfusion injury

Hawthorn extract has been shown to exhibit cardioprotective effects in both *in vitro* and *in vivo* models of ischemia/reperfusion[24,25]. Hawthorn extract WS® 1442 significantly reduced the infarct size and deterioration of contractile function in rat myocardium exposed to prolonged (240 minutes) ischemia followed by reperfusion[7]. In isolated rat heart, pretreatment with hawthorn extract significantly decreased the LDH release during ischemia and reperfusion[26]. Similarly, pretreatment with tincture of *Crataegus* (TCR), another hawthorn alcoholic extract isolated from the fruits, also exerts protective effect in the rat model of isoproterenol-induced myocardial infarction. Other than the reduction in creatinine kinase and LDH isoenzyme release, it also prevented the isoproterenol-induced decrease in antioxidant enzyme activity (e.g. glutathione peroxidase, superoxide dismutase, and catalase)[25]. In fact, it has been suggested that the protective effect hawthorn extract exerts against ischemia/reperfusion injury is related to its antioxidant activity.

Anti-arrhythmic effect

So far there have been few studies focusing on the anti-arrhythmic effects herbal medications like hawthorn may have. In fact, hawthorn appears to exhibit some cardioprotective effects resulting from its anti-arrhythmic properties. An early study showed that several species of the genus *Crataegus* may prevent cardiac arrhythmia induced by aconitine, calcium chloride, and adrenaline[27]. Recently it was further found that hawthorn extract WS® 1442 dose-dependently diminishes the incidence of ventricular tachycardia and fibrillation following left coronary artery ligation[7]. Moreover, it seems that long-term application is more effective. Though hawthorn extract may prevent reperfusion arrhythmia following 7 minutes of coronary occlusion either after short-term (7 days) pretreatment or acute treatment immediately prior to coronary occlusion[28], the effects seemed to be better in the chronic (3 months) treatment group in which there was a significant reduction in the prevalence of reperfusion arrhythmia despite an even longer duration (18 to 20 minutes) of global myocardial ischemia[29]. Similar results were also obtained from a rat myocardial ischemia model, which showed that an extract of *Crataegus meyeri* isolated from the flowering top significantly reduced the incidence and severity of ischemia-related arrhythmia[30].

The mechanism underlying the anti-arrhythmic effect of hawthorn, however, remains elusive. Electrophysiologic studies showed that *Crataegus* extract prolongs the refractory period in isolated perfused hearts and increases the action potential duration in guinea pig papillary muscle[31]. With the voltage-clamp technique, these effects were found to be related to the blocking of repolarizing potassium currents[21], an effect similar to that of the class III anti-arrhythmic drugs. This might be the pharmacophysiologic basis of the anti-arrhythmic effect described for hawthorn extract. On the other hand, there have been concerns regarding the roles of free radicals in the induction of reperfusion arrhythmia[32]. Hawthorn extract, with the active component flavonoids showing strong antioxidant activity, may scavenge free radicals and thus exhibit its anti-arrhythmic effect. To date, all the results of the hawthorn's anti-arrhythmic properties were obtained from animal studies. Electrophysiologic studies in humans are still unavailable.

Antihyperlipidemic effect

It is believed that oxidation of the low density lipoprotein (LDL)-cholesterol plays an important role in atherosclerosis. The oxidized LDL-cholesterol may induce endothelial injury and foam cell formation, leading to the development of atherosclerotic plaques. It has been shown that hawthorn extract possesses hypolipidemic activity and protects LDL-cholesterol from copper II- and peroxyl radical-induced oxidation[14,33]. Treatment with hawthorn extract TCR significantly decreases the plasma total cholesterol, LDL-cholesterol, very low-density lipoprotein (VLDL)-cholesterol, and the ratio of LDL plus VLDL to high-density lipoprotein (HDL)-cholesterol in rats fed an atherogenic diet. TCR also increases the binding of LDL-cholesterol to liver plasma membrane and prevents the accumulation of cholesterol in the liver by enhancing its excretion into bile acid, a significant route for removing cholesterol from the body[13]. Supplementation of hawthorn dry fruit powder lowers the serum levels of total cholesterol and triglyceride in rabbits fed for 12 weeks a high-cholesterol diet[34]. In human studies of hyperlipidemia, the reduction of total serum cholesterol was found mostly due to the reduction in LDL-cholesterol and triglyceride, with HDL-cholesterol completely unaffected[35].

The mechanisms by which hawthorn lowers LDL cholesterol are not fully understood, though a number of hypotheses have been raised. One possibility is the upregulation of LDL-receptors on the hepatic cell membrane. Typically, the serum cholesterol level is maintained at a steady state in which rate of entry into the blood stream equals that of removal from the blood stream. An upregulated system, either due to decrease in the rate of entry or increase in the rate of removal, would result in lowered LDL-cholesterol levels. Hawthorn extract TCR significantly increases the binding of LDL-cholesterol to hepatocyte membrane and promotes the influx of plasma cholesterol into the liver, indicating an enhancement in hepatic LDL-receptor activity[13]. On the other hand, in rabbits fed a high-cholesterol diet it was found that supplementation with hawthorn inhibited the intestinal acyl CoA: cholesterol 7α-hydroxylase (ACAT) activity instead of affecting the hepatic 3-hydroxy-3-methyl glutaryl CoA (HMG-CoA) reductase activity[34]. Being that the hepatic HMG-CoA reductase pathway is responsible for cholesterol biosynthesis and intestinal ACAT is believed to play a role in cholesterol absorption, this result suggests that hawthorn inhibits cholesterol absorption rather than cholesterol synthesis.

In addition, since hawthorn extract, rich in flavonoids (such as quercetin and epicatechin), has been shown to inhibit the oxidative modification of LDL-cholesterol[14] and thus prevent associated cytotoxicity[36], it is also possible that hawthorn exhibits its protective effects via this mechanism.

CLINICAL STUDIES

Though the inotropic, vasodilatory, lipid-lowering, and anti-arrhythmic effects of hawthorn extract have been demonstrated in experimental studies, there are, however, few randomized controlled trials evaluating its clinical efficacy. Up to now, most clinical studies were carried out in Europe, particularly in Germany, and focused on the treatment of mild to moderate congestive heart failure. Also, some studies tested its lipid lowering and blood pressure lowering effects.

Congestive heart failure

A number of studies evaluating the clinical effects of hawthorn extract in patients with congestive heart failure have emerged over the past two decades. Most of these studies used specialized hawthorn extract WS 1442 or LI 132 for standardization of its active components. The subjects were mostly NYHA functional class I–II heart failure patients, though in a few studies NYHA functional class III patients were included[37]. The clinical parameters most often employed included subjective symptoms, exercise capacity or tolerance, blood pressure, heart rate, and rate-pressure products. Direct evaluation of the cardiac function by echocardiogram was performed in some cases. Quality-of-life indicators were also included in some studies. With cardiac glycosides, beta-blockers, diuretics, and angiotensin-converting-enzyme inhibitors (ACE-I) currently being the standard treatment for congestive heart failure, hawthorn extract was usually evaluated as an adjunctive therapy. Other than the effects from standard pharmacologic therapy, additional benefits can often be demonstrated. Furthermore, in the rare studies directly comparing hawthorn with standard heart failure remedies such as angiotensin-converting enzyme inhibitors and diuretics, it was also not shown to be inferior[38].

Despite the numerous studies published, the strength of the evidence, however, was often limited by lack of controls or placebos, non-randomization, non-blinded design, or small number of patients. The dosage, frequency, duration of treatment, and the percentages of active components in extract preparations also varied. To better assess the beneficial effects hawthorn extract may have, a meta-analysis was performed including data from eight well-designed clinical trials that fulfilled the criteria of randomization, double-blindness, and placebo control[39]. In all these studies hawthorn extract was used in monopreparation, and in most it served as an adjunct to conventional therapy. With the 632 chronic heart failure patients included, the physiologic outcomes of maximal workload showed a beneficial increase in patients treated with hawthorn extracts, while the heart rate–blood pressure product showed a beneficial decrease. Subjective symptoms such as dyspnea and fatigue also improved significantly. Exercise tolerance revealed a marginal non-significant increase. Though there exist some controversies usually seen in meta-analysis (such as the clinical heterogeneity of the included patients, unequal distribution of the concomitant treatment, publication bias, etc.), this is probably the best evidence to date demonstrating hawthorn's beneficial effects in patients with congestive heart failure. Nevertheless, because the treatment (3 to 16 weeks) and follow-up durations in these studies are short, concerns have been raised regarding the long-term therapeutic effects hawthorn extract may confer. This is an issue worthy of notification, especially when many inotropic predecessors have been shown to improve the short-term symptoms and exercise tolerability at the expense of mortality in the long run[40].

To answer this question, an international, randomized, placebo-controlled, double-blinded study was conducted to investigate the long-term therapeutic effects of hawthorn extract WS 1442[41]. Up to 2300 NYHA class II/III heart failure patients with reduced left ventricular ejection fraction were enrolled from 120 investigation centers in seven European countries. With treatment consisting of WS 1442 at 900 mg per day for 24 months, the primary endpoints included cardiac death, non-lethal myocardial infarction, and hospitalization due to progression of heart failure. Secondary outcome measurements included total mortality, exercise duration, echocardiographic parameters, quality of life, and pharmacoeconomic parameters. With the study completed and data waiting to be published, it will be the largest prospective, placebo-controlled, randomized trial to date offering level I evidence for hawthorn's long-term cardiovascular effects.

Hypertension

Human studies investigating the pressure lowering effects of hawthorn extract in patients with hypertension are limited. One placebo-controlled study evaluated patients with mild hypertension treated with hawthorn extract or magnesium supplements. While the results showed a decline in both systolic and diastolic blood pressure in all groups, including placebo, there were non-significant trends in favor of the reduction in resting diastolic pressure and anxiety after 10 weeks of hawthorn extract supplementation (500 mg per day)[42]. However, this study tended to be limited by the small number of patients as well as the low dose and short duration of hawthorn extract supplementation. Further studies are still needed to verify the clinical efficacy of hawthorn as an antihypertension remedy.

Hyperlipidemia

While the lipid-lowering property of the hawthorn extract has been shown in a number of animal studies, there are still few studies focusing on evaluating its clinical application in patients with hyperlipidemia. Though reduction of serum lipid levels was mentioned in some heart failure studies described above, there was only one clinical trial designed to demonstrate its lipid-lowering effect[35]. Further placebo-controlled, randomized studies are needed to test what role hawthorn may have in the treatment of hyperlipidemia.

Ischemic heart disease

Studies evaluating the clinical efficacy of hawthorn extract in patients with ischemic heart disease are still limited, though the beneficial effects have been demonstrated in the animal models of myocardial ischemia[7]. Two studies evaluating the therapeutic effects of *Crataegus* extract in patients with angina pectoris were performed in the early 1980s[43,44]. Although the results showed some improvement in objective symptoms, the studies were basically small-scaled and non-randomized. Because coronary heart disease is one of the leading public health problems in modern society, it would be valuable to conduct a well-designed, prospective clinical trial to evaluate the anti-ischemic effect hawthorn extract may have.

Adverse effects

The adverse effects associated with hawthorn extract within the therapeutic dose range are usually mild and tolerable. These include rash, sweating, headache, dizziness, vertigo, palpitation, agitation, sleepiness, and gastro-intestinal symptoms. Larger doses in animal studies were reported to cause sedation, hypotension, and arrhythmia. In a clinical study evaluating the efficacy and safety of the hawthorn extract in NYHA functional class III heart failure, patients taking doses up to 1800 mg per day showed only mild and infrequent (1.4%) adverse events such as dizziness and vertigo, which were statistically no different from those on 900 mg per day (4.3%), and were even fewer than in those taking the placebo (10%)[37]. The post-marketing surveillance with recommended dose of 900 mg per day also revealed that the adverse reactions associated with hawthorn extract are usually mild and infrequent, with the incidence about 1.3–1.4%[45,46]. This suggests that hawthorn may serve as a safe and tolerable therapy for patients with various cardiovascular diseases. However, for older patients or those who have concomitant systemic diseases, then any adverse reactions should be given more consideration.

DRUG INTERACTIONS

Even though the adverse effects of hawthorn extract itself are infrequent and usually mild, attention has been raised concerning its interactions with other medications, especially those commonly employed in the treatment of congestive heart failure. It has been suggested that compounds in hawthorn extract (rutin, quercetin, etc.) might potentially alter the activity of several drug-metabolizing enzymes, although few studies have focused on this. Recent studies also showed that natural compounds containing flavonoids could alter the activity of P-glycoprotein, an efflux transporter found in high concentration in the gut and kidneys. Since hawthorn is rich in flavonoids, the activity of P-glycoprotein could be changed after long-term use. Thus, the co-administration of digoxin, a substrate of P-glycoprotein, in patients receiving hawthorn extract may lead to changes in the serum digoxin levels. However, a study evaluating the interaction between digoxin and hawthorn preparation showed no significant difference in the pharmacokinetics of digoxin after co-administration for 3 weeks[47]. This study, however, was carried out in healthy subjects. Whether the pharmacokinetic characteristics would be changed in chronic heart failure patients, warranting the adjustment of digoxin dose, is not yet clear. Studies are still needed for clarification of the interactions between hawthorn extract and other heart failure medications, both in healthy volunteers and clinical patients, for a better understanding of the pharmacokinetic changes that may occur when they are used in combination clinically.

CONCLUSIONS

The data from animal studies and clinical trials suggest that hawthorn extract may confer protection against various cardiovascular diseases. Antioxidant flavonoid components may be responsible for these beneficial effects. With increasing interest in applying hawthorn extract in preventing and treating cardiovascular diseases, continuing efforts are necessary for elucidating its pharmacologic activities as well as clinical usefulness.

References

1. Rao AV. Lycopene, tomatoes, and the prevention of coronary heart disease. Exp Biol Med (Maywood) 2002; 227: 908–13

2. Weisburger JH. Lycopene and tomato products in health promotion. Exp Biol Med (Maywood) 2002; 227: 924–7

3. Bagchi D, Sen CK, Ray SD, et al. Molecular mechanisms of cardioprotection by a novel grape seed proanthocyanidin extract. Mutat Res 2003; 523–4: 87–97

4. Kaufman DW, Kelly JP, Rosenberg L, et al. Recent patterns of medication use in the ambulatory adult population of the United States: the Slone survey. J Am Med Assoc 2002; 287: 337–44

5. Rigelsky JM, Sweet BV. Hawthorn: pharmacology and therapeutic uses. Am J Health Syst Pharm 2002; 59: 417–22

6. Hobbs C, Foster S. Hawthorn: a literature review. Herbalgram 1990; 22: 19–33

7. Veveris M, Koch E, Chatterjee SS. Crataegus special extract WS 1442 improves cardiac function and reduces infarct size in a rat model of prolonged coronary ischemia and reperfusion. Life Sci 2004; 74: 1945–55

8. Miller AL. Botanical influences on cardiovascular disease. Altern Med Rev 1998; 3: 422–31

9. Scalbert A, Williamson G. Dietary intake and bioavailability of polyphenols. J Nutr 2000; 130: 2073–85S

10. Chen JW, Zhu ZQ, Hu TX, Zhu DY. Structure–activity relationship of natural flavonoids in hydroxyl radical-scavenging effects. Acta Pharmacol Sin 2002; 23: 667–72

11. Manach C, Scalbert A, Morand C, et al. Polyphenols: food sources and bioavailability. Am J Clin Nutr 2004; 79: 727–47

12. Ness AR, Powles JW. Fruit and vegetables, and cardiovascular disease: a review. Int J Epidemiol 1997; 26: 1–13

13. Rajendran S, Deepalakshmi PD, Parasakthy K, et al. Effect of tincture of Crataegus on the LDL-receptor activity of hepatic plasma membrane of rats fed an atherogenic diet. Atherosclerosis 1996; 123: 235–41

14. Zhang Z, Chang Q, Zhu M, et al. Characterization of antioxidants present in hawthorn fruits. J Nutr Biochem 2001; 12: 144–52

15. Chang Q, Zuo Z, Harrison F, Chow MS. Hawthorn. J Clin Pharmacol 2002; 42: 605–12

16. Bahorun T, Trotin F, Pommery J, et al. Antioxidant activities of Crataegus monogyna extracts. Planta Med 1994; 60: 323–8

17. Shanthi RPK, Deepalakshmi PD, Niranjali DS. Protective effect of tincture of Crataegus on oxidant stress in experimental atherosclerosis in rats. J Clin Biochem Nutr 1996: 211–23

18. Dai YGC, Tian QL, Liu Y. Effect of extracts of some medicinal plants on superoxide dismutase activity in mice. Planta Med 1987: 309–10

19. Petkov E, Nikolov N, Uzunov P. Inhibitory effect of some flavonoids and flavonoid mixtures on cyclic AMP phosphodiesterase activity of rat heart. Planta Med 1981; 43: 183–6

20. Schwinger RH, Pietsch M, Frank K, Brixius K. Crataegus special extract WS 1442 increases force of contraction in human myocardium cAMP-independently. J Cardiovasc Pharmacol 2000; 35: 700–7

21. Muller A, Linke W, Klaus W. Crataegus extract blocks potassium currents in guinea pig ventricular cardiac myocytes. Planta Med 1999; 65: 335–9

22. Chen ZY, Zhang ZS, Kwan KY, et al. Endothelium-dependent relaxation induced by hawthorn extract in rat mesenteric artery. Life Sci 1998; 63: 1983–91

23. Kim SH, Kang KW, Kim KW, Kim ND. Procyanidins in cratagus extract evoke endothelium-dependent vasorelaxation in rat aorta. Life Sci 2000; 67: 121–31

24. Li LD, Liu JX, Shang XH, et al. Studies on hawthorn and its active principle. I. Effect on myocardial ischemia and hemodynamics in dogs. J Tradit Chin Med 1984; 4: 283–8

25. Jayalakshmi R, Niranjali Devaraj S. Cardioprotective effect of tincture of Crataegus on isoproterenol-induced myocardial infarction in rats. J Pharm Pharmacol 2004; 56: 921–6

26. Al Makdessi S, Sweidan H, Mullner S, Jacob R. Myocardial protection by pretreatment with Crataegus oxyacantha: an assessment by means of the release of lactate dehydrogenase by the ischemic and reperfused Langendorff heart. Arzneimittelforschung 1996; 46: 25–7

27. Ammon HP, Handel M. Crataegus, toxicology and pharmacology. Part II: Pharmacodynamics. Planta Med 1981; 43: 209–39

28. Krzeminski T, Chatterjee SS. Ischemia and early reperfusion arrhythmias: beneficial effects of an extract of Crataegus oxyacantha L. Pharm Pharmacol Lett 1993; 3: 45–8

29. Al Makdessi S, Sweidan H, Dietz K, Jacob R. Protective effect of Crataegus oxyacantha against reperfusion arrhythmias after global no-flow ischemia in the rat heart. Basic Res Cardiol 1999; 94: 71–7

30. Garjani A, Nazemiyeh H, Maleki N, Valizadeh H. Effects of extracts from flowering tops of Crataegus meyeri A. Pojark. on ischaemic arrhythmias in anaesthetized rats. Phytother Res 2000; 14: 428–31

31. Muller A, Linke W, Zhao Y, Klaus W. Crataegus extract prolongs action potential duration in guinea-pig papillary muscle. Phytomedicine 1996; 3: 257–61

32. Gaudel Y, Duvellerroy MA. Role of oxygen radicals in cardiac injury due to reoxyhenation. J Mol Cell Cardiol 1984: 459–70

33. Quettier-Deleu C, Voiselle G, Fruchart JC, et al. Hawthorn extracts inhibit LDL oxidation. Pharmazie 2003; 58: 577–81

34. Zhang Z, Ho WK, Huang Y, et al. Hawthorn fruit is hypolipidemic in rabbits fed a high cholesterol diet. J Nutr 2002; 132: 5–10

35. Chen JD, Wu YZ, Tao ZL, et al. Hawthorn (shan zha) drink and its lowering effect on blood lipid levels in humans and rats. World Rev Nutr Diet 1995; 77: 147–54

36. de Whalley CV, Rankin SM, Hoult JR, et al. Flavonoids inhibit the oxidative modification of low density lipoproteins by macrophages. Biochem Pharmacol 1990; 39: 1743–50

37. Tauchert M. Efficacy and safety of crataegus extract WS 1442 in comparison with placebo in patients with chronic stable New York Heart Association class-III heart failure. Am Heart J 2002; 143: 910–15

38. Schroder D, Weiser M, Klein P. Efficacy of a homeopathic Crataegus preparation compared with usual therapy for mild (NYHA II) cardiac insufficiency: results of an observational cohort study. Eur J Heart Fail 2003; 5: 319–26

39. Pittler MH, Schmidt K, Ernst E. Hawthorn extract for treating chronic heart failure: meta-analysis of randomized trials. Am J Med 2003; 114: 665–74

40. Baughman KL, Bradley DJ. Hawthorn extract: is it time to turn over a new leaf? Am J Med 2003; 114: 700–1

41. Holubarsch CJ, Colucci WS, Meinertz T, et al. Survival and prognosis: investigation of Crataegus extract WS 1442 in congestive heart failure (SPICE) – rationale, study design and study protocol. Eur J Heart Fail 2000; 2: 431–7

42. Walker AF, Marakis G, Morris AP, Robinson PA. Promising hypotensive effect of hawthorn extract: a randomized double-blind pilot study of mild, essential hypertension. Phytother Res 2002; 16: 48–54

43. Hanak T, Bruckel MH. Behandlung von leichtern atabilen Formen der Angina pectoris mit Crataegus novo. Therapiewoche 1983; 33: 4331–3

44. Weng WL, Zhang WQ, Liu FZ, et al. Therapeutic effect of Crataegus pinnatifida on 46 cases of angina pectoris – a double blind study. J Tradit Chin Med 1984; 4: 293–4

45. Schroder D, Hehmke B, Kloting I, et al. Humoral-mediated anti-islet cytotoxicity in diabetes-prone BB/OK rats – effect on beta-cell function and autologous islets. Exp Clin Endocrinol 1990; 95: 22–30

46. Tauchert M, Gildor A, Lipinski J. High-dose Crataegus extract WS 1442 in the treatment of NYHA stage II heart failure. Herz 1999; 24: 465–74

47. Tankanow R, Tamer HR, Streetman DS, et al. Interaction study between digoxin and a preparation of hawthorn (Crataegus oxyacantha). J Clin Pharmacol 2003; 43: 637–42

Obesity

18

L. Dey and C.-S. Yuan

INTRODUCTION

Obesity is defined as the presence of an abnormally high proportion of body fat. This condition poses a serious health risk and is a chronic disease. There is a genetic predisposition that is modified by the environment, lifestyle, or both, and behavior. Obesity is associated with increased morbidity and mortality. The National Health and Nutrition Examination Survey (NHANES) found that 55% of US adults were above their ideal weight range: 33% were overweight (body mass index (BMI) 25.0 to 29.9 kg/m^2, and 22% were obese (BMI > 30.0 kg/m^2)[1].

Obesity is the second leading cause of preventable death in the USA[2,3] and it causes or exacerbates many health problems, both independently and in association with other diseases. For example, it is associated with the development of coronary heart disease, type 2 diabetes, an increased incidence of several forms of cancer, respiratory complications (obstructive sleep apnea), and osteoarthritis[4,5].

The economic burden of the condition is substantial. The weight-loss industry accrues about $33 billion each year. The estimated medical costs of treating obesity are about $238 billion per year, of which approximately $100 billion covers the cost of treating co-morbid conditions[2].

Alternative therapies have often been used in chronic conditions that may be only partially alleviated by conventional treatment. Among 14 679 adults randomly surveyed by telephone from 1996 to 1998, 7% reported overall use of non-prescription weight-loss products, with 2% using phenylpropanolamine (which has since been withdrawn from any use in the United States by the FDA) and 1% using ephedra[6].

ALTERNATIVE THERAPIES

Medicinal herbs

Ma huang (ephedra)

Ma huang (Chinese name), also known as desert herb, contains ephedra, a compound that is similar to ephidrine. Dietary supplements that contain ephedra alkaloids (ma huang) are widely promoted and used in the USA as a means of losing weight and increasing energy.

Shekelle *et al.* published a meta-analysis of 22 studies of ephedrine or ephedrine and caffeine, ephedra or ephedra and herbs containing caffeine, each lasting 8 weeks to 4 months[7]. Rate of weight loss was 0.6–1.0 kg per month, and 21 of 22 studies found 5–11% weight loss at 4 months compared to placebo. However, ephedrine and ephedra had 2–3 times the risk of adverse effects, including psychiatric symptoms, autonomic symptoms, gastro-intestinal symptoms, and heart problems. Another reviewer reported that of ephedra-related adverse effects reported to the FDA, 47% were cardiovascular and 18% central nervous system symptoms. Hypertension was the most common adverse effect. A disproportionate number of adverse events due to ephedra were reported to poison control centers. Although effective, ephedra is not considered safe for use in obesity treatment.

In April 2004, the FDA banned the sale of dietary supplements containing ephedrine alkaloids because they present an 'unreasonable risk of illness or injury'[8]. This FDA action followed the publication of several studies that highlighted the potential dangers of ephedra[8–10]. Before the announcement of the FDA ban, it was estimated that approximately 2 million adults took ephedra-containing products daily[11].

Ma huang was previously available in dried branchlets and tablet form, in combination with guarana (see below). Some commercial weight-reduction products (e.g. Metabolife®) contained a combination of ma huang and guarana. The dose for ma huang used previously was 20 mg ephedrine equivalent, and for guarana is 200 mg caffeine equivalent, three times daily[12].

Citrus aurantium

In response to the ban of ephedra, many manufacturers changed their supplement formulations to 'ephedra-free' products by eliminating ephedra and substituting the herb citrus aurantium (also known as 'bitter orange' and 'sour orange'). Citrus aurantium extract contains m-synephrine (phenylephrine)[13], a sympathomimetic drug, which primarily stimulates α-1 adrenergic receptors[14]. The systematic review by Bent *et al.*, found no evidence that citrus aurantium is effective for weight loss[10]. Safety information is extremely limited, and, because citrus aurantium contains the drug m-synephrine, consumption of the herb may lead to increases in blood pressure and pulse, and the risk of adverse cardiovascular events.

Guarana

Guarana is derived from the seeds of *Paullinia cupana*, and is also known as Brazilian cocoa. It contains the chief alkaloid caffeine, in addition to small amounts of theophylline and theobromine. Guarana is used by Brazilian Indians in a stimulating beverage similar to coffee or tea. Several studies have shown that guarana may be effective in treating obesity when it is used with ma huang.

A controlled study of 180 obese patients showed significantly greater weight loss using guarana in combination with ma huang, over a 24-week period[14]. However, Breum *et al.*[15] reported that 54% of patients treated with the guarana and ma huang combination experienced central nervous system side-effects, especially agitation, but noted that these side-effects declined markedly after the first month of treatment. In another study, the hemodynamic side-effects, such as increased systolic, but not diastolic, blood pressure and increased heart rate, were transient, while the thermogenic effects on energy expenditure were persistent[16]. As mentioned above, the usual dose for guarana is 200 mg caffeine equivalent three times daily.

Garcinia cambogia and Garcinia indica

Garcinia cambogia and *Garcinia indica*, which is also known as brindleberry, are isolated from the fruit of the Malabar tamarind. The tamarind is native to southern India, where it is dried and used extensively in curries.

Garcinia cambogia and *Garcinia indica* are now incorporated into many commercial weight-loss products. Hydroxycitric acid is the active ingredient, which competitively inhibits the extramitochondrial enzyme adenosine triphosphate-citrate (pro-3S)-lyase. In many *in vitro* and *in vivo* studies, investigators have demonstrated that hydroxycitric acid not only inhibited the actions of the citrate cleavage enzyme and suppressed fatty acid synthesis[17], but also increased rates of hepatic glycogen synthesis[18], suppressed food intake[19], and decreased body weight gain[20].

Six published human studies have examined hydroxycitric acid in weight loss. Of these studies, five reported positive results, but all had experimental inadequacies[21]. A randomized controlled study over a 12-week period found no differences in weight loss between a group of obese individuals given 3000 mg of *Garcinia cambogia* (50% hydroxycitric acid) daily and a control group given placebo[21]. However, this study did not measure either the appetite-suppressant effect or the plasma concentration of hydroxycitric acid. Opponents of this study have postulated that the high-fiber diet used in the study may have limited the bioavailability, thus rendering the study ineffective and leading to the disappointing results[22]. It appears that hydroxycitrate may offer a safe, natural aid for weight loss when taken at a dose of 500 mg three times daily[23].

Green tea

Green tea has been widely consumed in China and Japan for many centuries. Using an *in vitro* intercapsular brown adipose tissue system, Dulloo *et al.*[24] showed that the effect of green tea on thermogenesis and fat oxidation may be attributed to an interaction between the high content of catechin polyphenols and caffeine[24]. In *in vivo* animal experiments, Kao *et al.*[25] demonstrated that green tea epigallocatechin gallate reduced food intake. Human studies by Dulloo *et al.*[26] observed that administration of capsules containing the green tea extract resulted in a significant increase in 24-h energy expenditure, thermogenesis, fat oxidation, and urinary noradrenalin relative to placebo. These findings could be of value in assisting the management of obesity. The dosage of green tea extract containing 50 mg caffeine and

90 mg epigallocatechin gallate was used in these clinical studies. No adverse effects have been reported.

Gymnema sylvestre (gurmar)

The leaves of *Gymnema sylvestre* have been highly valued as folk medicine for diabetes in India for more than 2000 years[27]. Gymnemic acid, a mixture of triterpene glycosides extracted from the leaves of *Gymnema sylvestre*, can improve glucose tolerance and decrease the blood glucose level in diabetic patients[28,29]. On the basis of this effect, gymnemic acid has been suggested as a useful agent in therapy for obesity[30], since overingestion of carbohydrates is a well-documented cause of obesity. Wang and associates[31] observed that gymnemic acid also potently inhibited oleic acid absorption in the rat intestine, dose-dependently and reversibly. To date, no controlled studies have been conducted to evaluate the efficacy of *Gymnema* extract on obesity.

The recommended dose of *Gymnema* extract is 400 mg/day. An undesirable effect of this agent is that it reduces or abolishes the taste sensation of sweetness and bitterness[32].

Ginseng

There are over a dozen articles reporting the effects of ginseng on animal body-weight changes. However, in most cases, the reports on ginseng's body-weight effects were based on one of the measurements in the study, rather than being the primary goal of the project. Interestingly, these results are highly variable: six articles showed an increase in body-weight effect, three showed a decreased effect, and another four showed no effect.

Several studies reported an increase in body weight after treatment with *Panax ginseng* root. Rats fed a diet containing purified ginseng saponin extract[33,34] and ginseng root extract[35,36] showed an increase in body weight. In addition, some studies reported that treatment with *Panax ginseng* extract or ginsenosides prevented stress-associated weight loss[37,38]. Other studies reported that *Panax ginseng* root had a body-weight-reducing effect. Park *et al.*[39] observed that red ginseng total saponins caused a significant drop in the body weight of rats. A single high dose of red ginseng total saponins significantly reduced the weight of rats and mice[40]. Administration of panaxatriol (isolated from *Panax ginseng* root) to healthy mice suppressed their maturity-associated increase in body weight[41]. Results of other studies failed to show an association between ginseng and body weight[42–45]. It is important to point out that these stud-

ies used different ginseng preparations and components in different animal species and models.

A clinical trial[46] that investigated antidiabetic effects of ginseng root reported that, in addition to an improvement in fasting blood glucose levels, the subjects experienced a reduction in body weight. In this study of patients with type 2 diabetes, patients in both the control and the ginseng-treated group were encouraged to reduce body weight by exercise and food intake control. Thus, patients in the ginseng-treated group as well as the placebo group lost weight. It appears that the anti-obesity effect of ginseng is inconclusive.

The recommended daily ginseng dose is 1–2 g of the crude root, or 200–600 mg of standardized extracts[47]. As the possibility of hormone-like or hormone-inducing effects cannot be ruled out, some authors suggest limiting treatment to 3 months[47].

Kelp

Kelp generically refers to seaweed species including *Laminaria*, *Macrocystis*, *Nereocystis*, and *Fucus*. It has been used as an anti-obesity agent, presumably by supplying iodine, hence increasing thyroid hormone production with consequent increased metabolism and removal of fat. Iodine content is different in kelp products. Hyperthyroidism has been reported after the use of a kelp product[48]. Potassium iodide content may result in hypersensitivity reactions in sensitive patients. Concomitant use of kelp with levothyroxine could result in excessive replacement, producing typical symptoms of hyperthyroidism[49]. Since kelp and related seaweed products contain sodium, they should consequently be avoided by those who must restrict their salt intake. In addition, using any thyroid hormone-related product to control body weight is inadvisable and should be discouraged.

Capsaicin

Capsaicin is the major pungent principle in various species of capsaicin fruits, such as hot chili peppers, and has long been globally used as an ingredient of spices, preservatives, and medicines (Figure 18.1)[50].

Dietary supplementation of capsaicin in high-fat diets lowered the peripheral adipose tissue weight and serum triglyceride concentration in rats, owing to enhancement of energy metabolism[51,52]. Watanabe *et al.*[53,54] have investigated the neurophysiologic functions of capsaicin and have demonstrated that capsaicin increases energy metabolism by catecholamine secretion from the adrenal medulla through sympathetic

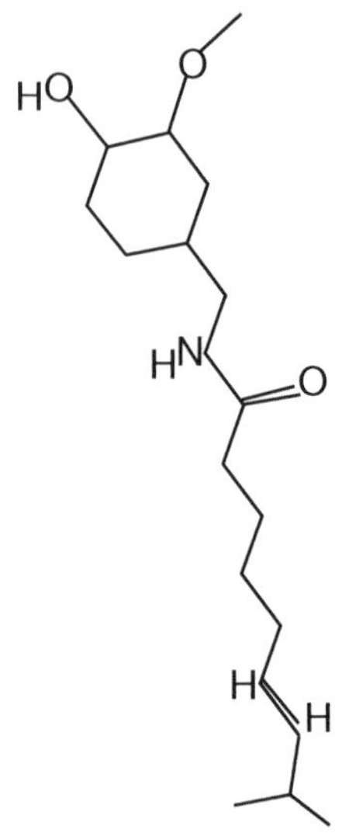

Figure 18.1   Chemical structure of capsaicin

activation via the central nervous system. In a human study, Yoshioka *et al.*[55] observed that energy expenditure increased immediately after a meal containing red pepper, whereas this enhancement of energy metabolism by a red pepper diet was inhibited after the administration of the β-adrenergic blocker propranolol. In a more recent human study, Matsumoto *et al.*[56] investigated the effect of capsaicin on sympathetic nervous system activity and energy metabolism in 16 lean and obese young women, matched for age and height. Their observation supported previous investigations and reinforced the finding that the altered specific sympathetic function related to thermogenic capacity may be a significant sign reflecting the autonomic state in human obesity. However, data from their study also indicated that the reduced sympathetic responsiveness to thermogenic perturbation such as that found in a diet including capsaicin, which may cause impaired diet-induced thermogenesis and further weight gain, could be an important etiologic factor leading to obesity in young women. The dose in the study was 3 mg of capsaicin in spicy yellow curry sauce.

Guggul gum (gugulipid)

This resin from the myrrh species, in addition to being used as a cholesterol-lowering agent, is found in some over-the-counter diet products. Gugulipid has been shown to stimulate the release of endogenous thyroid

hormone in rats[57], although there are no additional animal or human studies supporting this claim. Gugulipid is available in the extract form, powdered resin, and concentrated tablets.

Nutritional supplements

Chromium

Chromium has lately gained a great deal of public attention as an aid to weight loss. One of the key goals for enhancing weight loss is to increase insulin sensitivity of cells throughout the body, on the basis that chromium plays an important role in cellular sensitivity to insulin[58].

Preliminary studies with chromium demonstrated that chromium picolinate promoted an increase in percentage of lean body weight and a decrease in percentage of body fat, which may lead to weight loss[58,59]. Greater muscle mass has greater fat-burning potential. Chromium supplementation also improves blood sugar control and lowers cholesterol and triglyceride levels[60].

Several forms of chromium are available, such as chromium picolinate, chromium polynicotinate, chromium chloride, and chromium-enriched yeast. The recommended chromium dose is 200–400 μg daily[23]. There have been reports of possible tissue accumulation and damage to DNA and renal damage following long-term ingestion of large doses of chromium[61,62].

Conjugated linoleic acid

Conjugated linoleic acid is found in dairy products and beef and is thought to work by inhibiting lipoprotein lipase, an enzyme that breaks down fat for absorption, and increasing the breakdown of stored fat[63].

Three randomized clinical trials with a total of 126 patients used conjugated linoleic acid for weight loss. Typical doses were 3.0–3.6 g per day, in three divided doses with meals, for 12 weeks or less. None of these showed changes in weight or BMI, but did report significant decreases in abdominal diameter, body fat mass, and percent body fat. Adverse effects included mild gastro-intestinal symptoms, but were not different from placebo[63].

5-Hydroxytryptamine (serotonin)

There are three clinical studies with 5-hydroxytryptamine (5-HT) in overweight women[64–66] and these studies showed that 5-HT appeared to promote weight loss by promoting satiety, leading to fewer calories being consumed at meals. Besides mild nausea, no other side-effects were reported.

The recommended starting dose of 5-HT is 50–100 mg 20 min before meals for 2 weeks, and then double the dosage to a maximum of 300 mg if weight loss is less than 1 lb (0.45 kg) per week. Higher doses of 5-HT are associated with nausea, but this symptom disappears after 6 weeks of use[23].

L-Carnitine

L-Carnitine is an amino acid found in meat and dairy products; it is formed from the amino acids lysine and methionine, in the liver and kidney. Its proposed action is an increase in fat metabolism. Two studies have shown no changes in the rate of fat oxidation following L-carnitine supplementation[67,68]. Control studies examining the effects of l-carnitine on weight loss have not been published. Oral supplementation may cause diarrhea, but no other major adverse effects have been noted.

Medium-chain triglycerides

Medium-chain triglycerides are saturated fats (which can be extracted from coconut oil) whose chains range in length from six to 12 carbon atoms. Unlike regular fats and long-chain triglycerides, medium-chain triglycerides appear to promote weight loss rather than weight gain. They may promote weight loss by increasing thermogenesis[69]. A study demonstrated that oil of medium-chain triglycerides given over a 6-day period could increase diet-induced thermogenesis by 50%[70]. In order to gain the benefit from medium-chain triglycerides, a diet must remain low in long-chain triglycerides. Medium-chain triglycerides can be used as an oil for salad dressing or a bread spread, or simply be taken as a supplement. Dosage recommendation is 1–2 tablespoons per day. Diabetics and individuals with liver disease should be monitored very closely when using medium-chain triglycerides, as they may develop ketoacidosis.

Coenzyme Q10

Coenzyme Q_{10} is an essential compound required in the transport and breakdown of fatty acids into energy. In one study, coenzyme Q_{10} levels were found to be low in 52% of overweight subjects tested. In the study, nine subjects (five with low coenzyme Q_{10} levels and four with normal levels) were given 100 mg/day of coenzyme Q_{10} along with a low-calorie diet. After 9 weeks, mean weight loss in the coenzyme Q_{10}-deficient group was 29.7 lb (13.4 kg), compared with 12.8 lb (5.8 kg) in those with initially normal levels of coenzyme Q_{10}[71]. The recommended dose is 100–300 mg/day.

Chitosan

Chitosan is an amino polysaccharide derived from the powdered shells of marine crustaceans such as prawns and crabs. Some clinical studies have shown lipid-lowering effects[72], as well as weight loss[73–75]. The proposed action of chitosan is binding to dietary fat, preventing digestion and storage. However, in one controlled trial in 17 individuals, the weight-reduction effect of chitosan was not confirmed[76]. Risks such as steatorrhea and malabsorption of essential nutrients are possible.

Fiber

Increasing the amount of dietary fiber promotes weight loss. The best fiber sources for weight loss are psyllium, chitin, guar gum, glucumannan, gum karaya, and pectin, which are rich in water-soluble fibers. When taken with water before meals, these fiber sources bind to water in the stomach to form a gelatinous mass, which induces a sense of satiety[23]. Fiber supplements have been shown to enhance blood sugar control, decrease insulin levels, and reduce the number of calories absorbed by the body[77]. The most impressive results in studies of weight loss have been achieved with guar gum, a water-soluble fiber obtained from the Indian cluster bean (*Cyamopsis tetragonoloba*).

The starting dose should be between 1 and 2 g before meals and at bedtime, with gradual increase of the dose to 5 g[23]. Water-soluble fibers are fermented by intestinal bacteria; therefore, a great deal of gas can be produced, leading to increased flatulence and abdominal discomfort.

Acupuncture

One indication for acupuncture is obesity[78]. Ernst[79] reviewed the results of sham/placebo-controlled clinical trials of acupuncture/acupressure for obesity. His goal was to determine whether these therapies have specific effects on appetite and reduction of body weight. Two studies suggested a positive effect of acupuncture on appetite and body weight[80,81], whereas two other trials showed no effect of acupuncture or acupressure[82,83].

Richards and Marley[84] studied the effectiveness of transcutaneous electrical nerve stimulation of specific auricular acupuncture points on appetite suppression. They observed that frequent stimulation of a specific auricular acupuncture point was an effective method of appetite suppression, leading to weight loss. It has been postulated that acupuncture stimulation of certain parts of the ear can reduce appetite by activating the satiety center within the hypothalamus[85], or control stress and depression via endorphin and dopamine production[84].

CONCLUSIONS

In the USA, weight loss is a national obsession. Over one-third of all Americans are obese, and they spend over $30 billion annually to lose weight. Clinically, obesity is a serious medical disorder, because it can cause a myriad of health problems, such as heart disease, hypertension, and adult-onset diabetes. Alternative therapies, especially herbal medicines, are increasingly used by obese people and some non-obese people who want to lose weight. Most herbs and nutritional supplements are used in conjunction with prescription anti-obesity drugs. Potential adverse herb–drug interactions should also be kept in mind for patients who are receiving conventional pharmacologic agents. In addition, since a single herb may be used in different commercial anti-obesity dietary preparations, consumers should not take more than one product simultaneously, to avoid any undesirable additive effects.

References

1. Kuczmarski RJ, Carroll MD, Flegal KM, Troiano RP. Varying body mass index cutoff points to describe overweight prevalence among U.S. adults: NHANES III (1988–1994). Obes Res 1997; 5: 542–8

2. McGinnis JM, Forge WH. Actual causes of death in the United States. J Am Med Assoc 1993; 270: 2207–12

3. de Jonge L, Bray GA. The thermic effect of food and obesity: a critical review. Obes Res 1997; 5: 622–31

4. Bray GA. Drug treatment of obesity: don't throw the baby out with the bath water. Am J Clin Nutr 1998; 67: 1–4

5. Negro AD. It's Time to Treat Obesity. American Heart Association Scientific Sessions, 2000

6. Blanck HM, Khan LK, Serdula MK. Use of nonprescription weight loss products: results from a multistate survey. J Am Med Assoc 2001; 286: 930–5

7. Shekelle PG, Hardy ML, Morton SC, et al. Efficacy and safety of ephedra and ephedrine for weight loss and athletic performance: a meta-analysis. J Am Med Assoc 2003; 289: 1537–45

8. Final rule declaring dietary supplements containing ephedrine alkaloids adulterated because they present an unreasonable risk. Department of Health and Human Services, Food and Drug Administration 2004: 1–363. Available at: www.fda.gov/OHRMS/DOCKETS/98fr/1995n-0304-nfr0001.pdf

9. Haller CA, Benowitz NL. Adverse cardiovascular and central nervous system events associated with dietary supplements containing ephedra alkaloids. N Engl J Med 2000; 343: 1833–8

10. Bent S, Tiedt TN, Odden MC, Shlipak MG. The relative safety of ephedra compared with other herbal products. Ann Intern Med 2003; 138: 468–71

11. Kaufman DW, Kelly JP, Mitchell AA. Use of ephedra-containing products in the U.S. population. Data from the Sloane Survey 2003. FDA Docket Number 1995N-0304, emc126, Vol 297: 1–9

12. Morelli V, Zoorob RJ. Alternative therapies: Part 1. Depression, diabetes, obesity. Am Fam Physician 2000; 62: 1051–60

13. Penzak SR, Jann MW, Cold JA, et al. Seville (sour) orange juice: synephrine content and cardiovascular effects in normotensive adults. J Clin Pharmacol 2001; 41: 1059–63

14. Astrup A, Breum L, Toubro S, et al. The effect and safety of an ephedrine/caffeine compound compared to ephidrine, caffeine and placebo in obese subjects on an energy restricted diet. A double blind trial. Int J Obes Relat Metab Disord 1992; 16: 269–77

15. Breum L, Pedersen JK, Ahlstrom F, Frimodt-Moller J. Comparison of an ephedrine/caffeine combination and dexfluramine in the treatment of obesity. A double-blind multi-center trial in general practice. Int J Obes Relat Metab Disord 1994; 18: 99–103

16. Astrup A, Toubro S. Thermogenic, metabolic and cardiovascular responses to ephedrine and caffeine in man. Int J Obes Relat Metab Disord 1993; 17 (Suppl 1): S41–3

17. Lowenstein JM. Effect of (-)-hydroxycitrate on fatty acid synthesis by rat liver in vivo. J Biol Chem 1971; 246: 629–32

18. Sullivan AC, Triscari J, Neal Miller O. The influence of (-)-hydroxycitrate on in vivo rates of hepatic glycogenesis: lipogenesis and cholesterol genesis. Fed Proc 1974; 33: 656

19. Sullivan AC, Triscari J, Hamilton JG, Neal Miller O. Effect of (-)-hydroxycitrate upon the accumulation of lipid in the rat: appetite. Lipids 1973; 9: 129–34

20. Nageswara RR, Sakeriak KK. Lipid-lowering and antiobesity effect of (-) hydroxycitric acid. Nutr Res 1988; 8: 209–12

21. Heymsfield SB, Allison DB, Vasselli JR, et al. Garcinia cambogia (hydroxycitric acid) as a potential antiobesity agent: a randomized controlled trial. J Am Med Assoc 1998; 280: 1596–600

22. Firenzuoli F, Gori L. Garcinia cambogia for weight loss. J Am Med Assoc 1999; 282: 234

23. Murray MT, Pizzorno JE Jr. Obesity. In Pizzorno JE Jr, Murray MT, eds. Textbook of Natural Medicine, 2nd edn. Edinburgh: Churchill Livingstone, 1999: 429–39

24. Dulloo AG, Seydoux J, Girardier L, et al. Green tea and thermogenesis: interactions between catechin-polyphenols, caffeine and sympathetic activity. Int J Obes 2000; 24: 252–8

25. Kao YH, Hiipakka RA, Liao S. Modulation of endocrine systems and food intake by green tea epigallocatechin gallate. Endocrinology 2000; 141: 980–7

26. Dulloo AG, Duret C, Rohrer D, et al. Efficacy of a green tea extract rich in catechin polyphenols and caffeine in increasing 24-h energy expenditure and fat oxidation in humans. Am J Clin Nutr 1999; 70: 1040–5

27. Nadkarni KM. Gymnema sylvestre, R. Br. or Asclepias geminata. In Nadkarni KM, ed. Indian Materia Medica. Bombay: Popular Prakashan, 1982; 1: 596–9

28. Baskaran K, Kizar AB, Radha SK, Shanmugasundaram ER. Antidiabetic effect of a leaf extract from Gymnema sylvestre in non-insulin dependent diabetes mellitus patients. J Ethnopharmacol 1990; 30: 295–300

29. Shanmugasundaram ER, Rajeswari G, Baskaran K, et al. Use of Gymnema sylvestre leaf extract in the control of blood glucose in insulin dependent diabetes mellitus. J Ethnopharmacol 1990; 30: 281–94

30. Terasawa H, Miyoshi M, Imoto T. Effects of long term administration of Gymnema sylvestre watery-extract on variations of body weight, plasma glucose, serum triglyceride, total cholesterol and insulin in Wistar fatty rats. Yonago Acta Med 1994; 37: 117–27

31. Wang LF, Luo H, Imoto T, et al. Inhibitory effect of gymnemic acid on intestinal absorption of oleic acid in rats. Can J Physiol Pharmacol 1998; 76: 1017–23

32. Mozersky RP. Herbal products and supplemental nutrients used in the management of diabetes. J Am Osteopath Assoc 1999; 99: 54–9

33. Rhee DK, Lim CJ, Kim DH, et al. Studies on the acute and subacute toxicity of ginseng saponin. Yakhak Hoe Chi 1982; 26: 209–14

34. Rim KT, Choi JS, Lee SM, Cho KS. Effect of ginsenosides from red ginseng on the enzymes of cellular signal transduction system (Korean). Koryo Insam Hakhoechi 1997; 21: 19–27

35. Hong SA. Effects of Panax ginseng on the general behavioral activity and survival time of food deprivation in rats. Ch'oesin Uihak 1972; 15: 81–91

36. Eui S, Kim BY, Paik TH, Joo CN. The effect of ginseng on alcohol metabolism. Hanguk Saenghwa Hakhoe Chi 1978; 11: 1–15

37. Fujimoto K, Sakata T, Ishimaru T, et al. Attenuation of anorexia induced by heat or surgery during sustained administration of ginsenoside Rg1 into rat third ventricle. Psychopharmacology 1989; 99: 257–60

38. Zierer R. Prolonged infusion of Panax ginseng saponins into the rat does not alter the chemical and kinetic profile of hormones from the posterior pituitary. J Ethnopharmacol 1991; 34: 269–74

39. Park CW, Kim JG, Lee YS, et al. Subacute toxicity study of red ginseng total saponin in rats. J Toxicol Publ Health 1998; 14: 77–82

40. Kim JG, Park CW, Lee YS, et al. Acute toxicity study of red ginseng total saponin in rats and mice. J Toxicol Publ Health 1998; 14: 69–75

41. Kim YS, Kang KS, Kim S II. Effects of a cytotoxic substance, panaxytriol from Panax ginseng C.A. Meyer on the immune responses in normal mice. Korean J Toxicol 1990; 6: 13–19

42. Hong BJ, Kim CI, Kim UH, Rhee YC. Effect of feeding ginseng crude saponin on body weight gain and reproductive function in chicken. Hanguk Ch'uksan Hakhoe Chi 1976; 18: 355–61

43. Hess FG Jr, Parent RA, Cox GE, et al. Reproduction study in rats of ginseng extract G115. Food Chem Toxicol 1982; 20: 189–92

44. Hess FG Jr, Parent RA, Stevens KR, et al. Effects of subchronic feeding of ginseng extract G115 in beagle dogs. Food Chem Toxicol 1983; 21: 95–7

45. Murphy LL, Cadena RS, Chavez D, Ferraro JS. Effect of American ginseng (Panax quinquefolium) on male copulatory behavior in the rat. Physiol Behav 1998; 64: 445–50

46. Sotaniemi EA, Haapakoski E, Rautio A. Ginseng therapy in non-insulin-dependent diabetic patients. Diabetes Care 1995; 18: 1373–5

47. Schulz V, Hansel R, Tyler VE. Rational phytotherapy. In Schulz V, Hansel R, Tyler VE, eds. Agents that Increase Resistance to Diseases. New York, NY: Springer-Verlag, 1998: 269–72

48. Foster S, Tyler VE, eds. Tyler's Honest Herbal. A Sensible Guide to the Use of Herbs and Related Remedies, 4th edn. Binghamton, NY: Haworth Press, 1999

49. Miller LG. Herbal medications, nutraceuticals, and diabetes. In Miller LG, Murray WJ, eds. Herbal Medicinals, A Clinician's Guide. Binghamton, NY: Pharmaceutical Products Press, Imprint of Haworth Press, 1998: 115–33

50. Suzuki T, Iwai K. Constituents of red pepper spices: chemistry, pharmacology and food science of the pungent principle of Capsicum species. In Bross A, ed. The Alkaloids. New York, NY: Academic Press, 1984; 23: 227–9

51. Kawada T, Hagiharaa K, Iwai K. Effects of capsaicin on lipid metabolism in rats fed a high fat diet. J Nutr 1986; 116: 1272–8

52. Kawada T, Watanabe T, Takaishi T, et al. Capsaicin-induced β-adrenergic action on energy metabolism in rats: influence of capsaicin on oxygen consumption, the respiratory quotient, and substrate utilization. Proc Soc Exp Biol Med 1986; 183: 250–6

53. Watanabe T, Kawada T, Iwai K. Enhancement by capsaicin of energy metabolism in rats through secretion of catecholamine from adrenal medulla. Agric Biol Chem 1987; 51: 75–9

54. Watanabe T, Kawada T, Kurosawa M, et al. Adrenal sympathetic efferent nerve and catecholamine secretion excitation caused by capsaicin in rats. Am J Physiol 1988; 255: E23–7

55. Yoshioka M, Lim K, Kikuzato S, et al. Effects of red-pepper diet on the energy metabolism in men. J Nutr Sci Vitaminol 1995; 41: 647–56

56. Matsumoto T, Miyawaki C, Ue H, et al. Effects of capsaicin-containing yellow curry sauce on sympathetic nervous system activity and diet-induced thermogenesis in lean and obese young women. J Nutr Sci Vitaminol 2000; 46: 309–15

57. Tripathi YB, Malhotra OP, Tripathi SN. Thyroid stimulation action of Z-guggulsterone obtained from Commiphora mukul. Planta Med 1984; 1: 78–80

58. Anderson RA. Effects of chromium on body composition and weight loss. Nutr Rev 1998; 56: 266–70

59. Evans GW. Chromium picolinate is an efficacious and safe supplement. Int J Sport Nutr 1993; 3: 117–22

60. Press RI, Gellaer J, Evans GW. The effect of chromium picolinate on serum cholesterol and apolipoprotein fractions in human subjects. West J Med 1993; 152: 41–5

61. Stearns DM, Belbruno JJ, Wetterhahn KE. A prediction of chromium (iii) accumulation in humans from chromium dietary supplements. FASEB J 1995; 9: 1650–7

62. Cerulli J, Grabe DW, Gauthier L, et al. Chromium picolinate toxicity. Ann Pharmacother 1998; 32: 428–31

63. Lenz TL, Hamilton WR. Supplemental products used for weight loss. J Am Pharm Assoc (Wash DC) 2004; 44: 59–67

64. Ceci F, Cangiano C, Cairella M, et al. The effects of oral 5-hydroxytryptophan administration on feeding behavior in obese adult female subjects. J Neural Transm 1989; 76: 109–17

65. Cangiano C, Ceci F, Cairella M, et al. Effects of 5-hydroxytryptophan on eating behavior and adherence to dietary prescriptions in obese adult subjects. Adv Exp Med Biol 1991; 294: 591–3

66. Cangiano C, Ceci F, Cascino A, et al. Eating behavior and adherence to dietary prescriptions in obese adult subjects treated with 5-hydroxytryptophan. Am J Clin Nutr 1992; 56: 863–7

67. Sulkers EJ, Lafeber HN, Degenhart HJ, et al. Effects of high carnitine supplementation on substrate utilization in low-birth-weight infants receiving total parenteral nutrition. Am J Clin Nutr 1990; 52: 889–94

68. Vukovich MD, Costill DL, Fink WJ. Carnitine supplementation: effect on muscle carnitine and glycogen content during exercise. Med Sci Sports Exerc 1994; 26: 1122–9

69. Baba N, Bracco EF, Hashim SA. Enhanced thermogenesis and diminished deposition of fat in response to overfeeding with diet containing medium chain triglyceride. Am J Clin Nutr 1982; 35: 678–82

70. Hill JO, Peters JC, Yang D, et al. Thermogenesis in humans during over feeding with medium-chain triglycerides in man. Am J Clin Nutr 1986; 44: 630–4

71. Van Gaal L. Exploratory study of coenzyme Q10 in obesity. In Folkers K, Yamamura Y, eds. Biomedical and Clinical Aspects of Coenzyme Q10. Amsterdam: Elsevier Science, 1984; 4: 369–73

72. Ventura P. Lipid lowering activity of chitosan, a new dietary integrator. In Muzzarelli RAA, ed. Chitin Enzymology. Ancona, Italy: Atec Edizioni, 1996; 2: 55–62

73. Maezaki Y, Tsuji K. Hypochlosterolaemic effect of chitosan in adult males. Biosc Biochem Biotech 1993; 57: 1439–44

74. Abelin J, Lassus AL. 112 Bipolymar-Fat [Binder] as a Weight Reducer in Patients with Moderate Obesity. Medical research report. A study performed at Ars Medicinar, Helsinki, August–October, 1994

75. Veneroni G, Veneroni F, Contos S. Effect of a new chitoson on hyperlipidaemia and overweight in obese patients. In Muzzarelli RAA, ed. Chitin Enzymology. Ancona, Italy: Atec Edizioni, 1996; 2: 63–7

76. Pittler MH, Abbot NC, Harkness EF, Ernst E. Randomized, double-blind trial of chitosan for body weight reduction. Eur J Clin Nutr 1999; 53: 379–81

77. Spiller GA. Dietary Fiber in Health and Nutrition. Boca Raton, FL: CRC Press, 1994

78. Cassell DK, Larocca FE. The Encyclopedia of Obesity and Eating Disorders. New York, NY: Fact on File, 1994

79. Ernst E. Acupuncture/acupressure for weight reduction? A systemic review. Wien Klin Wochenschr 1997; 109: 60–2

80. Giller RM. Auricular acupuncture and weight reduction. A controlled study. Am J Acupuncture 1975; 3: 151–3

81. Shafshak TS. Electroacupuncture and exercise in body weight reduction and their application in rehabilitating patients with knee osteoarthritis. Am J Clin Med 1995; 13: 15–25

82. Mok MS, Parker LN, Voina S, Bray GA. Treatment of obesity by acupuncture. Am J Clin Nutr 1976; 29: 832–5

83. Allison DB, Krie K, Heshka S, Heymsfield SB. A randomised placebo-controlled clinical trial of an acupressure device for weight loss. Int J Obes 1995; 19: 653–8

84. Richards D, Marley J. Stimulation of auricular acupuncture points in weight loss. Aust Fam Physician 1998; 27 (Suppl 2): 73–7

85. Huang MH, Yang RC, Hu SH. Preliminary results of triple therapy for obesity. Int J Obes 1996; 20: 830–6

Type 2 diabetes

19

L. Dey and A. S. Attele

INTRODUCTION

Diabetes mellitus or diabetes is a serious chronic metabolic disorder that has a significant impact on the health, quality of life, and life expectancy of patients, as well as on the health-care system. In the USA, diabetes is the sixth leading cause of death[1]. Diabetes is divided into two major categories: type 1 and type 2. The overall prevalence of diabetes is approximately 6%, of which 90% is type 2 diabetes[2]. Treatment and care of diabetes represents a substantial portion of the national health-care expenditure. In 1992, for example, diabetes care cost 14.6% of every dollar spent on US health care[3].

PATHOPHYSIOLOGY AND COMPLICATIONS

Type 2 diabetes is known to have a strong genetic component, with contributing environmental determinants. The early stage of type 2 diabetes is characterized by insulin resistance in insulin-targeting tissues, mainly the liver, skeletal muscle, and adipocytes. Insulin resistance in these tissues is associated with excessive glucose production by the liver and impaired glucose utilization by peripheral tissues, especially the muscle. With increased insulin secretion to compensate for insulin resistance, baseline blood glucose levels can be maintained within normal ranges, but the patients may demonstrate impaired responses to prandial carbohydrate loading and to oral glucose tolerance tests. Thus, this early stage of diabetes features both insulin resistance and a relative insulin deficiency. The chronic overstimulation of insulin secretion gradually diminishes and eventually exhausts the islet β-cell reserve. A state of absolute insulin deficiency ensues and clinical diabetes becomes overt[4–6]. The transition of impaired glucose tolerance to type 2 diabetes can also be influenced by ethnicity, degree of obesity, distribution of body fat, sedentary lifestyle, aging, and other concomitant medical conditions[7].

The quality of life of type 2 diabetic patients with chronic and severe hypoglycemia is adversely affected. Characteristic symptoms of tiredness and lethargy can become severe and lead to a decrease in work performance in adults and an increase of falls in the elderly[8]. The most common acute complications are metabolic problems (hyperosmolar hyperglycemic non-ketotic syndrome (HHNS)) and infection. The long-term complications are macrovascular complications (hypertension, dyslipidemia, myocardial infarction, stroke), microvascular complications (retinopathy, nephropathy, diabetic neuropathy, diarrhea, neurogenic bladder, impaired cardiovascular reflexes, sexual dysfunction) and diabetic foot disorders[8].

CONVENTIONAL THERAPIES

The general consensus on treatment of type 2 diabetes is that lifestyle management remains a foremost therapy. In addition to exercise, weight control, and medical nutrition therapy, oral glucose-lowering drugs and injection of insulin are the conventional therapies for type 2 diabetes.

Pharmacologic treatment and limitations

Oral drug therapy

In the USA, five classes of oral agents are approved for the treatment of type 2 diabetes. Oral agent therapy is indicated in any patient with type 2 diabetes in whom diet and exercise fail to achieve acceptable glycemic control[9]. Although the initial responses have been good, oral hypoglycemic drugs may lose their effectiveness in a significant percentage of patients.

Sulfonylureas Both first-generation (e.g. tolbutamide) and second-generation (e.g. glyburide) sulfonylureas enhance insulin secretion from the pancreatic β-cells. A significant side-effect is hypoglycemia. Sulfonylurea therapy is also usually associated with weight gain due to hyperinsulinemia[10,11], which has been implicated as a cause of secondary drug failure[9–11].

Metformin Originally derived from a medicinal plant, *Galega officinalis*, metformin reduces plasma glucose by inhibiting hepatic glucose production and increasing muscle glucose uptake. It also enhances muscle glucose uptake and utilization. The most common side-effects are lactic acidosis and gastro-intestinal disturbances.

Glucosidase inhibitors These decrease postprandial glucose levels. They work by interfering with carbohydrate digestion and delaying gastro-intestinal absorption of glucose. The major side-effects are related to the gastro-intestinal tract such as flatulence and abdominal bloating.

Thiazolidinediones Rosiglitazone and pioglitazone have been approved for use. These are relatively expensive oral agents, which work by improving insulin sensitivity in muscle and by suppressing hepatic glucose production. Liver toxicity is a concern; therefore, monthly monitoring of liver function is required once therapy with the thiazolidinediones begins. Potential adverse effects are weight gain and volume expansion. These are contraindicated in congestive heart failure.

Meglitinides Repaglinide and nateglinide are non-sulfonylurea secretagogues in the meglitinide class. Their primary effect is to lower blood glucose levels by stimulating release of insulin in response to a glucose load (meal). Weight gain, hypoglycemia, and hypersensitivity are side-effects.

Insulin therapy

Insulin is usually added to an oral agent when glycemic control is suboptimal at maximal doses of oral medications. Some diabetologists prefer to initiate insulin therapy in patients with newly diagnosed type 2 diabetes[9]. Weight gain and hypoglycemia are common side-effects of insulin therapy[12–15]. Vigorous insulin treatment may also carry an increased risk of atherogenesis[13]. Table 19.1 summarizes some limitations of current drug therapies.

Exercise

Any exercise prescription should be individualized to account for patient interests, physical status, capacity,

Table 19.1 Limitations of some antidiabetic drugs

Antidiabetic drug	Major limitations
Sulfonylureas	hypoglycemia, weight gain
Metformin	gastro-intestinal disturbances
Acarbose	gastro-intestinal disturbances
Thiazolidinediones	liver toxicity, weight gain, high LDL-cholesterol, high cost
Meglitinides	hypoglycemia, weight gain
Insulin	hypoglycemia, weight gain

LDL, low-density lipoprotein

and motivation. Exercising five to six times per week enhances weight reduction. Because many people with diabetes have not been active and are deconditioned, exercise should be started at a low level and gradually increased to avoid adverse effects such as injury, hypoglycemia, or cardiac problems[16,17].

Diet therapy

Given the heterogeneous nature of type 2 diabetes, no single dietary approach is appropriate for all patients. Meal plans and diet modifications should be individualized by a registered dietitian to meet a patient's unique needs and lifestyle.

ALTERNATIVE THERAPIES

Tremendous effort has been spent in searching for alternative therapies with antidiabetic activity. Ideal therapies should have a similar degree of efficacy without the troublesome side-effects associated with conventional treatments. Some alternative therapies, which claimed to alleviate or cure diabetes, have become increasingly popular over the past several years[15]. Among them, medicinal herbs, nutritional supplementation, acupuncture, and hot-tub therapy may be effective.

Medicinal herbs

Many conventional drugs have been derived from prototypic molecules in medicinal plants. Metformin exemplifies an efficacious oral glucose-lowering agent, and its development was based on the use of *Galega officinalis* to treat diabetes[18]. *Galega officinalis* is rich in guanidine, the hypoglycemic component[19–21]. Because guanidine is too toxic for clinical use, the alkyl diguanides synthalin A and synthalin B were introduced as oral antidiabetic agents in Europe in the 1920s, but were discontinued after insulin became more widely available. However, experience with guanidine and diguanides prompted the development of metformin[22,23].

To date, over 400 traditional plant treatments for diabetes have been reported[20], although only a small number of these have received scientific and medical evaluation to assess their efficacy. A hypoglycemic effect resulting from the treatment of some herbal extracts has been confirmed in animal models of type 2 diabetes. The World Health Organization Expert Committee on Diabetes has recommended that traditional medicinal herbs be further investigated[18]. The following is a summary of several of the most studied and commonly used medicinal herbs.

Ginseng

The root of ginseng has been used for over 2000 years in the Far East for its health-promoting properties. In recent years, it has consistently been one of the ten top-selling herbs in the USA. Of the several species of ginseng, *Panax ginseng* (Asian ginseng) and *Panax quinquefolius* (American ginseng) are commonly used. Constituents of all ginseng species include ginsenosides, polysaccharides, peptides, polyacetyleinic alcohol, and fatty acids[24]. Most pharmacologic actions of ginseng are attributed to ginsenosides, a family of steroids named steroidal saponins[25,26]. The chemical composition of ginseng products and their potency may vary with the plant extract derivative, the age of the root, the location where it was grown, the season when it was harvested, and the methods of drying[27,28].

Data from animal studies indicate that both Asian ginseng[29,30] and American ginseng[31,32] have significant hypoglycemic action. This blood-glucose-lowering effect might be attributed to ginsenoside Rb_2 and, more specifically, to panaxans I, J, K, and L in type 1 diabetic models[33–37]. Whether these constituents would have a similar effect on type 2 diabetes is still unknown.

There is some clinical evidence of ginseng's hypoglycemic activity. Sotaniemi *et al.* demonstrated a reduction in the levels of fasting blood glucose and hemoglobin A_{1c} in type 2 diabetics treated with a small dose (100–200 mg) of ginseng relative to placebo[38]. Ginseng also elevated mood, improved psychophysiologic performance and physical activity, and reduced body weight[38]. Recently, Vuksan *et al.* also demonstrated that 3 g of American ginseng, when given 40 min prior to the test meal, significantly lowered blood glucose in non-diabetic subjects and type 2 diabetic patients[39]. However, when ginseng was given together with meals, this effect did not persist in non-diabetic subjects. Vuksan *et al.*[39] proposed several plausible hypotheses that may work independently or in concert: first, ginseng may slow the digestion of food, decreasing the rate of carbohydrate absorption into the portal hepatic circulation[28,40]; second, ginseng may affect glucose transport, which is mediated by nitric oxide (NO)[30,41–43]; third, ginseng may modulate NO-mediated insulin secretion[44]. It was recently shown that NO stimulated glucose-dependent secretion of insulin in rat islet cells[45].

The most commonly reported side-effects are nervousness and excitation, but these diminish with continued use or dosage reduction[46]. However, there are few reports of noticeable adverse effects of ginseng, despite the fact that over 6 million ingest it regularly in the USA[46]. Ginseng may exert an estrogen-like effect in postmenopausal women, resulting in diffuse mammary nodularity and vaginal bleeding[47,48]. Ginseng may inhibit the effects of warfarin[49], and interact with the monoamine oxidase inhibitor phenelzine[50]. Often, such case reports failed to provide sufficient details concerning the type or quality of ginseng used, or whether the preparation actually contained ginseng or ginsenoside[51,52]. Massive overdose can bring about ginseng abuse syndrome, which is characterized by hypertension, insomnia, hypertonia, and edema[46].

The recommended daily ginseng dosage is 1–2 g of the crude root, or 200–600 mg of standardized extracts[52]. As the possibility of hormone-like or hormone-inducing effects cannot be ruled out, some authors suggest limiting treatment to 3 months[53].

Momordica charantia

Momordica charantia (bitter melon), also known as balsam pear or karela, has been referred to as both a vegetable and a fruit and is widely cultivated in Asia, Africa, and South America (Figure 19.1). It has been used extensively in folk medicines as a remedy for diabetes. The blood-sugar-lowering action of the fresh juice or unripe fruit has been established in animal experimental models as well as human clinical trials[54,55].

Bitter melon contains several compounds with confirmed antidiabetic properties. Alcohol-extracted charantin from *Momordica charantia* consists of mixed steroids and is more potent than the oral hypoglycemic agent tolbutamide[56]. Bitter melon also contains an insulin-like polypeptide, polypeptide-P, which decreases

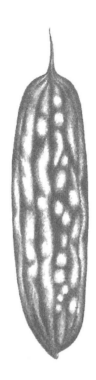

Figure 19.1 *Momordica charantia*, the bitter melon

blood sugar levels when injected subcutaneously into type 1 diabetics, and it appears to have fewer side-effects than insulin. The oral administration of bitter melon preparations has also shown satisfactory results in clinical trials in type 2 diabetic patients. Welihinda *et al.*[54] showed that glucose tolerance was improved in 73% of type 2 diabetics given 57 g of the juice. In another study, 15 g of the aqueous extract of bitter melon produced a 54% decrease in postprandial blood sugar levels and a 17% reduction in glycosylated hemoglobin in six patients[55]. The mechanism of bitter melon's activity in lowering blood glucose is unknown, but in diabetic rabbit models it has been proposed to possess a direct action similar to that of insulin[57]. Karela was also found to be effective in lowering blood glucose in alloxan-treated rabbits[58]. Bailey and Day[18] reported that karela appeared to inhibit the effect of gluconeogenesis.

The recommended bitter melon dosage is 5 ml of tincture two to three times a day, with a total as high as 50 ml/day[59]. However, bitter melon juice is very difficult to make palatable, since it is quite bitter. To avoid the bitter taste, the Indians and Chinese crush karela and form tablets. In Central America, it is prepared as an extract or decoction. Hepatic portal inflammation and testicular lesions in dogs have been reported with excessive administration of cerasee (a component of the wild variety of bitter melon)[60].

Trigonella foenumgraecum

Trigonella foenumgraecum (fenugreek) has been used as a folk remedy for diabetes[61]. The active principle is in the defatted portion of the seed and contains the alkaloid trigonelline, nicotinic acid, and coumarin. Administration of the defatted seed (1.5–2.0 g/kg daily) to both normal and diabetic dogs reduced fasting and postprandial blood levels of glucose, glucagon, somatostatin, insulin, total cholesterol, and triglycerides, and increased high-density lipoprotein (HDL)-cholesterol levels[62]. Human studies have confirmed these effects[56]. Of the seeds, 50–60% is fiber, and this may constitute another potential mechanism of fenugreek's beneficial effect in diabetic patients[63].

In type 2 diabetics, the ingestion of 15 g of powdered fenugreek seed soaked in water significantly reduced postprandial glucose levels during a glucose tolerance test[65]. The dosage of fenugreek is 625 mg in capsule form two to three times a day[59].

Gymnema sylvestre

Gymnema sylvestre (gurmar), a plant native to the tropical forests of India, has long been used as a treatment for diabetes. *Gymnema sylvestre* appeared on the US market several years ago, and it was promoted as a 'sugar blocker'[56]. In a study of type 2 diabetes, 22 patients were given *Gymnema sylvestre* extract along with their oral hypoglycemic drugs. All patients demonstrated improved blood sugar control; 21 out of the 22 were able to reduce their oral hypoglycemic drug dosage considerably, and five patients were able to discontinue their oral medication and maintain blood sugar control with the gurmar extract alone[59]. It was postulated that *Gymnema sylvestre* enhances the production of endogenous insulin[64].

The dosage of *Gymnema sylvestre* extract is 400 mg/day. One of its side-effects is that it reduces or abolishes the taste sensation of sweetness and bitterness[59].

Allium cepa and Allium sativum

Allium cepa (onions) and *Allium sativum* (garlic) have demonstrated a blood-sugar-lowering action in several studies[65,66]. Volatile oils in raw onion and garlic cloves have been shown to lower fasting glucose concentration in diabetic animals and in human subjects[67]. The active components are believed to be sulfur-containing compounds, allyl propyl disulfide (APDS) and diallyl disulfide (allicin), although other constituents such as flavonoids may play a role as well. Experimental and clinical evidence has suggested that the active components lower glucose levels by competing with insulin for insulin-inactivating sites in the liver[56]. This results in an increase of free insulin.

There is a marked fall in blood glucose levels and an increase in serum insulin level when a dose of 125 mg/kg of APDS is administered to humans. Allicin at doses of 100 mg/kg produces a similar effect[56]. Onion extracts also reduce blood sugar levels in a dose-dependent manner[65]. The dosage of *Allium cepa* is one standardized capsule of 400 mg/day. Excessive amounts can cause liver toxicity[68]. The general daily dosage of garlic is 4 g of fresh garlic or 8 mg of essential oil[69].

Pterocarpus marsupium and other epicatechin-containing plants

Pterocarpus marsupium has a long history of use in India as a treatment for diabetes. The flavanoid, (-)-epicatechin, extracted from the bark of this plant, has been shown to prevent β-cell damage in rats[58]. In addition, both epicatechin and a crude alcohol extract of *Pterocarpus marsupium* have been shown to regenerate functional pancreatic β-cells in diabetic animals[70,71].

Epicatechin and catechin consist of glycosides and esters. They are flavan-3-ols, a group of flavanols which have antidiabetic properties[72]. Also, *Camellia sinensis* (green tea polyphenols) and *Acacia catechu* (Burma cutch) are a good source of flavan-3-ols. Since *Pterocarpus* is not very common in the USA, green tea may be the suitable alternative for *Pterocarpus*. The recommended dose of green tea is two 120-ml cups daily or roughly 240 mg of green tea daily. Side-effects of green tea have not been reported.

Vaccinium myrtillus

Vaccinium myrtillus (bilberry or European blueberry) is a shrubby plant that grows in Europe. Leaves of *Vaccinium myrtillus* were widely used as a treatment for diabetes before the availability of insulin[18]. Oral administration of bilberry leaf tea reduced blood sugar level in normal and diabetic dogs, even when glucose was concurrently injected intravenously[73]. Bilberry also has a beneficial effect in microvascular abnormalities of diabetes[74,75]. The anthocyanoside myrtillin is the most active constituent of bilberry.

The standard dose of bilberry extract is based on its anthocyanoside content and is 80–160 mg three times daily[56]. Animal data suggest that *Vaccinium myrtillus* administration may be associated with renal and hepatic carcinogenicity[18,76,77].

Atriplex halimu

Atriplex halimu (salt bush) is a branchy woody shrub native to the Mediterranean, North Africa, and Southern Europe. Salt bush is rich in fiber, protein, and numerous trace minerals including chromium. Human studies with salt bush conducted in Israel demonstrated improved blood glucose regulation and glucose tolerance in type 2 diabetic patients[56]. The dose used in the trial was 3 g/day.

Soybeans

Soybeans are legumes that contain a large dietary source of isoflavones. Soybeans are known to be high in soluble fiber and delay glucose absorption. This mechanism of action is similar to acarbose[78]. Studies showed soy intake may slow the deterioration of renal function and lead to a decrease in proteinuria, in diabetic patients[79]. Soybeans also improved blood lipid levels in both diabetic and non-diabetic subjects. In a randomized double-blind study, 20 type 2 diabetic subjects participated in a cross trial with soy proteins versus placebo. The results showed significant decrease in low-density lipoprotein, triglycerides, and homocysteine, but no change in high-density lipoprotein, glucose, or hemoglobin A1C[80]. Well-designed randomized controlled trials with larger sample sizes are warranted.

Nutritional supplements

The treatment of diabetes requires nutritional supplementation, as these patients have a greatly increased need for many nutrients. Supplying the diabetic with additional key nutrients has been shown to improve blood sugar control as well as helping to prevent or ameliorate many major complications of diabetes.

Chromium

Chromium is an essential micronutrient for humans. Considerable experimental and epidemiologic evidence now indicates that chromium levels are the major determinant of insulin sensitivity, and that chromium functions as a co-factor in all insulin-regulating activities[81]. Chromium works closely with insulin in facilitating the uptake of glucose into cells. Supplemental chromium has been shown to decrease fasting glucose levels, improve glucose tolerance, lower insulin levels, and decrease total cholesterol and triglyceride levels while increasing HDL-cholesterol levels in normal, elderly, and type 2 diabetic patients[82,83]. Without chromium, insulin's action is blocked, and glucose levels are elevated[82].

Chromium picolinate, a trivalent chromium (Cr^{3+}), is the only form of chromium that exhibits biologic activity[84], and is an integral component of the so-called 'glucose tolerance factor' (GTF) when combined with two molecules of nicotinic acid. Chromium deficiency may be an underlying contributing factor in a large number of Americans suffering from diabetes, hypoglycemia, and obesity, and marginal chromium deficiency is common in the USA[52].

A large clinical study in 180 diabetics clearly documented the benefit of chromium for type 2 diabetics. In the study, while patients continued their normal medication, they were placed in one of three groups: placebo group, group receiving 100 µg chromium picolinate twice a day, and group receiving 500 µg chromium picolinate twice a day. There were significant dose- and time-dependent decreases in glycosylated hemoglobin, fasting glucose, 2-h postprandial glucose levels, fasting and 2-h postprandial insulin values, and total cholesterol[85]. Supplementing the diet with chromium also lowers body weight while increasing lean body mass, and these chromium effects appear to be due to an increased insulin sensitivity. However, not all studies on chromium have yielded positive results. In a controlled 6-month study to determine the effect of chromium picolinate on individuals with type 2 diabetes, Lee and Reasner[86] reported an improvement in triglyceride level but no statistical difference between control and chromium-treated subjects with respect to measured parameters of glucose control. Joseph *et al.*[87] also found no added benefit of chromium supplementation when it was provided in addition to resistance training.

Although no recommended daily allowance (RDA) has been established for chromium, over 200 µg/day appears to be necessary for optimal blood sugar regulation[51]. A good supply of chromium is assured by adequate daily intake of about 50–200 µg[88], and the best dietary sources are brewer's yeast[61] and barley flour[89]. Interestingly, some aromatic plants, which are utilized by diabetics as medicinal plants, contain a high level of chromium[89]. Refined sugars, white-flour products, and lack of exercise can deplete chromium levels. In addition

to the regular consumption of chromium-rich foods, diabetics and hypoglycemics should supplement their diet with chromium polynicotinate, chromium picolinate, and chromium-enriched yeast[89]. Recently, Cefalu and Hu reviewed previous human clinical trials, and their data indicated that chromium picolinate supplementation can improve both glucose and insulin metabolism in patients with diabetes[90].

Trivalent chromium has long been considered to be a safe nutritional supplement[91]. Although the hexavalent form of chromium is a known human respiratory tract carcinogen in high-exposure industrial use, there is no evidence of any carcinogenesis in humans from the trivalent form of chromium found in chromium picolinate[92,93]. However, concerns about possible chromosomal damage from long-term, high-dose chromium picolinate have been raised[94,95]. Further evaluation of the safety and efficacy of trivalent chromium in diabetes treatment is warranted.

Magnesium

Magnesium is involved in several areas of glucose metabolism and there is considerable evidence that diabetics need supplemental magnesium. It has been reported that magnesium deficiency is common in diabetics and magnesium may prevent some of the complications of diabetes, such as retinopathy and heart disease[96]. Because most Americans consume a diet high in refined foods, meat, and dairy products, low magnesium levels are common. The best dietary sources of magnesium are tofu, legumes, seeds, nuts, whole grains, and green leafy vegetables. In addition to a diet high in magnesium, supplementation with 300–500 mg of magnesium as aspartate or citrate is recommended for non-diabetic adults, and diabetics may need twice this amount. Diabetics should also take at least 50 mg/day of vitamin B_6, as intracellular vitamin B_6 appears to be intricately linked to the magnesium of the cell[56].

Zinc

Zinc is involved in synthesis, secretion, and utilization of insulin. Zinc also has a protective effect against β-cell destruction and has an antiviral effect[58]. Diabetics typically excrete excessive amounts of zinc in the urine and thus require supplementation[97]. It has been shown that zinc can improve insulin levels in both type 1 and type 2 diabetes[98]. In addition, zinc helps to improve wound healing in diabetics[99]. Zinc is found in good amounts in whole grains, legumes, nuts, and seeds. The recommended level of zinc supplementation for diabetics should be over 30 mg/day[56].

Besides chromium, magnesium, and zinc, there are a number of other minerals such as calcium, potassium, and vanadium that appear to improve insulin sensitivity. Some amino acids, such as L-carnitine, taurine, and L-arginine may also play a role in the reversal of insulin resistance. Vitamins E, C, B$_6$, and biotin are also effective in diabetic patients. Other nutrients, such as glutathione, fish oils (omega-3 essential fatty acids), co-enzyme Q$_{10}$ and lipoic acid may also have therapeutic potential for diabetics[100]. Nutrients used in type 2 diabetes are summarized in Table 19.2.

Fiber

Supplementation with plant fibers (e.g. guar gum at a dosage of 5 g/meal and pectin 10 g/meal) has demonstrated a positive impact on diabetes control[56]. Guar gum or cluster bean is the powder extracted by milling *Cyamopsis tetragonoloba*[71]. It has been reported to decrease fasting blood glucose and postprandial glucose, and to improve insulin sensitivity[101–103]. Many experts in diabetes are now using these fiber supplements, along with the standard American Diabetic Association diet[104]. When diabetic patients ate between 14 and 26 g/day of guar, they required less insulin and had less glycosuria[105,106]. However, fiber-supplemented diets are not as effective as the high-carbohydrate, high-plant-fiber diet and they are reserved for the type 2 diabetics who are unwilling to implement the more difficult dietary change[56].

Interactions between supplements and conventional medications

There are potential interactions between some dietary supplements and conventional antidiabetic medications. For example, there are possible interactions between oral hypoglycemics and *Momordica charantia* and ginseng, and between insulin and chromium and ginseng[107]. Thus, patients using oral hypoglycemic medications or insulin should consult their physicians before using dietary supplements.

Acupuncture

Acupuncture is best known in the USA as an alternative therapy for chronic pain. However, considerable progress has been made in the treatment of diabetes by acupuncture since 1970[108]. There are numerous publications in

Table 19.2 Supplemental nutrients used in type 2 diabetes

Nutrient	Effect
Chromium picolinate	improves glucose tolerance
Magnesium	improves glucose metabolism
Zinc	improves glucose metabolism
Calcium	improves insulin sensitivity
Potassium	may improve insulin sensitivity
Vanadyl sulfate	improves insulin sensitivity
L-Carnitine	improves insulin sensitivity after intravenous infusion
Taurine	may improve insulin sensitivity
L-Arginine	improves insulin sensitivity after intravenous infusion
Vitamin E	reduces glycosylation and antioxidant activity
Vitamin C	reduces glycosylation and antioxidant activity
Vitamin B$_6$	improves glucose metabolism and nerve function
Biotin	improves glucose metabolism and nerve function
Glutathione	improves insulin sensitivity after intravenous infusion
Omega-3 essential fatty acids	improves insulin sensitivity
Coenzyme Q$_{10}$	improves insulin sensitivity
Lipoic acid	improves insulin sensitivity
Inositol	improves glucose metabolism

Chinese on the use of acupuncture for diabetes, but only those published in English are cited here. It is believed that acupuncture is effective not only in treating diabetes, but also in preventing and managing complications of the disease[108].

The effects of acupuncture on diabetes have been observed experimentally and clinically[109]. Animal experiments have shown that acupuncture can activate glucose-6-phosphatase, an important enzyme in carbohydrate metabolism, and affect the hypothalamus to a certain extent[110]. Acupuncture can act on the pancreas to enhance insulin synthesis, increase the number of receptors on target cells, accelerate the utilization of glucose, and, thus, help to lower the blood sugar[109]. Data from another study showed the beneficial anti-obesity effect of acupuncture[111], which is the most modifiable risk factor for type 2 diabetes. It appears that the therapeutic effect of acupuncture on diabetes was not the result of its action on a single organ, but on multiple systems.

The four commonly used points are:

(1) *Zusanli* point, located 3 in (8 cm) below the lateral knee depression, one finger width from the lateral side of the anterior crest of the tibia;

(2) *Sanyinjiao* point, located 3 in above the tip of the inner ankle, on the posterior margin of the metatarsal bone;

(3) *Feishu* point, located 1.5 in (4 cm) lateral and inferior to the spinous process of the third thoracic vertebra in a prone position;

(4) *Shenshu* point, located 1.5 in lateral to the posterior midline, lateral and inferior to the spinous process of the second lumbar vertebra in a prone position.

The selection of acupuncture points was based on Traditional Chinese Medicine theory. During the treatment, other points can be added according to symptoms and signs[108]. Other methods have also been employed such as point injection with normal saline, a small dose of insulin or Chinese herbal medicine extracts. Treatment is generally given once a day or once every other day as a course of 14–21 treatments. It is believed that the longer the course of treatment, the more marked the effect. Effects of acupuncture usually appear after 25 treatments and the therapy generally lasts 2–5 months[108].

Acupuncture is more effective when the course is mild or moderate, and less effective in severe cases with a prolonged course. It is often very effective in treating diabetic complications, usually with marked improvement in clinical symptoms. However, in patients with ketoacidosis, the therapeutic results are poor[108]. Patients with a strong needling sensation often show a better therapeutic effect than those with a weak needling sensation. Usually obese patients have better therapeutic results. Results of treatment are often unsatisfactory in depressed or emotionally unstable individuals. Better therapeutic results are obtained in patients with dietary control than in those without it. Proper physical exercises, breathing exercises, and massage can help improve the therapeutic effect.

Although acupuncture shows some effectiveness in treating diabetes, its mechanisms of action are still obscure. Integration of scientific advances and research methods would further develop acupuncture treatment for diabetes.

Hot-tub therapy

Since hot-tub therapy can increase blood flow to skeletal muscles, it has been recommended for patients with type 2 diabetes who are unable to exercise[112]. A study reported that eight patients were asked to sit in a hot tub for 30 min daily for 3 weeks. During the study period, the patients' weight, mean plasma glucose level, and mean glycosylated hemoglobin decreased[113]. Proper water sanitation and appropriate guidance should be considered when prescribing hot-tub therapy for diabetic patients.

CONCLUSIONS

Type 2 diabetes is a chronic metabolic disease that has a significant impact on the health, quality of life, and life expectancy of patients, as well as on the health-care system. Exercise, diet, and weight control continue to be essential and effective means of improving glucose homeostasis. However, these lifestyle management measures may be insufficient, and conventional drug therapies (oral-glucose-lowering agents and insulin injection) are indicated in most of the patients. In addition to adverse effects, drug treatments are not always satisfactory in maintaining euglycemia and avoiding late-stage diabetic complications. Alternative therapies have often been used in chronic conditions that may be only partially alleviated by conventional treatment. Herbal medication is the most commonly used alternative therapy, but its safety and hypoglycemic effects need to be further evaluated via carefully planned animal research, and well-designed controlled clinical studies. Lastly, potential adverse herb–drug interactions should be kept in mind for patients also receiving conventional antidiabetic medications.

References

1. National Institutes of Diabetes and Digestive and Kidney Diseases. Diabetes Statistics. NIH publication no. 96-3926. Bethesda, MD: NIDDK, 1995

2. American Diabetes Association. Diabetes 1996 Vital Statistics. Alexandria, VA: American Diabetes Association, 1996

3. Rubin RJ, Altman WM, Mendelson DN. Health care expenditures for people with diabetes mellitus, 1992. J Clin Endocrinol Metab 1994; 78: 809A–F

4. DeFronzo RA. The triumvirate: B-cell, muscle, liver. A collusion responsible for NIDDM. Diabetes 1988; 37: 667–87

5. Seely BL, Olefsky JM. Potential cellular and genetic mechanisms for insulin resistance in common disorders of obesity and diabetes. In Moller D, ed. Insulin Resistance and its Clinical Disorders. London: John Wiley & Sons, 1993: 187–252

6. Olefsky JM. Insulin resistance and pathogenesis of non insulin dependent diabetes mellitus: cellular and molecular mechanisms. In Efendic S, Ostenson CG, Vranic M, eds. New Concepts in the Pathogenesis of NIDDM. NewYork, NY: Plenum Publishing, 1999

7. Clark CM Jr. The burden of chronic hyperglycemia. Diabetes Care 1998; 21(Suppl 3): C32–4

8. Davidson MB. Diabetes Mellitus: Diagnosis and Treatment, 3rd edn. New York, NY: Churchill Livingstone, 1991

9. DeFronzo RA. Pharmacologic therapy for type 2 diabetes mellitus. Ann Intern Med 1999; 131: 281–303

10. Parving HH, Gall MA, Skott MA, et al. Prevalence and causes of albuminuria in non-insulin dependent diabetic patients. Kidney Int 1992; 41: 758–62

11. Kelley DE. Effects of weight loss on glucose homeostasis in NIDDM. Diabetes Rev 1995; 3: 366–77

12. United Kingdom Prospective Diabetes Study 24 (UKPDS 24). A 6-year, randomized, controlled trial comparing sulfonylurea, insulin, and metformin therapy in patients with newly diagnosed type 2 diabetes that could not be controlled with diet therapy. United Kingdom Prospective Diabetes Study Group. Ann Intern Med 1998; 128: 165–75

13. United Kingdom Prospective Diabetes Study 33 (UKPDS 33). Intensive blood-glucose control with sulphonylureas or insulin compared with conventional treatment and risk of complications in patients with type 2 diabetes. United Kingdom Prospective Diabetes Study Group. Lancet 1998; 352: 837–53

14. United Kingdom Prospective Diabetes Study 34 (UKPDS 34). Effect of intensive blood-glucose control with metformin on complications in overweight patients with type 2 diabetes. UK Prospective Diabetes Study Group. Lancet 1998; 352: 854–65

15. Sinha A, Formica C, Tsalamandris C, et al. Effect of insulin on body composition in patients with insulin-dependent and non-insulin-dependent diabetes. Diabetes Med 1996; 13: 40–6

16. American Diabetes Association. Medical Management of Non-insulin-dependent (Type ll) Diabetes, 3rd edn. Alexandria, VA: American Diabetes Association, 1994: 22–39

17. American Diabetes Association. Clinical practice recommendations 1995. Position statement: diabetes mellitus and exercise. Diabetes Care 1995; 18 (Suppl 1): 28

18. Bailey CJ, Day C. Traditional plant medicines as treatments for diabetes. Diabetes Care 1989; 12: 553–65

19. British Herbal Medicine Association. British Herbal Pharmacopoeia. Keighley, UK: British Herbal Medicine Association, 1971

20. Hermann M. Herbs and Medicinal Flowers. New York, NY: Galahad, 1973

21. Petricic J, Kalogjera Z. Bestimmung des Galegins und die Antidiabetische Wirkung der Droge Herba Galegae. Planta Med 1982; 45: 140

22. Sterne J. Pharmacology and mode of action of the hypoglycemic agents. In Campbell GD, ed. Oral Hypoglycemic Agents: Pharmacology and Therapeutics. New York, NY: Academic, 1969: 193–245

23. Bailey CJ. Metformin revisited: its action and indications for use. Diabetic Med 1988; 5: 315–20

24. Lee FC. Facts about Ginseng, the Elixir of Life. Elizabeth, NJ: Hollyn International, 1992

25. Huang KC. The Pharmacology of Chinese Herbs. Boca Raton, FL: CRC Press, 1999

26. Attele AS, Wu JA, Yuan CS. Ginseng pharmacology, multiple constituents and multiple actions. Biochem Pharm 1999; 58: 1685–93

27. Reis CA, Sahud MA. Agranulocytosis caused by Chinese herbal medicine: dangers of medications containing aminopyrine and phenylbutazone. J Am Med Assoc 1975; 231: 352

28. Yuan CS, Wu JA, Lowell T, Gu M. Gut and brain effects of American ginseng root on brainstem neuronal activities in rats. Am J Chin Med 1998; 26: 47–55

29. Liu CX, Xiao PG. Recent advances on ginseng research in China. J Ethnopharmacol 1992; 36: 27–38

30. Ohnishi Y, Takagi S, Miura T, et al. Effect of ginseng radix on GLUT2 protein content in mouse liver in normal and epinephrine-induced hyperglycemic mice. Biol Pharm Bull 1996; 19: 1238–40

31. Oshima Y, Sato K, Hikino H. Isolation and hypoglycemic activity of quinquefolans A, B, and C, glycans of Panax quinquefolium roots. J Nat Prod 1987; 50: 188–90

32. Martinez B, Staa EJ. The physiological effects of Aralia, Panax and Eleutherococcus on exercised rats. Jpn J Pharmacol 1984; 35: 79–85

33. Tomoda M, Shimada K, Konno C, et al. Partial structure of Panaxan A: a hypoglycemic glycan of Panax ginseng roots. Planta Med 1984; 50: 436–8

34. Konno C, Sugiyama K, Kano M, et al. Isolation and hypoglycemic activity of panaxans A, B, C, D, and E: glycans of Panax ginseng roots. Planta Med 1984; 50: 434–6

35. Konno C, Murakani M, Oshima Y, Hikino H. Isolation and hypoglycemic activity of panaxans Q, R, S, R, and U: glycans of Panax ginseng roots. J Ethnopharmacol 1985; 14: 69–74

36. Yokozawa T, Kobayashi T, Oura H, Kawashima Y. Studies on the mechanism of the hypoglycemic activity of ginsenoside-Rb2 in streptozotocin-diabetic rats. Chem Pharm Bull 1985; 33: 869–72

37. Oshima Y, Konno C, Hikino H. Isolation and hypoglycemic activity of panaxans I, J, K and L, glycans of Panax ginseng roots. J Ethnopharmacol 1985; 14: 255–9

38. Sotaniemi EA, Happakoski E, Rautio A. Ginseng therapy in non-insulin dependent diabetic patients. Diabetes Care 1995; 18: 1373–5

39. Vuksan V, Sievenpiper JL, Koo VY, et al. American ginseng (Panax quinquefolius L) reduces postprandial glycemia in non-diabetic subjects and subjects with type 2 diabetes mellitus. Arch Intern Med 2000; 60: 1009–13

40. Suzuki Y, Ito Y, Konno C, Furuya T. Effects of tissue culture of ginseng on gastric secretion and pepsin activity [in Japanese]. Yakugaku Zasshi 1991; 111: 770–4

41. Hasegawa H, Matsumiya S, Murakami C, et al. Interaction of ginseng extract, ginseng seperated fractions, and some triterpenoid saponins with glucose transporters in sheep erythrocytes. Planta Med 1994; 60: 153–7

42. Gills CN. Panax ginseng pharmacology: a nitric oxide link? Biochem Pharmacol 1997; 54: 1–8

43. Roy D, Perrault M, Marette A. Insulin stimulation of glucose uptake in skeletal muscle and adipose tissue in vivo is NO dependent. Am J Physiol 1998; 274: E692–9

44. Kimura M, Waki I, Chujo T, et al. Effects of hypoglycemic components in ginseng radix on blood insulin level in alloxan diabetic mice and on insulin release from perfused rat pancreas. J Pharmacobiodyn 1981; 4: 410–17

45. Spinas GA, Laffranchi R, Francoys I, et al. The early phase of glucose-stimulated insulin secretion requires nitric oxide. Diabetologia 1998; 41: 292–9

46. Punnonen R, Lukola A. Oestrogen-like effect of ginseng. Br Med J 1980; 281: 1110

47. Palmer BV, Montgomery ACV, Monteiro JCMP. Ginseng and mastalgia. Br Med J 1978; 1: 1284

48. Hammond TG, Whitworth JA. Adverse reactions to ginseng. Med J Aust 1981; 1: 492

49. Janetzky K, Morreale AP. Probable interaction between warfarin and ginseng. Am J Health Syst Pharm 1997; 54: 692–3

50. Jones BD, Runkis AM. Interaction of ginseng with phenelzine. J Clin Psychopharmacol 1987; 7: 201–2

51. Cui J, Garle M, Eneroth P, Bjorkhem I. What do commercial ginseng preparations contain? Lancet 1994; 344: 134

52. Awang DVC. Maternal use of ginseng and neonatal androgenization. J Am Med Assoc 1991; 266: 363

53. Schulz V, Hansel R, Tyler VE, eds. Rational phytotherapy. In Agents that Increase Resistance to Diseases. New York, NY: Springer-Verlag, 1998: 269–72

54. Welihinda J, Karunanaya EH, Sherrif MHR, Jayasinghe KSA. Effect of Momordica charantia on the glucose tolerance in maturity onset diabetes. J Ethnopharmacol 1986; 17: 277–82

55. Srivastava Y, Venkatakrishna-Bhatt H, Verma Y, et al. Antidiabetic and adaptogenic properties of Momordica charantia extract. An experimental and clinical evaluation. Phytother Res 1993; 7: 285–9

56. Murray MT, Pizzorno JE Jr. Diabetes mellitus. In Pizzorno JE Jr, Murray MT, eds. Textbook of Natural Medicine, 2nd edn. Edinburgh: Churchill Livingstone, 1999: 1193–218

57. Akhtar MS, Athar MA, Yaqub M. Effect of Momordica charantia on blood glucose level of normal and alloxan diabetic rabbits. Planta Med 1981; 42: 205–12

58. Larner J, Haynes C. Insulin and hypoglycemia drugs, glycogen. In Gilman GG, Goodman LS, Rall TW, Murad F, eds. The Pharmacological Basis of Therapeutics, 5th edn. New York, NY: Macmillan Publishing, 1975: 1507–28

59. Mozersky RP. Herbal products and supplemental nutrients used in the management of diabetes. J Am Osteopath Assoc 1999; 99: S4–9

60. Dixit VP, Khanna P, Bhargava SK. Effects of Momordica charantia L fruit extract on the testicular function of dog. Planta Med 1978; 34: 280–6

61. Miller LG. Herbal medications, nutraceuticals, and diabetes. In Miller LG, Murray WJ, eds. Herbal Medicinals, A Clinician's Guide. Binghamton, NY: Pharmaceutical Products Press, Imprint of the Haworth Press, 1998: 115–33

62. Ribes G, Sauvaire Y, Baccou JC, et al. Effects of fenugreek seeds on endocrine pancreatic secretions in dogs. Ann Nutr Metab 1984; 28: 37–43

63. Madar Z, Abel R, Samish S, Arad J. Glucose-lowering effect of fenugreek in non-insulin dependent diabetes. Eur J Clin Nutr 1988; 42: 51–4

64. Shanmugasundaram ERB, Rajeswara G, Baskaran K, et al. Use of Gymnema sylvestre leaf extract in the control of blood glucose in insulin-dependent diabetes mellitus. J Ethnopharmacol 1990; 30: 281–94

65. Sharma KK, Gupta S, Samuel KC. Antihyperglycemic effect of onion: effect on fasting blood sugar and induced hyperglycemia in man. Ind J Med Res 1977; 65: 422–9

66. Sheela CG, Augusti KT. Antidiabetic effects of S-allyl cysteine sulphoxide isolated from garlic (Allium sativum, Linn.). Ind J Exp Biol 1992; 30: 523–6

67. Jain RC, Vyas CR, Mahatama OP. Hypoglycemic action of onion and garlic [letter]. Lancet 1973; 2: 1491

68. Augusti KT, Benaim ME. Effect of essential oil of onion (allyl propyl disulphide) on blood glucose, free fatty acid and insulin levels of normal subjects. Clin Chim Acta 1975; 60: 121–3

69. Herbal monographics. In Gruenwald J, Brendler T, Jaenicke C, eds. PDR for Herbal Medicines, 2nd edn. Montvale, NJ: Medical Economics Company, 2000: 376–8

70. Chakravarthy BK, Gupa S, Gambhir SS, Gode KD. Pancreatic beta-cell regeneration in rats by (-)-epicatechin. Lancet 1981; 2: 759–60

71. Chakravarthy BK, Gupa S, Gode KD. Functional beta cell regeneration in the islets of pancreas in alloxan induced diabetic rats by (-)-epicatechin. Life Sci 1982; 31: 2693–7

72. Subramanian SS. (-)Epicatechin as an antidiabetic drug. Ind Drugs 1981; 18: 259

73. Allen FM. Blueberry leaf extract. Physiological and clinical properties in relation in carbohydrate metabolism. J Am Med Assoc 1927; 89: 1577–81

74. Scharrer A, Ober M. Anthocyanosides in the treatment of retinopathies. Klin Monatsbl Augenheikd 1981; 178: 386–9

75. Caselli L. Clinical and electroretinographic study on activity of anthocyanosides. Arch Med Int 1985; 37: 29–35

76. Devillers J, Boule P, Vasseur P, et al. Enviromental and health risks of hydroquinone. Ecotoxicol Environ Safety 1990; 19: 327–54

77. Shibata MA, Hirose M, Tanaka H, et al. Induction of renal cell tumors in rats and mice, and enhancement of hepatocellular tumor development in mice after long-term hydroquinone treatment. Jpn J Cancer Res 1991; 82: 1211–19

78. Anderson JW, Blake JE, Turner J, Smith BM. Effects of soy protein on renal function and proteinuria in patients with type 2 diabetes. Am J Clin Nutr 1998; 68: 1347S–53S

79. Anderson JW Smith BM, Washnock CS. Cardiovascular and renal benefits of dry bean and soybean intake. Am J Clin Nutr 1999; 70: 464S–74S

80. Hermansen K, Sondergaard M, Hoie L, et al. Beneficial effects of a soy-based dietary supplement on lipid levels and cardio-

vascular risk markers in type 2 diabetic subjects. Diabetes Care 2001; 24: 228–33

81. Offenbacher E, Stunyer F. Beneficial effect of chromium-riched yeast on glucose tolerance and blood lipids in elderly patients. Diabetes 1980; 29: 919–25

82. Mooradian AD, Failla M, Hoogwerf B. Selected vitamin and mineral in diabetes. Diabetes Care 1994; 17: 464–79

83. Baker B. Chromium supplements tied to glucose control. Fam Practice News 1996; 15: 5

84. Mertz M. Chromium occurrence and function in biologic systems. Physiol Rev 1969; 49: 163–237

85. Anderson R, Cheng N, Chi J, Feng J. Beneficial effect of chromium for people with type 2 diabetes. Diabetes 1996; 45: 124A/454

86. Lee NA, Reasner CA. Beneficial effect of chromium supplementation on serum triglyceride levels in NIDDM. Diabetes Care 1994; 17: 1449–52

87. Joseph LJ, Farrell PA, Davey SL, et al. Effect of resistance training with or without chromium picolinate supplementation on glucose metabolism in older men and women. Metabolism 1999; 48: 546–53

88. Anderson RA, Bryden NA, Polansky M. Dietary chromium intake. Freely chosen diets, institutional diet, and individual foods. Biol Trace Element Res 1992; 32: 117

89. Castro VR. Chromium in a series of Portuguese plants used in the herbal treatment of diabetes. Biol Trace Element Res 1998; 62: 101–6

90. Cefalu WT, Hu FB. Role of chromium in human health and in diabetes. Diabetes Care 2004; 27: 2741–51

91. Nielsen FH. Chromium. In Shils ME, Olson JA, Shike M, eds. Modern Nutrition in Health and Disease, 8th edn. Philadelphia, PA: Lea & Febiger, 1994: 264–8

92. Reading SA, Wecker L. Chromium picolinate. J Fla Med Assoc 1996; 83: 29–31

93. Stearns DM, Wetterhahn KE. Chromium (iii) picolinate [letter, author's reply]. FASEB J 1996; 10: 367–9

94. Stearns DM, Belbruno JJ, Wetterhahn KE. A prediction of chromium (iii) accumulation in humans from chromium dietary supplements. FASEB J 1995; 9: 1650–7

95. Stearns DM, Wise JP Sr, Patierno SR, Wetterhahn KE. Chromium (iii) picolinate produces chromosome damage in Chinese hamster ovary cells. FASEB J 1995; 9: 1643–8

96. White JR, Campbell RK. Magnesium and diabetes. A review. Ann Pharmacother 1993; 27: 775–80

97. Mooradian AD, Morley JE. Micronutrient status in diabetes mellitus. Am J Clin Nutr 1987; 45: 877–95

98. Hegazi SM. Effect of zinc supplementation on serum glucose, insulin, glucose-6-phosphatase, and mineral levels in diabetics. J Clin Biochem Nutr 1992; 12: 209–15

99. Engel ED, Erlich NE, Davis RH. Diabetes mellitus. Impaired wound healing from zinc deficiency. J Am Pediatr Assoc 1981; 71: 536–44

100. Kelly GS. Insulin resistance: lifestyle and nutritional interventions. Altern Med Rev 2000; 5: 109–32

101. Tagliaferro V, Cassader M, Bozzo C, et al. Moderate guar-gum addition to usual diet improves peripheral sensitivity to insulin and lipaemic profile in NIDDM. Diabetes Metab 1985; 11: 380–5

102. Landin K, Holm G, Tengborn L, Smith U. Guar gum improves insulin sensitivity, blood lipids, blood pressure, and fibrinolysis in healthy men. Am J Clin Nutr 1992; 56: 1061–5

103. Fairchild RM, Ellis PR, Byrne AJ, et al. A new breakfast cereal containing guar gum reduces postprandial plasma glucose and insulin concentrations in normal-weight human subjects. Br J Nutr 1996; 76: 63–73

104. Vahouny G, Kritchevsky D. Dietary Fiber in Health and Disease. New York, NY: Plenum Press, 1982

105. Jenkins DJA, Wolever TMS, Bacon S, et al. Diabetic diets: high carbohydrate combined with high fiber. Am J Clin Nutr 1980; 33: 1729–33

106. Jenkins DJA, Wolever TMS, Taylor RH, et al. Glycemic index of foods: a physiological basis for carbohydrate exchange. Am J Clin Nutr 1981; 24: 362–6

107. AACE Nutrition Guidelines Task Force. American association of clinical endocrinologists medical guidelines for the clinical use of dietary supplements and nutraceuticals. Endocr Pract 2003; 9: 417–70

108. Hui H. A review of treatment of diabetes by acupuncture during the past forty years. J Tradit Chin Med 1995; 15: 145–54

109. Chen JF, Wei J. Changes of plasma insulin level in diabetics treated with acupuncture. J Tradit Chin Med 1985; 5: 79–84

110. Wateri N. Reviews of presentation of the 7th World Congress of Acupuncture, 1982: 74

111. Lei ZP. Treatment of 42 cases of obesity with acupuncture. J Tradit Chin Med 1988; 8: 125–6

112. Hooper PL. Hot-tub therapy for type 2 diabetes mellitus. N Engl J Med 1999; 341: 924–5

113. Hooper PL. Hot-tub therapy for type 2 diabetes mellitus. N Engl J Med 2000; 342: 218–19

Osteoporosis

20

F. A. Yao, T. T. Brown and A. S. Dobs

INTRODUCTION

Osteoporosis is the most common metabolic bone disease in the United States, with recent prevalence estimates of approximately 10% of the national population[1]. About 17–20% of older non-Hispanic white women in the United States have osteoporosis[1]. Of the men older than 50 years of age, 5% have osteoporosis[2]. Osteoporosis accounts for about 1.5 million fractures annually, including 700 000 vertebral fractures, 250 000 distal forearm fractures, 300 000 hip fractures, and 300 000 fractures at other sites[3]. The lifetime risk for fractures of spine, hip, and distal radius is 40% for white women after the age of 50[3].

Osteoporosis is currently defined as 'a skeletal disorder characterized by compromised bone strength predisposing a person to an increased risk of fracture'[4]. The World Health Organization considers a bone density value of 2.5 standard deviations less than the young adult mean value, or a T-score of less than –2.5, to be diagnostic of osteoporosis[5]. Clinically, osteoporosis is recognized by characteristic low trauma fractures that typically arise at the hip, spine, and distal forearm, and there is increased relative risk of subsequent fractures associated with decreased bone mineral density (BMD) at both the hip and spine[1].

Those who are female, Caucasian, thin, of advanced age, postmenopausal, have amenorrhea, and use excessive alcohol are at risk for osteoporosis. Estrogen deficiency is strongly associated with recognized risk factors[6]. Men who have had prostate cancer treatment with androgen deprivation therapy may be at a higher risk of osteoporosis[2].

Because drugs that are used to treat osteoporosis have documented negative side-effects, a variety of synthetic and natural products are now being examined for potential use. This chapter describes existing evidence for common complementary and alternative medicine therapies that are hypothesized to be effective in the management of osteoporosis.

PATHOPHYSIOLOGY OF OSTEOPOROSIS

The continual remodeling of bone involves old bone being resorbed by osteoclasts and new bone being formed by osteoblasts. The balance between the two processes is dependent on a variety of factors including age, hormonal milieu, and calcium intake. Osteoporosis is characterized by an imbalance between bone resorption and bone formation, which results in a progressive decrease in bone mass[7].

Women begin losing bone around age 35 at a rate of 0.5% to 1% per year, but begin to lose bone at an accelerated rate of 3% to 5% per year in the decade after menopause. The gradual loss of BMD accounts for the increased risk of fracture that accompanies increased age[8].

CURRENT STANDARD THERAPIES FOR OSTEOPOROSIS

The National Osteoporosis Foundation (NOF) recommends that physicians initiate therapy to reduce the fracture risk in women who have BMD T-scores below –2.0 by hip dual X-ray absorptiometry (DXA) with no risk factors, BMD T-scores below –1.5 by hip DXA with one or more risk factors, or a prior vertebral or hip fracture. The pharmacologic options approved by the United States Food and Drug Administration for the prevention and treatment of postmenopausal osteoporosis include estrogen replacement therapy, bisphosphonates, calcitonin, parathyroid hormone, and selective estrogen receptor modulators. Calcium and vitamin D supplementation are also included in standard therapies for osteoporosis[9].

Estrogen

It is well established that estrogen supplied orally, transdermally, or intramuscularly in postmenopausal women is osteoprotective and diminishes the rate of bone loss that ensues after the loss of ovarian steroid production[10]. Estrogen has been demonstrated to reduce bone resorption, improve BMD at vertebral sites, and reduce fracture rates by about 50% in postmenopausal women[11,12]. The exact mechanism of how estrogen decreases bone loss is unclear[8]. Despite the potential health benefits of estrogens, they have the disadvantage of being tissue agonists for breast and endometrial tissue[11,12]. Potential side-effects of long-term estrogen replacement as a part of hormone replacement therapy include increased breast cancer, endometrial carcinoma, thromboembolism, and occlusive arterial disease, as demonstrated by recent randomized trials including the Women's Health Initiative[13,14].

Bisphosphonates

Bisphosphonates are analogs of pyrophosphate that bind to hydroxyapatite in bone and may reduce bone resorption by disabling or killing osteoclasts[13]. The best studied bisphosphonate, alendronate, appears to exert an anti-resorptive potency similar to that of estrogen when used at low doses such as 5 mg/day[15]. Well-designed trials have shown that alendronate is effective at preventing vertebral and non-vertebral fractures when compared to placebo. Bisphosphonates are generally well tolerated, although they have been reported to cause gastrointestinal side-effects[9].

Selective estrogen receptor modulators

Selective estrogen receptor modulators (SERMs) like raloxifene have been shown to decrease the risk of new vertebral fractures in postmenopausal women with osteoporosis. Raloxifene is a non-steroidal compound that can inhibit bone resorption without stimulating uterine or breast tissue. Studies have shown the ability of raloxifene to increase BMD in the femoral neck and spine[9] and to increase total hip BMD to a similar extent as observed with estrogen or bisphosphonate treatment[14]. Raloxifene has been associated with hot flashes and thromboembolism, and the effect of SERMs on heart disease is uncertain[16].

Calcitonin

Calcitonin is a peptide hormone that is documented to inhibit BMD loss in postmenopausal women with much less efficacy than alendronate or HRT regimens. Calcitonin inhibits bone resorption by decreasing osteoclast activity[17]. However, it is used to treat severe bone pain frequently associated with more severe osteoporosis. It may be best suited as an adjuvant therapy[9].

Parathyroid hormone

Unlike other therapies for treating osteoporosis, parathyroid hormone (PTH) has an anabolic effect on bone[14]. PTH can increase the proliferation of osteoblast progenitor cells, reduce the death rate of mature osteoblasts, and enhance the function of mature osteoblasts[12]. Men and women experience similar increases in BMD and reductions in fracture risk in response to PTH treatment[18]. Reports of minor side-effects to PTH include occasional nausea and headache[15].

Calcium and vitamin D

Calcium and vitamin D supplementation are incorporated into the treatment of osteoporosis. Calcium is a necessary nutrient for bone growth and provides mechanical rigidity to bone[19]. Insufficient calcium intake results in a net loss of calcium from bone, thus increasing susceptibility to fractures[7]. It is recommended to consume calcium with vitamin D, which has a major role in calcium absorption[17]. Vitamin D deficiency can influence the development of osteoporosis[2]. Vitamin D can be obtained by sunlight activation of 7-dehydrocholesterol in the skin and can be absorbed through dietary sources[7]. The NOF recommends that women over age 50 consume at least 1200 mg/day of elemental calcium and 800 IU/day of vitamin D[9].

CAM THERAPIES

Various complementary therapies have been advocated to treat osteoporosis. This section describes some of the exercise, dietary, and orthomolecular medicine therapies that have been investigated, as outlined in Table 20.1.

Exercise

Exercise may be effective in preventing and treating osteoporosis and its sequelae through multiple

Table 20.1   CAM therapies investigated for their role in maintaining bone health

Therapies and interventional study references	*Possible action on bone*
Exercise Tai-chi chuan[21], balance training[23], weight-bearing exercise[28], non-impact exercise[26]	promotes bone turnover[2,8], enhances bone strength[26]
Reducing animal protein in the diet	reduces acidemia and resulting bone resorption[31]
Herbal supplements Essential oils Safflower seeds Traditional Chinese Medicine[37] Black cohosh[39]	inhibit bone resorption[35] unknown
Phytoestrogens[11,54]	promote calcium absorption ↑ insulin growth factor-1[44] inhibit bone resorption[46]
Omega-3 fatty acids	increase calcium absorption from gut increases bone formation decrease bone resorption[67]
Vitamin K[74]	promotes bone mineralization via osteocalcin[72]
Reducing dietary vitamin A (animal derived)	minimizes vitamin A-mediated bone resorption and vitamin D antagonism[7,75]
Vitamin C	may increase bone formation[77]

mechanisms such as modifying the risk of falling due to muscle weakness, improving balance, lessening pain, improving quality of life, and preserving bone mass[20,21]. The extent to which exercise directly affects bone is controversial. During exercise, bone undergoes a certain amount of strain, which is hypothesized to result in a biochemical signal that initiates the formation of new bone and the removal of damaged bone[2,8]. Several types of exercise that have been evaluated for the treatment of osteoporosis include Tai chi chuan and other balance training programs, impact training, non-impact calisthenics, stretching, and weight-bearing exercise.

Tai chi chuan and other balance training programs

Tai chi chuan (TCC) is a low-impact, weight-bearing exercise that requires no jumping and involves well-coordinated sequences of movements in the trunk and four extremities, neuromuscular coordination, and low-velocity muscle contraction[22]. As a result, TCC has been recommended as a suitable exercise for patients with osteoporotic conditions. One explanation for the observed beneficial effects of TCC exercise on reducing

bone loss may be the association of the TCC intervention with an active lifestyle[21].

A recent randomized controlled trial involving 132 early postmenopausal women revealed beneficial effects of TCC exercise intervention on the deceleration of bone loss. Postmenopausal Chinese women with no hormone replacement therapy or drug treatment and no regular participation in physical exercise attended supervised *Yang* style TCC for 1 hour/day, 4.2 times/week over 12 months. There was a significant 2.6 to 3.6-fold slower rate of bone loss at the distal tibia in the TCC group as compared to the control group when volumetric bone mineral density (BMD) was measured by peripheral quantitative computerized tomography. One explanation for the inability to increase or maintain BMD in postmenopausal women after 12 months of TCC may be a diminished responsiveness of bone to weight-bearing or muscle contraction stimuli induced by increased age[21].

Balance training programs other than TCC can improve problems with dynamic balance and knee extension strength, which are two outcome variables that are independent risk factors for fracture[23]. In a small randomized controlled trial, 93 osteoporotic women aged

65 to 75 years who underwent 40 minutes of a community-based intervention that emphasized improving posture and balance twice a week for 20 weeks improved their dynamic balance and knee extension strength when compared to the control group[23].

Impact exercise, non-impact calisthenics, stretching

Impact exercise in postmenopausal women has been shown to increase hip and spine BMD. The efficacy of a 24-week aerobic exercise program consisting of treadmill walking followed by stepping exercises increased spine and femoral BMD in osteopenic postmenopausal women with a mean age of 64[24]. Other investigators reported a 1.54% increased BMD of the femoral neck in those who engaged in jumping exercises three times a week for 32 weeks each year, over a total period of 5 years[25].

In a separate study, early postmenopausal women who participated in stretching and non-impact exercise such as calisthenics for 40 minutes daily, three times a week, during a 12-month randomized study did not observe any changes in vertebral or femoral neck bone mass, but observed thickening of the bone cortex. It was concluded that the non-impact exercise was effective in increasing the mechanical properties of bone at some of the most loaded bone sites while improving participants' muscular performance and dynamic balance[26].

Weight-bearing exercises

Weight-bearing exercise has been shown to have mixed effects on BMD in postmenopausal women. A 6-month exercise program designed to maximize stress on the wrist was implemented by 250 postmenopausal women aged 52 to 72 for 30 minutes daily at home, and for 70 minutes twice per week with an instructor. These site-specific moderate physical exercises did not increase total bone mineral content (BMC) significantly at the ultra-distal radius and there was no increase in spine or femoral BMD[20].

In a study of 35 postmenopausal women who regularly participated in less than 30 minutes of weight-bearing exercise per week, completing weight-bearing exercises such as walking, jogging, and stair-climbing for 9-month and 22-month periods led to 5.2% and 6.1% increases in BMC[27]. However, in a trial assessing the benefits of walking, 255 women were randomized into a control group or a walking group. The walking group met twice a week with the goal of walking three miles per session. After 3 years, BMD changes in the cross-sectional dimensions of the radius did not differ significantly between the two groups[28].

In summary, there have been few prospective controlled trials that have examined effects of physical training on changes in bone density. Some studies have shown that regular physical activity can increase BMD and that the bone preserving action of exercise in postmenopausal women may contribute to the prevention of osteoporotic fractures[29]. Others have shown a limited increase in BMD due to physical exercise[20]. The conflicting results may be due to differences in exercise regimen or in the characteristics of volunteer participants[30].

Dietary measures

Reduced animal protein

The breakdown of high animal protein diets by the body produces metabolic acidosis, which can mobilize calcium from bone. In young women, high protein diets increase renal calcium excretion and maintain markers of bone formation at a steady concentration, suggesting that bone resorption is increased while bone formation is unaffected. The increased bone resorption may be exaggerated in older persons, who may have decrements in renal clearance of acid[31].

Some epidemiologic evidence suggests that high intakes of protein may decrease bone density and increase the incidence of bone fracture. A strong, positive correlation was found between the incidence of hip fracture and high dietary animal protein intake by a study that reviewed 34 published surveys in 16 countries[32]. Similarly, a 12-year prospective investigation of diet and bone fractures in 121 700 women found that higher protein consumption contributes to increased incidence of adult bone fractures. While a small significant increase in the risk of forearm fracture was observed, there was no corresponding increase in the risk of hip fracture[33].

The high prevalence of spinal osteoporosis in females living in countries that have a low animal protein intake, like Japan and India, may reflect low calcium rather than low protein intake[34]. Overall, epidemiologic studies of association between dietary protein intake and BMD and risk of hip fracture have been inconclusive and no intervention trials have been published[33].

Herbal treatments

Certain herbs have been effective in reducing bone loss in animal models, although little evidence is available to support the use of herbal treatments for osteoporosis in humans. Essential oil constituents of herbs like sage, rosemary, and thyme are efficient inhibitors of bone resorption when added to rat diets. The mechanism by which essential oils inhibit bone resorption is not known at present[35]. In Korea, safflower (*Carthamus tinctoris* L.) seeds are prescribed to promote bone formation and to prevent osteoporosis. Feeding safflower seeds to ovariectomized rats partially prevents bone loss caused by estrogen deficiency, without causing an increase in uterine weight. The bone-protecting effects of safflower seeds may be attributable to phytoestrogen components[36].

Herbs in Traditional Chinese Medicine

Herbal osteoporosis treatments in Traditional Chinese medicine (TCM) are available in many prepared formulae in China, and data from Chinese studies demonstrate that they can be effective in relieving some of the symptoms of osteoporosis. In a non-randomized trial, 74 post-menopausal women with osteoporosis were treated with a Chinese medicine identified as 'strong bone capsules' or with calcium. After 3 months, bone markers of formation were significantly increased in the treatment group when compared to levels in the calcium control group[37].

The traditional Chinese herbal medicine hochu-ekki-to is composed of ten herbal compunds including black cohosh (*Cimicifugae rhizoma*). Hochu-ekki-to prevented bone loss in rats that manifested a temporary clinical menopausal pattern, and it maintained BMD similar to that in estradiol treated and intact animals[38].

A randomized three-armed, double-blind clinical trial found that black cohosh exerted identical effects to those of conjugated estrogens in producing a statistically significant improvement in bone metabolism when compared to placebo-treated women[39]. Reported side-effects were gastro-intestinal discomfort, headache, dizziness, weight gain, heaviness in legs, and cramping. Black cohosh does not appear to be mutagenic, teratogenic, or carcinogenic[40].

In general, the formulae, mechanisms, and safety of herbal therapies for bone turnover need to be studied further in different populations.

Phytoestrogens

Phytoestrogens are non-steroidal, plant-derived compounds that bind to estrogen receptors and can mimic or modulate actions of endogenous estrogens[41]. Three major classes of phytoestrogens are the lignans, isoflavones, and coumestans. Lignans are widely distributed in flaxseed, whole grains, beans, and fruits, but have not been studied as much because of difficulties in isolation and analysis[42]. Coumestans do not play a major role in the human diet[40]. Isoflavones are the most extensively studied and are found in soybean products, chickpeas, and other legumes[42]. Concentrations of isoflavones in tofu and soymilk vary considerably between types and brands.

Isoflavones have estrogenic activity that is 100 to 10 000 times weaker than the activity of estradiol[42]. However, isoflavones can potentially exert biologic effects *in vivo* because plasma levels of isoflavones may exceed endogenous estrogen levels by several orders of magnitude[43]. Phytoestrogens may affect bone metabolism by promoting calcium absorption and increased production of insulin growth factor-1 (IGF-1), which is known to enhance osteoblastic activity and correlate with bone formation[44,45]. Additionally, *in vitro* studies of rat osetoblasts and osteoclasts have demonstrated that phytoestrogens decrease bone loss by inhibiting osteoclast recruitment and function and enhancing osteoblast cell proliferation and differentiation[46].

Observational studies on phytoestrogens and bone health   In a US study, the daily intake of isoflavones in Caucasian and African American women was estimated to be less than 2 mg/day, but the intakes in Japanese or Chinese women living in similar geographic regions ranged from 35 to 70 mg/day[47]. The incidence of hip fractures is lower in Asia than in most Western communities, but these differences in osteoporosis-related fractures may be accounted for by skeletal size and other factors, and not differing phytoestrogen intakes[42].

A number of cross-sectional studies have observed that a high intake of dietary isoflavones is associated with increased bone mass in postmenopausal Chinese and Japanese women[48,49]. In one analysis of postmenopausal Chinese women, an intake of 20 g/day soy protein with roughly 40 mg/day isoflavones was associated with significantly higher hip BMD and total body BMD in women after the first 4 years of menopause[50]. Among women eating a Western diet, habitual, unsupplemented consumption of isoflavones was positively correlated with increased bone density at the spine and negatively correlated with a marker of bone resorption, as reported by a cross-sectional study in Southern California[51].

However, a cross-sectional study of 87 post-menopausal Japanese women found no association of BMD with soy or isoflavone intake or serum isoflavone levels; similar results have also been reported from Australia[52,53].

Interventional studies on phytoestrogens and bone health   The results of previous studies of isoflavones and bone metabolism have been inconsistent. In a 12-month randomized clinical trial of healthy post-menopausal women, an isoflavone dose of 54 mg/day from genistein, a major isoflavone found in soy foods, increased BMD by 3.6% at the femur and 3% at the lumbar spine compared to a less than 1% loss of bone at both sites in the placebo-treated group[54]. In contrast, in a randomized double-blind study of postmenopausal women comparing dietary soy protein supplementation to casein placebo, soy supplementation with an isoflavone amount equivalent to a high Asian dietary intake, or 118 mg/day for 3 months, had no effect on indices of bone resorption[11].

The only phytoestrogen intervention trials that have evaluated fracture reduction in addition to bone metabolism and density as an endpoint have employed a synthetic derivative of isoflavones, called ipriflavone. According to two multicenter, double-blind, placebo-controlled studies, consuming 200 mg of ipriflavone three times a day for 2 years maintained bone mass, while BMD significantly decreased in the placebo group[55]. However, a large European randomized, placebo-controlled trial reported that ipriflavone supplementation in postmenopausal osteoporotic women for 3 years did not provide a statistically significant difference between the treatment and placebo groups for the measured biochemical markers of bone metabolism, annual percentage change from baseline in BMD of lumbar spine, or incidental vertebral fractures[56].

Isoflavone dosage   The dose of isoflavones may influence the effects of isoflavones on bone. A 6-month, double-blind, and placebo-controlled study in 40 post-menopausal women reported that subjects consuming 90 mg/day of isoflavones contained in soy protein had a significant 2% increase in bone density in the lumbar spine compared with no increase in those taking 56 mg/day of isoflavones at the same protein level[57]. However, doses of isolated isoflavones from red clover at levels between 58 mg/day and 85 mg/day produced a non-dose-dependent increase of BMD of 3% to 4% at the proximal radius and ulna in a single-blind, 6-month study in postmenopausal women. Limitations of the study include the absence of a simultaneously studied control group[58].

Soy protein   Soy protein supplementation without isoflavones may not have bone-sparing effects. In a 2-year study of 108 postmenopausal women, consumption of 18 g/day of soy protein in soy milk containing 85 mg

isoflavones prevented bone loss in the lumbar spine, and BMD and BMC showed 1.1% and 2.2% increases. Those who consumed the same amount of soy protein lacking isoflavones lost 4.2% and 4.3%, respectively, in lumbar spine BMD and BMC[59].

Phytoestrogen safety   Given their long tradition of consumption in Asian countries, phytoestrogens from soy products are generally regarded as safe. Currently there are no long-term safety data for food-free phytoestrogens classified as dietary supplements, and there is no scientific basis to assume that these plant compounds would be any safer than traditional pharmaceuticals[60]. Side-effects of consuming powdered soy protein include constipation, bloating, and nausea[61]. Phytoestrogen supplementation does not appear to be associated with any significant adverse effect on the breast and uterus[42,54]. Overconsumption of phytoestrogens should be avoided in postmenopausal females due to reported cases of vaginal bleeding after consumption of large quantities of different types of phytoestrogens[62].

Additionally, 29 out of 234 women who were being treated with ipriflavone developed subclinical lymphocytopenia. This lymphocytopenia took more than 24 months to resolve in some women. The mechanism and health consequences of the lymphocytopenia observed in association with ipriflavone treatment remain unknown[56].

Data interpretation   The interpretation of phytoestrogen data from human trials is difficult because of their short duration. Studies that cover a minimum of one bone remodeling cycle lasting 30 to 80 weeks should be conducted. Variability in findings on soy may be attributable to the types of soy products used, preparation of soy, frequency of consumption, and isoflavone content[52]. In addition, the biologic effects of phytoestrogens are dependent on factors like dosage, duration of use, protein binding affinity, individual metabolism, and the intrinsic estrogenic state of the patient. Future clinical studies should evaluate the risk of fracture with soy isoflavones[63].

In sum, observational studies in postmenopausal women indicate that soy isoflavone intake levels of about 50 mg/day can allow preservation of bone mass through decrease in bone resorption. Short-term intervention studies are inconsistent in indicating impact on either BMD or bone turnover, and the findings of these studies need to be confirmed by longer studies of 2 to 3 years[57]. The most recent studies lasting 6 months show moderate positive effects of phytoestrogens on bone, with few negative side-effects[41].

Orthomolecular medicine

Orthomolecular medicine employs molecules normally present in the body for the prevention and treatment of disease. In some cases, natural substances are used in doses beyond those normally required to correct a deficiency[64].

Omega-3 fatty acids

Omega-3 fatty acids are essential nutrients that can be derived from either plant or animal sources. α-Linolenic acid is a principal constituent of canola and soy bean oils, and is also found in high abundance in flaxseed and walnuts. Marine fish, such as salmon and mackerel, are the principal sources of the longer chain omega-3 fatty acids, eicosapentanoic acid (EPA) and docosahexanoic acid (DHA)[65]. To a limited extent, α-linolenic acid can be converted to DHA. In the US diet, the consumption of omega-3 fatty acids is much less compared to that of other fatty acids, including omega-6 fatty acids, which are found in corn oils, cereal grains, poultry, and meats.

Epidemiologic evidence suggests that higher consumption of omega-3 fatty acids is associated with higher bone density. In a study of 1532 women and men aged 45 to 90 years, a higher ratio of omega-6 to omega-3 fatty acid consumption was associated with a lower BMD, independent of age, body mass index, or lifestyle factors[66].

While it is not possible to discern from these data, whether this association is due to a detrimental effect of omega-6 fatty acids or a beneficial effect of omega-3 fatty acids, other evidence would suggest that omega-3 fatty acids have multiple effects on bone and calcium metabolism which may lead to higher BMD. In animal models, omega-3 fatty acids have been shown to increase calcium absorption from the gut, increase bone formation, and reduce bone resorption[67], likely through the inhibition of inflammatory cytokines and prostaglandins. Bone strength has been shown to increase with omega-3 fatty acid supplementation in ovariectomized rats, an animal model of high bone turnover osteoporosis[68].

The clinical trial data in humans are limited. In a pilot study of 80 elderly females supplemented with omega-3 fatty acids (EPA 6 g/day) or coconut oil for 18 months those who received omega-3 fatty acids showed improvements or stabilization of bone density, whereas BMD declined in the control group[69]. Another study in postmenopausal women showed no effect of omega-3 fatty acid supplementation[70]. None of the studies investigated the effect on fracture risk. Further investigation of the effects of omega-3 fatty acid supplementation on bone and calcium metabolism is required.

Vitamin K

Low concentrations of vitamin K have been associated with bone fractures. Vitamin K_1, derived from green vegetables, and vitamin K_2, derived from meat and fermented foods, are the two most important forms of vitamin K[71]. Vitamin K is a cofactor required for synthesis of osteocalcin, the bone protein that promotes mineralization of bone. Vitamin K may also influence bone metabolism through its reduction of urinary calcium excretion[72]. Cross-sectional and retrospective epidemiologic studies of vitamin K_1 have found lower dietary vitamin K_1 intakes and mean serum vitamin K_1 concentrations in patients with a history of vertebral crush fractures than in age-matched controls[73].

Vitamin K has also been shown to reduce the rate of bone loss. In one intervention study in 132 postmenopausal women with osteoporosis, supplementation with 45 mg/day vitamin K_2 for 2 years resulted in new vertebral fractures in 14% of the women, while 26% of the women in the control group developed new vertebral fractures. Supplementation with vitamin K_2 had modest effects on reducing the rate of bone loss[74].

Vitamin A

It has been hypothesized that dietary vitamin A may negatively affect bone strength. The highest incidence of osteoporotic fractures is found in regions where dietary intake of vitamin A, or retinol, is unusually high. In laboratory animals, hypervitaminosis A results in accelerated bone resorption, bone fragility, and spontaneous fractures[75]. High levels of retinol also interfere with vitamin D activity, which is necessary for calcium absorption[7].

A case–control study in Swedish women 40 to 76 years old found an inverse correlation between retinol intake and BMD. Women with retinol intakes in excess of 1500 μg/day had a reduced BMD and a two-fold increased risk for hip fracture compared to those with intakes of retinol less than 500 μg/day[7]. Similarly, the Nurses Health Study, which had 18 years of follow-up, reported that postmenopausal women with retinol intakes of about 2000 μg/day or more had an almost doubled risk of hip fracture compared with those with intakes of less than 500 μg/day[76].

The source of retinol in the diet, whether from dietary supplementation or conversion from dietary beta-carotene, appeared to have differing effects on bone. Excessive dietary intake of beta-carotene from brightly colored fruits and vegetables did not seem to increase the risk of hip fracture[76].

These studies may provide further evidence that chronic intake of excessive vitamin A from retinol may contribute to the development of osteoporotic hip fractures in women.

Vitamin C

In vitro studies in rat osteoblastic cells suggest that vitamin C, or ascorbic acid, is required for bone mineralization and may be associated with increased bone formation[77]. Few studies in human populations have examined the relationship between ascorbic acid and bone mass. In a study of women aged 45 to 64, 1 to 10 years postmenopausal, there was a significant positive correlation found between dietary vitamin C and femoral and hip BMD[77]. However, a cross-sectional study of Swedish women aged 25–74 showed that there was no statistically significant association between vitamin C and BMD of the total body, lumbar spine, and femoral neck[77].

CONCLUSIONS

To date, the most extensive research on CAM therapy and osteoporosis has focused on phytoestrogens. Although a number of short-term studies in postmenopausal women show beneficial effects of isoflavone supplementation on biochemical markers of bone turnover, BMC and BMD, it is undetermined whether these data will translate into long-term effects[42]. Because there have been few prospective controlled trials that have examined effects of physical training and herbal formulae on changes in bone density in postmenopausal women, the efficacy of these therapies is unclear. The pathogenesis and treatment of osteoporosis clearly involves nutrients like calcium, vitamin D, protein, and vitamins A, C, and K. Many of the mentioned dietary supplements are commercially available, and more research will aid in the clarification of which CAM therapies are safe and can lower the risk of osteoporotic fracture.

ACKNOWLEDGMENT

This work is supported in part by NIH 1K23AT 002862-01 (TTB).

References

1. Harkness L. Soy and bone. Where do we stand? Orthop Nurs 2004; 23: 12–17
2. Moyad MA. Complementary therapies for reducing the risk of osteoporosis in patients receiving luteinizing hormone-releasing hormone treatment/orchiectomy for prostate cancer: a review and assessment of the need for more research. Urology 2002; 59 (4 Suppl 1): 34–40
3. Riggs BL, Melton LJ III. The worldwide problem of osteoporosis: insights afforded by epidemiology. Bone 1995; 17 (5 Suppl): 505S–11S
4. Wehren LE. The epidemiology of osteoporosis and fractures in geriatric medicine. Clin Geriatr Med 2003; 19: 245–58
5. Cooper C. Epidemiology of osteoporosis. In Favus MJ, ed. Primer on the Metabolic Bone Diseases and Disorders of Mineral Metabolism, 5th edn. Washington, DC: American Society for Bone and Mineral Research, 2003: 307–13
6. Setchell KD, Lydeking-Olsen E. Dietary phytoestrogens and their effect on bone: evidence from in vitro and in vivo, human observational, and dietary intervention studies. Am J Clin Nutr 2003; 78 (3 Suppl): 593S–609S
7. Advani S, Wimalawansa SJ. Bones and nutrition: common sense supplementation for osteoporosis. Curr Womens Health Rep 2003; 3: 187–92
8. Chilibeck PD. Exercise and estrogen or estrogen alternatives (phytoestrogens, bisphosphonates) for preservation of bone mineral in postmenopausal women. Can J Appl Physiol 2004; 29: 59–75
9. Osteoporosis: Review of the Evidence for Prevention, Diagnosis and Treatment and Cost-Effectiveness Analysis. Osteoporosis International, 1998
10. Cohen DP. Anti-osteoporotic medications: traditional and non-traditional. Clin Obstet Gynecol 2003; 46: 341–8
11. Dalais FS, Ebeling PR, Kotsopoulos D, et al. The effects of soy protein containing isoflavones on lipids and indices of bone resorption in postmenopausal women. Clin Endocrinol (Oxf) 2003; 58: 704–9
12. Warren MP, Shortle B, Dominguez JE. Use of alternative therapies in menopause. Best Pract Res Clin Obstet Gynaecol 2002; 16: 411–48

13. Bonn D. New ways with old bones. Osteoporosis researchers look for drugs to replace hormone replacement therapy. Lancet 2004; 363: 786–7

14. Nikander E, Metsa-Heikkila M, Ylikorkala O, Tiitinen A. Effects of phytoestrogens on bone turnover in postmenopausal women with a history of breast cancer. J Clin Endocrinol Metab 2004; 89: 1207–12

15. Pinkerton JV, Santen R. Use of alternatives to estrogen for treatment of menopause. Minerva Endocrinol 2002; 27: 21–41

16. Register TC, Jayo MJ, Anthony MS. Soy phytoestrogens do not prevent bone loss in postmenopausal monkeys. J Clin Endocrinol Metab 2003; 88: 4362–70

17. Stafford RS, Drieling RL, Hersh AL. National trends in osteoporosis visits and osteoporosis treatment, 1988–2003. Arch Intern Med 2004; 164: 1525–30

18. Orwoll ES. Treatment of osteoporosis in men. Calcif Tissue Int 2004; 75: 114–19

19. Weaver CM, Liebman M. Biomarkers of bone health appropriate for evaluating functional foods designed to reduce risk of osteoporosis. Br J Nutr 2002; 88 (Suppl 2): S225–32

20. Adami S, Gatti D, Braga V, et al. Site-specific effects of strength training on bone structure and geometry of ultradistal radius in postmenopausal women. J Bone Min Res 1999; 14: 120–4

21. Chan K, Qin L, Lau M, et al. A randomized, prospective study of the effects of Tai Chi Chun exercise on bone mineral density in postmenopausal women. Arch Phys Med Rehabil 2004; 85: 717–22

22. Lao L. Traditional Chinese Medicine. In Jonas WE, Levin JS, eds. Essentials of Complementary and Alternative Medicine. Philadelphia: Lippincott Williams & Wilkins, 1999: 216–32

23. Carter ND, Khan KM, McKay HA, et al. Community-based exercise program reduces risk factors for falls in 65- to 75-year-old women with osteoporosis: randomized controlled trial. CMAJ 2002; 167: 997–1004

24. Chien MY, Wu YT, Hsu AT, et al. Efficacy of a 24-week aerobic exercise program for osteopenic postmenopausal women. Calcif Tissue Int 2000; 67: 443–8

25. Snow CM, Shaw JM, Winters KM, Witzke KA. Long-term exercise using weighted vests prevents hip bone loss in postmenopausal women. J Gerontol A Biol Sci Med Sci 2000; 55: M489–M491

26. Uusi-Rasi K, Kannus P, Cheng S, et al. Effect of alendronate and exercise on bone and physical performance of postmenopausal women: a randomized controlled trial. Bone 2003; 33: 132–43

27. Dalsky GP, Stocke KS, Ehsani AA, et al. Weight-bearing exercise training and lumbar bone mineral content in postmenopausal women. Ann Intern Med 1988; 108: 824–8

28. Sandler RB, Cauley JA, Hom DL, et al. The effects of walking on the cross-sectional dimensions of the radius in postmenopausal women. Calcif Tissue Int 1987; 41: 65–9

29. Mayoux-Benhamou MA, Roux C, Perraud A, et al. Predictors of compliance with a home-based exercise program added to usual medical care in preventing postmenopausal osteoporosis: an 18-month prospective study. Osteo Int 2005; 16: 325–31

30. Heinonen A, Kannus P, Sievanen H, et al. Randomised controlled trial of effect of high-impact exercise on selected risk factors for osteoporotic fractures. Lancet 1996; 348: 1343–7

31. Kerstetter JE, Mitnick ME, Gundberg CM, et al. Changes in bone turnover in young women consuming different levels of dietary protein. J Clin Endocrinol Metab 1999; 84: 1052–5

32. Abelow BJ, Holford TR, Insogna KL. Cross-cultural association between dietary animal protein and hip fracture: a hypothesis. Calcif Tissue Int 1992; 50: 14–18

33. Feskanich D, Willett WC, Stampfer MJ, Colditz GA. Protein consumption and bone fractures in women. Am J Epidemiol 1996; 143: 472–9

34. Nordin BE. International patterns of osteoporosis. Clin Orthop Relat Res 1966; 45: 17–30

35. Muhlbauer RC, Lozano A, Palacio S, et al. Common herbs, essential oils, and monoterpenes potently modulate bone metabolism. Bone 2003; 32: 372–80

36. Kim HJ, Bae YC, Park RW, et al. Bone-protecting effect of safflower seeds in ovariectomized rats. Calcif Tissue Int 2002; 71: 88–94

37. Xu H, Lawson D. Theories and practice in prevention and treatment principles in relation to Chinese herbal medicine and bone loss. J Tradit Chin Med 2004; 24: 88–92

38. Sakamoto S, Sassa S, Kudo H, et al. Preventive effects of a herbal medicine on bone loss in rats treated with a GnRH agonist. Eur J Endocrinol 2000; 143: 139–42

39. Wuttke W, Seidlova-Wuttke D, Gorkow C. The Cimicifuga preparation BNO 1055 vs. conjugated estrogens in a double-blind placebo-controlled study: effects on menopause symptoms and bone markers. Maturitas 2003; 44 (Suppl 1): S67–S77

40. Roemheld-Hamm B, Dahl NV. Herbs, menopause, and dialysis. Semin Dial 2002; 15: 53–9

41. Branca F. Dietary phyto-estrogens and bone health. Proc Nutr Soc 2003; 62: 877–87

42. Cassidy A. Potential risks and benefits of phytoestrogen-rich diets. Int J Vitam Nutr Res 2003; 73: 120–6

43. Setchell KD, Brown NM, Desai P, et al. Bioavailability of pure isoflavones in healthy humans and analysis of commercial soy isoflavone supplements. J Nutr 2001; 131 (4 Suppl): 1362S–75S

44. Arjmandi BH, Khalil DA, Hollis BW. Soy protein: its effects on intestinal calcium transport, serum vitamin D, and insulin-like growth factor-I in ovariectomized rats. Calcif Tissue Int 2002; 70: 483–7

45. Arjmandi BH, Khalil DA, Smith BJ, et al. Soy protein has a greater effect on bone in postmenopausal women not on hormone replacement therapy, as evidenced by reducing bone resorption and urinary calcium excretion. J Clin Endocrinol Metab 2003; 88: 1048–54

46. Gao YH, Yamaguchi M. Suppressive effect of genistein on rat bone osteoclasts: involvement of protein kinase inhibition and protein tyrosine phosphatase activation. Int J Mol Med 2000; 5: 261–7

47. Greendale GA, FitzGerald G, Huang MH, et al. Dietary soy isoflavones and bone mineral density: results from the study of women's health across the nation. Am J Epidemiol 2002; 155: 746–54

48. Mei J, Yeung SS, Kung AW. High dietary phytoestrogen intake is associated with higher bone mineral density in postmenopausal but not premenopausal women. J Clin Endocrinol Metab 2001; 86: 5217–21

49. Somekawa Y, Chiguchi M, Ishibashi T, Aso T. Soy intake related to menopausal symptoms, serum lipids, and bone mineral density in postmenopausal Japanese women. Obstet Gynecol 2001; 97: 109–15

50. Ho SC, Woo J, Lam S, et al. Soy protein consumption and bone mass in early postmenopausal Chinese women. Osteo Int 2003; 14: 835–42

51. Kritz-Silverstein D, Goodman-Gruen DL. Usual dietary isoflavone intake, bone mineral density, and bone metabolism in postmenopausal women. J Womens Health Gend Based Med 2002; 11: 69–78

52. Gallagher JC, Satpathy R, Rafferty K, Haynatzka V. The effect of soy protein isolate on bone metabolism. Menopause 2004; 11: 290–8

53. Nagata C, Shimizu H, Takami R, et al. Soy product intake and serum isoflavonoid and estradiol concentrations in relation to bone mineral density in postmenopausal Japanese women. Osteo Int 2002; 13: 200–4

54. Morabito N, Crisafulli A, Vergara C, et al. Effects of genistein and hormone-replacement therapy on bone loss in early post-menopausal women: a randomized double-blind placebo-controlled study. J Bone Min Res 2002; 17: 1904–12

55. Gennari C, Adami S, Agnusdei D, et al. Effect of chronic treatment with ipriflavone in postmenopausal women with low bone mass. Calcif Tissue Int 1997; 61 (Suppl 1): S19–22

56. Alexandersen P, Toussaint A, Christiansen C, et al. Ipriflavone in the treatment of postmenopausal osteoporosis: a randomized controlled trial. J Am Med Assoc 2001; 285: 1482–8

57. Potter SM, Baum JA, Teng H, et al. Soy protein and isoflavones: their effects on blood lipids and bone density in postmenopausal women. Am J Clin Nutr 1998; 68 (6 Suppl): 1375S–9S

58. Clifton-Bligh PB, Baber RJ, Fulcher GR, et al. The effect of isoflavones extracted from red clover (Rimostil) on lipid and bone metabolism. Menopause 2001; 8: 259–65

59. Lydeking-Olsen E, Beck-Jensen JE, Setchell KD, Holm-Jensen T. Soymilk or progesterone for prevention of bone loss – a 2 year randomized, placebo-controlled trial. Eur J Nutr 2004; 43: 246–57

60. Strauss L, Santti R, Saarinen N, et al. Dietary phytoestrogens and their role in hormonally dependent disease. Toxicol Lett 1998; 102–3: 349–54

61. Albertazzi P, Pansini F, Bonaccorsi G, et al. The effect of dietary soy supplementation on hot flushes. Obstet Gynecol 1998; 91: 6–11

62. Fitzpatrick LA. Soy isoflavones: hope or hype? Maturitas 2003; 44 (Suppl 1): S21–9

63. Morin S. Isoflavones and bone health. Menopause 2004; 11: 239–41

64. Gaby AR. Orthomolecular medicine and megavitamin therapy. In Jonas WE, Levin JS, eds. Essentials of Complementary and Alternative Medicine. Philadelphia: Lippincott Williams & Wilkins, 1999: 459–71

65. Kris-Etherton PM, Harris WS, Appel LJ. Fish consumption, fish oil, omega-3 fatty acids, and cardiovascular disease. Circulation 2002; 106: 2747–57

66. Weiss LA, Barrett-Connor E, von Muhlen D. Ratio of n-6 to n-3 fatty acids and bone mineral density in older adults: the Rancho Bernardo Study. Am J Clin Nutr 2005; 81: 934–8

67. Watkins BA, Li Y, Lippman HE, Feng S. Modulatory effect of omega-3 polyunsaturated fatty acids on osteoblast function and bone metabolism. Prost Leuk Ess Fatty Acids 2003; 68: 387–98

68. Sakaguchi K, Morita I, Murota S. Eicosapentaenoic acid inhibits bone loss due to ovariectomy in rats. Prost Leuk Ess Fatty Acids 1994; 50: 81–4

69. Kruger MC, Coetzer H, de Winter R, et al. Calcium, gamma-linolenic acid and eicosapentaenoic acid supplementation in senile osteoporosis. Aging (Milano) 1998; 10: 385–94

70. Bassey EJ, Littlewood JJ, Rothwell MC, Pye DW. Lack of effect of supplementation with essential fatty acids on bone mineral density in healthy pre- and postmenopausal women: two randomized controlled trials of Efacal v. calcium alone. Br J Nutr 2000; 83: 629–35

71. Braam LA, Knapen MH, Geusens P, et al. Vitamin K1 supplementation retards bone loss in postmenopausal women between 50 and 60 years of age. Calcif Tissue Int 2003; 73: 21–6

72. Feskanich D, Weber P, Willett WC, et al. Vitamin K intake and hip fractures in women: a prospective study. Am J Clin Nutr 1999; 69: 74–9

73. Hart JP, Shearer MJ, Klenerman L, et al. Electrochemical detection of depressed circulating levels of vitamin K1 in osteoporosis. J Clin Endocrinol Metab 1985; 60: 1268–9

74. Ishida Y, Kawai S. Comparative efficacy of hormone replacement therapy, etidronate, calcitonin, alfacalcidol, and vitamin K in postmenopausal women with osteoporosis: The Yamaguchi Osteoporosis Prevention Study. Am J Med 2004; 117: 549–55

75. Melhus H, Michaelsson K, Kindmark A, et al. Excessive dietary intake of vitamin A is associated with reduced bone mineral density and increased risk for hip fracture. Ann Intern Med 1998; 129: 770–8

76. Feskanich D, Singh V, Willett WC, Colditz GA. Vitamin A intake and hip fractures among postmenopausal women. J Am Med Assoc 2002; 287: 47–54

77. Hall SL, Greendale GA. The relation of dietary vitamin C intake to bone mineral density: results from the PEPI study. Calcif Tissue Int 1998; 63: 183–9

Male and female sexual dysfunction

21

H. H. Aung and V. Rand

INTRODUCTION

Sexual dysfunction is characterized by disturbances in sexual desire and in the psychophysiologic changes associated with the sexual response cycle[1]. Prevalent in both genders, it ranges from 10 to 52% of men and 25 to 63% of women, based on several studies[2–4]. It has been reported that the incidence of sexual dysfunction in the United States is greater in women (43%) than in men (31%)[5].

Advances have occurred in the understanding of the neurovascular mechanisms of sexual response in both men and women[6–8]. Several new classes of drugs have been identified that offer significant therapeutic potential for the treatment of male erectile disorder[9–11], while other agents are indicated for sexual desire and orgasm disorders[10,12,13]. In addition to conventional therapies, however, individuals with sexual dysfunction often seek alternative therapies.

SEXUAL DYSFUNCTION IN MEN

Penile erection is mediated by the parasympathetic nervous system, which, when stimulated, can cause arterial dilatation and relaxation of the cavernosal smooth muscle. Increased blood flow into the corpora cavernosa in association with reduced venous outflow results in penile rigidity. Nitric oxide (NO), a chemical mediator of erection, is released from nerve endings and vascular endothelium. This causes smooth muscle relaxation, resulting in venous engorgement and penile tumescence.

Erectile dysfunction is defined as the inability to achieve and maintain an erection sufficient to permit satisfactory sexual intercourse[14], and has been estimated to affect 20–30 million men in the United States[15,16]. Erectile dysfunction can be classified as psychogenic, organic (neurogenic, hormonal, arterial, cavernosal, or drug-induced), or mixed psychogenic and organic[17]. Treatment options have progressed from psychosexual therapy and penile prostheses (1970s), through revascularization, vacuum constriction devices, and intracavernous injection therapy (1980s), to transurethral and oral drug therapy (1990s). The discovery that the nitric oxide–cyclic GMP pathway affects erectile function and the development of sildenafil citrate (Viagra®) are recent advances[17].

Medicinal herbs

Yohimbine

Yohimbine is an alkaloid derived from the bark of the central African tree *Corynanthe yohimbe*. It may cause penile vasodilatation via alpha-2-receptor antagonism. The results from a meta-analysis suggest yohimbine is effective for erectile dysfunction. No trials have been conducted to compare yohimbine with sildenafil citrate, but indirect comparison of placebo-controlled trials suggests that yohimbine is less effective but relatively safer[18]. The combination of yohimbine and L-arginine is in early phase III development[19]. A double-blind, cross-over trial of 4 weeks' duration was used to evaluate the efficacy of yohimbine in reversing anorgasmia; 10–15 mg dosage did not cause any worsening of patients' obsessive compulsive (depression) symptoms[20].

In addition, one case report showed that yohimbine is effective in the treatment of antidepressant medication (selective serotonin reuptake inhibitors, clomipramine, and tricyclic antidepressants) induced sexual dysfunction, anorgasmia, and difficulty obtaining and maintaining an erection. It has been shown that a clomipramine dosage of up to 150 mg/day inhibited the patient's orgasmic ability and a dosage of 200 mg/day inhibited the ability to obtain an erection[21].

Oral doses of yohimbine of 5–10 mg three times daily are generally well tolerated. The side-effects of yohimbine are clearly dose dependent[22], with doses over 30 mg occasionally causing small increases in blood pressure and doses of 50 mg or higher associated with increased heart rate in normotensive subjects[22].

Ginkgo biloba

Ginkgo biloba, or ginkgo, facilitates microvascular circulation that may physiologically lead to improvement in sexual function, according to animal studies[23]. There is evidence that ginkgo extract may directly elucidate smooth muscle relaxation, likely via effects on the NO pathway. The extract has an effect in both human and rabbit corpus cavernosum tissue, using organ bath and electric field stimulation[24]. An open-label clinical trial used ginkgo extract to treat arterial erectile dysfunction. Sixty patients who had not improved with papaverine injections up to 50 mg were treated with ginkgo extract 60 mg/day for 12 to 18 months. The penile blood flow was re-evaluated by duplex sonography every 4 weeks. Fifty percent of patients had regained potency[25].

Another open-label trial showed that ginkgo is effective in treating antidepressant-induced sexual dysfunction. Ginkgo generally had a positive effect on all four phases of the response cycle (i.e. desire, excitement, erection, and lubrication), orgasm, and resolution[26].

Ginseng

Ginseng has been an essential herbal in Traditional Chinese Medicine (TCM) for many years. The principal active constituents in ginseng are ginsenosides. Over 20 different ginsenosides have been identified from ginseng root extracts of different ginseng species. Ginseng is commonly used for the treatment of sexual dysfunction[27,28].

Effects of American ginseng on copulatory behavior have been shown in adult male rats. Ginseng-treated rats demonstrated a significant decrease in mount, intromission, and ejaculation latencies compared to vehicle controls. Hormone analyses revealed no difference in plasma luteinizing hormone or testosterone levels between ginseng- and vehicle-treated animals. However, plasma prolactin levels were significantly reduced by all doses of ginseng tested, suggesting ginseng-induced alterations in dopaminergic neurotransmission may play a role in the ability of ginseng to stimulate copulatory behavior[29]. One study showed that both Asian ginseng and American ginseng enhance libido and copulatory performance. These effects of ginseng may not be due to changes in hormone secretion, but to direct effects of ginseng, or its ginsenoside components, on the central nervous system and gonadal tissues. Ginsenosides can facilitate penile erection by directly inducing the vasodilatation and relaxation of penile corpus cavernosum. In addition, the effects of ginseng on the corpus cavernosum appear to be mediated by the release and/or modification of release of nitric oxide from endothelial cells and perivascular nerves[28].

Clinically, ginseng is believed to have aphrodisiac effects for patients with sexual dysfunction[30]. One placebo-controlled study assessed 90 patients for 3 months. Among them, 30 patients were treated with Korean red ginseng extract 1.8 g, 30 were treated with placebo, and the remaining 30 patients received trazodone 25 mg. Although no intergroup differences were reported for frequency of intercourse, the results suggested superiority of ginseng for penile rigidity, girth, libido, and satisfaction[31]. Ginsenosides, have been shown to increase NO production in endothelial cells in *in vitro* studies, possibly due to upregulation of NO synthase activity by the compounds[32,33]. Thus, the effects of ginsenosides on NO production have implications for improved sexual function.

Ginseng was also demonstrated to increase spermatozoa count and motility in infertility patients. In a study with a total of 66 participants, 30 were oligoastenospermic sine causa, 16 were oligoastenospermic with idiopathic varicocele, and the remaining 20 age-matched volunteers were used as controls. Ginseng extract showed an increase in spermatozoa number per ml and progressive oscillating motility, an increase in plasma total and free testosterone, DHT, FSH, and LH, but a decrease in mean prolactin. It is suggested that ginsenosides may have an effect at different levels of the hypothalamus–pituitary–testes axis[34].

Tribulus terrestris/protodioscin

Protodioscin is a phytochemical agent derived from the *Tribulus terrestris* plant, which has been clinically proven to improve sexual desire and enhance erection via the conversion of protodioscin to DHEA (dehydroepiandrosterone)[35]. In a double-blind, placebo-controlled multicenter study on 45 subfertile couples with idiopathic oligo-astheno-terato-zoosperma, the husbands were treated with Tribestan (a protodioscin phytochemical compound) 500 mg/day for 12 weeks. Eight pregnancies were noted after 4 months[36]. Another controlled study enrolled 40 subjects (20 in a DHEA group and 20 in a placebo group), age range 43–68 years old, for 24 weeks. A DHEA daily dose of 50 mg has been found to be effective in increasing fertility in subfertile males and improving erectile dysfunction in both diabetic and non-diabetic men[36,37].

Damiana

Damiana (*Turnera diffusa*, *Turnera aphrodisiaca*) has been traditionally used as a tonic for the central nervous system and hormonal system in Latin America[38]. It has been shown that damiana has progestin receptor-binding activity and is considered a phyto-progestin, a progesterone derived from plants[39]. In an *in vivo* study, high progestin-binding activity of damiana has been demonstrated, based on the effect on alkaline phosphatase, an endproduct of progestin action[39]. Sexually impaired rats treated with damiana increased their rates of copulatory performance[40].

Others

Eurycoma longifolia, *Pimpinella pruacen*, and *Muara puama* are also believed to enhance sexual functions[35]. In addition to botanicals, vitamins and minerals may also possess abilities to enhance sexual function[41–45]. More research studies are needed to prove their efficacy.

Vitamins and minerals

There is evidence that vitamins and minerals enhance sexual function. B-complex vitamins are important for the activity of many enzymes and for energy metabolism. Low levels of circulating folate and vitamin B_6 increase the risk of peripheral vascular disease, leading to potential reduction of sexual function[45]. Vitamin B_{12} injections have increased sperm counts in men[42,43]. Vitamin E supplementation has been shown to increase fertility in men[41].

Zinc is a fundamental mineral in the maintenance of human reproductive function. Low zinc levels have been shown to cause sexual dysfunction, and are associated with infertility in males[44].

Herb formulations

Herbal formulae constitute an important aspect of TCM treatment. Individual herbs are organized into broad therapeutic TCM categories according to the principal action observed by its administration. Each herb has a primary effect on one or more organ systems[46].

Gosyajinki-gan

Gosyajinki-gan is a traditional Chinese medicine formulation composed of ten herbs[47]. One study compared the effect of limaprost, an oral prostaglandin E_1 (PGE_1) derivative, to that of gosyajinki-gan. The study comprised 50 patients with mild erectile dysfunction who showed a good erectile response to intracavernosal injection of 20 mg of PGE_1. Limaprost was administered to the first 25 patients (30 mg three times daily), and gosyajinki-gan (7.5 g three times daily) to the next 25 patients, for 8 consecutive weeks. Patients were evaluated by their ability to achieve vaginal penetration and by a subjective assessment of erectile functions (i.e. penile rigidity and maintenance of erection) before and after the treatment, using a self-administered questionnaire. Objective measurements (e.g. nocturnal penile tumescence) were also evaluated. Four of the 24 taking gosyajinki-gan succeeded in vaginal penetration. However, these positive responders did not experience a full erection[47].

Ryu-wei-ti-huang-wan

Ryu-wei-ti-huang-wan is a Chinese herbal formulation composed of extracts from six plants[48]. It is used in the clinical treatment of male diabetic impotence. On evaluation of diabetic impotence, adult male rats were divided into three groups:

(1) Rats rendered diabetic with a single intraperitoneal injection of streptozotocin (60 mg/kg body weight);

(2) Rats with streptozotocin-induced diabetes treated with a ryu-wei-ti-huang-wan powder 30 mg/kg twice a day; and

(3) Control rats.

Each male rat was caged with an adult ovariectomized female rat during the dark cycle. Infra-red-light-illuminated video recording was utilized to evaluate the sexual performance. The diabetic rats exhibited depressed mounting activity and no intromission or ejaculation. After ryu-wei-ti-huang-wan treatment, either for 1 day or 2 weeks, the diabetic rats showed significant improvement in mounting performance, with preservation of intromission and ejaculation. No significant difference in the blood sugar level was noted between the treatment and non-treatment groups[48].

Another Chinese herbal medicine formulation

This formulation was composed of 18 herbs including ginseng, dioscoreae, and paeoiae alba[49]. The formulation showed an effective response in hypercholesterolemic erectile dysfunction male rats. In a study with 32 rats, 8 control animals were fed a normal diet and the remaining 24 were fed a cholesterol diet for 4 months. After 2 months, herbal medicine was added to the drinking water of the treatment group of 16 rats, but not the cholesterol only group. Serum cholesterol levels were measured at 2 and 4 months. At 4 months erectile function was evaluated with cavernous nerve electrostimulation in all animals. Penile tissues were collected for electron microscopy, and to perform Western blot for endothelial nitric oxide synthase, neuronal nitric oxide synthase, basic fibroblast growth factor (bFGF), and caveolin-1. Erectile response was significantly better in the Chinese herbal treated group. High levels of bFGF and caveolin-1 expression in the treated group may protect the cavernous smooth muscle and endothelial cells from the harmful effect of high serum cholesterol[49].

Mustong

An uncontrolled study assessed the potential of mustong, an Oriental herbal preparation containing mainly *Mucuna pruriens* and *Withania somnifera*, as an option for male sexual dysfunction[50]. The report suggests improvement of sexual function in 16 out of 25 diabetic patients with impotency. Mustong was given in two tablets, twice daily for 7–8 weeks. After mustong administration, there was an increased desire to have sexual intercourse, strong erection, hardness, and increased duration of coitus[50]. No adverse effects were observed.

L-Arginine

L-Arginine is an amino acid that functions as a precursor to the formation of NO, which mediates the relaxation of vascular and non-vascular smooth muscle. In a double-blind, placebo-controlled study, a high oral dose of L-arginine (5 g/day) was given for 6 weeks, and the treatment induced significant improvement in sexual function in men with organic erectile dysfunction[51]. A combination of L-arginine and yohimbine was used for individuals with sexual dysfunction[52]. One controlled, three-way cross-over clinical trial was conducted to compare the efficacy and safety among 6 g L-arginine plus 6 mg yohimbine, 6 mg yohimbine alone, and placebo,

for the treatment of erectile dysfunction. The primary endpoint was a change in the erectile function domain score of the International Index of Erectile Function. The secondary endpoints were patient and investigator assessments of treatment success. Forty-five patients were enrolled in this 2-week cross-over study, and the drug was orally administered 1 to 2 hours before intended sexual intercourse. This study showed that administration of L-arginine plus yohimbine is effective in improving erectile function in patients with mild to moderate erectile dysfunction[53]. However, data from another controlled study reported that, compared to placebo, low-dose oral L-arginine (1.5 g/day) for 17 days did not show any improvement in the mixed type of erectile dysfunction[54].

Acupuncture

One randomized controlled trial evaluated acupuncture as a treatment for patients with non-organic erectile dysfunction[55]. Nine patients were treated with acupuncture points and six received placebo acupuncture twice weekly for 6 weeks. Improvements in sexual function were reported in the treatment group, but were not significantly different from the control group. Data from uncontrolled studies indicate some positive effects on the quality of erection and sexual activity in erectile dysfunction due to non-organic[56] and mixed[57] etiologies. In another study with 52 patients, improvement of impotence was seen in the majority of cases[58].

Biofeedback

A controlled trial of biofeedback training assessed 30 patients with psychogenic erectile dysfunction. There were 10 patients in each group. The first group received feedback plus the viewing of segments of erotic film. The second group viewed film segments without feedback, and the third group received no feedback and no film. There were no intergroup differences in erectile functioning during a one-month follow-up period[59]. It was concluded that the therapeutic value of erectile feedback remains undemonstrated.

Hypnotherapy

A randomized controlled trial assessed the effects of hypnotic suggestion on sexual function in patients with sexual dysfunction with no detectable organic cause[55,60]. In the study, the first group received testosterone, the second group received trazodone, the third group underwent hypnosis therapy, and the last group served as control. After 4, 6, and 8 weeks, the effects were verified by interviews with their partners. The study found some obvious improvements in sexual function by hypnosis therapy.

Pelvic floor exercise

Pelvic floor exercises apply pressure on the glans penis to trigger reflex contractions of the ischiocavernosus and perineal muscles. The exercise may reinforce the strength of perineal muscles and facilitate penile rigidity during erection[61]. One controlled trial compared a pelvic floor exercise program with surgery[62]. One hundred and fifty patients with erectile dysfunction and with leakage from the corpora cavernosa as diagnosed by dynamic infusion cavernosometry were included; 78 were randomized to the training program. Prior to the study, pelvic floor exercises were demonstrated to the patients, who also underwent general muscle consciousness training to help them differentiate between abdominal, gluteal, femoral adductor, and pelvic floor muscles. Patients were also instructed in a home exercise program in the prone, sitting, and standing positions. Training was given in five once-weekly sessions and was supervised by a trained physiotherapist. In this context, the mechanism of penile erection focused on the muscular and vascular role, for increasing arterial inflow and restricting venous outflow[63–65]. The study data suggested that in mild-to-moderate cases of venous leakage, pelvic floor exercises might provide benefit and eliminate the need for surgery. However, surgical intervention was recommended for severe venous leakage cases.

SEXUAL DYSFUNCTION IN WOMEN

Female sexual response consists of a three-phase model: desire, arousal, and orgasm[66]. In female sexual function, neurotransmitter-mediated vascular smooth muscle relaxation results in increased vaginal lubrication, vaginal wall engorgement, and vaginal luminal diameter expansion, as well as increased clitoral length and diameter[67]. Female sexual dysfunction is characterized by decreased libido, vaginal dryness, pain and discomfort with intercourse, decreased genital sensation, decreased arousal, and difficulty in achieving orgasm. These dysfunctions are due to vasculogenic, neurogenic, hormonal, or psychogenic etiologies[52]. For example, atherosclerotic vascular disease can result in conditions such as insufficient vaginal engorgement and clitoral erectile syndromes.

In the rat, vaginal atrophy and decreased sexual interest often occur during menopause. It is believed that NO is involved in both of these conditions[68], as estrogen withdrawal appears to play a role in the regulation of vaginal NO synthase expression and apoptosis in nerves, smooth muscle, vascular endothelium, and epithelium of the vagina, implying an NO-related mechanism in female sexual function. As an NO precursor, L-arginine has been shown to be essential to sexual maturation in the female rat[69].

Female sexual dysfunction is a complex result of psychologic and physiologic factors and no efficacious pharmaceutical therapies are currently available. Administration of sildenafil citrate to 30 postmenopausal women did not significantly improve sexual function, although there was some increase in vaginal lubrication and clitoral sensitivity[70].

Herbal therapies

Some herbal medicines have been tested for treating sexual dysfunction in women. In a study of women with a low sex drive, yohimbine had no significant effect on improving sexual desire, although it increased plasma 3-methoxy-4-hydroxyphenylglycol, the major central nervous system metabolite of norepinephrine, to a plasma level similar to that seen in men[63,71].

In an open-label trial, ginkgo seemed efficacious in the treatment of antidepressant-induced sexual dysfunction, particularly in women[26]. In the study with 33 women and 30 men, subjects were given an average dose of 207 mg per day for 4 weeks. After 4 weeks, over 80% of women had symptom relief in antidepressant-induced sexual dysfunction. The data also showed that women were more responsive to sexually enhancing effects of gingko than men, with relative success rates of 91% versus 76%[26].

A nutritional supplement containing ginseng (30% ginseng extract), ginkgo (24% flavone glycosides, 6% terpene lactones), damiana leaf, L-arginine, along with vitamins A, B_6, B_{12}, biotin, folate, niacin, pantothenic acid, riboflavin, thiamin, antioxidant vitamins (C and E), calcium, iron, and zinc, was tested in a double-blind placebo-controlled trial for enhancement of female sexual function. The study enrolled 77 women over the age of 21 years with an interest in improving their sexual function. In these subjects, 34 received the nutritional supplement and 43 received placebo. After 4 weeks, 74% of the nutritional supplement group had improvement in satisfaction with their sex life. Notable improvements were observed in sexual desire, reduction in vaginal dryness, frequency of sexual intercourse and orgasm, and clitoral sensation without significant side-effects[72].

CONCLUSIONS

There is convincing evidence for the effectiveness of yohimbine for male erectile dysfunction from organic or non-organic causes. Comparative studies with conventional oral medication, such as sildenafil citrate, are not available at present, but it has been suggested that yohimbine is less effective but probably safer. Whether yohimbine is safe for long-term use remains to be tested in future controlled studies. There are some data supporting ginkgo's use for impotency due to arterial insufficiency and selective serotonin reuptake inhibitors. However, patients on blood thinners, such as warfarin and aspirin, should be cautious in using ginkgo as it may potentiate the blood thinning effects. Despite the huge popularity of ginseng for centuries, there is a lack of solid data to support its use for sexual concerns. Since L-arginine is a precursor to the formation of NO, it may play a role in treating male and female sexual dysfunction. Other approaches, such as hypnotherapy, although the evidence is not compelling, may be beneficial for some patients.

References

1. American Psychiatric Association. Diagnostic and Statistical Manual of Mental Disorders, 4th edn. Washington, DC: American Psychiatric Association, 1994
2. Frank E, Anderson C, Rubinstein D. Frequency of sexual dysfunction in 'normal' couples. N Engl J Med 1978; 299: 111–15
3. Spector IP, Carey MP. Incidence and prevalence of the sexual dysfunctions: a critical review of the empirical literature. Arch Sex Behav 1990; 19: 389–408
4. Rosen RC, Taylor JF, Leiblum SR, Bachmann GA. Prevalence of sexual dysfunction in women: results of a survey study of 329 women in an outpatient gynecological clinic. J Sex Marital Ther 1993; 19: 171–88
5. Laumann EO, Paik A, Rosen RC. Sexual dysfunction in the United States: prevalence and predictors. J Am Med Assoc 1999; 281: 537–44
6. Rajfer J, Aronson WJ, Bush PA, et al. Nitric oxide as a mediator of relaxation of the corpus cavernosum in response to nonadrenergic, noncholinergic neurotransmission. N Engl J Med 1992; 326: 90–4
7. Burnett AL. Role of nitric oxide in the physiology of erection. Biol Reprod 1995; 52: 485–9
8. Park K, Goldstein I, Andry C, et al. Vasculogenic female sexual dysfunction: the hemodynamic basis for vaginal engorgement insufficiency and clitoral erectile insufficiency. Int J Impot Res 1997; 9: 27–37
9. Heaton JP, Morales A, Adams MA, et al. Recovery of erectile function by the oral administration of apomorphine. Urology 1995; 45: 200–6
10. Morales A, Heaton JP, Johnston B, Adams M. Oral and topical treatment of erectile dysfunction. Present and future. Urol Clin N Am 1995; 22: 879–86
11. Boolell M, Gepi-Attee S, Gingell JC, Allen MJ. Sildenafil, a novel effective oral therapy for male erectile dysfunction. Br J Urol 1996; 78: 257–61
12. Rosen RC, Ashton AK. Prosexual drugs: empirical status of the 'new aphrodisiacs'. Arch Sex Behav 1993; 22: 521–43
13. Segraves RT, Saran A, Segraves K, Maguire E. Clomipramine versus placebo in the treatment of premature ejaculation: a pilot study. J Sex Marital Ther 1993; 19: 198–200
14. NIH. NIH Consensus Conference. Impotence. NIH Consensus Development Panel on Impotence. J Am Med Assoc 1993; 270: 83–90
15. Feldman HA, Goldstein I, Hatzichristou DG, et al. Impotence and its medical and psychosocial correlates: results of the Massachusetts Male Aging Study. J Urol 1994; 151: 54–61
16. Benet AE, Melman A. The epidemiology of erectile dysfunction. Urol Clin N Am 1995; 22: 699–709
17. Lue TF. Erectile dysfunction. N Engl J Med 2000; 342: 1802–13
18. O'Leary M. Erectile dysfunction. In Godlee F, ed. Clinical Evidence. London: BMJ Books, 1999
19. Padma-Nathan H, Giuliano F. Oral drug therapy for erectile dysfunction. Urol Clin N Am 2001; 28: 321–34
20. Segraves RT. Treatment emergent sexual dysfunction in affective disorder. J Clin Psychiatry 1993; 11: 1–4
21. Price J, Grunhaus LJ. Treatment of clomipramine-induced anorgasmia with yohimbine: a case report. J Clin Psychiatry 1990; 51: 32–3
22. Tam SW, Worcel M, Wyllie M. Yohimbine: a clinical review. Pharmacol Ther 2001; 91: 215–43
23. Welt K, Weiss J, Koch S, Fitzl G. Protective effects of Ginkgo biloba extract EGb 761 on the myocardium of experimentally diabetic rats. II. Ultrastructural and immunohistochemical investigation on microvessels and interstitium. Exp Toxicol Pathol 1999; 51: 213–22
24. Paick JS, Lee JH. An experimental study of the effect of Ginkgo biloba extract on the human and rabbit corpus cavernosum tissue. J Urol 1996; 156: 1876–80
25. Richard S, Michael S, Friedrich JD, et al. Ginkgo biloba extract in therapy for erectile dysfunction. J Urol 1989; 141: 188A
26. Cohen AJ, Bartlik B. Ginkgo biloba for antidepressant-induced sexual dysfunction. J Sex Marital Ther 1998; 24: 139–43

27. Attele AS, Wu JA, Yuan CS. Ginseng pharmacology: multiple constituents and multiple actions. Biochem Pharmacol 1999; 58: 1685–93

28. Murphy LL, Lee TJ. Ginseng, sex behavior, and nitric oxide. Ann NY Acad Sci 2002; 962: 372–7

29. Murphy LL, Cadena RS, Chavez D, Ferraro JS. Effect of American ginseng (Panax quinquefolium) on male copulatory behavior in the rat. Physiol Behav 1998; 64: 445–50

30. Vogler BK, Pittler MH, Ernst E. The efficacy of ginseng. A systematic review of randomised clinical trials. Eur J Clin Pharmacol 1999; 55: 567–75

31. Choi HK, Seong DH, Rha KH. Clinical efficacy of Korean red ginseng for erectile dysfunction. Int J Impot Res 1995; 7: 181–6

32. Chen X, Lee TJ. Ginsenosides-induced nitric oxide-mediated relaxation of the rabbit corpus cavernosum. Br J Pharmacol 1995; 115: 15–18

33. Han SW, Kim H. Ginsenosides stimulate endogenous production of nitric oxide in rat kidney. Int J Biochem Cell Biol 1996; 28: 573–80

34. Salvati G, Genovesi G, Marcellini L, et al. Effects of Panax ginseng C.A. Meyer saponins on male fertility. Panminerva Med 1996; 38: 249–54

35. Adimoelja A. Phytochemicals and the breakthrough of traditional herbs in the management of sexual dysfunctions. Int J Androl 2000; 23 (Suppl 2): 82–4

36. Moeloek N, Pangkahila W, Tanojo TD, Adimoelja A. Trials on Tribulus terrestris on idiopathic ologo-asthenoteratozoosperms. Paper presented at 6th National Congress Indonesian Society of Andrology and 3rd International Symposium of Andrology, Manado, Indonesia, 1994

37. Morales AJ, Nolan JJ, Nelson JC. Effects of replacement dose of dehydroepiandrosterone in men and women of advancing age. J Clin Endocrinol Metab 1994; 78: 1360–7

38. Foster S. Herbs and sex: separating fact from fantasy. Health Food Bus 1991; 74: 573–80

39. Zava DT, Dollbaum CM, Blen M. Estrogen and progestin bioactivity of foods, herbs, and spices. Proc Soc Exp Biol Med 1998; 217: 369–78

40. Arletti R, Benelli A, Cavazzuti E, et al. Stimulating property of Turnera diffusa and Pfaffia paniculata extracts on the sexual-behavior of male rats. Psychopharmacology (Berl) 1999; 143: 15–19

41. Bayer JR. Treatment of infertility with vitamin E. Int J Fertility 1960; 5: 70–8

42. Sandler B, Faragher B. Treatment of oligospermia with vitamin B12. Infertility 1984; 7: 133–8

43. Kumamoto Y, Maruta H, Ishigami J, et al. Clinical efficacy of mecobalamin in the treatment of oligozoospermia – results of double-blind comparative clinical study. Hinyokika Kiyo 1988; 34: 1109–32

44. Mohan H, Verma J, Singh I, et al. Inter-relationship of zinc levels in serum and semen in oligospermic infertile patients and fertile males. Ind J Pathol Microbiol 1997; 40: 451–5

45. Robinson K, Arheart K, Refsum H, et al. Low circulating folate and vitamin B_6 concentrations: risk factors for stroke, peripheral vascular disease, and coronary artery disease. European COMAC Group. Circulation 1998; 97: 437–43

46. Crimmel AS, Conner CS, Monga M. Withered Yang: a review of traditional Chinese medical treatment of male infertility and erectile dysfunction. J Androl 2001; 22: 173–82

47. Sato Y, Horita H, Adachi H, et al. Effect of oral administration of prostaglandin E_1 on erectile dysfunction. Br J Urol 1997; 80: 772–5

48. Tong YC, Hung YC, Lin SN, Cheng JT. Treatment effect of 'ryu-wei-ti-huang-wan' (a Chinese herbal prescription) on the sexual performance of male rats with streptozotocin-induced diabetes. Urol Int 1996; 57: 230–4

49. Bakircioglu ME, Hsu K, El-Sakka A, et al. Effect of a Chinese herbal medicine mixture on a rat model of hypercholesterolemic erectile dysfunction. J Urol 2000; 164: 1798–801

50. Ojha JK, Roy CK, Bajpai HS. Clinical trial of mustong on secondary sexual impotence in male married diabetics. J Med Assoc Thai 1987; 70 (Suppl 2): 228–30

51. Chen J, Wollman Y, Chernichovsky T, et al. Effect of oral administration of high-dose nitric oxide donor L-arginine in men with organic erectile dysfunction: results of a double-blind, randomized, placebo-controlled study. BJU Int 1999; 83: 269–73

52. Berman JR, Berman LA, Werbin TJ, Goldstein I. Female sexual dysfunction: anatomy, physiology, evaluation and treatment options. Curr Opin Urol 1999; 9: 563–8

53. Lebret T, Hervé J-M, Gorny P, et al. Efficacy and safety of a novel combination of L-arginine glutamate and yohimbin hydrochloride: a new oral therapy for erectile dysfunction. Eur J Clin Pharmacol 2002; 41: 608–13

54. Klotz T, Mathers MJ, Braun M, et al. Effectiveness of oral L-arginine in first-line treatment of erectile dysfunction in a controlled crossover study. Urol Int 1999; 63: 220–3

55. Aydin S, Ercan M, Caskurlu T, et al. Acupuncture and hypnotic suggestions in the treatment of non-organic male sexual dysfunction. Scand J Urol Nephrol 1997; 31: 271–4

56. Kho HG, Sweep CG, Chen X, et al. The use of acupuncture in the treatment of erectile dysfunction. Int J Impot Res 1999; 11: 41–6

57. Yaman LS, Kilic S, Sarica K, et al. The place of acupuncture in the management of psychogenic impotence. Eur Urol 1994; 26: 52–5

58. Zhu Y, Ni L. Treatment of impotence by Chinese herbs and acupuncture. J Tradit Chin Med 1997; 17: 226–37

59. Reynolds BS. Biofeedback and facilitation of erection in men with erectile dysfunction. Arch Sex Behav 1980; 9: 101–13

60. Aydin S, Odabas O, Ercan M, et al. Efficacy of testosterone, trazodone and hypnotic suggestion in the treatment of non-organic male sexual dysfunction. Br J Urol 1996; 77: 256–60

61. Lavoisier P, Proulx J, Courtois F. Reflex contractions of the ischiocavernosus muscles following electrical and pressure stimulations. J Urol 1988; 139: 396–9

62. Claes H, Baert L. Pelvic floor exercise versus surgery in the treatment of impotence. Br J Urol 1993; 71: 52–7

63. Newman HF, Northup JD. Mechanism of human penile erection: an overview. Urology 1981; 17: 399–408

64. Wagner G. Erection physiology and endocrinology. In Wagner G, Green RP, eds. Impotence: Physiological, Psychological, Surgical Diagnosis and Treatment. New York: Plenum Press, 1981

65. Junemann KP, Luo JA, Lue TF. Further evidence of venous outflow restriction during erection. Br J Urol 1986; 58: 320–4

66. Kaplan HS. The New Sex Therapy. London: Bailliere Tindall, 1974

67. Goldstein I, Berman JR. Vasculogenic female sexual dysfunction: vaginal engorgement and clitoral erectile insufficiency syndromes. Int J Impot Res 1998; 10 (Suppl 2): S84–90; discussion S98–101

68. Berman JR, McCarthy MM, Kyprianou N. Effect of estrogen withdrawal on nitric oxide synthase expression and apoptosis in the rat vagina. Urology 1998; 51: 650–6

69. Pau MY, Milner JA. Dietary arginine and sexual maturation of the female rat. J Nutr 1982; 112: 1834–42

70. Kaplan SA, Reis RB, Kohn IJ, et al. Safety and efficacy of sildenafil in postmenopausal women with sexual dysfunction. Urology 1999; 53: 481–6

71. Piletz JE, Segraves KB, Feng YZ, et al. Plasma MHPG response to yohimbine treatment in women with hypoactive sexual desire. J Sex Marital Ther 1998; 24: 43–54

72. Ito TY, Trant AS, Polan ML. A double-blind placebo-controlled study of ArginMax, a nutritional supplement for enhancement of female sexual function. J Sex Marital Ther 2001; 27: 541–9

Insomnia

22

A. S. Attele and C.-S. Yuan

INTRODUCTION

Insomnia is the most commonly reported sleep problem, not only in the United States, but also in industrialized nations worldwide. Approximately 35% of the adult population has insomnia during the course of a year[1]. Up to 17% indicate that the insomnia is chronic, severe, or both[2,3]. It currently affects more than 60 million Americans, and this figure is expected to grow to 100 million by the middle of the twenty-first century[4].

Insomnia is the subjective complaint of impaired duration, depth, or restful quality of sleep. It is characterized by one or more of the following: difficulty falling asleep, difficulty maintaining sleep, early morning wakening, and unrefreshing sleep[5,6]. It is a symptom associated with a number of medical, psychiatric, and sleep disorders. In contrast to the occasional sleepless night experienced by most people, insomnia may be a persistent or recurrent problem with serious complications such as anxiety and depression[7].

Insomnia has a significant impact on quality of life, work performance, and utilization of medical resources. Poor sleep may be associated with a perceived decrease in quality of life, an increase in physical complaints, and economic repercussions including decreased work productivity[8].

ETIOLOGY AND CLASSIFICATION

Insomnia is classified as primary or secondary, as well as acute or chronic. It occurs more frequently with aging and in women.

Primary insomnia is sleeplessness that is not attributable to a medical, psychiatric, or environmental cause. The etiology of primary insomnia relates in part to psychologic conditioning processes. Secondary insomnia is a symptom caused by medical, psychiatric,

or environmental factors[9]. In secondary insomnia the target of treatment is the underlying disorder.

Acute insomnia is often caused by emotional or physical discomfort, such as stressful life events, or medical problems of recent onset. Various substances (caffeine, nicotine, alcohol, steroids, etc.) can impair both falling asleep and staying asleep[10]. Chronic insomnia is more complex and often results from a combination of factors, including underlying physical or mental disorders. A common cause of chronic insomnia is depression. Chronic insomnia may also be due to behavioral factors, including misuse of caffeine, alcohol, shift work, and chronic stress[11].

ALTERNATIVE THERAPIES

Over-the-counter sleep aids are becoming popular as an alternative to prescription hypnotics. Surveys of young adults indicate that approximately 10% used non-prescription medications in the past year to improve sleep[12]. Patients report self-medicating with herbs, hormones, and amino acids in an effort to improve sleep and avoid the unacceptable side-effects of prescription medications. The most commonly used botanical sleep aids are valerian and hops; physiologic substances include melatonin and L-tryptophan. In addition, acupuncture and 'low-energy emission therapy' (LEET) are also utilized.

Medicinal herbs

Valerian (Valeriana officinalis)

This is a perennial plant native to Europe and Asia and naturalized in North America. The use of the rhizome and roots of *Valeriana officinalis* as an anxiolytic and sleep aid dates back 1000 years[13]. The US Food and

Drug Administration (FDA) categorizes valerian as a GRAS (generally recognized as safe) herb. It is widely used as a hypnotic and daytime sedative[14]. Commercial preparations are made from its roots, rhizomes, and stolons (horizontal stems).

Valerian contains valepotriates, valerenic acid, and unidentified aqueous constituents that may contribute to its sedative properties[15]. Valepotriates, a 0.5–2% mixture of unstable irridoid compounds, have been identified in valerian. The rhizome and root also contain 0.3–0.7% of a potent-smelling volatile oil containing bornyl acetate and the sesquiterpene derivatives of valerenic acid[14]. The proportion of these constituents can vary greatly between and within species[16]. The primary active ingredient of valerian has not been identified. It is likely that valerian's effects result from multiple constituents acting independently or synergistically.

Valerian has been shown to have sleep-inducing, anxiolytic, and tranquilizing effects in clinical trials. An earlier placebo-controlled, cross-over trial of 128 volunteers reported that 400 mg of valerian extract at bedtime led to improved sleep quality and decreased sleep latency, and reduced the number of night awakenings[17]. However, the participants of this study did not have a diagnosis of insomnia. Two other clinical studies using 400–900 mg of valerian before sleep improved insomnia[18,19]. An EEG study reported that 135 mg of aqueous, dried extract of valerian, taken three times daily, improved delta sleep and decreased stage 1 sleep[20]. In a more recent randomized, double-blind, placebo-controlled cross-over study, the researchers utilized polysomnographic techniques to objectively monitor sleep stages, sleep latency, and total sleep time. After 14 days of treatment with valerian, although sleep efficiency increased with both valerian and placebo, valerian showed significant improvement over placebo on parameters for slow-wave sleep[21]. In general, clinical studies with valerian extracts show that the mild hypnotic effects of valerian may decrease sleep latency and improve sleep quality.

Valerian extracts cause both central nervous system (CNS) depression and muscle relaxation. Sedation may result from an interaction of valerian constituents with central type A γ-aminobutryric acid (GABA) receptors[22]. Valerenic acid has been shown to inhibit enzyme-induced breakdown of GABA in the brain, resulting in sedation[23]. Aqueous extracts of the root contain appreciable amounts of GABA, which could directly cause sedation, but there is uncertainty about its availability[24]. A recent study on the GABAergic effects of valerian extract and valerenic acid on rat brainstem neuronal activity suggests that the pharmacologic effects of valer-ian extract and valerenic acid are mediated through modulation of GABA A receptor function[25].

Although valerian is effective in producing depression of the CNS, neither valepotriates nor valerenic acid have activity alone. It is possible that a combination of volatile oil, valepotriates, and other constituents is involved.

Valerian is generally recommended for the treatment of patients with mild psychophysiologic insomnia. One or two tablets or capsules (200–1000 mg *V. officinalis* root) are taken 30–60 min before bedtime[14]. While valerian has been shown to be generally safe, there are concerns about its quality and efficacy[23]. Reports on the cytotoxicity of valepotriates as well as the possible carcinogenicity of epoxide groups that act as alkylating agents warrant further investigation[26]. Patients using large doses over several years can experience serious withdrawal symptoms following abrupt discontinuation[27].

Ginseng

The effect of ginseng in the treatment of insomnia may be, at least in part, related to maintaining normal sleep and wakefulness. Of the several species of ginseng, *Panax ginseng* (Asian ginseng), *Panax quinquefolius* (American ginseng), and *Panax vietnamensis* (Vietnamese ginseng) are reported to have sleep-modulating effects[28].

Constituents of most ginseng species include ginsenosides, polysaccharides, peptides, polyacetyleinic alcohols, and fatty acids[29]. *Panax vietnamensis* contains ocotillol-type saponins, the major one being majonoside-R2 (MR2). Most pharmacologic actions of ginseng are attributed to ginsenosides[30]. Except for ginsenoside Ro, more than 20 ginsenosides that have been isolated belong to a family of steroids named steroidal saponins[31]. There is a wide variation (2–20%) in ginsenoside content of different ginseng species[32]. Furthermore, within a single species cultivated in two different locations, pharmacologic differences have been reported[32].

Ginseng has an inhibitory effect on the CNS and may modulate neurotransmission. *Panax ginseng* extract decreased the amount of wakefulness during a 12-h light period and increased the amount of slow-wave sleep[33]. Ginseng is known as an 'adaptogen', capable of normalizing physiologic disturbances. For example, *Panax ginseng* extract normalized the disturbances caused by food deprivation in sleep–waking states in rats[34]. MR2, a major ocotillol-type saponin, isolated exclusively from *Panax vietnamensis*, restored the hypnotic activity of pentobarbital that was decreased by two models of psychologic stress[35,36]. A recent double-blind study investigating the influence of ginseng on the quality of life of city dwellers revealed that a daily dose of 40 mg of ginseng extract for 12 weeks significantly improved the quality of life, including sleep[37].

There is evidence to suggest that one mechanism for the CNS-depressant action of ginseng extract and ginsenosides is via regulation of GABA-ergic neurotransmission. Ginsenosides have been reported to compete with agonists for binding to $GABA_A$ and $GABA_B$ receptors[38]. Neuronal discharge frequency in the nucleus tractus solitarius was inhibited by *Panax quinquefolius* extract[38] and the $GABA_A$ receptor agonist muscimol[32]. The reversal effect of MR2 and diazepam on the psychologic stress-induced decrease in pentobarbital sleep was antagonized by flumazenil, a selective benzodiazepine antagonist[36].

Several side-effects of ginseng have been reported. Ginseng lowers blood glucose in patients with type 2 diabetes and without diabetes[39]. Ginsenosides inhibit platelet aggregation *in vitro* and in laboratory rats, and prolong both coagulation time of thrombin and activated thromboplastin[40]. The most commonly reported side-effects are nervousness and excitation, but these diminish with continued use or dosage reduction[37].

The recommended daily dose is 1–2 g of the crude root, or 200–600 mg of extracts[41]. As the possibility of hormone-like or hormone-inducing effects cannot be ruled out, some authors suggest limiting treatment to 3 months of extracts[41].

Kava kava (Piper methysticum)

Kava kava or kava is a large shrub cultivated in the Pacific islands. Therapeutically, the rhizome of this herb is used to treat anxiety, stress, and restlessness[41], the underlying causes of insomnia.

The CNS activity of kava is due to a group of resinous compounds known as kavalactones and kavapyrones. Sedative, anticonvulsive, antispasmodic, and central muscular relaxant effects are attributed to kava[42]. While the underlying mechanism is not entirely clear, it is possible that kava acts on GABA and benzodiazepine-binding sites in the brain[42]. A recent meta-analysis of double-blind, randomized, placebo-controlled trials reported that kava extract was superior to placebo as a symptomatic treatment for anxiety[43]. Several relatively short-term clinical studies have also provided favorable evidence that kava is effective in treating anxiety and insomnia[44].

As a sleep aid, 180–210 mg of kavalactones are recommended daily[41]. It is important to note that ethanol and other CNS depressants can potentiate the effects of kava[45].

Passion flower (Passiflora incarnata)

The herb consists of the dried flowering and fruiting top of a perennial climbing vine (family Passifloraceae) (Figure 22.1). While studies proving its effectiveness are lacking, it has been traditionally used for insomnia[16]. Active components of passion flower may be harmala-type indole alkaloids, maltol and ethyl-maltol, and flavonoids[46]. When administered intraperitoneally to rats, passion flower extract significantly prolonged sleeping time[47]. The principal flavonoid, chrysin, was demonstrated to have benzodiazepine-receptor activity.

The usual daily dose is 4–8 g taken as a tea[41]. Since harmala compounds are uterine stimulants, passion flower extract is not recommended in pregnant women. Reports on the side-effects of passion flower are lacking.

Hops (Humulus lupulus)

The dried strobile with its glandular trichomes of *Humulus lupulus* is a popular sleep aid. Hops has been used for centuries in the treatment of intestinal ailments, but its use as a sedative–hypnotic is more recent. Active ingredients in hops include a volatile oil, valerianic acid, estrogenic substances, tannins, and flavonoids[45]. The

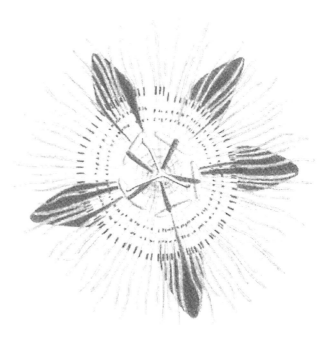

Figure 22.1 The passion flower, *Passiflora incarnata*

sedative effects of hops have been demonstrated to induce sleep.

The use of hops for insomnia as an infusion in tea was reported to have a calming effect within 20–40 min of ingestion[48]. The recommended dose is 0.5 g of the dried herb, or its equivalent in extract-based products, taken one to several times daily[41]. Side-effects are uncommon, and large doses have been ingested safely. It is not recommended for pregnant women or women with estrogen-dependent breast cancer[48]. The use of hops is generally regarded to be safe by the FDA[45].

Physiologic agents

Melatonin

Melatonin, a hormone secreted by the pineal gland, is considered to be a remedy for insomnia caused by circadian schedule changes, such as jet lag and shift work[49]. Rapid travel across several time zones results in a desynchronization between intrinsic human circadian rhythm and the local environmental photoperiod. The severity and duration of the resulting sleep disturbance vary, depending on the number of time zones crossed, direction of travel, departure time, and age. A clinical study with flight-crew members who completed a 9-day New Zealand–Los Angeles–England round trip reported that subjects who received melatonin only after arrival had significantly less jet lag overall[50].

Night-shift workers, during their nights off, have problems falling asleep. Folkard *et al.*[51] reported that melatonin increased sleep quality compared with baseline and placebo in night-shift workers. Melatonin has also been shown to have a beneficial effect on the quality of sleep for elderly patients with insomnia[52]. Delayed sleep phase syndrome, a circadian rhythm disorder, is a chronic condition characterized by the persistent inability to fall asleep and rise at conventional times. A randomized, double-blind, placebo-controlled, cross-over study showed that a 4-week treatment with melatonin decreased sleep onset latency without altering sleep architecture[53]. Adverse effects of melatonin most commonly reported in the clinical trials include sedation, headache, depression, tachycardia and pruritus[54].

Variable melatonin dosages (0.3–5 mg) and drug timing administrations have been studied[55], but the optimal effective dosing is still unclear. The exact means by which melatonin induces its soporific effects have not been fully elucidated. It has been suggested that the hypothermic action of melatonin may underlie its soporific effects[56], but as yet only a temporal relationship

between increased melatonin levels, decreased core temperature, and initiation of sleep has been demonstrated. However, a randomized, placebo-controlled, cross-over clinical trial with the melatonin agonist β-methyl-6-chloromelatonin showed a direct soporific effect[57]. A randomized, double-blind, placebo-controlled study that assessed the toxic effects of 10 mg melatonin for 28 days reported that, while there was a significant reduction of stage 1 sleep, there were no toxicologic effects that might compromise the use of melatonin[58].

L-Tryptophan and 5-hydroxytryptophan

L-Tryptophan and 5-hydroxytryptophan are precursors of 5-hydroxytryptamine (serotonin). Experimental data and clinical observations indicate that the serotonergic system plays an important role in sleep regulation. Pharmacologic manipulations in humans and animals, that have affected the serotonergic system, have resulted in profound alterations in sleep[59]. However, the precise role of the serotonergic system in sleep regulation is not fully understood.

L-Tryptophan is an essential amino acid that occurs in plants and animals in concentrations of 1–2%. A dose of 1 g of L-tryptophan has been reported to reduce sleep latency by increasing subjective 'sleepiness' and also decreasing waking time[60]. It may function by increasing serotonin in certain brain cells, thus inducing sleep. Although never approved as a drug, L-tryptophan was widely sold as a sleep aid in health-food stores until 1989. That year, following the deaths of 37 healthy people of eosinophilia–myalgia syndrome after consuming contaminated L-tryptophan, the FDA recalled the product[16].

5-Hydroxytryptophan, the immediate precursor of serotonin, is still being used as a sleep aid. A daily dose of 100 mg/day was found to increase slow-wave sleep[61]. Its clinical efficacy has yet to be confirmed by controlled therapeutic studies.

Others

Acupuncture

Acupuncture is best known in the USA as an alternative therapy for chronic pain. However, in Traditional Chinese Medicine, it is commonly employed for the treatment of insomnia. There are numerous publications in Chinese on the use of acupuncture for insomnia. The literature cited in this review, however, is restricted to articles in English.

Clinical reports on acupuncture therapy verify its efficacy in the treatment of insomnia in psychiatric patients[62,63]. Controlled, clinical trials demonstrating acupuncture's effect on insomnia are rare. Many studies provide only subjective evaluations of sleep. Since acupuncture is an individualized treatment, controlled studies are difficult to execute.

Using scalp, body, and ear acupuncture points, positive effects appeared almost immediately after treatment[63]. The mechanisms by which acupuncture treatment modulates insomnia may be understood in terms of the general mechanism by which it produces analgesia. In addition, acupuncture treatment increased nocturnal melatonin secretion and reduced insomnia and anxiety[64]. Additional clinical studies are necessary to elucidate how acupuncture can reharmonize a disturbed sleep–wake cycle.

Low-energy emission therapy

LEET is a method of delivering low levels of amplitude-modulated radio-frequency electromagnetic fields to humans. The LEET device consists of a signal generator, microprocessor, and amplifier. The signal generator is connected to a mouthpiece, which is held between the tongue and palate for the duration of the treatment[65]. Results of some investigations have suggested that LEET may be a potential alternative therapy for chronic insomnia that is refractory to conventional treatment. In healthy volunteers, 15 min of LEET treatment induced EEG changes, and was associated with objective and subjective feelings of relaxation[66]. A double-blind, placebo-controlled study showed that 12 LEET treatments over a 4-week period improved the sleep of chronic insomniacs[67].

The mechanism underlying the effect of LEET is poorly understood. Low levels of electromagnetic field, such as those to which the brain is exposed during LEET, affect *in vitro* and *in vivo* calcium release from neural cells[68], modify the release of GABA, and change benzodiazepine receptor concentration in rat brains[69]. In addition, low levels of electromagnetic field modify the release of melatonin in mammals[65]. So far, the administration of LEET treatment is confined to sleep-disorder centers. Unlike conventional therapies, LEET may be administered on an every-other-day basis, and discontinuation does not appear to induce rebound insomnia[67]. LEET therapy-related side-effects have not been reported.

CONCLUSIONS

Insomnia is the most common sleep disorder. It is often associated with significant medical, psychologic and social disturbances. The inability to attain restful sleep in adequate amounts exacts a heavy toll. Conventional treatment for insomnia includes psychologic therapy and drugs that exert a depressant effect on the CNS. Most of the drugs prescribed for insomnia involve some risk of overdose, tolerance, and addiction. Long-term use of frequently prescribed medications can lead to habituation and problematic withdrawal symptoms. As alternative therapies, herbal products and other agents with sedative–hypnotic effects are increasingly sought after by the general population. The herbs commonly used for their sedative–hypnotic effects are less likely to have the drawbacks of conventional drugs. How alternative therapies compare to conventional therapies warrants further investigation.

References

1. Quan SF. SLEEP year in review 2003 – insomnia, sleep in psychiatric disorders, periodic limb movement disorder/restless legs syndrome, sleep in medical disorders. Sleep 2004; 27: 1205–8

2. Johnson EO, Roehrs T, Roth T, Breslau N. Epidemiology of alcohol and medication as aids to sleep in early adulthood. Sleep 1998; 21: 178–86

3. Stoller MK. Economic effects of insomnia. Clin Ther 1994; 16: 873–97

4. Hossain JL, Shapiro CM. The prevalence, cost implications, and management of sleep disorders: an overview. Sleep Breathing 2002; 6: 85–102

5. Walsh JK, Benca RM, Bonnet M, et al. Insomnia: assessment and management in primary care. Am Family Physician 1999; 59: 3029–38

6. Vgontzas AN, Kales A. Sleep and its disorders. Annu Rev Med 1999; 50: 387–400

7. Mendelson WB. Long-term follow-up of chronic insomnia. Sleep 1995; 18: 698–701

8. Leger D, Guilleminault C, Bader G, et al. Medical and socio-professional impact of insomnia. Sleep 2002; 25: 625–9

9. Eddy M, Walbroehl GS. Insomnia. Am Fam Physician 1999; 59: 1911–15

10. Sharpley AL, Cowen PJ. Effect of pharmacologic treatments on the sleep of depressed patients. Biol Psychiatry 1995; 37: 85–8

11. Sateia MJ, Doggramji K, Hauri PJ, et al. Evaluation of chronic insomnia. Sleep 2000; 23: 243–50

12. Johnson EO, Roehrs T, Roth T, Breslau N. Epidemiology of alcohol and medication as aids to sleep in early adulthood. Sleep 1998; 21: 178–86

13. Foster S, Tyler VE. Valerian. In Roberts JE, Tyler VE, eds. Tyler's Honest Herbal. New York, NY: Haworth Press, 1999: 377–8

14. Wagner J, Wagner ML, Hening WA. Beyond benzodiazepines: alternative pharmacologic agents for the treatment of insomnia. Ann Pharmacother 1998; 32: 680–91

15. Castleman M. The Healing Herbs: The Ultimate Guide to the Curative Power of Nature's Medicines. Emmaus, PA: Rodale Press, 1991

16. Robbers JE, Tyler VE. Nervous system disorders. In Roberts JE, Tyler VE, eds. Tyler's Herbs of Choice. New York, NY: Haworth Press, 1999: 154–7

17. Leathwood PD, Chauffard F, Heck E, Munoz-Box R. Aqueous extract of valerian root (Valeriana offiinalis L.) improves sleep quality in man. Pharmacol Biochem Behav 1982; 17: 65–71

18. Leathwood PD, Chauffard F. Aqueous extract of valerian reduces latency to fall asleep in man. Planta Med 1985; 51: 144–8

19. Lindahl O, Lindwall L. Double blind study of a valerian preparation. Pharmacol Biochem Behav 1989; 32: 1065–6

20. Schulz H, Stolz C, Muller J. The effect of valerian extract on sleep polygraphy in poor sleepers: a pilot study. Pharmacopsychiatry 1994; 27: 147–51

21. Donath F, Quispe S, Diefenbach K, et al. Critical evaluation of the effects of valerian extract on sleep structure and sleep quality. Pharmacopsychiatry 2000; 33: 47–53

22. Mennini T, Bernasconi P, Bombardelli E, Morazzoni P. In vitro study on the interaction of extracts and pure compounds from Valeriana officinalis roots with GABA, benzodiazepine and barbiturate receptors in rat brain. Fitoterapia 1993; 64: 291–300

23. Houghton PJ. The scientific basis for the reputed activity of valerian. J Pharm Pharmacol 1999; 51: 505–12

24. Santos MS, Ferreira F, Faro C, et al. The amount of GABA present in aqueous extracts of valerian is sufficient to account for [3H]GABA release in synaptosomes. Planta Med 1994; 60: 2475–6

25. Yuan CS, Mehendale S, Xiao Y, et al. The gamma-aminobutyric acidergic effects of valerian and valerenic acid on rat brainstem neuronal activity. Anesthes Analges 2004; 98: 353–8

26. Tortarolo M, Braun R, Hubner GE, Maurer HR. In vitro effects of epoxide-bearing valepotriates on mouse early hematopoietic progenitor cells and human T-lymphocytes. Arch Toxicol 1982; 51: 37–42

27. Garges HP, Varia I, Doraiswamy PM. Cardiac complications and delirium associated with valerian root withdrawal [letter]. J Am Med Assoc 1998; 280: 1566–7

28. Attele AS, Wu JA, Yuan CS. Multiple pharmacological effects of ginseng. Biochem Pharmacol 1999; 58: 1685–93

29. Lee FC. Facts about Ginseng, the Elixir of Life. Elizabeth, NJ: Hollyn International, 1992

30. Huang KC. The Pharmacology of Chinese Herbs. Boca Raton, FL: CRC Press, 1999

31. Kim YS, Kim DS, Kim SI. Ginsenoside Rh2 and Rh3 induce differentiation of HL-60 cells into granulocytes: modulation of protein kinase C isoforms during differentiation by ginsenoside Rh2. Int J Biochem Cell Biol 1998; 30: 327–38

32. Yuan CS, Wu JA, Lowell T, Gu M. Gut and brain effects of American ginseng root on brainstem neuronal activities in rats. Am J Chin Med 1998; 26: 47–55

33. Rhee YH, Lee SP, Honda K, Inoue S. Panax ginseng extract modulates sleep in unrestrained rats. Psychopharmacol 1990; 101: 486–8

34. Lee SP, Honda K, Rhee YH, Inoue S. Chronic intake of Panax ginseng extract stabilizes sleep and wakefulness in food-deprived rats. Neurosci Lett 1990; 111: 217–21

35. Huong NTT, Matsumoto K, Yamasaki K, Watanabe H. Majonoside-R2 reverses social isolation stress-induced decrease in pentobarbital sleep in mice: possible involvement of neuroactive steroids. Life Sci 1997; 61: 395–402

36. Huong NTT, Matsumoto K, Watanabe H. The antistress effect of majonoside-R2, a major saponin component of Vietnamese ginseng: neuronal mechanism of action. Meth Find Exp Clin Pharmacol 1998; 20: 65–76

37. Marasco AC, Ruiz RV, Villagomex AS, Infante CB. Double-blind study of a multivitamin complex supplemented with ginseng extract. Drugs Exp Clin Res 1996; 22: 323–9

38. Kimura T, Saunders PA, Kim HS, et al. Interactions of ginsenosides with ligand-bindings of GABAA and GABAB receptors. Gen Pharm 1994; 25: 193–9

39. Vuksan V, Sievenpiper JL, Koo VY, et al. American ginseng (Panax quinquefolius L) reduces postprandial glycemia in nondiabetic subjects and subjects with type 2 diabetes mellitus. Arch Intern Med 2000; 160: 1009–13

40. Park HJ, Lee JH, Song YB, Park KH. Effects of dietary supplementation of lipophilic fraction from Panax ginseng on cGMP and cAMP in rat platelets and on blood coagulation. Biol Pharm Bull 1996; 19: 1434–9

41. Schulz V, Hansel R, Tyler VE. Rational phytotherapy. In Hansel R, Schulz V, eds. Agents that Increase Resistance to Diseases. New York, NY: Springer-Verlag, 1998: 269–72

42. Singh YN. Kava: an overview. J Ethnopharmacol 1992; 37: 38

43. Davies LP, Drew CA, Duffield P, et al. Kava pyrones and resin: studies on GABAA, and GABAB, and benzodiazepine binding sites in rodent brain. Pharmacol Toxicol 1992; 71: 120

44. Pittler MH, Edzard E. Efficacy of kava extract for treating anxiety: systematic review and meta-analysis. J Clin Psychopharmacol 2000; 20: 84–9

45. Murray MT. The Healing Power of Herbs, 2nd edn. Rocklin, CA: Prima Publishing, 1995: 210–19

46. Miller LG, Murrey WJ. Herbal medications, nutraceuticals, and anxiety and depression. In Herbal Medicine: A Clinician's Guide. New York, NY: Pharmaceutical Products Press, 1998: 211–12

47. Speroni E, Minghetti A. A neuropharmacological activity of extracts from Passiflora incarnata. Planta Med 1988; 54: 488–91

48. Mowrey DB. The Scientific Validation of Herbal Medicine. New Canaan, CT: Keats Publishing, 1986

49. Chase JE, Gidal BE. Melatonin: therapeutic use in sleep disorders. Ann Pharmacother 1997; 31: 1218–26

50. Petrie K, Dawson AG, Thompson L, Brook R. A double-blind trial of melatonin as a treatment for jet lag in international cabin crew. Biol Psychiatry 1993; 33: 526–30

51. Folkard S, Arendt J, Clark M. Can melatonin improve shift workers' tolerance of the night shift? Some preliminary findings. Chronobiol Int 1993; 10: 315–20

52. Garfunkel D, Laundon M, Nof D, Zisapel N. Improvement of sleep quality in elderly people by controlled release of melatonin. Lancet 1990; 346: 541–3

53. Kayumov L, Brown G, Jindal R, et al. A randomized, double-blind, placebo-controlled crossover study of the effect of exogenous melatonin on delayed sleep-phase syndrome. Psychosom Med 2001; 63: 40–8

54. Haimov I, Laudon M, Zisapel N, et al. Sleep disorders and melatonin rhythms in elderly people. Br Med J 1994; 309: 167

55. Chase JE, Gidal BE. Melatonin: therapeutic use in sleep disorders. Ann Pharmacother 1997; 31: 1218–26

56. Cajochem C, Krauchi K, Wirz-Justice A. Role of melatonin in the regulation of human circadian rhythms and sleep. J Neuroendocrinol 2003; 15: 432–7

57. Zemlan FP, Mulchahey J, Scharf MB, et al. The efficacy and safety of the melatonin agonist β-methyl-6-chloromelatonin in primary insomnia: a randomized, placebo-controlled, crossover clinical trial. J Clin Psychiatry 2005; 66: 384–90

58. de Lourdes M, Seabra V, Bignotto M, et al. Randomized, double-blind clinical trial, controlled with placebo, of the toxicology of chronic melatonin treatment. J Pineal Res 2000; 29: 193–200

59. Adriene J. The serotonergic system and sleep–wakefulness regulation. In Kales A, ed. The Pharmacology of Sleep. Berlin: Springer Verlag, 1995: 91–116

60. Reynolds JEF. Martindale: The Extra Pharmacopoeia, 31st edn. London: Royal Pharmaceutical Society of Great Britain, 1996: 336–7

61. Soulairac A, Lambinet H. The effects of 5-hydroxy-tryptophan, a precursor of serotonin, on sleep disorder. Ann Med Psychol (Paris) 1977; 1: 792–7

62. Shi ZX, Tan MZ. An analysis of the therapeutic effect of acupuncture in 500 cases of schizophrenia. J Tradit Chin Med 1986; 6: 99

63. Romoli M, Giommi A. Ear acupuncture in psychosomatic medicine: the importance of Sanjiao (triple heater) area. Acupunct Electrother Res 1993; 18: 185–94

64. Spence DW, Kayumov L, Chen A, et al. Acupuncture increases nocturnal melatonin secretion and reduces insomnia and anxiety: a preliminary report. J Neuropsychiatry Clin Neurosci 2004; 16: 19–28

65. Reiter RS. Electromagnetic fields and melatonin production. Biomed Pharmacother 1993; 51: 394–403

66. Higgs L, Reite M, Barbault A. Subjective and objective relaxation effects of low energy emission therapy. Stress Med 1994; 10: 5–14

67. Pasche B, Erman M, Hayduk R, et al. Effects of low energy emission therapy in chronic psychophysiological insomnia. Sleep 1996; 19: 327–36

68. Blackman CF. Calcium release from nervous tissue: experimental results and possible mechanisms. In Norden B, Ramel C, eds. Interaction Mechanisms of Low-level Electromagnetic Fields in Living Systems. Oxford: Oxford University Press, 1992: 107–29

69. Lai H, Corino MA, Horita A, Guy AW. Single vs repeated microwave exposure: effects on benzodiazepine receptors in the brain of the rat. Bioelectromagnetics 1992; 13: 57–66

Natural products and cancer

23

W. Sampson

DEFINITIONAL AND HISTORICAL PROBLEMS OF HERBAL THERAPIES IN CANCER

Some questions of definition arise when considering the roles of herbs and other natural substances in cancer. First, natural products may be sources for specific chemical compounds, which may be extracted and used in purified form. Other natural substances may be consumed as a tea, the rough equivalent of an aqueous extract. Others are consumed whole, as foods, in the normal diet. Some whole foods are wild species, but most modern food varieties have been cultivated, selected and bred over centuries for qualities of taste and appearance. Cultivated varieties may or may not be considered 'natural'. For purposes here, all plant foods and herbs are considered, but only those of considerable interest are described in detail.

Many differentiate herbs from other natural products. According to the *Random House College Dictionary*, an herb is 'a flowering plant whose stem above ground does not become woody' and 'such a plant valued for its medicinal properties, flavor, scent…'. Some authors include the property of being an annual plant. It is implied that the herb plant is not a common food source, and is not commonly known to be particularly toxic – at least in its folklore. Taste and trial and error over millennia probably eliminated many toxic plants from medicinal use.

Most would consider an herb to be taken in small quantities for either medicinal purpose or to impart flavor. This chapter considers relations of cancer to herbs, whole foods, and specific products derived from them.

NATURAL PRODUCT HISTORICAL PERSPECTIVE

Most traditional uses as recorded in standard references were for conditions no longer common, or for which the definitions have been changed, for instance, the disorders quinsy, erysipelas, and inflammatory rheumatism. Some disorders, such as smallpox and polio, have been practically eliminated, and the frequency of rheumatic fever has been markedly diminished. Some conditions, such as systemic lupus and other autoimmune disorders, were not recognized or accurately defined a century ago. Pernicious (megaloblastic) anemia was found to have three or four different causes, and those not due to vitamin B_{12} deficiency have been renamed and have different specific treatments.

Until one and a half centuries ago, cancer was identifiable in life only through changes visible on the body surface. Internal cancers were unknown before formal body dissections were carried out in the sixteenth century, and leukemias were not classified until the twentieth century. Diagnoses were made on gross appearance only – the microscope and tissue slides not being in common use until the 1800s. Radiographs appeared in the twentieth century. Traditional diagnoses were frequently erroneous or lacked relevance to modern classification, and some were based mainly on symptoms. Therefore, traditional observations of herb and natural product effects were also erroneous or are irrelevant to modern disease concepts.

In addition, older uses were based on almost uniformly faulty observations. Spontaneous recovery from self-limited illness was often misinterpreted as caused by whichever herb or other remedy was applied at the time.

This mistaken attribution is a common source of error made by unsystematic observation.

Finally, controlled clinical trials were not routinely performed until after World War II, and many refinements have been made only in the past two decades. All of these considerations have rendered traditional uses close to meaningless. The historical conclusion, then, is that there is little to no rational historical foundation on which to base any human study, which in turn makes it unlikely for new controlled trials to uncover significant effects of traditional herbs and plants. Endpoints for controlled trials on traditional natural products are essentially equal to randomly chosen ones. Most meaningful studies will have been devised from modern understanding of herb and plant components, or on recently discovered properties such as antioxidant, enzyme-inhibiting, or enzyme-inducing properties, or neutralizing of pathways of cell differentiation, growth, and apoptosis.

PRINCIPLES OF CANCER

General principles regarding the nature of cancer also set limits on the possibilities for treatment with natural substances. First, cancer cells closely resemble normal cells from the tissue from which they are derived. This fact makes it unlikely that any particular substance would have an effect on cancer cells markedly different from that on normal cells. In fact, most anticancer agents have a narrow therapeutic ratio, meaning that the dosage difference between the desired anticancer effect and undesirable or toxic effects is quite small. Doses have to be carefully drawn, and unwanted effects monitored (hence the poor reputation of anticancer chemotherapy even with purified, standardized materials). The use of raw, impure, and combined materials, with variable and uncontrollable contents, has potential for producing more harm than good. Natural substances do not contain any beneficent or other property that confers special qualities of effectiveness in cancer.

Since cancer cell metabolism differs only slightly and in special circumstances from normal cell metabolism, substances necessary for normal cell growth are also necessary for cancer cell growth. This principle makes it possible for any natural herb or food substance even to stimulate cancer cell growth.

The complexities of natural substances magnify the problems. Some natural substances interfere with pharmaceuticals by several different mechanisms. Some, such as St John's wort, induce enzymes (e.g. cytochrome P450) that metabolize drugs, causing the drugs to be removed more rapidly from circulation. This mechanism is responsible for the diminished effect of cyclosporin, an immune suppressant used in organ transplants and in autoimmune diseases, and of protease inhibitors in HIV disease.

Other substances reduce the effectiveness of those enzymes, thus increasing the amount of circulating drug, as in the interaction between grapefruit and statin drugs for cholesterol lowering. Other substances displace drugs from circulating binding proteins, releasing free drug, thus increasing the activity. Many substances displace warfarin, increasing the concentration of free drug, causing that anticoagulant's dosage to be difficult to control. On the other hand, vitamin K in the diet counters the effects of warfarin. Not much is known about botanical interactions with anticancer medications.

Herbal contents vary depending on several factors. All plant contents vary according to season or time of year of planting; time of harvest; soil, moisture, heat and sun conditions; conditions of manufacture; conditions of storage; length of storage; and degree of insect, mold, and bacterial infestation. One method attempting to create more consistency is being developed at the University of Guelph, through cloning of plant cells and using constant growing conditions[1].

Because of lax oversight, contamination and adulteration are a source of morbidity, as illustrated by the epidemic of renal failure in hundreds of Belgian women who took a Chinese herbal tea for weight loss. The herbal mixture contained the wrong herb, mistakenly substituted for another because of similar sounding names. Many of the women later developed renal pelvis cancers[2]. Another type of contamination, adulteration, probably occurred in the herbal mixture PC-SPES, in which added pharmaceuticals were found to be responsible for its anticancer actions (described below.) Often, the particular active materials are unknown, further complicating evaluation.

In regard to increasing resistance or anticancer immunity, no such activity has been described as being due to a natural product, despite references to such properties in some of the literature on natural products. In fact, no material, natural or synthetic, has properties of increasing any form of host resistance to cancer. This is an important principle to keep in mind, as several herbs such as echinacea and ginseng (*Panax*) as well as other substances have been used for presumed stimulation of the immune system or other unspecified form of resistance.

Nevertheless, a number of whole herbal and whole plant materials have been proposed as treatments for cancer. None of them has succeeded in clinical trials, or has been shown to have enough activity in experimental animal or tissue culture systems to warrant further investigation in human trials.

Some products proposed as active cancer-fighting agents are echinacea, evening primrose oil, St John's wort, and turmeric[3]. Another reference lists 32 botanicals that have been proposed or have been studied for their effect on cancer[4].

Whole herbal and other natural plant materials have been proposed as cancer preventives based largely on antioxidant qualities (Table 23.1).

Others have been proposed as having anticancer, antiproliferative activity. The evidence for antioxidant activity is adequate for some, but antioxidant activity is limited to a preventive role (Table 23.2).

As mentioned, the products were selected mainly because of known or presumed antioxidant properties. However, there is no known activity of antioxidants on established cancers, and there is no plausible mechanism for such action. Therefore, it is not surprising that researchers have not found herbs to have activity against established human cancer. One should note that antioxidant natural products can neutralize effects of anticancer agents such as bleomycin and alkylating agents, actions of which depend partially on their oxidant properties.

DIETARY APPROACHES

Soy-based diets

Soy is the focus of study because of the lower incidence of breast and other cancers (prostate, colon) in Asian countries, where soy is a major component of many diets. Observational studies of diets in different cultures show a negative correlation between soy-containing diets

Table 23.1 Herbal remedies with antioxidant qualities

Adrographis (*Andrographis panniculus*)
Arnica (*Arnica montana*)
Bilberry fruit (*Chelidonium majus*)
Ginseng (*Panax ginseng*)
Licorice (*Glycyrrhiza*)
Melilotus (*Melilotus officinalis*)
Pau d'arco

Table 23.2 Evidence for effects of herbal remedies

Botanical	Claimed action	Evidence (quality)
Aloe	marrow stimulation	none
	anticancer	none
Astragalus	anticancer	none
Barberry	marrow stimulation	none
	anticancer	none
Beetroot	anticancer	none
	'detoxification'	none
Bromelain	anticancer	none
Burdock	anticancer	none
Chapparal	anticancer	none
Chlorella	anticancer	none
Cottonseed	anticancer	none
Essiac	anticancer	none
Garlic	anticancer	none
	antioxidant (adequate)	some
Goldenseal	marrow stimulation	none
	anticancer	none
Green tea	antioxidant (prevention)	conflicting
	anticancer	none
Hoxsey formula	anticancer	none
Milk thistle	anti-liver toxicity	poor
	anticancer	none
Mistletoe	anticancer	none
Noni juice	marrow stimulation	none
	anticancer	none
Pau d'arco	anticancer	none
PC-SPES	anticancer (prostate)	none
Soy	anticancer (breast, prevention)	some (adequate)
Red clover	anticancer	none
Saw palmetto	anticancer (prostate)	poor
Siberian ginseng	anticancer	none
Turmeric	antioxidant	some
	anticancer	none
Wheatgrass	'detoxification'	none
	anticancer	none

and breast cancer incidence. Studies on soy-based diets show that soy may have an inhibitory effect on breast cancer generation if the diet is consumed from an early age. There is no good evidence that a soy diet affects an established cancer.

Isoflavones, genistein

Isoflavones and lignans are subtypes of phytoestrogens. Genistein, one of the isoflavones, is abundant in many legumes, especially soybeans.

Studies on phytoestrogens range from comparative observational studies on the diets of whole populations, analyses of the proportions of isoflavones and soy, to studies of isoflavones and specific compounds such as genistein in animals and cells. Phytoestrogens may, like other hormone analogs and response modifiers such as tamoxifen and raloxifene, demonstrate either mild estrogenic activity or inhibitory activity, depending on the conditions of the experiment, the clinical situation, the target tissue and perhaps the types and amounts of other isoflavonoids in the diet. Activity is difficult to predict, and must be determined by observation and experiment.

Studies on genistein in animal breast cancers and on breast cancer cells show a complex of actions. Some studies show a negative influence on cancer incidence, but a few show stimulation of established breast cancer cells[5]. The genistein precursor genistin also shows stimulation of breast cancer cell growth[6].

In males, phytoestrogens have an antitestosterone action, as might be anticipated from the mild estrogenic activity of these compounds. Substrates of lignans and isoflavonoid phytoestrogens inhibit the conversion of testosterone to dihydrotestosterone, and inhibit 5α-reductase activity[7].

Overall, the anticarcinogenic mechanisms of dietary genistein and soy products seem to predominate, favoring some degree of breast cancer prevention, possibly if the diet is begun before maturity. It is uncertain whether effects are due directly to soy or to reduced intake of other carcinogen-containing foods. Evidence is incomplete for prevention of other cancers. Evidence warrants caution in the presence of established breast cancer, especially estrogen and progesterone receptor-positive tumor[8].

A few studies have tried to assess the value of vegetable- and fruit-based diets in established cancer. One such study used a vegetable mixture plus herbs, and claimed to have shown increased survival in lung cancer. However, these claims were based on a non-randomized, small number of subjects, with the treatment group affected by one long-term survivor[9].

At the same time, researchers in nutrition and biochemistry are discovering specific food component compounds and their mechanisms of cancer prevention. At this point in time, most authorities agree that a few simple actions can optimize the reduction in likelihood of cancer development. They involve a diet predominantly of grains, leafy and pigmented vegetables and fruits, especially tomato products and cruciferous vegetables, moderate fish and meat intake, and minimizing intake of charcoal-broiled meats. No known supplement adds to the effects of this simple dietary approach.

NATURAL SUBSTANCES IDENTIFIED WITH ANTICARCINOGENIC ACTIONS

Carotenes

Carotenoids are pigment compounds that have antioxidant and other chemical properties, and are found mainly in vegetables and fruits. Beta-carotene is a precursor of vitamin A. Because of its antioxidant property and because foods containing it were associated negatively with cancer incidence, beta-carotene supplements were tested prospectively. Several studies found paradoxically that cancer incidence increased with carotene supplementation, especially in smokers[10]. The mechanisms for these results are not known, although some antioxidants act as pro-oxidants under some circumstances (see ascorbate, below).

In addition, in ferrets, whose cellular processes closely resemble those of humans, there is evidence of changes in other intracellular processes. Daily pharmacologic doses of beta-carotene reduced (beneficial) levels of retinoic acid, and the retinoic acid receptor-beta declined in lung tissues. Indicators of cell proliferation (gene products) increased. Lung tissues showed precancerous squamous metaplasia that increased with added daily exposure to cigarette smoke[11]. These changes might help explain the increase in cancer incidence in the human beta-carotene trials.

Lycopenes

Lycopenes are carotenoids also found in red and yellow vegetables, especially in tomatoes. The amount of available lycopene is increased by cooking and the richest sources are in tomato paste. In a prospective controlled trial, prostate cancer patients preparing for surgery received 3 weeks of lycopene supplement and at surgery showed reduced cancer markers and microscopic evidence of cell regression and apoptosis when compared to controls[12]. This treatment period seems short for the surprising amount of changes found.

Lycopene blood levels were inversely correlated with breast cancer as well[13]. As with other findings on botanic approaches, such intriguing results have to be verified. Other carotenes, such as lutein, have not been tested extensively.

Cruciferous plants and sulforaphane

Other classes of fruits and vegetables have become objects of study. Population studies seem to point to the genus *Brassica* of the Crucifera family (broccoli and cauliflower) as cancer inhibitors. The search began for agents that neutralize highly reactive oxygen free radicals, natural carcinogens, and chemicals resulting from oxidant processes, and resulted in finding large amounts of isothiocyanates, especially sulforaphane.

Instead of directly neutralizing oxygen and other free radicals, the isothiocyanate compounds were found in a variety of animal models to work indirectly. Two mechanisms are involved. First, they inhibit phase 1 enzymes involved in carcinogen activation. Second, they induce enzymes that accelerate the inactivation or metabolism of carcinogens (phase 2 enzymes).

These isothiocyanates have variable potencies as enzyme inducers, depending partly on their intracellular concentrations and area under the curve (integral of concentration and duration of presence)[14].

The matter is further complicated because of natural compounds in brassica vegetables that themselves act as inducers or promoters of carcinogenesis. Indole glucosinolates, which predominate in the mature vegetable, may give rise to degradation products (e.g. indole-3-carbinol) that can enhance tumorigenesis[15].

Small quantities of cruciferous sprouts may protect against the risk of cancer as effectively as much larger quantities of mature vegetables of the same variety. In a series of experiments on plants of various ages, Talalay and his group found that 3-day-old sprouts of cultivars of broccoli and cauliflower contained 10–100 times higher levels of glucoraphanin (the glucosinolate of sulforaphane) than did the corresponding mature plants[16]. This finding has launched a search for methods to prolong high quantities of sulforaphane in mature plants.

Curcumin

These are a lesser known series of naturally occurring compounds, derived from plants of the ginger family.

They are also inducers of phase 2 enzymes. A number of natural and synthetic structural analogs of the dietary constituent also capably induce phase 2 detoxification enzymes[17].

Green tea

In 1992, Japanese researchers reported on epidemiologic findings of a reduced incidence of esophageal and gastric cancer in one Western Japanese prefecture. They found the most marked reduction in areas where green tea was habitually produced and drunk, with frequent refreshing of the tea leaves. Residents had decreased incidence of death from other cancers also. Subsequent animal experiments showed that both initiation and promotion and growth were slowed by administration of a tannin component of the tea, catechin[18–20].

However, subsequent studies failed to find similar relationships. 'In a population-based, prospective cohort study in Japan, we found no association between green-tea consumption and the risk of gastric cancer'[21]. Because of conflicting reports, the effects of green tea remain unknown.

PC-SPES

The history of PC-SPES serves as a warning example of how difficult it is to evaluate a material's true nature by following strictly defined evidence-based guidelines. PC-SPES enjoyed a period of scientific legitimacy before it was found to be inactive or misrepresented.

Clinicians' interest in the herbal supplement PC-SPES flared after a 1998 report in the *New England Journal of Medicine* showed the herb's therapeutic effect on prostate cancer[22]. The popularity was unusual, given the product's known existence of only 10 years. PC-SPES is a mixture of seven Asian herbs and one North American herb, including chrysanthemum, isatis, licorice, *Ganoderma lucidum*, *Panax pseudoginseng*, *Rabdosia rubescens*, saw palmetto (*Serenoa repens*), and skullcap. The herbs contain a range of plant chemicals including flavonoids, alkanoids, polysaccharides, amino acids, and trace minerals.

PC-SPES was developed in the early 1990s by Chen, who claimed to have created the formula by integrating modern science and ancient Chinese herbal wisdom. However, there is not much rationale given for why the specific herbs were selected. By the mid-1990s, the formula became widely promoted in the USA and was named PC-SPES[23]. PC stands for prostate cancer and SPES comes from the Latin root for hope.

Chinese herbs are used for conditions defined in Traditional Chinese Medicine (TCM), which do not relate or conform to modern scientific or tissue diagnoses. Therefore, PC-SPES had no historic use in prostate cancer. Before systematic identification of the contents began, clinical trials studied the herbal mixture. Most clinical trials use identified and purified compounds. The PC-SPES materials were produced in Taiwan, from sources in mainland China without effective regulation. Nevertheless, earlier studies demonstrated anticancer activity in animals and in *in vitro* experiments on human tissue. Early and later clinical trials showed activity against both hormone-sensitive and hormone-resistant prostate cancer[24].

By 2001 researchers had identified a number of cellular mechanisms through which the herbal combination apparently worked[25]. None of the individual herbs had the same magnitude or variety of effects as did the mixture. Taken singly, three herbs inhibited cell activity, and five of the eight stimulated cancer cell activity *in vitro*. 'Our results show that the cytotoxic and cytostatic properties of PC SPES are not entirely dependent on the presence of AR (androgen receptor). The antitumor mechanism of PC SPES is complex. It involves multiple metabolic pathways, such that the whole extract acts on redundant mechanisms, which otherwise will permit cell survival if a single-target agent is used.' Three herbs lowered intracellular and secreted prostate-specific antigen (PSA), while the remaining herbs actually increased PSA expression[26]. It is 'unlikely that the activity of a single herb can account for the overall effects of PC-SPES'. The authors implied that the whole mixture was required for full effect and that the contents interacted in a yet undetermined way.

In October 2001, researchers reported bleeding in a patient on PC-SPES. Warfarin was found in the blood, as well as in the PC-SPES mixture. On 9 February 2002, the Food and Drug Administration (FDA) issued a recall of PC-SPES and recommended that all people cease taking it. Californian authorities also found the companion supplement, SPES, to be contaminated with the sedative alprazolam (Xanax®).

In 2002 independent research oncologist Nagourney, who followed the PC-SPES reports from 1996, reported finding varying amounts of diethylstilbestrol in samples which decreased over 4 years, during which warfarin levels increased[27]. He also identified the anti-inflammatory drug indomethacin in the herb mixture. Anti-inflammatory, cyclooxygenase-2 inhibitors are a

class of drugs effective against colon and prostate cancer[27]. PC-SPES activity against prostate cancer was apparently found to be due to adulteration with pharmaceuticals.

UNPROVED AND DISPROVED SUBSTANCES

The following are a number of diet- and plant-based cancer treatments that are promoted by a few individuals and have large followings from time to time. Advocates synthesize claims without experimental or epidemiologic evidence. The claims lack plausibility, have not been evaluated, or have been disproved by surveys or clinical trials. Nevertheless, many non-research-based dietary approaches to cancer have been claimed by their advocates to prevent, slow the growth of, or cure cancer. Most involve strict adherence to food and supplement plans and other lifestyle methods.

Laetrile

Laetrile is the commercial name given to an extract of fruit pits: amygdalin from apricots, prunasin, linamarin, and other cyanogenic glycosides from other fruits and cassava root. Laetrile marketed in the 1970s was mainly amygdalin. Its structure is a benzene molecule with a side arm of two sequential glycosides and a CN moiety on the adjacent carbon. It contains 6% cyanide by weight[28]. The proposed theory of action was an invention of E.T. Krebs Jr, a one-time medical student, who tried to find an explanation for his father's claim to have found a cancer cure in these compounds. He theorized that amygdalin's cyanide, released by the enzyme β-glucosidase in cancer tissue, would kill the cancer cell. He claimed that the neutralizing enzyme rhodanese would protect normal cells by converting cyanide to thiocyanate. The major error was that human tissue, including cancer, does not contain significant amounts of β-glucosidase. Glucosidase occurs naturally in the amygdalin-containing food and intestinal bacteria. The glucosidase in the gut cleaves the sugar from the benzene moiety, and hydrolysis releases cyanide on further digestion. Cyanide released by ingested food in the gut is absorbed, and both cancer cells and normal cells are affected equally.

The theory was invented to give plausibility to a fraudulent stock investment scheme on Canadian stock exchanges and in the USA. The promoters were convicted of fraud in Canadian and US courts in the 1970s. Two FDA-sponsored studies showed insignificant Laetrile activity in human cancer[29,30].

Iscador (*Viscum album*, mistletoe)

Iscador is an extract of the common parasitic vine, mistletoe. An early twentieth century spiritual philosopher, Rudolph Steiner, theorized that mistletoe would be effective against cancer by using the doctrine of signatures (like cures like – a principle of homeopathy). He conceived mistletoe to share qualities of parasitism similar to the role of a cancer to its host. Mistletoe became part of his methods called anthroposophical medicine. Mistletoe is popular in Germany, where many citizens believe in natural and philosophic approaches to treatment, although most regular physicians do not prescribe it. Certain extracts have been shown to have some effect on cancer cells *in vitro*[31]. However, no convincing evidence of effect in humans has been forthcoming[32]. The effectiveness of adjuvant mistletoe treatment was shown in a controlled trial in reseected head and neck cancer patients[33,34]. Some components of Iscador have been shown to function as oxidants[35].

Ascorbate (vitamin C)

Ascorbate was proposed and popularized as having anticancer activity by biochemist Linus Pauling, based on the theory that it strengthened connective tissue, which would prevent cancer from spreading. The strength of connective tissue has not been shown to affect cancer growth or spread.

Ascorbate is a powerful antioxidant and may have some role, along with other food constituents, in reducing cancer development by neutralizing DNA damage by oxygen free radicals. However, in some circumstances ascorbate is a pro-oxidant, and acts to augment oxidation, resulting in DNA damage[36]. Ascorbate's most beneficial effects are found through intake of foods high in ascorbate rather than in supplement form. Pauling's anticancer theory lacked plausibility and the action was disproved in two clinical trials at the Mayo Clinic[30,37].

Essiac

Essiac (Caisse backwards) is an herbal mixture introduced by nurse R. Caisse, who obtained the formula from a patient who attributed it to a Canadian Chippewa medicine man. The tea is made from the following contents: burdock root, sheep sorrel, Turkish rhubarb, slippery elm bark; blessed thistle, red clover and kelp, added to later formulations. It has been tested in humans with no effect found[38].

Hoxsey formula

Hoxsey formula is a water extract of a mixture of pokeweed, burdock root, licorice, barberry, buckthorn, stillingia, red clover, prickly ash, and sometimes other materials. The promoter, Harry Hoxsey, claimed that a poultice of the herbs cured a cancer on his grandfather's horse's leg. (A microscopic diagnosis of cancer was not possible at the time.) Lacking any plausibility, it has not been studied seriously. It was declared fraudulent by the US FDA, although it is marketed through clinics in Mexico and somewhat clandestinely in the USA.

Gerson therapy

Gerson therapy is a mix of strict vegetarian and juice diet, supplements, and coffee enemas. Available in Mexico, it has no demonstrable effect.

Other nutrition-based methods include the Kelley (grape) and Gonzales methods, wheatgrass, Di Bella (Italy), and other varieties of dieting.

COMPLEMENTARY METHODS

True complementary methods are not treatments or therapies[39]. They are a variety of unrelated methods that satisfy esthetic or 'spiritual' needs of people or help to integrate a philosophy, ideology, or other set of ideas into a psychologic heuristic system that either makes sense for or adds meaning to the person whose humanity and existence are threatened. The methods may be as simple as exercise and relaxation or as complex as a religion. The practical help these methods supply includes reduction of symptoms, increase in life quality, aid in traversing difficult treatments, and aid in adjustment to illness and death.

No measurement of effectiveness is necessary for these methods. Claims of effectiveness are few, and would be difficult to prove, because they are not used alone, but in conjunction with measurable and proved treatments. There is little to prove, as each person may find one or a combination of methods attractive and useful, and the intent is to offer qualitative support. They include the following.

Knowledge

This is often forgotten as a means of psychologic support, but knowledge of the disease process and of one's clinical status reduces uncertainty, and thus decreases anxiety.

Arts

These include drawing and painting, music, dance, and poetry (reading and composition). These have the benefit of being practiced without the aid of others. Groups and instructors can also be used, of course.

Self-help groups

Psychologic support groups are increasingly popular. Some meet in person, others such as Internet discussion groups may serve the same purpose for those who are unable, or do not desire, to travel to meeting places. A drawback of unsupervised groups is the dissemination of false and sometimes harmful suggestions. Initial studies showing increased survival by participating in groups failed in subsequent trials and were shown to have been incorrectly devised[40].

Massage

Massage requires a helper or a professional, but even lay helpers or relatives can learn basic techniques quickly and be of help. Massage may provide relaxation, relief of tension and anxiety, and even an opportunity to open discussion of concerns that might otherwise be kept private.

Occupational and physical therapies

These services are supplied at most hospitals and in many medical groups, using trained and sometimes specialty-educated and licensed personnel. They are important during recovery from surgery and other debilitating procedures.

Stress reduction, relaxation, and meditation techniques

These are relatively recently developed techniques intended, as named, to reduce stress and induce a more relaxed state in order to reduce perception of pain and other uncomfortable symptoms, and provide a sense of control. They were developed in recent decades, and are associated with some New Age and other philosophies, and Eastern (Asian) religious practices. They may not appeal to everyone. Some techniques are accompanied by music or recorded voice tapes.

Hospice

The hospice movement developed in the 1970s and includes home care, and attention to relief of pain and other symptoms. The concept was not new, as home symptom care for dying patients had been in use before and had simply not been given a name.

Humanistic, patient-centered approaches

The idea that the patient could be in charge of his own care and that one might choose among treatment options and supportive measures was also not new, or a manifestation of complementary medicine. The concept became more formalized and was given a name in the late twentieth century.

CONCLUSIONS

Regional and cultural differences in cancer incidence suggest strongly that environmental factors are important determinants of carcinogenesis. The diet is the most common vehicle for carcinogen transport into the body – the other routes being inhalation and skin absorption (including radiation.) Along with other environmental differences, nutritional factors may account for as much as 30% or more of cancer incidence. Despite the difficulties in determining the roles of individual compounds and specific conditions, research on natural products will remain a fertile field for decades, and will have potential for making a significant contribution to human health. Nutrition will also lead into unavoidable, unproductive cul-de-sacs and will be a fertile field for unfounded claims.

References

1. Murch SJ, KrishnaRaj, S, Saxena P. Phytopharmaceuticals: mass production, standardization, and conservation. Sci Rev Altern Med 2000; 4: 39–43

2. Betz W. Herbal crisis in Europe: a review of the epidemic of renotoxicity from Chinese herbal remedies. Sci Rev Altern Med 2000; 4: 23–8

3. Mills S, Bone K. Principles and Practice of Phytotherapy. London: Churchill Livingstone, 2000: 614

4. Labriola D. Complementary Cancer Therapies. Roseville, CA: Prima Publishing, 2000: 173–4

5. Allred CD, Allred KF, Ju YH, et al. Soy diets containing varying amounts of genistein stimulate growth of estrogen-dependent (MCF-7) tumors in a dose dependent manner. Cancer Res 2001; 61: 5045–50

6. Allred CD, Ju YH, Allred KF, et al. Dietary genistin stimulates growth of estrogen-dependent breast cancer tumors similar to that observed with genistein. Carcinogenesis 2001; 10: 1667–73

7. Evans BF, Griffith K, Morton MS. Inhibition of 5α-reductase in genital skin fibroblasts and prostate tissue by dietary lignans and isoflavonoids. J Endocrinol 1995; 147: 295–302

8. Tham DM, Gardner CD, Haskell WL. Potential health benefits of dietary phytoestrogens: a review of the clinical, epidemiological, and mechanistic evidence. J Clin Endocrinol Metab 1999; 83: 2223–35

9. Sun AS, Yeh HC, Wang LH, et al. Pilot study of a specific dietary supplement in tumor-bearing mice and in stage IIIB and IV non-small cell lung cancer patients. Nutr Cancer 2001; 39: 85–95

10. Omenn G, Goodman GE, Thornquist MD, et al. Effects of a combination of beta carotene and vitamin A on lung cancer and cardiovascular disease. N Engl J Med 1996; 334: 1150–5

11. Wolf G. The effect of low and high doses of beta-carotene and exposure to cigarette smoke on the lungs of ferrets. Nutr Rev 2002; 60: 88–90

12. Kucuk O, Sarkar FH, Sakr W, et al. Phase II randomized clinical trial of lycopene supplementation before radical prostatectomy. Cancer Epidemiol Biomarkers Prev 2001; 10: 861–8

13. Hulten K, Van Kappel AL, Winkvist A, et al. Carotenoids, alpha-tocopherols, and retinol in plasma and breast cancer risk in northern Sweden. Cancer Causes Control 2001; 12: 529–37

14. Zhang Y, Talalay P. Mechanism of differential potencies of isothiocyanates as inducers of anticarcinogenic Phase 2 enzymes. Cancer Res 1998; 58: 4632–9

15. Bjeldanes L, Kim J, Grose KR, et al. Receptor agonists generated from indole-3-carbinol in vitro and in vivo. Proc Natl Acad Sci 1991; 88: 9534–47

16. Fahey J, Zhang Y, Talalay P. Broccoli sprouts: an exceptionally rich source of inducers of enzymes that protect against chemical carcinogens. Proc Natl Acad Sci USA 1997; 94: 10367–72

17. Dinkova-Kostova AT, Talalay P. Relation of structure of curcumin analogs to their potencies as inducers of Phase 2 detoxification enzymes. Carcinogenesis 1999; 20: 911–14

18. Sano M, Ozeki K, Taguchi M, Oguni I. Effects of green tea and tea catechins on the development of mammary gland. Biosci Biotechnol Biochem 1996; 60: 169–70

19. Yamane T, Nakatani H, Kikuoka N, et al. Inhibitory effects and toxicity of green tea polyphenols for gastrointestinal carcinogenesis. Cancer 1996; 77 (Suppl 8): 1662–7

20. Mabe K, Yamada M, Oguni I, Takahashi T. In vitro and in vivo activities of tea catechins against Helicobacter pylori. Antimicrob Agents Chemother 1999; 43: 1788–91

21. Tsubono Y, Nishino Y, Komatsu S, et al. Green tea and the risk of gastric cancer in Japan. N Engl J Med 2001; 344: 632–6

22. DiPaola RS, Zhang H, Lambert GH, et al. Clinical and biologic activity of an estrogenic herbal combination (PC-SPES) in prostate cancer. N Engl J Med 1998; 339: 785–91

23. Anon. Complementary and Alternative Cancer Methods. Atlanta, GA: American Cancer Society, 2000: 251–2

24. Small EJ, Frohglich MW, Bok R, et al. Prospective trial of the herbal PC-SPES in progressive cancer of the prostate. J Clin Oncol 2000; 18: 3595–603

25. De La Taille A, Hayek OR, Buttyan R, et al. Effects of phytotherapeutic agent, PC-SPES, on prostate cancer: a preliminary investigation on human cell lines and patients. Br J Urol Int 1999; 84: 845–50

26. Hsieh TC, Wu JM. Mechanism of action of herbal supplement PC-SPES: elucidation of effects of individual herbs of PC-SPES on proliferation and prostate specific gene expression in androgen-dependent LNCaP cells. Int J Oncol 2002; 3: 583–8

27. Sovak M, Seligson AL, Konas M, et al. PC-SPES in prostate cancer: an herbal mixture currently containing warfarin and previously diethylstilbestrol and indomethacin. Trans Am Assoc Cancer Res 2002; LB152 [http://aacr02.agora.com/planner/displayabstract.asp? presentationid=10056]

28. Herbert V, Barrett S. Vitamins and Health Foods. Amherst, NY: Prometheus Books, 1980: 12–15

29. Ellison NM, Byar DP, Newell GR. Special report on Laetrile: the NCI Laetrile review. N Engl J Med 1978; 299: 549–52

30. Moertel CG, Fleming TR, Rubin J, et al. A clinical trial of amygdalin (Laetrile) in the treatment of human cancer. N Engl J Med 1982; 306: 201–6

31. Kutton G, Menon LG, Antony S, Kuttan R. Anticarcinogenic and antimetastatic activity of Iscador. Anticancer Drugs 1997; 1: S15–16

32. Steuer-Vogt MK, Bonkowsky V, Ambrosch P, et al. The effect of an adjuvant mistletoe treatment programme in resected head and neck cancer patients: a randomized controlled clinical trial. Eur J Cancer 2001; 37: 23–31

33. Kaegi E. Unconventional therapies for cancer: 3. Iscador. CMAJ 1998; 158: 1157–9

34. Maier G, Fiebig HH. Absence of tumor growth stimulation in a panel of 16 human tumor cell lines by mistletoe extracts in vitro. Anticancer Drugs 2002; 13: 373–9

35. Bussing A, Schaller G, Pfuller U. Generation of reactive oxygen intermediates (ROI) by the thionins from Viscum album L. Anticancer Res 1998; 18: 4291–6

36. Saltman P. Oxidative stress; a radical view. Semin Hematol 1989; 26: 249–56

37. Moertel CG, Fleming TR, Creagan ET, et al. High-dose vitamin C versus placebo in the treatment of patients with advanced cancer who have had no prior chemotherapy. A randomized double-blind comparison. N Engl J Med 1985; 312: 137–41

38. Kaegi E. Unconventional therapies for cancer. 1. Essiac. The task force on alternative therapies of the Canadian Breast Cancer Research Initiative. CMAJ 1998; 158: 897–902

39. Bruss K, ed. American Cancer Society Guide to Complementary and Alternative Cancer Methods. Atlanta, GA: American Cancer Society, 2000

40. Sampson W. Contoversies in cancer and the mind: effects of psychosocial support. Semin Oncol 2002; 29: 595–600

Chemotherapy-induced nausea and vomiting

24

S. R. Mehendale, H. H. Aung and C.-S. Yuan

INTRODUCTION

Chemotherapy and radiotherapy administered for cancer treatment produce severe adverse effects. Among others, nausea and vomiting are considered significant effects experienced by 30–90% of patients undergoing chemotherapy and about 40% of patients undergoing radiotherapy[1]. These symptoms reduce the quality of life and could lead to severe complications such as dehydration, electrolyte imbalance, and esophageal tears from retching (Mallory Weiss syndrome)[2]. Patients who have experienced these symptoms are more likely to refuse further chemotherapy or to experience anticipatory emesis during subsequent chemotherapy. Therefore, to achieve adequate control of nausea and vomiting would be an important step towards improving tolerability and effectiveness of cancer treatment. Herbal medicines may play an important role in the management of these adverse effects.

PATHOGENESIS OF CHEMOTHERAPY-INDUCED EMESIS

Chemotherapy-induced nausea and vomiting has been arbitrarily described to occur in two phases, the acute and the chronic phase, lasting for up to 24 hours and from 24–120 hours, respectively[3,4]. Overall, chemotherapy (and radiation)-induced nausea and vomiting are caused by either stimulation of receptors in the gastro-intestinal tract or direct stimulation of the chemoreceptor trigger zone (CTZ)[5].

The acute phase, in particular, appears to be mediated largely by serotonin (5-HT) release from the enterochromaffin cells in the gut, which contain high 5-HT concentrations[6]. Oxidative injury to gut cells is proposed to occur following administration of chemothera-peutic agents like cisplatin[7–9]. The released 5-HT acts via activation of 5-HT$_3$ receptors in the gastro-intestinal tract to stimulate vagal afferent sensory nerves that relay to the CTZ in the brainstem to cause emesis[8,10,11]. Thus, antagonists of 5-HT$_3$ receptors significantly decrease emesis[12,13].

The delayed emesis following cisplatin chemotherapy cannot be inhibited by 5-HT$_3$ antagonists, but can be relieved by a substance P antagonist (or neurokinin antagonist)[14–17]. Substance P is present in the enteric neurons[18–20] and may be released during the oxidant gut injury. Substance P is also released in the brainstem following vagal input from the gastro-intestinal tract and is initiated by 5-HT release[21]. Thus an initial insult causing 5-HT release in the gut may mediate the acute emetic phase and stimulation of substance P release, which, in turn, is responsible for the delayed phase of chemotherapy-induced emesis[21].

CURRENTLY AVAILABLE ANTI-EMETICS

Several classes of anti-emetic drugs such as dopamine antagonists, anticholinergics, steroids, and various combinations of these drugs have shown limited efficacy in chemotherapy-induced nausea and vomiting[22]. A newer class of anti-emetic drugs, 5HT$_3$ receptor antagonists, like ondansetron, is significantly more effective in the treatment of chemotherapy-induced nausea and vomiting, but only in treating the early symptoms[3,22,23]. The more recently developed drug aprepitant, a substance P antagonist, showed efficacy in treating the delayed emetic phase of cisplatin[24,25]. Studies have shown that these new classes of medications, when administered as a combination with supplemental dexamethasone, treat both the acute and delayed phase of emesis induced by chemotherapy[24,25].

POTENTIAL USE OF ANTIOXIDANT HERBS IN DRUG-INDUCED EMESIS

Consumption of several additional anti-emetic drugs for controlling nausea and vomiting results in an increased probability of drug-induced side-effects and increased cost of treatment. More importantly, these drugs may reduce the efficacy of chemotherapy. For example, pretreatment with dexamethasone may reduce the tumoricidal activity of chemotherapeutic agents[26]. Using safe and efficacious herbal medications could reduce the costs, reduce side-effects, and improve overall health. Since an estimated 30–50% of cancer patients already choose to use complementary and alternative medicine in addition to their conventional medications[27–29], this population may be more inclined to use well-researched herbal alternatives that do not interfere with chemotherapy.

Chemotherapeutic agents such as cisplatin are known to produce oxidative gut damage leading to release of neurohumoral mediators and emesis[8,9,14,30–32]. The pathogenetic mechanism of oxidative injury is further validated by studies that demonstrate exaggeration of cisplatin-induced emesis by ferric chloride, which catalyzes production of free radicals[7]. Also, treatment with antioxidants, such as ascorbic acid, alpha tocopherol, or *N*-(2-mecaptopropionyl)glycine, ameliorates the cisplatin-induced emetic response[7,8,33]. In our animal studies, we have therefore focused on researching herbs with known antioxidant activity in preventing chemotherapy induced-emesis.

ANTIOXIDANT HERBS REDUCE CHEMOTHERAPY-INDUCED EMESIS

We previously evaluated the effects of the antioxidant herbs *Scutellaria baicalensis*[34,35] (a Chinese herbal medicine that is also discussed in Chapter 26), American ginseng[36–38], and *Ganoderma lucidum* for chemotherapy-induced emesis in a rat pica model. The chemotherapeutic agent cisplatin induces a severe emetic response in some animals similar to humans[14,15]. We used a rat model; although the rat does not vomit, it increases kaolin or clay consumption (also known as pica) in response to several emetic stimuli, including chemotherapy and radiotherapy[39–41]. Further validation of the pica model is demonstrated by treatment of pica with conventional anti-emetic drugs[42].

We have confirmed the findings of other researchers that cisplatin induces pica in rats[35,40]. We observed that

rats consumed significant amount of kaolin at 24 h following 3 mg/kg cisplatin injection compared to the vehicle control. Additionally, we observed that the rats continued to consume kaolin up to 120 h[35]. This rat pica model therefore demonstrated that the emetic response correlates with clinical phases of cisplatin-induced nausea and vomiting[4,25,43,44].

We evaluated whether *S. baicalensis* extract (SbE) attenuates cisplatin-induced pica. As shown in Figure 24.1, we observed that pretreatment with intraperitoneal SbE 1 mg/kg or 3 mg/kg, 30 min prior to 3 mg/kg cisplatin injection, significantly decreased kaolin consumption, suggesting that both acute and delayed emetic effects of cisplatin in the pica model can be attenuated by *S. baicalensis*[35].

Similar to the antioxidant properties of *S. baicalensis*[34], our previous studies demonstrated the antioxidant properties of American ginseng berry extract (AGBE) in cultured cardiomyocytes exposed to acute oxidant injury[45]. We also demonstrated that AGBE is efficacious in treating cisplatin-induced kaolin consumption. Figure 24.2 shows that pretreatment with AGBE dose-dependently reduced pica at all time points, reflecting the significant effects of AGBE on both acute and delayed emesis. In addition, we observed that pretreatment with AGBE may also improve food consumption that is significantly reduced after cisplatin treatment.

Recently, we also evaluated the effects of *Ganoderma lucidum* (SunRecome®) in attenuating cisplatin-induced nausea and vomiting in the rat pica model. *Ganoderma*

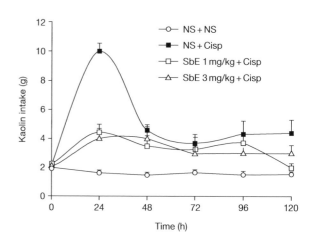

Figure 24.1   Effect of cisplatin and *Scutellaria baicalensis* extract (SbE) on kaolin intake in rats. Cisplatin-induced increased kaolin intake was attenuated by 1 mg/kg and 3 mg/kg SbE administration ($p < 0.01$). NS, normal saline; Cisp, cisplatin 3 mg/kg

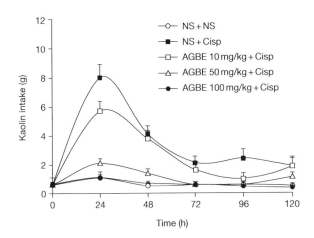

Figure 24.2 Effects of pretreatment with American ginseng berry extract (AGBE) on kaolin intake induced by cisplatin in rats. Increased kaolin intake induced by cisplatin was reduced dose-dependently with AGBE pretreatment ($p < 0.01$). NS, normal saline; Cisp, cisplatin 3 mg/kg

lucidum, or Reishi mushroom, or Lingzhi[46] has been recognized as a remedy in treating a number of medical conditions, including balancing immunity and decreasing drug-induced side-effects, possibly linked to its antioxidant property. We observed that cisplatin-induced kaolin intake dose-dependently decreased significantly after 1 mg/kg, 3 mg/kg, and 10 mg/kg SunRecome administration. The reduced food intake after cisplatin also improved significantly after SunRecome treatment, suggesting that nausea may also have improved.

Another antioxidant herb that appears to show promise as an anti-emetic is ginger (*Zingiber officinale*), which is beneficial in treating nausea and vomiting in various populations[47]. Ginger may exert the anti-emetic effects by blocking 5-HT$_3$ receptors and by scavenging free radicals[48], suggesting that it may be beneficial in reducing both the incidence and severity of chemotherapy-induced emesis. This possible effect of ginger, however, needs to be verified in clinical trials[49]. An ongoing clinical trial, sponsored by NIH/NCCAM, will assess the efficacy and safety of two oral dose levels (1.0 g or 2.0 g per day) of ginger extract (standardized for 5% gingerols) in patients undergoing chemotherapy (cisplatin or adriamycin) who have experienced at least one episode of chemotherapy-induced nausea and vomiting despite optimal conventional medical therapy[50]. Data obtained from this study should clarify whether ginger is efficacious in treating chemotherapy-induced emesis.

DO ANTIOXIDANTS INTERFERE WITH THE DRUGS' TUMORICIDAL EFFECTS?

Consumption of antioxidants concurrently during chemotherapy may hamper or help the tumoricidal activity of chemotherapeutic agents[51]. When the free radical producing activity of chemotherapeutic drugs is not the primary mechanism of action of the tumoricidal activity, antioxidants may not interfere with the pharmacologic activity. For example, cisplatin exerts its primary tumoricidal activity by forming cross-links between DNA strands, thus inhibiting growth in rapidly developing tissues[52]. Scavenging free radicals released incidentally during chemotherapy by antioxidants should, in most instances, mitigate the free radical mediated toxicity without compromising tumoricidal activity[53–55].

Individual antioxidants, however, need to be studied to rule out interactions with chemotherapeutic agents. Interactions of cisplatin with the antioxidant *N*-acetyl cysteine demonstrated an inhibition of antitumor activity by blocking the mitochondrial apoptotic pathway, which is activated downstream after cisplatin-induced DNA cross-linking[56]. In contrast, other antioxidants, like quercetin and glutathione, showed a trend towards greater tumor response or antitumor activity[51]. L-Carnitine protected from cisplatin mediated oxidant injury, while preserving tumoricidal activity *in vivo*[54].

Of the antioxidant herbs we studied for treating cisplatin-induced anti-emetic effects, *S. baicalensis* is known to boost immunity (see Chapter 26); however, whether it interferes with tumoricidal activity needs evaluation. Ginseng, on the other hand, has been researched extensively. Ginseng extracts have demonstrated tumoricidal properties against cancer cell lines[57,58]. Ginsenosides such as Rh$_2$ potentiate the anticancer effects of cisplatin against human ovarian cancer cells[59,60]. Since the antitumor activities of ginseng seem to be mediated through growth inhibition, and possibly through apoptotic mechanisms such as activation of caspase-3[61], they may not interfere with cisplatin's antitumor activity. Also, there is significant evidence, in terms of retrospective epidemiologic studies, that demonstrate a decreased incidence of cancer or improved prognosis with ginseng[62–64], and suggest that interaction between ginseng and cisplatin may be complementary.

CONCLUSIONS

Nausea and vomiting caused by cancer therapy greatly reduce the quality of life and adversely affect continuation of the therapy in cancer patients. An efficacious herbal anti-emetic therapy could potentially have a role in the management of cancer patients who experience chemotherapy- and radiotherapy-induced emesis. Antioxidant herbs like ginseng that possess tumoricidal activity could thus play a dual role by complementing chemotherapy, in addition to their anti-emetic effects.

Herbal remedies can be equally effective, low-cost alternatives to conventional anti-emetics, which can reduce drug-induced side-effects while improving patients' quality of life. Controlled clinical trials are required to test these potential anti-emetic antioxidant herbs in order to offer safe and effective herbal alternatives to cancer patients[27–29,65]. The candidate antioxidant herbs, however, need to be carefully chosen after ensuring non-interference with the tumoricidal actions of chemotherapeutic drugs.

References

1. Kovac AL. Benefits and risks of newer treatments for chemotherapy-induced and postoperative nausea and vomiting. Drug Safety 2003; 26: 227–59

2. Schnell FM. Chemotherapy-induced nausea and vomiting: the importance of acute antiemetic control. Oncologist 2003; 8: 187–98

3. Hesketh PJ, Van Belle S, Aapro M, et al. Differential involvement of neurotransmitters through the time course of cisplatin-induced emesis as revealed by therapy with specific receptor antagonists. Eur J Cancer 2003; 39: 1074–80

4. Roila F. Prevention of delayed nausea and emesis induced by chemotherapy. In Donnerer J, ed. Antiemetic Therapy. New York: J Karger, 2003: 169–78

5. Meyer M. Palliative care and AIDS: 2–Gastrointestinal symptoms. Int J STD AIDS 1999; 10: 495–505

6. Endo T, Minami M, Monma Y, et al. Emesis-related biochemical and histopathological changes induced by cisplatin in the ferret. J Toxicol Sci 1990; 15: 235–44

7. Matsuki N. [Mechanisms of cytotoxic drug-induced emesis and its prevention.] Yakugaku Zasshi 1996; 116: 710–18

8. Torii Y, Mutoh M, Saito H, Matsuki N. Involvement of free radicals in cisplatin-induced emesis in Suncus murinus. Eur J Pharmacol 1993; 248: 131–5

9. Sodhi A, Gupta P. Increased release of hydrogen peroxide (H_2O_2) and superoxide anion (O^{2-}) by murine macrophages in vitro after cisplatin treatment. Int J Immunopharmacol 1986; 8: 709–14

10. Fukui H, Yamamoto M, Ando T, et al. Increase in serotonin levels in the dog ileum and blood by cisplatin as measured by microdialysis. Neuropharmacology 1993; 32: 959–68

11. Yuan CS, Barber WD. Area postrema: gastric vagal input from proximal stomach and interactions with nucleus tractus solitarius in cat. Brain Res Bull 1993; 30: 119–25

12. Andrews PL, Bhandari P. The 5-hydroxytryptamine receptor antagonists as antiemetics: preclinical evaluation and mechanism of action. Eur J Cancer 1993; 29: S11–16

13. Gale JD. Serotonergic mediation of vomiting. J Pediatr Gastroenterol Nutr 1995; 21 (Suppl 1): S22–8

14. Cubeddu LX. Mechanisms by which cancer chemotherapeutic drugs induce emesis. Semin Oncol 1992; 19: 2–13

15. Watson JW, Gonsalves SF, Fossa AA, et al. The anti-emetic effects of CP-99,994 in the ferret and the dog: role of the NK1 receptor. Br J Pharmacol 1995; 115: 84–94

16. Cocquyt V, Van Belle S, Reinhardt RR, et al. Comparison of L-758,298, a prodrug for the selective neurokinin-1 antagonist, L-754,030, with ondansetron for the prevention of cisplatin-induced emesis. Eur J Cancer 2001; 37: 835–42

17. Tanihata S, Oda S, Kakuta S, Uchiyama T. Antiemetic effect of a tachykinin NK1 receptor antagonist GR205171 on cisplatin-induced early and delayed emesis in the pigeon. Eur J Pharmacol 2003; 461: 197–206

18. Holzer P, Holzer-Petsche U. Tachykinin receptors in the gut: physiological and pathological implications. Curr Opin Pharmacol 2001; 1: 583–90

19. Holzer P, Holzer-Petsche U. Tachykinins in the gut. Part I. Expression, release and motor function. Pharmacol Ther 1997; 73: 173–217

20. Hockerfelt U, Franzen L, Forsgren S. Substance P (NK1) receptor in relation to substance P innervation in rat duodenum after irradiation. Regul Peptides 2001; 98: 115–26

21. Stahl SM. The ups and downs of novel antiemetic drugs, part 1: substance P, 5-HT, and the neuropharmacology of vomiting. J Clin Psychiatry 2003; 64: 498–9

22. Pendergrass KB. Options in the treatment of chemotherapy-induced emesis. Cancer Pract 1998; 6: 276–81

23. Tsukada H, Hirose T, Yokoyama A, Kurita Y. Randomised comparison of ondansetron plus dexamethasone with dexamethasone alone for the control of delayed cisplatin-induced emesis. Eur J Cancer 2001; 37: 2398–404

24. Martin AR, Carides AD, Pearson JD, et al. Functional relevance of antiemetic control. Experience using the FLIE questionnaire in a randomised study of the NK-1 antagonist aprepitant. Eur J Cancer 2003; 39: 1395–401

25. Herrstedt J. Risk-benefit of antiemetics in prevention and treatment of chemotherapy-induced nausea and vomiting. Expert Opin Drug Saf 2004; 3: 231–48

26. Wu W, Chaudhuri S, Brickley DR, et al. Microarray analysis reveals glucocorticoid-regulated survival genes that are associated with inhibition of apoptosis in breast epithelial cells. Cancer Res 2004; 64: 1757–64

27. Ernst E. The role of complementary and alternative medicine in cancer. Lancet Oncol 2000; 1: 176–80

28. Bernstein BJ, Grasso T. Prevalence of complementary and alternative medicine use in cancer patients. Oncology (Huntingt) 2001; 15: 1267–72; discussion 72–8, 83

29. Shumay DM, Maskarinec G, Kakai H, Gotay CC. Why some cancer patients choose complementary and alternative medicine instead of conventional treatment. J Fam Pract 2001; 50: 1067

30. Schworer H, Racke K, Kilbinger H. Cisplatin increases the release of 5-hydroxytryptamine (5-HT) from the isolated vascularly perfused small intestine of the guinea-pig: involvement of 5-HT3 receptors. Naunyn Schmiedebergs Arch Pharmacol 1991; 344: 143–9

31. Dumontet C, Drai J, Thieblemont C, et al. The superoxide dismutase content in erythrocytes predicts short-term toxicity of high-dose cyclophosphamide. Br J Haematol 2001; 112: 405–9

32. Berrigan MJ, Struck RF, Gurtoo HL. Lipid peroxidation induced by cyclophosphamide. Cancer Biochem Biophys 1987; 9: 265–70

33. Yang Y, Kinoshita K, Koyama K, et al. Novel experimental model using free radical-induced emesis for surveying antiemetic compounds from natural sources. Planta Med 1999; 65: 574–6

34. Shao ZH, Li CQ, Vanden Hoek TL, et al. Extract from Scutellaria baicalensis Georgi attenuates oxidant stress in cardiomyocytes. J Mol Cell Cardiol 1999; 31: 1885–95

35. Aung HH, Dey L, Mehendale S, et al. Scutellaria baicalensis extract decreases cisplatin-induced pica in rats. Cancer Chemother Pharmacol 2003; 52: 453–8

36. Gillis CN. Panax ginseng pharmacology: a nitric oxide link? Biochem Pharmacol 1997; 54: 1–8

37. Attele AS, Wu JA, Yuan CS. Ginseng pharmacology: multiple constituents and multiple actions. Biochem Pharmacol 1999; 58: 1685–93

38. Mehendale S, Aung H, Wang A, et al. American ginseng berry extract and ginsenoside Re attenuate cisplatin-induced kaolin intake in rats. Cancer Chemother Pharmacol 2005; 56: 63–9

39. Mitchell D, Wells C, Hoch N, et al. Poison induced pica in rats. Physiol Behav 1976; 17: 691–7

40. Takeda N, Hasegawa S, Morita M, Matsunaga T. Pica in rats is analogous to emesis: an animal model in emesis research. Pharmacol Biochem Behav 1993; 45: 817–21

41. Takeda N, Hasegawa S, Morita M, et al. Neuropharmacological mechanisms of emesis. I. Effects of antiemetic drugs on motion- and apomorphine-induced pica in rats. Methods Find Exp Clin Pharmacol 1995; 17: 589–90

42. Takeda N, Hasegawa S, Morita M, et al. Neuropharmacological mechanisms of emesis. II. Effects of antiemetic drugs on cisplatin-induced pica in rats. Methods Find Exp Clin Pharmacol 1995; 17: 647–52

43. Kris MG, Gralla RJ, Clark RA, et al. Incidence, course, and severity of delayed nausea and vomiting following the administration of high-dose cisplatin. J Clin Oncol 1985; 3: 1379–84

44. Kris MG, Roila F, De Mulder PH, Marty M. Delayed emesis following anticancer chemotherapy. Support Care Cancer 1998; 6: 228–32

45. Shao ZH, Xie JT, Vanden Hoek TL, et al. Antioxidant effects of American ginseng berry extract in cardiomyocytes exposed to acute oxidant stress. Biochim Biophys Acta 2004; 1670: 165–71

46. Bensky D, Gamble A, Stoger E. Chinese Herbal Medicine: Materia Medica. Seattle: Eastland Press, 2004

47. Anon. Zingiber officinale (ginger). Monograph. Altern Med Rev 2003; 8: 331–5

48. Jagetia G, Baliga M, Venkatesh P. Ginger (Zingiber officinale Rosc.), a dietary supplement, protects mice against radiation-induced lethality: mechanism of action. Cancer Biother Radiopharm 2004; 19: 422–35

49. Ernst E, Pittler MH. Efficacy of ginger for nausea and vomiting: a systematic review of randomized clinical trials. Br J Anaesth 2000; 84: 367–71

50. www.clinicaltrials.gov/show/NCT00065221, accessed July, 2005

51. Lamson DW, Brignall MS. Antioxidants in cancer therapy; their actions and interactions with oncologic therapies. Altern Med Rev 1999; 4: 304–29

52. Zamble DB, Lippard SJ. Cisplatin and DNA repair in cancer chemotherapy. Trends Biochem Sci 1995; 20: 435–9

53. Yokozawa T, Liu ZW. The role of ginsenoside-Rd in cisplatin-induced acute renal failure. Renal Fail 2000; 22: 115–27

54. Chang B, Nishikawa M, Sato E, et al. L-Carnitine inhibits cisplatin-induced injury of the kidney and small intestine. Arch Biochem Biophys 2002; 405: 55–64

55. Liu SJ, Zhou SW. Panax notoginseng saponins attenuated cisplatin-induced nephrotoxicity. Acta Pharmacol Sin 2000; 21: 257–60

56. Wu YJ, Muldoon LL, Neuwelt EA. The chemoprotective agent N-acetylcysteine blocks cisplatin-induced apoptosis through caspase signaling pathway. J Pharmacol Exp Ther 2005; 312: 424–31

57. Park IH, Piao LZ, Kwon SW, et al. Cytotoxic dammarane glycosides from processed ginseng. Chem Pharm Bull (Tokyo) 2002; 50: 538–40

58. Mochizuki M, Yoo YC, Matsuzawa K, et al. Inhibitory effect of tumor metastasis in mice by saponins, ginsenoside-Rb2, 20(R)- and 20(S)-ginsenoside-Rg3, of red ginseng. Biol Pharm Bull 1995; 18: 1197–202

59. Nakata H, Kikuchi Y, Tode T, et al. Inhibitory effects of ginsenoside Rh2 on tumor growth in nude mice bearing human ovarian cancer cells. Jpn J Cancer Res 1998; 89: 733–40

60. Karikura M, Miyase T, Tanizawa H, et al. Studies on absorption, distribution, excretion and metabolism of ginseng saponins. VII. Comparison of the decomposition modes of ginsenoside-Rb1 and -Rb2 in the digestive tract of rats. Chem Pharm Bull (Tokyo) 1991; 39: 2357–61

61. Lee SJ, Ko WG, Kim JH, et al. Induction of apoptosis by a novel intestinal metabolite of ginseng saponin via cytochrome c-mediated activation of caspase-3 protease. Biochem Pharmacol 2000; 60: 677–85

62. Suh SO, Kroh M, Kim NR, et al. Effects of red ginseng upon postoperative immunity and survival in patients with stage III gastric cancer. Am J Chin Med 2002; 30: 483–94

63. Yun TK, Choi SY. Preventive effect of ginseng intake against various human cancers: a case-control study on 1987 pairs. Cancer Epidemiol Biomarkers Prev 1995; 4: 401–8

64. Yun TK. Experimental and epidemiological evidence of the cancer-preventive effects of Panax ginseng C.A. Meyer. Nutr Rev 1996; 54: S71–81

65. Ott MJ. Complementary and alternative therapies in cancer symptom management. Cancer Pract 2002; 10: 162–6

Cachexia associated with cancer and AIDS

25

M.-Y. Song, A. S. Dobs and T. T. Brown

INTRODUCTION

Weight loss is a common feature of many chronic diseases in their advanced stages. Patients with diseases as diverse as cancer, AIDS, congestive heart failure, and chronic obstructive pulmonary disease often experience weight loss, muscle atrophy, and anorexia as the disease progresses. Unintentional weight loss can also be detected in the elderly without obvious disease[1]. This process, which has been termed cachexia, is associated with a poor prognosis and decreased survival[2]. An estimated 20% of cancer-related deaths is attributable to cachexia[3].

There is no definition of cachexia that has been universally accepted. The word originates from Greek, meaning 'bad condition'. It has been operationally defined as a greater than 10% unintentional weight loss in 1 year or after 5 years of follow-up[1,4]. The weight loss in cachexia, however, cannot be fully reversed by increasing caloric intake[5]. In this way, cachexia differs from simple starvation or malnutrition.

Cachexia also differs from starvation in the type of tissues involved. Whereas fat is preferentially catabolized in starvation and whole body protein is relatively preserved[6], cachexia is marked by a loss of both lean body mass and fat mass[1,4]. For this reason, simple body weight measurements, which cannot differentiate loss between body compartments, are limited in the assessment of cachexia.

This chapter will focus on complementary and alternative medicine (CAM) treatments of cachexia mainly associated with cancer and AIDS, two diseases in which cachexia is an important cause of morbidity and mortality. The extent to which findings of research studies can be extrapolated to other causes of cachexia is not clear.

IMPACT OF CACHEXIA

Cachexia has a broad impact on the lives of those affected. Symptoms of cachexia in cancer patients include severe weakness, weight loss, anorexia, and muscle wasting[7]. Eighty percent of upper gastro-intestinal cancers and 60% of lung cancer patients are reported to experience weight loss upon diagnosis[8]. Patients who lose weight involuntarily also respond poorly to chemotherapy[9].

Loss of lean body mass in cachexia causes muscle weakness which contributes to frailty and limits independent living, resulting in immobility and death[10]. Similarly, in HIV-infected patients, the risk of death increases by 11% for each 1% loss in body weight[11], and an intentional weight loss of 5–10% over a 4-month period increases the risk of death by over 2-fold[12]. HIV wasting adversely affects quality of life, leading to declines in physical function, psychologic comfort, and social function[13]. In its advanced stage, neurologic complications of HIV can further reduce muscle tone, strength, balance, and coordination[13,14], contributing to frailty[15].

PATHOPHYSIOLOGY OF CACHEXIA

Cancer cachexia

Cachexia results from a complicated interaction between the tumor and the host's response. This process includes multiple cytokines, tumor-specific products, and hormonal factors which lead to increased metabolism and anorexia (Figure 25.1). Gastro-intestinal problems such as physical obstruction, nausea, and constipation, and psychologic factors including depression may contribute

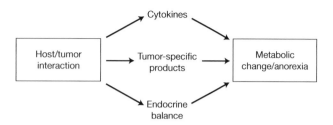

Figure 25.1 Potential mechanisms of cachexia. Reprinted from reference 16 with permission from Elsevier

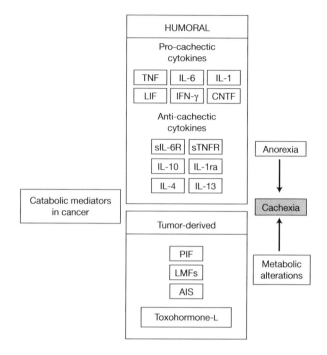

Figure 25.2 Catabolic mediators in cancer. Both tumor-derived and humoral (cytokines) factors are involved in mediating anorexia and metabolic changes, characteristic of the cachectic state. Reprinted from reference 21 with permission from Elsevier

to the loss of appetite[16]. However, after controlling for these factors, cancer patients with cachexia experience poor appetite, changes in taste, and early satiety[17].

In addition to decreased energy intake, patients with cachexia have an increased metabolic rate. Resting energy expenditure (REE), which normally accounts for about 70% of total energy expenditure, tends to be higher in cachectic patients. One source of caloric expenditure is the acute phase response (APR), which is an elaboration of inflammatory proteins involved in modulating host defense and promoting tissue repair[18,19]. This process is activated by pro-inflammatory cytokines[1]. Increased energy expenditure may also be due to the effects of uncoupling proteins (UCPs), mitochondrial proteins which increase thermogenesis by uncoupling the processes of oxidation and phosphorylation[20]. UCPs are activated by pro-inflammatory cytokines and, during tumor growth, both UCP2 and UCP3 mRNAs in skeletal muscle are increased[21]. These findings suggest that UCPs may be a major mechanism by which tumor growth and the host response lead to muscle wasting[22].

Two groups of mediators play a role in cachexia: pro-inflammatory cytokines and cancer-specific cachectic factors. The first group includes cytokines, such as TNF-α, interleukin (IL)-1, IL-6, and interferon-γ[23]. In colon adenocarcinoma-bearing mice, anti-mouse IL-6 antibody treatment inhibits cancer-related wasting[24], suggesting that IL-6 plays a central role in cachexia. The role of cytokines, however, is complicated since procachetic cytokines are often balanced by anti-cachetic cytokines, such as IL-4, IL-10, IL-13, and soluble receptor of TNF (sTNFR) and IL-6 (sIL-6R) (Figure 25.2)[21]. Procachectic cytokines might affect feeding behavior through modulation of hypothalamic signaling. Leptin is secreted from adipose tissue and is a major regulator of long-term body composition, through its influence on food intake and energy expenditure. With weight loss,

leptin concentrations decrease in proportion to body fat lost. Low leptin levels will stimulate feeding and suppress energy expenditure[25]. In cachexia, several cytokines like TNF-α and IL-1 inhibit normal compensatory mechanisms by stimulating the release of leptin. In mice, administration of TNF and IL-1 increased leptin mRNA expression in fat[26]. The effects of cytokines may also be mediated by neuropeptide Y (NPY), a hypothalamic peptide which stimulates feeding behavior. Chronic intracerebroventricular administration of IL-1 beta in rats induces anorexia and down-regulates NPY mRNA expression in the hypothalamus[27].

Lipid-mobilizing factor (LMF) and proteolysis-inducing factor (PIF) are two tumor products that have been isolated from the urine of cancer cachexia patients, but not from the other patients with wasting from other causes[28]. These tumor-derived factors may also directly lead to protein breakdown and hypermetabolism.

HIV-associated wasting

The up-regulation of pro-inflammatory cytokines also underlies the wasting process in HIV[29,30]. Elevation of resting energy expenditure and altered lipid metabolism also play a role in this process[31]. HIV wasting usually produces lean body mass loss and increased protein degradation[32,33]. Hormonal factors, such as hypogonadism, may also contribute to the catabolic state[34,35].

EPIDEMIOLOGY OF THE USE OF CAM AMONG CANCER AND AIDS PATIENTS

Cancer

Use of CAM in cancer patients is prevalent around the world. According to a systematic review of data from 13 countries, 31% of cancer patients use CAM. The most frequently used CAM modalities are vitamins, antioxidants, alternative diets, and herbal medicine[36]. CAM users are likely to be female, young, and more educated[37]. An estimated 2% of all health-care expenditures among cancer patients come from CAM use[38]. The extent to which CAM is used among cancer patients to prevent or ameliorate cachexia is unknown.

HIV/AIDS

Among HIV patients, use of CAM is more prevalent than among the general population, with estimates ranging from 30 to 68%[39–43]. In one study, 23% of patients used CAM to treat weight loss, nausea, and diarrhea, and most of them reported CAM as helpful[44].

CAM THERAPIES

While not always an option, the most effective treatment of cachexia in cancer and AIDS is the treatment of the underlying disease. Mainstream therapies for cachexia, such as megesterol, are limited and marginally effective. Few data using rigorous scientific methodology to investigate the safety and efficacy of the proposed treatment have been reported. In this part, focus will be on the most prevalent CAM therapies which have some effects on cachexia. In addition, we will also review CAM treatments which have been proposed for immunomodulation and nausea. Both of these processes may contribute to cachetic symptoms. Table 25.1 shows proposed CAM therapies for cachexia-related conditions.

Treatment for cachexia

In patients with cachexia, the effect of conventional nutritional support is controversial. However, some specific nutritional components have been reported to improve the metabolic response.

Fish oil

There has been an increasing number of studies focused on fish oil for the prevention and treatment of various conditions, including weight loss associated with chronic illness. Fish oil contains the essential omega-3 fatty acids such as eicosapentanoic acid (EPA) and docosahexanoic acid (DHA), as well as various types of other polyunsaturated fatty acids (PUFAs). Research investigating the effect of fish oil in cachexia has been inconsistent. While some studies have suggested that fish oil administration can decrease the inflammatory response and maintain lean body mass, thereby exerting an anti-cachetic effect, other studies have demonstrated no benefit.

Omega-3 fatty acids may have anti-inflammatory properties. In both *in vivo* and *in vitro* studies, fish oil supplementation down-regulates pro-inflammatory cytokine production. In an animal study using immunogen injected chicks, dietary fish oil decreased interleukin-1 release, which suggests a down-regulated inflammatory response[45]. *In vitro* studies, using human monocyte THP-1 cells, have shown that pre-incubation with EPA attenuates expression of TNF-α when exposed to the lipopolysaccharide, a potent inducer of inflammation[46]. This effect on inflammation has also been seen in human studies. In a small, uncontrolled study, EPA supplementation for a month with escalating dose (1 g/day in the first week to a maximum of 6 g over the final week, total dose 91 g in divided doses over 1 month) in six weight-losing cancer patients with cachexia down-regulated APR as well as suppressed interleukin-6[47]. Given the importance of the inflammatory response in the pathogenesis of cachexia, the down-regulation of pro-inflammatory mediators may represent the mechanism through which fish oils may prevent muscle wasting.

The results of clinical studies using fish oil to treat weight loss, however, are not consistent. In a single-arm study, administration of fish oil (18% EPA and 12% DHA) to weight-losing pancreatic cancer patients who had a median weight loss of 2.9 kg/month at baseline gained an average of 0.3 kg/month after 3 months' fish oil supplementation and showed significant down-regulation of APR and stabilization of energy expenditure at a maximum dose of 12 g/day[48]. In another single-arm study, omega-3 fatty acid supplementation (2 cans/day, 2.2 g EPA, 0.96 g DHA) to 20 weight-losing, pancreatic cancer patients for 7 weeks (median weight loss 2.9 kg/month) resulted in a weight gain of 2 kg, which

Table 25.1   Proposed CAM modalities for cachexia-related conditions

	CAM modality	Proposed mechanism	Maximum suggested dose	RCT (Y/N)	Strength of evidence out of 4 stars
Dietary supplement	*n*-3 (omega-3) fatty acid; EPA and DHA	suppression of pro-inflammatory cytokine	0.3 g/kg per day	Y	***
Herb	*Panax ginseng*	restores NK cell activity	100–200 mg extract (4% ginsenoids) 1–2/day up to 12 weeks	N	*
	Rhizoma coptidis	down-regulation of IL-6	N/A	N	
Others	melatonin	direct cytotoxic effect stimulating IL-2 secretion and activity; inhibitor of cytokines	20 mg/day during the dark	Y	**

EPA, eicosapentanoic acid; DHA, docosahexanoic acid; RCT, randomized controlled trial

included significantly increased lean body mass by bio-electrical impedance analysis[49]. However, since 7 of the original 20 patients dropped out because of disease progression, selection bias may have influenced the results[50].

In addition to these single-arm studies, several randomized, controlled trials have been conducted. In a randomized study of 60 patients with a variety of solid tumors, fish oil supplementation (18 g/day, 17% EPA, 11.5% DHA) increased survival time significantly and physical function when compared with the placebo group[51]. Results from subsequent studies in this area have been generally disappointing. In a randomized, multi-center trial of 200 patients with advanced pancreatic cancer and weight loss, fish oil supplementation (2 cans/day, 2.2 g EPA) for 8 weeks did not show a therapeutic advantage when compared with a placebo group receiving nutritional supplementation alone. However, poor compliance with the assigned treatment arm, i.e. treatment cross-overs, may have affected the results. The authors note that weight gain or stabilization was associated with the erythrocyte concentration of omega-3 fatty acids. This observation leaves open the possibility of a benefit from fish oil supplementation, but requires confirmation[52].

Another randomized trial, however, also failed to show a benefit of fish oil supplementation. In this multi-center study, 421 cancer patients with wasting were randomized to either fish oil (2.018 g EPA/0.92 g DHA), megesterol acetate (600 mg/day), or both therapies for a median of 3 months. On average, those given

fish oil supplementation did not show weight improvements when compared to megesterol alone or when given in combination with megesterol[53]. Discrepancies between the outcomes of various studies could be due to differences between populations, the dosages used, and other design features. Additional controlled trials of longer duration will be able to address this issue with more clarity.

The optimal dose of omega-3 fatty acids for the treatment of cachexia is not clearly established. Although the maximum dose was reported as 0.3 g/kg per day in a single-arm trial[54], 12 g/day also resulted in weight gain and significant reduction of APR production in a single-arm trial in patients with pancreatic cancer[49]. In most trials, fish oil was well tolerated at all doses used without unanticipated adverse reactions. The most common adverse effects include nausea, diarrhea, and fish belching[55]. However, these side-effects generally decrease over time and usually do not limit treatment.

As with all dietary supplements, the Food and Drug Administration does not regulate the composition or purity of fish oil products[50]. There is widespread concern about contamination with organochlorides in farm-raised fish, and mercury exposure from fish obtained from their natural habitats[56,57]. In 44 fish oil products from 15 countries, all products, with the exception of two, were reported to contain detectable organochloride residues[56]. However, Melanson *et al.* reported no detectable amount of organochlorides in five US over-the-counter fish oil preparations[58].

Mercury contamination is also a concern. In a case–control study of 684 men with a history of myocardial infarction and 724 matched controls, mercury measured in the toenail and DHA measured in the adipose tissue were significantly correlated. In addition, higher mercury levels were found in myocardial infarction patients, which may have limited the beneficial effect of fish consumption[57]. In children and pregnant and nursing women, excessive exposure to mercury should be avoided[59].

Melatonin

Melatonin is a hormone which is released from pineal grand, an endocrine gland at the base of the skull whose function is not clearly understood. Melatonin release is regulated by an endogenous circadian clock and may be involved in the regulation of the sleep cycle. Melatonin concentrations are very low during the daytime, increase during the night time hours, and then decrease to baseline levels by dawn. In addition, melatonin secretion is suppressed by light and may be influenced by other factors, such as age[60,61].

Melatonin supplementation has also been investigated for the treatment of cachexia. In a large randomized, clinical trial, 1440 advanced cancer patients were randomized to either supportive care alone or supportive care plus melatonin (20 mg/day at night for at least 2 months). According to this report, 5% of those who were randomized to melatonin reported symptoms of cachexia compared to 20% in the control group. In addition, the one-year survival rate in the melatonin supplementation group was significantly lower than in the supportive care group (20% vs 10%)[62]. Although seemingly promising, the findings are difficult to interpret, because the control group did not receive a placebo. The behavior of those who received melatonin may have differed in other ways from the control group, (i.e. diet, motivation, expectations, etc.) which may have contributed to the observed outcome. Furthermore, the methodology used to ascertain symptoms of cachexia was not clearly presented.

The mechanism through which melatonin may reduce the frequency of cachexia has not been elucidated, but may be related to its anti-inflammatory properties. One uncontrolled, single-arm study by the same authors as the above study showed that melatonin (20 mg/day) administered to 14 patients with evidence of immune activation (nine with solid tumor and five with autoimmune disease) on seven consecutive nights significantly decreased IL-6 levels, suggesting a possible

inhibition of the acute inflammatory response[63]. However, because there was no untreated comparison group, the clinical significance of this observation cannot be determined.

Melatonin may also have antineoplastic activity, which may indirectly impact on cachectic symptoms. In one study, 250 patients with metastatic disease were randomized to melatonin of 20 mg/day on seven consecutive days before chemotherapy or chemotherapy alone. The mean progression period was longer (8.9 ± 1.3 versus 4.2 ± 0.8 months) and the one-year survival rate was significantly higher in the melatonin plus chemotherapy group (51% survival rate) compared with chemotherapy alone group (23% survival rate). The authors conclude that melatonin may enhance the effect of chemotherapy and prevent chemotherapy-induced toxicity[64]. These intriguing findings require replication by other investigators before melatonin can be embraced as an effective adjunctive therapy. In addition, its mechanism of action requires further investigation. No adverse effects have been reported in clinical trials using melatonin and there are limited toxicity data[65].

Combination of fish oil and melatonin

The combination of fish oil and melatonin has also been investigated. Persson *et al.* compared 30 ml/day of fish oil (18% EPA and 12% DHA) with 18 mg/day of melatonin (in the evening) in 24 patients with advanced gastro-intestinal cancer for 4 weeks, after which both interventions were given simultaneously for an additional 4 weeks. After the first intervention period, the mean weight change was similar in the fish oil and melatonin groups (–0.6 kg and –1.8 kg). The authors note that there were five responders (gain or stabilized weight) in the fish oil group and three in the melatonin group. When both treatments were combined for an additional 4 weeks, 63% of patients ($n = 15$) showed a response. However, the median weight in both groups remained unchanged[66].

Because the study lacked a control group receiving usual care alone, the incremental benefit of fish oil and melatonin could not be fully assessed. The authors note that similar patients receiving supportive care alone usually lose approximately 3 kg/month. Interestingly, there were no changes in inflammatory markers including cytokines, CRP, and fibrinogen in either group, which suggests a non-inflammatory mechanism of action. The combination of these two agents requires further investigation.

Marijuana

Marijuana (*Cannabis sativa*) is used widely as a recreational drug for its psychotropic effect, but also has appetite stimulating properties[67]. The active component of marijuana, Δ9-tetrahydrocannabinol (THC), has been approved by the FDA in an oral preparation (dronabinol, Marinol) for the treatment of nausea and loss of appetite. Smoked or vaporized marijuana is also used as a complementary treatment to stimulate appetite in patients with cachexia[68].

According to a recent British survey, 27% of HIV patients reported using cannabis to treat symptoms related to HIV, most importantly lack of appetite. According to this uncontrolled study, 97% of patients reported improved appetite, 93% of patients reported improvement of nausea, and 69% of patients reported improvement of weight loss among individuals who had used cannabis[69].

There have been few studies published investigating the efficacy of marijuana in cachexia, in part because of the political controversy regarding its use for medical purposes. In a randomized-controlled clinical trial in 30 HIV patients who smoked marijuana at least twice a week for the previous 4 weeks, the effect of smoked marijuana (0.0, 1.8, 2.8, 3.9% Δ9-THC) and oral dronabinol (0, 10, 20, 30 mg) were compared to a placebo group over the 3–4 weeks. Both marijuana and dronabinol significantly increased calorie intake in patients with HIV wasting. However, the 30 mg dose of dronabinol was not tolerated in some participants[70]. To our knowledge, there has been no reported clinical studies of marijuana in cancer cachexia.

About 10% of people who ever used marijuana experience dependence[71]. In addition, smoking marijuana can have adverse effects on the respiratory system, similar to that seen with tobacco use[72]. The appropriate dosage needed to balance efficacy and safety has not yet been determined in clinical trials.

Rhizoma coptidis

Rhizoma coptidis is an herb which contains high amount of berberian. It has long been used in Eastern Asia as well as Europe to reduce inflammation[73,74]. It also has been reported as having direct antitumor effects in esophageal cancer cells[75]. In a mouse model of human cancer, *Rhizoma coptidis* supplementation prevented weight loss and down regulated IL-6 levels significantly when compared with control mice. Given these results, it is suggested that *Rhizoma coptidis* or berberian itself could be

useful in the prevention and treatment of cancer cachexia[76,77]. However, there have been no reported human trials to date.

Although a variety of herbal mixtures are used in East Asian medicine for the amelioration of cachetic symptoms associated with chronic illness[78], none have been evaluated with rigorous methodology and further investigation is required.

Treatment for immunomodulation

Since pro-inflammatory cytokines play a central role in the process of cachexia, compounds that modulate the immune response may also be beneficial.

Amino acids

Arginine and glutamine are considered as essential amino acids under conditions of stress[5] and may have immunomodulatory effects[79,80]. Supplementation of the amino acids can modulate the cachetic process through their effects on the inflammatory response. Further studies are required to determine the optimal use of immunonutrition for cachexia.

Micronutrients

It has been shown that enteral or parenteral nutritional support does not reduce morbidity and mortality associated with cachexia[81]. However, several micronutrients have been investigated which may slow the progression of the underlying disease, thereby preventing further wasting. Vitamin E, for example, has been shown to be deficient in advanced HIV infected patients and its supplementation has been associated with slower disease progression[82,84]. Low levels of beta-carotene and vitamins E and C have been reported in cancer patients of various types when compared with control groups[84]. However, the effects of these antioxidant vitamins are not clear[85]. While selenium and zinc have also been regarded as antioxidants, their effectiveness in cancer treatment is not consistent[86].

Panax ginseng

The root and rhizome of *Panax ginseng*, commonly called Korean or Chinese ginseng, has been used in Eastern Asia for more than 2000 years. The active compounds are thought to be plant steroids of the saponin class, called ginsenosides, and it has been extensively used for cancer chemoprevention and therapy throughout Asia[87]. Immunomodulatory properties of *Panax ginseng*, primarily associated with NK cell activity, have also been reported[88]. In a double-blind, randomized, placebo-controlled trial in healthy volunteers, ginseng root (100 mg extract, twice a day) showed a significant increase in the total number of T lymphocytes and activity of leukocytes after 8 weeks compared with baseline[89]. The effect of ginseng on immunomodulation in patients with cancer and HIV is not known.

Several herbal mixtures containing *Panax ginseng* have been reported to be effective in preventing weight loss in cancer patients in China and Korea, including Shi-quan-da-bu-tang[90], Hangammyunyouk[91], and Bojungikkeehpdaechilkitang[92]. Although 100 to 200 mg of standardized ginseng extract (4% ginsenosides) once or twice a day up to 12 weeks has been suggested[93], many different doses have been used in traditional East Asian medicine. Since there are no randomized, placebo-controlled clinical trials, the findings should be interpreted carefully and further investigation is necessary.

Treatment for nausea

Chronic nausea may limit calorie intake and contribute to weight loss in patients with advanced chronic disease.

Ginger rhizome

Ginger rhizome is the root of *Zingiber officinale* and its major activity is from the active ingredients of ginserol and shagoal which have various effects including an antiemetic effect[94]. In a randomized, double-blind trial in 120 pregnant women, 125 mg ginger extract (equivalent to 1.5 g of dried ginger), four times per day for 4 days, reduced the nausea experience score significantly when compared to a placebo group from the first day of treatment, and this difference continued throughout the treatment period[95]. Its effect in patients with cachexia is not known.

Acupuncture

Acupuncture may also be an adjunctive treatment for nausea, especially using the acupuncture point pericardium 6 (P6). In a single-blind, randomized-controlled trial, traditional acupuncture, P6 acupuncture, sham acupuncture, and no acupuncture groups were compared weekly for 4 weeks, in pregnant women of less than 14 weeks' gestation. Women in the

traditional acupuncture group reported less frequent nausea at the end of the first week when compared with the no acupuncture group. In the second week, both the traditional acupuncture and P6 acupuncture groups reported significantly reduced nausea compared with the no acupuncture group, which continued until the end of the study. However, the sham acupuncture group also reported a lower nausea score from the third week, which underscores the role of a strong placebo effect[96].

Another randomized, double-blind trial was done to determine the effect of acupuncture at P6 before or after the anesthesia in gynecologic or breast surgery patients. Both the acupuncture and placebo groups had two subgroups according to intervention time (before or after the anesthesia). Within 24 hours after surgery, vomiting was significantly decreased in the acupuncture group compared with the placebo group, regardless of intervention time[97]. However, during high-dose chemotherapy, P6 acupuncture 30 min before and the day after chemotherapy did not show an additional effect compared with the placebo group in a randomized-controlled trial[98].

Although there are no reported trials on the effect of acupuncture on cachexia per se, additional high-quality randomized trials need to be performed to verify the effect and mechanism of action of acupuncture on cachexia and its related conditions.

CONCLUSIONS

In cancer and AIDS, cachexia is an important cause of morbidity and mortality. While CAM use is prevalent in both of these diseases for the prevention or treatment of disease-related complications, such as cachexia, there have been few trials that have rigorously evaluated these treatments. The two best studied treatments, fish oil and melatonin, have had inconsistent and somewhat disappointing results. Further investigation is needed to study the safety and efficacy of CAM therapy in this important condition in which few therapies are effective.

ACKNOWLEDGMENTS

This work was partially supported by the 2005 Research Fund, Kyung Hee University (MYS) and the National Center for Complementary and Alternative Medicine (TTB 1 K23 AT002862-01).

References

1. Kotler DP. Cachexia. Ann Intern Med 2000; 133: 622–34

2. Harvey KB, Bothe A Jr, Blackburn GL. Nutritional assessment and patient outcome during oncological therapy. Cancer 1979; 43 (5 Suppl): 2065–9

3. Warren S. The immediate causes of death in cancer. Am J Med 1932; 184: 610–15

4. www.answers.com/topic/cachexia, accessed on 30 August 2005

5. Barber MD, Fearon KC, Delmore G, Loprinzi CL. Should cancer patients with incurable disease receive parenteral or enteral nutritional support? Eur J Cancer 1998; 343: 279–85

6. Cahill GF Jr. Starvation in man. Clin Endocrinol Metab 1976; 5: 397–415

7. Argiles JM, Alvarez B, Lopez-Soriano FJ. The metabolic basis of cancer cachexia. Med Res Rev 1997; 17: 477–98

8. Bruera E. ABC of palliative care. Anorexia, cachexia, and nutrition. Br Med J 1997; 315: 1219–22

9. Rosenbaum K, Wang J, Pierson RN Jr, Kotler DP. Time-dependent variation in weight and body composition in healthy adults. JPEN 2000; 24: 52–5

10. van den Beld AW, Lamberts SW. The male climacterium: clinical signs and symptoms of a changing endocrine environment. Prostate Suppl 2000; 10: 2–8

11. Tang AM, Forrester J, Spiegelman D, et al. Weight loss and survival in HIV-positive patients in the era of highly active antiretroviral therapy. J Acquir Immune Defic Syndr 2002; 31: 230–6

12. Wheeler DA, Gibert CL, Launer CA, et al. Weight loss as a predictor of survival and disease progression in HIV infection. Terry Beirn Community Programs for Clinical Research on AIDS. J Acq Imm Def Synd Hum Retrovirol 1998; 18: 80–5

13. Roubenoff R. Acquired immunodeficiency syndrome wasting, functional performance, and quality of life. Am J Manag Care 2000; 69: 1003–16

14. Rao VK, Thomas FP. Neurological complications of HIV/AIDS. BETA 2005; 17: 37–46

15. Gilmer WS. Neurologic conditions affecting the lower extremities in HIV infection. J Am Podiatr Med Assoc 1995; 85: 352–61

16. Barber MD, Ross JA, Fearon KC. Cancer cachexia. Surg Oncol 1999; 8: 133–41

17. Fearon KC, Moses AG. Cancer cachexia. Int J Cardiol 2002; 85: 73–81

18. Baumann H, Gauldie J. The acute phase response. Immunol Today 1994; 15: 74–80

19. Falconer JS, Fearon KC, Plester CE, et al. Cytokines, the acute-phase response, and resting energy expenditure in cachectic patients with pancreatic cancer. Ann Surg 1994; 219: 325–31

20. Tisdale MJ. Cachexia in cancer patients. Nat Rev Cancer 2002; 2: 862–71

21. Argiles JM, Moore-Carrasco R, Fuster G, et al. Cancer cachexia: the molecular mechanisms. Int J Biochem Cell Biol 2003; 35: 405–9

22. Bessesen DH, Faggioni R. Recently identified peptides involved in the regulation of body weight. Semin Oncol 1998; 25 (2 Suppl 6): 28–32

23. Inui A. Cancer anorexia–cachexia syndrome: are neuropeptides the key? Cancer Res 1999; 59: 4493–501

24. Strassmann G, Fong M, Freter CE, et al. Suramin interferes with interleukin-6 receptor binding in vitro and inhibits colon-26-mediated experimental cancer cachexia in vivo. J Clin Invest 1993; 92: 2152–9

25. Friedman JM, Halaas JL. Leptin and the regulation of body weight in mammals. Nature 1998; 395: 763–70

26. Sarraf P, Frederich RC, Turner EM, et al. Multiple cytokines and acute inflammation raise mouse leptin levels: potential role in inflammatory anorexia. J Exp Med 1997; 185: 171–5

27. Gayle D, Ilyin SE, Plata-Salaman CR. Central nervous system IL-1 beta system and neuropeptide Y mRNAs during IL-1 beta-induced anorexia in rats. Brain Res Bull 1997; 44: 311–17

28. Todorov P, Cariuk P, McDevitt T, et al. Characterization of a cancer cachectic factor. Nature 1996; 379: 739–42

29. Nelson KA, Walsh D, Sheehan FA. The cancer anorexia–cachexia syndrome. J Clin Oncol 1994; 12: 213–25

30. Tisdale MJ. Metabolic abnormalities in cachexia and anorexia. Nutrition 2000; 16: 1013–14

31. Kotler DP, Grunfeld C. Pathophysiology and treatment of the AIDS wasting syndrome. AIDS Clin Rev 1995; 229–75

32. Yarasheski KE, Zachwieja JJ, Gischler J, et al. Increased plasma gln and Leu Ra and inappropriately low muscle protein synthesis rate in AIDS wasting. Am J Physiol 1998; 275 (4 Pt 1): E577–83

33. Macallan DC, McNurlan MA, Milne E, et al. Whole-body protein turnover from leucine kinetics and the response to nutrition in human immunodeficiency virus infection. Am J Clin Nutr 1995; 61: 818–26

34. Grinspoon S, Corcoran C, Lee K, et al. Loss of lean body and muscle mass correlates with androgen levels in hypogonadal men with acquired immunodeficiency syndrome and wasting. J Clin Endocrinol Metab 1996; 81: 4051–8

35. Grinspoon S, Corcoran C, Miller K, et al. Body composition and endocrine function in women with acquired immunodeficiency syndrome wasting. J Clin Endocrinol Metab 1997; 82: 1332–7

36. Chrystal K, Allan S, Forgeson G, Isaacs R. The use of complementary/alternative medicine by cancer patients in a New Zealand regional cancer treatment centre. NZ Med J 2003; 116: U296

37. Molassiotis A, Fernadez-Ortega P, Pud D, et al. Use of complementary and alternative medicine in cancer patients: a European survey. Ann Oncol 2005; 16: 655–63

38. Lafferty WE, Bellas A, Corage BA, et al. The use of complementary and alternative medical providers by insured cancer patients in Washington State. Cancer 2004; 100: 1522–30

39. Fairfield KM, Eisenberg DM, Davis RB, et al. Patterns of use, expenditures, and perceived efficacy of complementary and alternative therapies in HIV-infected patients. Arch Intern Med 1998; 158: 2257–64

40. Anderson W, O'Connor BB, MacGregor RR, Schwartz JS. Patient use and assessment of conventional and alternative therapies for HIV infection and AIDS. AIDS 1993; 7: 561–5

41. Ostrow MJ, Cornelisse PG, Heath KV, et al. Determinants of complementary therapy use in HIV-infected individuals receiving antiretroviral or anti-opportunistic agents. J Acq Imm Def Synd Hum Retrovirol 1997; 15: 115–20

42. Singh N, Squier C, Sivek C, et al. Determinants of nontraditional therapy use in patients with HIV infection. A prospective study. Arch Intern Med 1996; 156: 197–201

43. Eisenberg DM, Davis RB, Ettner SL, et al. Trends in alternative medicine use in the United States, 1990–1997: results of a follow-up national survey. J Am Med Assoc 1998; 280: 1569–75

44. Fairfield KM, Eisenberg DM, Davis RB, et al. Patterns of use, expenditures, and perceived efficacy of complementary and alternative therapies in HIV-infected patients. Arch Intern Med 1998; 158: 2257–64

45. Korver DR, Klasing KC. Dietary fish oil alters specific and inflammatory immune responses in chicks. J Nutr 1997; 127: 2039–46

46. Zhao Y, Joshi-Barve S, Barve S, Chen LH. Eicosapentaenoic acid prevents LPS-induced TNF-alpha expression by preventing NF-kappaB activation. J Am Coll Nutr 2004; 23: 71–8

47. Wigmore SJ, Fearon KC, Maingay JP, Ross JA. Down-regulation of the acute-phase response in patients with pancreatic cancer cachexia receiving oral eicosapentaenoic acid is mediated via suppression of interleukin-6. Clin Sci (Lond) 1997; 92: 215–21

48. Wigmore SJ, Ross JA, Falconer JS, et al. The effect of polyunsaturated fatty acids on the progress of cachexia in patients with pancreatic cancer. Nutrition 1996; 12 (Suppl): S27–30

49. Barber MD, Ross JA, Voss AC, et al. The effect of an oral nutritional supplement enriched with fish oil on weight-loss in patients with pancreatic cancer. Br J Cancer 1999; 81: 80–6

50. Brown TT, Zelnik DL, Dobs AS. Fish oil supplementation in the treatment of cachexia in pancreatic cancer patients. Int J Gastrointest Cancer 2003; 34: 143–50

51. Gogos CA, Ginopoulos P, Salsa B, et al. Dietary omega-3 polyunsaturated fatty acids plus vitamin E restore immunodeficiency and prolong survival for severely ill patients with generalized malignancy: a randomized control trial. Cancer 1998; 82: 395–402

52. Fearon KC, Von Meyenfeldt MF, Moses AG, et al. Effect of a protein and energy dense N-3 fatty acid enriched oral supplement on loss of weight and lean tissue in cancer cachexia: a randomised double blind trial. Gut 2003; 52: 1479–86

53. Jatoi A, Rowland K, Loprinzi CL, et al. An eicosapentaenoic acid supplement versus megestrol acetate versus both for patients with cancer-associated wasting: a North Central Cancer Treatment Group and National Cancer Institute of Canada collaborative effort. J Clin Oncol 2004; 22: 2469–76

54. Burns CP, Halabi S, Clamon GH, et al. Phase I clinical study of fish oil fatty acid capsules for patients with cancer cachexia: cancer and leukemia group B study 9473. Clin Cancer Res 1999; 5: 3942–7

55. Jatoi A. Fish oil, lean tissue, and cancer: is there a role for eicosapentaenoic acid in treating the cancer anorexia/ weight loss syndrome? Crit Rev Oncol Hematol 2005; 55: 37–43

56. Jacobs MN, Santillo D, Johnston PA, et al. Organochlorine residues in fish oil dietary supplements: comparison with industrial grade oils. Chemosphere 1998; 37: 1709–21

57. Guallar E, Sanz-Gallardo MI, van't VP, et al. Mercury, fish oils, and the risk of myocardial infarction. N Engl J Med 2002; 347: 1747–54

58. Melanson SF, Lewandrowski EL, Flood JG, Lewandrowski KB. Measurement of organochlorines in commercial over-the-counter fish oil preparations: implications for dietary and therapeutic recommendations for omega-3 fatty acids and a review of the literature. Arch Pathol Lab Med 2005; 129: 74–7

59. Kris-Etherton PM, Harris WS, Appel LJ. Omega-3 fatty acids and cardiovascular disease: new recommendations from the American Heart Association. Arterioscler Thromb Vasc Biol 2003; 23: 151–2

60. Herljevic M, Middleton B, Thapan K, Skene DJ. Light-induced melatonin suppression: age-related reduction in response to short wavelength light. Exp Gerontol 2005; 40: 237–42

61. Zeitzer JM, Dijk DJ, Kronauer R, et al. Sensitivity of the human circadian pacemaker to nocturnal light: melatonin phase resetting and suppression. J Physiol 2000; 5263: 695–702

62. Lissoni P. Is there a role for melatonin in supportive care? Support Care Cancer 2002; 10: 110–16

63. Lissoni P, Rovelli F, Meregalli S, et al. Melatonin as a new possible anti-inflammatory agent. J Biol Regul Homeost Agents 1997; 11: 157–9

64. Lissoni P, Barni S, Mandala M, et al. Decreased toxicity and increased efficacy of cancer chemotherapy using the pineal hormone melatonin in metastatic solid tumour patients with poor clinical status. Eur J Cancer 1999; 35: 1688–92

65. Vijayalaxmi, Thomas CR Jr, Reiter RJ, Herman TS. Melatonin: from basic research to cancer treatment clinics. J Clin Oncol 2002; 20: 2575–601

66. Persson C, Glimelius B, Ronnelid J, Nygren P. Impact of fish oil and melatonin on cachexia in patients with advanced gastrointestinal cancer: a randomized pilot study. Nutrition 2005; 21: 170–8

67. Di Marzo, V, Matias I. Endocannabinoid control of food intake and energy balance. Nat Neurosci 2005; 8: 585–9

68. Watson SJ, Benson JA Jr, Joy JE. Marijuana and medicine: assessing the science base: a summary of the 1999 Institute of Medicine report. Arch Gen Psychiatry 2000; 57: 547–52

69. Woolridge E, Barton S, Samuel J, et al. Cannabis use in HIV for pain and other medical symptoms. J Pain Symptom Manage 2005; 29: 358–67

70. Haney M, Rabkin J, Gunderson E, Foltin RW. Dronabinol and marijuana in HIV+ marijuana smokers: acute effects on caloric intake and mood. Psychopharmacology (Berl) 2005; 181: 170–8

71. Budney AJ, Kandel DB, Cherek DR, et al. College on problems of drug dependence meeting, Puerto Rico (June 1996) marijuana use and dependence. Drug Alcohol Depend 1997; 45: 1–11

72. Polen MR, Sidney S, Tekawa IS, et al. Health care use by frequent marijuana smokers who do not smoke tobacco. West J Med 1993; 158: 596–601

73. Fukutake M, Yokota S, Kawamura H, et al. Inhibitory effect of Coptidis Rhizoma and Scutellariae Radix on azoxymethane-induced aberrant crypt foci formation in rat colon. Biol Pharm Bull 1998; 21: 814–17

74. Ivanovska N, Philipov S. Study on the anti-inflammatory action of Berberis vulgaris root extract, alkaloid fractions and pure alkaloids. Int J Immunopharmacol 1996; 18: 553–61

75. Iizuka N, Miyamoto K, Okita K, et al. Inhibitory effect of Coptidis Rhizoma and berberine on the proliferation of human esophageal cancer cell lines. Cancer Lett 2000; 148: 19–25

76. Iizuka N, Miyamoto K, Hazama S, et al. Anticachectic effects of Coptidis rhizoma, an anti-inflammatory herb, on

esophageal cancer cells that produce interleukin 6. Cancer Lett 2000; 158: 35–41

77. Iizuka N, Hazama S, Yoshimura K, et al. Anticachectic effects of the natural herb Coptidis rhizoma and berberine on mice bearing colon 26/clone 20 adenocarcinoma. Int J Cancer 2002; 99: 286–91

78. Kiyohara H, Matsumoto T, Yamada H. Combination effects of herbs in a multi-herbal formula: expression of Juzen-taiho-to's immuno-modulatory activity on the intestinal immune system. Evidence Based Comp Altern Med 2004; 1: 83–91

79. Garcia-de-Lorenzo A, Zarazaga A, Garcia-Luna PP, et al. Clinical evidence for enteral nutritional support with glutamine: a systematic review. Nutrition 2003; 19: 805–11

80. Brittenden J, Heys SD, Ross J, et al. Natural cytotoxicity in breast cancer patients receiving neoadjuvant chemotherapy: effects of L-arginine supplementation. Eur J Surg Oncol 1994; 20: 467–72

81. Cohn SH, Vartsky D, Vaswani AN, et al. Changes in body composition of cancer patients following combined nutritional support. Nutr Cancer 1982; 4: 107–19

82. Coodley GO, Coodley MK, Nelson HD, Loveless MO. Micronutrient concentrations in the HIV wasting syndrome. AIDS 1993; 7: 1595–600

83. Malvy DJ, Richard MJ, Arnaud J, et al. Relationship of plasma malondialdehyde, vitamin E and antioxidant micronutrients to human immunodeficiency virus-1 seropositivity. Clin Chim Acta 1994; 224: 89–94

84. Torun M, Yardim S, Gonenc A, et al. Serum beta-carotene, vitamin E, vitamin C and malondialdehyde levels in several types of cancer. J Clin Pharm Ther 1995; 20: 259–63

85. Brown BG, Crowley J. Is there any hope for vitamin E? J Am Med Assoc 2005; 293: 1387–90

86. Strain JJ. Putative role of dietary trace elements in coronary heart disease and cancer. Br J Biomed Sci 1994; 51: 241–51

87. Helms S. Cancer prevention and therapeutics: Panax ginseng. Altern Med Rev 2004; 9: 259–74

88. Kim JY, Germolec DR, Luster MI. Panax ginseng as a potential immunomodulator: studies in mice. Immunopharmacol Immunotoxicol 1990; 12: 257–76

89. Scaglione F, Ferrara F, Dugnani S, et al. Immunomodulatory effects of two extracts of Panax ginseng C.A. Meyer. Drugs Exp Clin Res 1990; 16: 537–42

90. Zee-Cheng RK. Shi-quan-da-bu-tang (ten significant tonic decoction), SQT. A potent Chinese biological response modifier in cancer immunotherapy, potentiation and detoxification of anticancer drugs. Methods Find Exp Clin Pharmacol 1992; 14: 725–36

91. Yoo HS, Cho CK. Clinical study in 40 cases for patients with stomach cancer taken Hangammyunyouk 1. J Kor Orient Oncol 1998; 4: 1

92. Lee YH, Kim BS, Oh JH, et al. The anti-tumor effect of Bojungikkeehapdaechilkitang with doxorubicin in MKN-45. Kor J Orient Int Med 2004; 25: 1

93. Ulbricht CE, Basch EM. Natural Standard Herb & Supplement Reference Evidence-based Clinical Reviews. St Louis: Elsevier Mosby, 2005

94. Langner E, Greifenberg S, Gruenwald J. Ginger: history and use. Adv Ther 1998; 15: 25–44

95. Willetts KE, Ekangaki A, Eden JA. Effect of a ginger extract on pregnancy-induced nausea: a randomised controlled trial. Aust NZ J Obstet Gynaecol 2003; 43: 139–44

96. Smith C, Crowther C, Beilby J. Acupuncture to treat nausea and vomiting in early pregnancy: a randomized controlled trial. Birth 2002; 29: 1–9

97. Streitberger K, Diefenbacher M, Bauer A, et al. Acupuncture compared to placebo-acupuncture for postoperative nausea and vomiting prophylaxis: a randomised placebo-controlled patient and observer blind trial. Anaesthesia 2004; 59: 142–9

98. Streitberger K, Friedrich-Rust M, Bardenheuer H, et al. Effect of acupuncture compared with placebo-acupuncture at P6 as additional antiemetic prophylaxis in high-dose chemotherapy and autologous peripheral blood stem cell transplantation: a randomized controlled single-blind trial. Clin Cancer Res 2003; 9: 2538–44

Boost AIDS patients' immune systems   26

J. A. Wu and C.-S. Yuan

INTRODUCTION

The acquired immunodeficiency syndrome (AIDS) is a result of human immunodeficiency virus (HIV) infection which subsequently leads to significant suppression of immune functions. AIDS is an unprecedented threat to nations as well as to global health[1,2]. Approximately 40 million people worldwide are living with HIV/AIDS. In 2004 alone, an estimated 5 million people worldwide were newly infected with HIV – about 14 000 each day[3]. Therefore, effective therapies to treat AIDS are urgently needed. In order to combat HIV, a colossal amount of money and manpower has been dedicated to searching for compounds that can be developed as therapeutic agents. In the past two decades, several chemical anti-HIV agents have been developed. The current strategy for the treatment of HIV infection is called highly active antiretroviral therapy (HAART) and is based on cocktails of drugs that are currently approved by the US Food and Drug Administration (FDA). However, besides the high cost, there are adverse effects and limitations associated with using chemotherapy for the treatment of HIV infection[4]. Herbal medicines are frequently used as an alternative medical therapy by HIV-positive individuals and AIDS patients. The aim of this chapter is to summarize research findings for herbal medicines that are endowed with the ability to inhibit HIV. In this chapter, we emphasize a Chinese herbal medicine, *Scutellaria baicalensis* Georgi, and its identified components (i.e. baicalein and baicalin), which have been shown to inhibit infectivity and replication of HIV.

CONVENTIONAL CHEMOTHERAPY FOR HIV INFECTION

According to De Clercq, the replicative cycle of HIV is composed of ten steps that may be adequate targets for chemotherapeutic intervention[5,6]. Most of the substances that have been identified as anti-HIV agents can be assigned to one of these ten classes of HIV inhibitors based on the stage at which they interfere with the HIV replicative cycle. These ten steps are:

(1) Viral adsorption to the cell membrane;

(2) Fusion between the viral envelope and the cell membrane;

(3) Uncoating of the viral nucleocapsid;

(4) Reverse transcription of the viral RNA to proviral DNA;

(5) Integration of the proviral DNA to the cellular genome;

(6) DNA replication;

(7) Transcription of the proviral DNA to RNA;

(8) Translation of the viral precursor mRNA to mature mRNA;

(9) Maturation of the viral precursor proteins by proteolysis, myristoylation, and glycosylation;

(10) Budding, virion assembly, and release.

Step 4, a key step in the replicative cycle of retroviruses, which makes it distinct from the replicative cycle of other viruses, is the reverse transcription catalyzed by reverse transcriptase. Another target for therapeutic intervention is step 9, particularly the proteolysis of precursor proteins by HIV protease. The majority of chemotherapeutic strategies have, therefore, focused on the development of retroviral enzyme inhibitors.

Table 26.1 lists the anti-HIV drugs approved by the FDA for clinical use[7]. However, these medications have limitations such as high cost, peripheral neuropathy, and decreased sensitivity due to the rapid emergence of drug-resistant mutant virus strains, and adverse effects such as bone marrow suppression and anemia[8,9]. Therefore,

Table 26.1 Antiviral drugs approved for the treatment of HIV infections*

Antiviral drug	Trade name	Mechanism of action
Zidovudine or AZT	Retrovir	NRTI
Didanosine or ddI	Videx	NRTI
Zalcitabine or ddC	Hivid	NRTI
Stavudine or d4T	Zerit	NRTI
Lamivudine or 3TC	Epivir	NRTI
Abacavir or ABC	Ziagen	NRTI
Tenofovir	Viread	NRTI
Nevirapine	Viramune	NNRTI
Delavirdine	Rescriptor	NNRTI
Efavirenz	Sustiva	NNRTI
Saquinavir	Invirase, Fortovase	PI
Ritonavir	Norvir	PI
Indinavir	Crixivan	PI
Nelfinavir	Viracept	PI
Amprenavir	Agenerase	PI
Lopinavir	Kaletra**	PI
Enfuvirtide	Fuzeon	FI

*The drugs are classified into four groups according to their mechanism of action: (1) nucleoside reverse transcriptase inhibitors (NRTIs), (2) non-nucleoside reverse transcriptase inhibitors (NNRTIs), (3) protease inhibitors (PIs), and (4) fusion inhibitors (FIs).

**In combination with ritonavir

more effective and less toxic anti-HIV agents are still needed. In addition, alternative approaches, including herbal therapies, long-term screening of plant extracts, particularly anti-infective or immunomodulating medicinal herbs, and the structural modification of leading compounds, have been attempted.

STUDIES OF MEDICINAL HERBS ON HIV INFECTION

Screening and use of herbs in Asia and North America

Herbal medicine has been used in China for centuries. Even after opening its doors to Western medicine two centuries ago, China still relies heavily on Traditional Chinese Medicine (TCM) and herbal therapies because of their efficacy. Indeed, the recent focus of the Chinese

government has been to propel research at its institutes and universities towards developing efficacious herbal drugs, particularly as anti-cancer, anti-cardiovascular disease, and immunomodulating agents[10].

Screening

Since 1987, the US National Cancer Institute has worked with the Chinese Academy of Sciences to study Chinese medicinal herbs for anti-AIDS application. Over 1000 Chinese traditional medicines were screened using different solvent extraction forms, and more than 140 different herbs were found to have HIV inhibitory activity. Among them, more than 20 herbs have exhibited significant HIV inhibitory activity[11].

In the USA, experimental studies are in progress to isolate anti-HIV agents from medicinal plants and their natural products. In one such study, conducted by the National Cancer Institute, approximately 4500 plant samples are currently screened per year for *in vitro* anti-HIV activity, based on a random selection of plants[12].

At the University of Illinois at Chicago[13], a simple *in vitro* method has been developed for screening the HIV type 1 (HIV-1) reverse transcriptase inhibitory potential of natural products. More than 100 plant extracts have been evaluated, and 15 of these extracts show significant inhibitory activity. A total of 156 natural products has been examined in this system[14].

In China, over 1000 traditional herbs were screened using aqueous and methanol extraction methods by the Chinese Academy of Sciences in Shanghai[15], Beijing[16], and Kunming[17,18]. Over a hundred different herbs and several hundred extract products were found to have HIV inhibitory activity. In addition, two multiple screening approaches have been applied to aqueous extracts of 19 herbs in Hong Kong[19,20] and in Taipei[21] in order to detect antiviral agents.

Scientists from both Thailand and Japan have worked together to screen the anti-HIV activity of 413 plants grown in Thailand. Significant inhibitory activity has been found in 81 of these plants[22].

Anti-HIV reverse transcriptase and protease activity have also been identified in extracts of Indian herb[23], Japanese herbs[24,25], Korean medicinal plants[26], Mongolian herbs[27], and New Zealand plants[28].

Use of single herbs

Studies on treating HIV with Chinese herbs have had mixed results. However, these studies usually used Chinese herbs as antiviral treatments. More recently, herbs are being combined with antiviral medications. Some herbalists believe that the best use of herbs will be to help deal with the side-effects of strong antiviral drugs, and to generally strengthen the immune system.

In China, medicinal herbs are being used in the treatment of HIV-positive subjects and AIDS patients. One example is the traditional Chinese medicinal herb Tian-Hua-Fen (*Trichosanthes kirilowii*), which appears in the classical Chinese medical reference work *Compendium of Materia Medica*, from the late fourteenth century. Tian-Hua-Fen has been used in China for hundreds of years to reset menstruation and expel retained placentas. Trichosanthin, an active protein component isolated from Tian-Hua-Fen, has been shown to inhibit HIV infection and has been used in the clinical treatment of AIDS[29–33].

The most interesting ingredient in licorice is the chemical glycyrrhizin (a word derived from the biologic name of the licorice plant, *Glycyrrhiza glabra*). Glycyrrhizin, 50 times sweeter than sugar, is responsible for the sweet taste of the infusions, tinctures, or other preparations made from the licorice root. (The Chinese name for licorice is *gan cao*, meaning 'sweet weed'.) With HIV itself, licorice appears to do four things:

(1) It slows HIV reproduction in infected white blood cells (monocytes, macrophages, and other cell populations);

(2) It interferes with cell-to-cell infection;

(3) It interferes with virus-to-cell infection; and

(4) It severely limits the clumping (syncytia) of HIV-infected white blood cells.

As an antiviral and antibacterial, licorice attacks fat-coated microorganisms like HIV, and other fat-coated AIDS cofactors such as tuberculosis, cytomegalovirus, herpes, hepatitis, and various parasites. In people with HIV, licorice increases T cells, and improves the T helper/T suppressor ratio, both important markers in HIV disease status[24,34–37].

Chinese herbs do not cure HIV infection. Many people, however, believe that the herbs have helped them improve their overall energy, or helped deal with the side-effects of antiviral medications. Some people have used herbs to reduce the upset stomach or diarrhea caused by their medications. In general, an herbalist makes up a personalized mixture for each patient, based on that person's particular energy flows and imbalances. However, some practitioners of Chinese medicine have noticed a consistent 'toxic heat' pattern of energy imbalances in people with advanced HIV disease. Due to

Chinese medicine's emphasis on long life and immune enhancement, they feel that some herbal preparations will probably help anybody with HIV. Studies on treating HIV with Chinese herbs have had mixed results. However, these studies usually used Chinese herbs as antiviral treatments. More recently, herbs are being combined with antiviral medications.

In the USA, the use of herbs as an alternative medical treatment for many illnesses has increased steadily over the past decade. Because herbs are categorized as natural food products or dietary supplements, they are not currently subject to strict control by the FDA[10]. However, many patients with AIDS are using herbal medical therapies in addition to conventional treatment. One study reported that, in 1991, 22% of AIDS patients had used one or more herbs for medicinal purposes in the previous 3 months[38]. Recently, this percentage has increased[39]. A recent nationwide survey of HIV-positive individuals in the USA found that up to 68% of participants admitted to using complementary and alternative medicine (CAM) therapy within the previous 12 months[40].

Use of polyherbal medicine

An Oriental remedy called Xiao-Chai-Hu-Tang (Chinese name) or Sho-saiko-to (SST or TJ9, Japanese name), which consists of a mixture of aqueous extracts from seven commonly used herbs, has been used in AIDS patients in China and Japan[41–43].

Qian-kun-nin is a Chinese herbal formulation considered to have anti-infection, anti-tumor and immuno-enhancing properties. Data from previous investigations showed that qian-kun-nin causes HIV growth inhibition and immunomodulation *in vitro*, suggesting that this formula has the ability to inhibit HIV and modulate impaired immune functions in humans. Qian-Qun-Ning, which consists of a mixture of aqueous extracts from 14 different herbs, showed efficacy in a pilot clinical trial of HIV-positive subjects[44,45]. Chinese and Thai scientists have worked out a new anti-AIDS drug that has proven effective in 89% of patients in a recent clinical trial. The compound 'SH', an herbal formula, was developed by the Kunming Institute of Botany of the Chinese Academy of Sciences in collaboration with Thai experts. The clinical trials have been conducted by Thai hospitals on 120 HIV-positive patients and proven effective in 89% of the patients[46].

A Chinese polyherbal medicine formula Zhongyan-2 recipe (ZY-2) has been discovered and developed by the China Academy of Traditional Chinese Medicine in

Beijing. After clinical treatment in 29 patients for 3 months, the total effective rate was 42.28 % on the basis of comprehensive assessment of viral load, immune function, body weight, and symptom signs. Thus the indications are that ZY-2 is an effective Chinese recipe in treating HIV-infected patients[47].

The antiretroviral activity and safety of a new poly-herbal drug named Immu-25 in patients with HIV infection have been evaluated in India. Thirty-six patients with confirmed HIV infection with a CD4 count < 500 cells/µl, received two capsules of the test drug twice daily for 1.8 months in this open-label, pilot study. Immu-25 showed a favorable effect, with a decrease in the mean viral load, which was associated with good symptomatic improvement, and an increase in the mean CD4 cell count[48].

A Chinese herbal medicine, bu-zhong-yi-qi-tang, with the Japanese name hochu-ekki-to (HET), a mixture of a spray-dried powder made from 10 medicinal plants, is widely used in China and Japan as an effective medication against some disorders of the human body such as renal ptosis and male infertility. The oral administration of HET increased both the number of leukocytes in the spleen and liver and the splenic NK cell cytotoxicity associated with the increased induction of serum IFN-α/β after a murine cytomegalovirus (MCMV) infection, but it had no effect on liver NK cells. Thus HET is useful in the treatment of human cytomegalovirus infection which commonly occurs in HIV-infected AIDS patients[49].

In addition, in the United States, some polyherbal medicines involving at least two Chinese herbal medicines or peptide components have been developed by different companies or research groups. The US patents of the methods and *in vitro* antiviral activities against HIV have been approved and published[50–52].

Bioactive components from the herbs

Many research groups are exploring the biodiversity of the plant kingdom to find new and better anti-HIV drugs. A number of articles that discuss the HIV inhibitory activity of herbs and their natural products[11,12,17,53–64] suggest that a variety of chemically disparate molecules, produced by species distributed across the plant kingdom, such as algae, pine trees, and flowering plants, are effective at inhibiting the activity of HIV. These compounds are composed of aliphatic ketones and aldehydes; terpenoids; alkaloids; coumarin derivatives; flavonoids; xanthone; flavone-xanthone

C-glucoside; hyperlein; tannins; gossypol acetic acid; polysaccharides; and proteins.

Some plant substances with an interesting anti-HIV activity according to the viral target(s) with which they interact have been discussed by Cos *et al.*[64] (Table 26.2). Because of their potential systemic effects and prophylactic action against HIV infection, plant-derived antiviral agents are prime study candidates. They may also be useful as topical agents to inactivate newly formed viruses, or as adjuvants with other antiviral drugs.

In the isolation of natural products, it is essential to adhere to the following steps. First, the plant kingdom as a source of new antiviral leading compounds should continue to be explored. Second, leading compounds that have been shown to inhibit HIV activity should be developed through modern pharmacologic methods to increase activity and decrease toxicity. Finally, herbal medicines or natural products as part of drug combination regimens for the treatment of HIV infections should be encouraged and continued[56].

Anti-HIV activity of flavonoids and *Scutellaria baicalensis* Georgi

Various flavonoids have been shown, *in vitro*, to inhibit the reverse transcriptase of certain retroviruses, including HIV (step 4 of the replicative cycle), as well as cellular DNA polymerases. These products exhibited selective anti-HIV-1 activity[65–68], whereas baicalein (5,6,7-trihydroxyflavone), a constituent isolated from *Scutellaria baicalensis* Georgi (Huang Qin in Chinese, Worgon in Japanese), specifically inhibited HIV reverse transcriptase[10,69,70].

In AIDS treatment, the inhibition of HIV reverse transcriptase is currently considered a useful approach, therefore natural products that show inhibitory activity have been extensively explored[54].

Effects of baicalein and baicalin

Oho *et al.* showed the effects of baicalein on the activity of various reverse transcriptases. They demonstrated that 1 µg/ml baicalein inhibited 90% of the activity of MLV-reverse transcriptase, and that 2 µg/ml baicalein inhibited 90% of the activity of HIV-reverse transcriptases[71].

Tang *et al.*[33] found that baicalin, which is isolated from *Scutellaria baicalensis* Georgi, inhibited HIV-reverse transcriptase, with an IC_{50} value of 22 µmol/l. Lee *et al.* reported that IC_{50} baicalein and baicalin for endonucleolytic activities of HIV-1 integrase were 4.4 ± 3.3 and 25.9 ± 4.0 µmol/l[72]. Some pharmacologic

Table 26.2 Potential anti-HIV targets for plant-derived substances*

Compound	Entry	RT	Integrase	Trans-cription
Betulinic acid derivatives	X			
Calanolides/ inophyllums		X		
DCQA/DCTA (chicoric acid)	X		X	
Flavonoids	X	X	X	X
Mannose-specific plant lectins	X			
Sulfated polysaccharides	X			X
Trichosanthin, MAP30, GAP31			X	

*The main mechanism of action is indicated by X; RT, reverse transcriptase; DCQA/DCTA, dicaffeoylquinic acid/ dicaffeoyltartaric acid

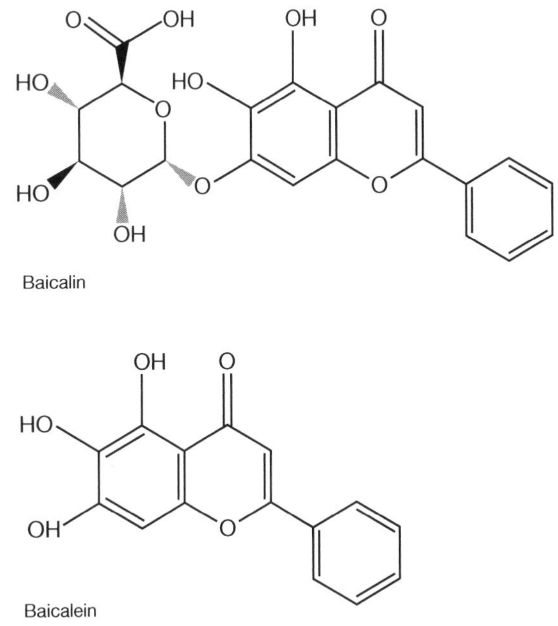

test results have demonstrated non-competitive inhibition of retroviral reverse transcriptase activity in HIV-1-infected H9 cells[73,74], HIV-1 specific core antigen p24 expression, and quantitative focal syncytium formation on CEM-SS monolayer cells[75]. Baicalin and its derivative 7-glucuronic acid 5,6-dihydroxyflavone was also efficacious in inhibiting reverse transcriptase of other retroviruses[76]. The difference in HIV-1 reverse transcriptase inhibitory activity between baicalein and baicalin has been examined[77]. The results show that the HIV-1 reverse transcriptase inhibitory activity of baicalein was four times higher than that of baicalin. The inhibition of HIV-1 integration (step 5 of the replicative cycle) by baicalein was investigated biochemically and by means of structure–activity relationships. It was reported that the IC_{50} for HIV integrase inhibition by baicalein was 4.3 μmol/l[78].

The *in vitro* anti-HIV-1 activity of baicalin was compared with its zinc complex (BA–Zn). The results suggested that BA–Zn has lower cytoxicity and higher anti-HIV-1 activity *in vitro* compared with those of BA. The CC_{50} of BA–Zn and BA was 221.52 and 101.73 μmol/l, respectively. BA–Zn was more effective than baicalin in inhibiting the entry of recombinant RT and VIV-1 into host cells[79].

Baicalin

Baicalein

Figure 26.1 Chemical structures of baicalin and baicalein

An investigation into the metabolism of baicalin has been published[80]. The results indicated that baicalin is first metabolized into baicalein (Figure 26.1), and the final metabolite was identified as baicalein 6-*O*-sulfate by comparing its retention time in high-performance liquid chromatography (HPLC) and electrospray ionization mass spectra (ESI-MS)/MS methods with that of an authentic sample.

Mechanisms of action

As for the mechanism of the anti-HIV-1 effect of baicalin, it was found that baicalin and baicalein have an inhibitory effect on various cellular DNA and RNA polymerases[69,81]. In the case of baicalein, the mode of inhibition was of the competitive type (murine leukemia virus reverse transcriptase and HIV-1 reverse transcriptase) with respect to the template primer ((rA)n•(dT)12-18), or mixed type, suggesting that baicalein also inhibits HIV-1 reverse transcriptase activity by interfering with the binding of viral RNA to the reverse transcriptase molecule near the active site of the enzyme. Baicalin does not inhibit the activity of HIV-2 reverse transcriptase, nor murine leukemia virus reverse transcriptase. Furthermore, baicalin neither inhibited the binding of OKT4A monoclonal antibody to the gp 120 binding site of CD4, nor interfered with the gp 120–CD4 binding. This rules out the possibility that baicalin interferes with the virus adsorption step (step 1 of the replicative cycle). It may interact with HIV-1 Env domains and interfere with their interaction with chemokine co-receptors and block HIV-1 at the early stage of infection[82]. Flavonoids such as gardennin, myricetin, and baicalein were found to inhibit HIV-1 protease. However, the IC_{50} value of baicalein was 480 µmol/l, almost 44 times that of gardennin (IC_{50} = 11 µmol/l)[83].

Efficacy of herbal formulation

As mentioned above, Xiao-Chai-Hu-Tang or Sho-saiko-to consists of a mixture of aqueous extracts from seven different plants, 7.5 g of this contains 4.5 g dried extract, which is prepared from boiled water extracts of seven herbs: 7.0 g of *Bupleurum* root, 5.0 g of *Pinellia* tuber, 3.0 g of *Scutellaria* root, 3.0 g of *Jujube* fruit, 3.0 g of *Ginseng* root, 2.0 g of *Glycyrrhiza* root, and 1.0 g of ginger rhizome[84,85]. Some research groups have demonstrated that, among the active components of Sho-saiko-to, baicalein and baicalin were found to be mainly responsible for the antioxidative[84,86], anti-tumor[65,87–91], antiproliferative[92–94], and anti-HIV[41,80] activities.

It is interesting to note that comparative data on antioxidative activity of Sho-saiko-to and *Scutellaria* root using MeOH extracts were very similar[84]. Our group and other researchers have shown that the water extracts of *Scutellaria* root also have significant antioxidant activity[95]. In the four major constituents, the order of antioxidant activity is baicalein > baicalin >> worgonin > wogonoside[96]. Antioxidant and other mechanisms may also play a role in the anti-HIV effects of baicalin and baicalein[69]. An oral dose toxicity study of Sho-saiko-to in rats has been reported[97]. Two oral doses (2 and 6.4 g/kg) of Sho-saiko-to were administered to the animal after overnight fasting, and no death was observed.

Combination of herbal medicine and chemotherapy

Combination therapy for AIDS patients has been applied, discussed, and standardized. Synergistic anti-HIV-1 effects of baicalin with 3′-azido-2′,3′-dideoxythymidine (AZT) have been reported[98], suggesting that baicalin might be potentially useful as part of a drug combination regimen for the treatment of HIV-1 infections. The use of Sho-saiko-to as an adjuvant with other antiviral drugs such as 3TC has been published[43]. A patent for anti-AIDS-virus effect-enhancing agents containing Sho-saiko-to or baicalein has been approved in Japan[99].

Discovery and development of plant-derived natural products and their analogs as anti-HIV agents

Although the history of Chinese herbal medicine dates back thousands of years, herb–drug interactions should not be overlooked[100–103]. With any anti-AIDS drug, attention must be paid to adverse effects, long-term sustainable effects, and increased toxicity due to drug–drug interactions in a person receiving multiple drug therapies.

The search for effective and less toxic anti-AIDS agents of single structure still continues. One approach is to modify novel, leading compounds derived from plants. Some promising research developments from different groups have been reported[8,11,62–64,104–108].

A successful example is the study by Lee and Morris-Natschke[8]. Through a bioactivity-directed search for plant-derived, naturally occurring compounds, the leading compound sukudorfin was isolated from the fruit of *Lomatium suksorfii* and its structure was identified. Sukudorfin inhibited HIV-1 replication in H9 lymphocytes with an *in vitro* IC_{50} value of 1.3 µmol/l and a therapeutic index (TI; TI = LD_{50}/IC_{50}) value of over 40. The discovery of sukudorfin led to the synthesis of 42 khellactone derivatives by structure modification. Among these synthetic compounds, the most promising lead compound was 3′, 4′-di-*O*-(*S*)-(-)-camphanoyl-(3′R, 4′R)-(+)-cis-khellactone (or DCK) (Figure 26.2), which showed

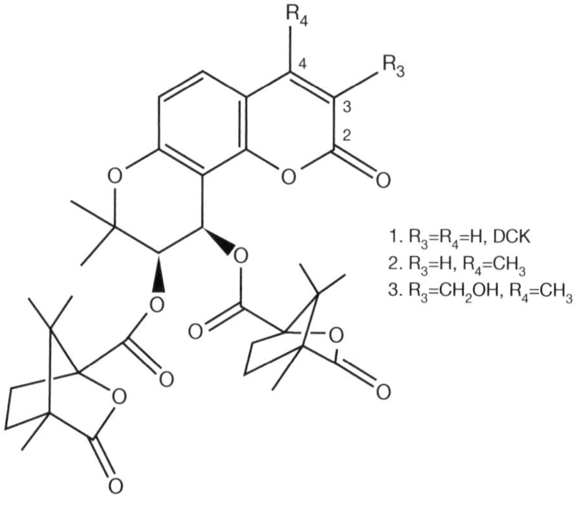

1. $R_3=R_4=H$, DCK
2. $R_3=H$, $R_4=CH_3$
3. $R_3=CH_2OH$, $R_4=CH_3$

Figure 26.2   3′, 4′-Di-*O*-(*S*)-(-)-camphanoyl-(3′R, 4′R)-(+)-cis-khellactone (DCK) (1), 4-methyl DCK (2), and hydroxymethyl DCK analog (3)

extremely potent activity (EC_{50} 2.56×10^{-4} µmol/l) ($IC_{50} = 0.00041$ µmol/l) against HIV-1 replication in the H9 cell line, and had a remarkable TI value of 1.37×10^5. In comparison, the values of AZT in the same assays were 0.15 µmol/l and 12 500, respectively. As an anti-HIV chemotherapeutic agent, DCK is a candidate for an anti-AIDS clinical trial[8,104,105]. Further research studies indicated that 3-methyl DCK, 40-methyl DCK and 5-methyl DCK were much more potent than DCK and AZT in the same assay, with EC_{50} and TI values ranging from 5.25×10^{-5} µmol/l to 2.39×10^7 µmol\l and 2.15×10^6 to 3.97×10^8 [109,110]. These compounds could be used to functionally dissect HIV-1 RT and might have the potential to be clinically useful[111].

When baicalein was first found to be a strong inhibitor of reverse transcriptase activity, the question arose as to the necessary structural requirements of the flavonoid for such activity. It is believed that number, position of the putative functional groups (hydroxyl groups), and flavone or flavonoid structure[112] are important. Research on structural modification and structure–activity relationships of baicalin and baicalein has been reported. The results indicated that the flavonoids with hydroxyl groups at C-5 and C-7 in the A-ring, and with a C-2–C-3 double bond, were the most potent inhibitors of HIV growth. In general, the presence of substituents (hydroxyl and halogen) in the B-ring increased toxicity and/or decreased activity[65,113,114].

According to the above information on structure–activity relationships, structure modification methods can also be used for flavonoid leading compounds, which are derived from plants with possible anti-HIV activity. As a potential target, the heteroatom in position 1 of the C-ring of the flavonoid compounds has been considered. Therefore, similar or even new biologic activities could be anticipated when the oxygen of bioactive flavonoids is replaced by another atom such as nitrogen or sulfur, which is closely aligned with oxygen in the periodic table. Thus, a series of 5,6,7,8-substituted 2-phenylthio-chromen-4-ones have been synthesized and evaluated for anti-HIV activity[65]. Among them, one new compound was the most active (IC_{50} value of 0.65 µmol/L) against HIV in acutely infected H9 lymphocytes, and had a TI of approximately 5.

Many research groups are exploring the biodiversity of the herb kingdom to find new and better anti-HIV drugs, as shown in Table 26.2. In addition to flavonoids and trichosanthin, several plant substances have been reported and reviewed. For example, betulinic acid derivatives[115–117], calanolides[118–120], L-chicoric acid[121–124], mannose-specific plant lectins[125], and sulfated polymannuroguluronate[126].

CONCLUSIONS

Medicinal herbs may have practical value as an alternative medical therapy in the inhibition of HIV activity. There is considerable evidence that sukudorfin, baicalin, and baicalein are important lead compounds for the development of antiviral and/or virucidal drugs against HIV. Presently, baicalin and baicalein might be useful as topical agents to deactivate a newly formed virus, or act as an adjuvant with other antiviral drugs. However, it is essential that the herbal medicine kingdom, as a source of new anti-HIV leads, should be explored further.

References

1. Fauci AS, Masur H, Gelmann EP, et al. NIH Conference. The acquired immunodeficiency syndrome: an update. Ann Intern Med 1985; 102: 800–13

2. Fauci AS, Artlett JG. Guideline for the use of antiretroviral agents in HIV-infected adults and adolescents. Ann Intern Med 1998; 128: 1079–100

3. Fauci AS. NIAID in 2004: The year in review. US Med 2005: 24

4. Witvrouw M, VanMaele B, Vercammen J, et al. Novel inhibition of HIV-1 integration. Curr Drug Metab 2004; 5: 291–304

5. De Clercq E. Antiviral therapy for human immunodeficiency virus infections. Clin Microbiol Rev 1995; 8: 200–39

6. De Clercq E. Toward improved anti-HIV chemotherapy: therapeutic strategies for intervention with HIV infections. J Med Chem 1995; 38: 2491–517

7. De Clercq E. HIV-chemotherapy and -prophylaxis: new drugs, lead and approaches. Int J Biochem Cell Biol 2004; 36: 1800–22

8. Lee KH, Morris-Natschke SL. Recent advances in the discovery and development of plant-derived natural products and their analogs as anti-HIV agents. Pure Appl Chem 1999; 71: 1045–51

9. Vandamme AM, Van Vaerenbergh K, De Clercq E. Anti-human immunodeficiency virus drug combination strategies. Antivir Chem Chemother 1998; 9: 187–203

10. Huang KC. The Pharmacology of Chinese Herbs. Boca Raton, FL: CRC Press, 1999

11. Luo SD, Chen JJ, Wang HY. Natural compounds with anti-HIV activity. Chin Tradit Herb Drug (Suppl) 1999; 30: 40–3

12. Vlietinck AJ, De Bruyne T, Vanden Berghe DA. Plant substances as antiviral agents. Curr Org Chem 1997; 1: 307–44

13. Tan GT, Pezzuto JM, Kinghorn AD. Evaluation of natural products as inhibitors of human immunodeficiency virus type 1 (HIV-1) reverse transcriptase. J Nat Prod 1991; 54: 143–54

14. Tan GT, Miller JF, Kinghorn AD, et al. HIV-1 and HIV-2 reverse transcriptases: a comparative study of sensitivity to inhibition by selected natural products. Biochem Biophys Res Commun 1992; 185: 370–8

15. Xu RS. Some bioactive natural products from Chinese medicinal plants. Studies Nat Prod Chem 2000; 21 (Bioactive Natural Products (Part B)): 729–72

16. Tang XS, Chen HS, Zhang XQ. Inhibition of human immunodeficiency virus reverse transcriptase by Chinese medicines in vitro. Proc CAMS PUMC 1990; 5: 140–4

17. De LS. Study on Anti-AIDS Activity of the Traditional Chinese Folk Herbs. Kunming: Yunnan Science and Technology Press, 1998

18. Wang JH, Zheng YT. Natural peptides and proteins with anti-HIV activity. Zhongguo Tianran Yaowu 2004; 2: 321–7

19. Collins RA, Ng TB, Fong WP, et al. A comparison of human immunodeficiency virus type 1 inhibition by partially purified aqueous extracts of Chinese medicinal herbs. Life Sci 1997; 60: 345–51

20. Au TK, Lam TL, Ng TB, et al. A comparison of HIV-1 integrase inhibition by aqueous and methanol extracts of Chinese medicinal herbs. Life Sci 2001; 68: 1687–94

21. Wu JH, Morris-Natschke SL, Lee KH. Progress in the recent discovery and development of promising anticancer and anti-HIV agents from natural products in the United States. J Chin Chem Soc 2003; 50: 11–22

22. Yamamoto T, Takahashi H, Sakai K, et al. Screening of Thai plants for anti-HIV-1 activity. Nature Med 1997; 51: 541–6

23. Kusmoto IT, Nakabayashi T, Kida H, et al. Screening of various plant extracts used in Ayurvedic medicine for inhibitory effects on human immunodeficiency virus type (HIV-1) protease. Phytother Res 1995; 9: 180–4

24. Xu HX, Wan M, Loh BN, et al. Screening of traditional medicines for their inhibitory activity against HIV-1 protease. Phytother Res 1996; 10: 207–10

25. Kusumoto IT, Hattori M. Pharmacological Research on Traditional Herbal Medicines. Amsterdam, Netherlands: Harwood Academic Publishers, 1999

26. Yamasaki K, Nakano M, Kawahata T, et al. Anti-HIV-1 acitivity of herbs in Labiatae. Biol Pharmaceut Bull 1998; 21: 829–33

27. Ma CM, Nakamura N, Miyashiro H, et al. Screening of Chinese and Mongolian herbal drugs for anti-human immunodeficiency virus type 1 (HIV-1) activity. Phytother Res 2002; 16 (S1): 186–9

28. Wan M, Bloor S, Foo LY, Loh BN. Screening of New Zealand plant extracts for inhibitory activity against HIV-1 protease. Phytother Res 1996; 10: 589–95

29. Zhao J, Ben LH, Wu YL, et al. Anti-HIV agent trichosanthin enhances the capabilities of chemokines to stimulate chemotaxis and G protein activation, and this is mediated through interaction of trichosanthin and chemokine receptors. J Exp Med 1999; 190: 101–11

30. Wang JH, Nie HL, Tam SC, et al. Anti-HIV-1 property of trichosanthin correlates with its ribosome inactivating activity. FEBS Lett 2002; 531: 295–8

31. Wang JH, Nie HL, Tam SC, et al. Independency of anti-HIV-1 activity from ribosome-inactivating activity of trichosanthin. Biochem Biophys Res Comm 2003; 302: 89–94

32. Wang JH, Tam SC, Huang H, et al. Side-directed PEGylation of trichosanthin retained its anti-HIV activity with reduced potency in vitro. Biochem Biophys Res Comm 2004; 317: 965–71

33. Au TK, Collins RA, Lam TL, et al. The plant ribosome inactivating proteins luffin and saporin are potent inhibitors of HIV-1 integrase. FEBS Lett 2000; 471: 169–72

34. Lin JC. Mechanism of action of glycyrrhizic acid in inhibition of Epstein-Barr virus replication in vitro. Antivir Res 2003; 59: 41–7

35. Sasaki H, Takei M, Kobayashi M, et al. Effect of glycyrrhizin, an active component of licorice roots, on HIV replication in cultures of peripheral blood mononuclear cells from HIV-seropositive patients. Pathobiology 2002–2003; 70: 229–36

36. Xing GX, Lin N, Wang T, Yao MY. Advances in studies on flavonoids of licorice. Zhongguo Zhong Yao Za Zhi 2003; 28: 593–7

37. Manfredi KP, Vallurupalli V, Demidova M, et al. Isolation of an anti-HIV diprenylated bibenzyl from Glycyrrhiza lepidota. Phytochemistry 2001; 58: 153–7

38. Kassler WJ, Blanc P, Greenlatt R. The use of medicinal herbs by human immunodeficiency virus-infected patients. Arch Intern Med 1991; 151: 2281–8

39. Phillips LG, Nichols MH, King WD. Herbs and HIV: the health food industry's answer. South Med J 1995; 88: 911–13

40. Leonard B, Huff H, Merryweather B, et al. Knowledge of safety and herb–drug interactions amongst HIV+ individuals: a focus group study. Can J Clin Pharmacol 2004; 11: e227–31

41. Buimovici-Klein E, Mohan V, Lange M, et al. Inhibition of HIV replication in lymphocyte cultures of virus-positive subjects in the presence of Sho-saiko-to, an oriental plant extract. Antivir Res 1990; 14: 279–86

42. Wu XS, Akatsu H, Okada H. Apoptosis of HIV-infected cells following treatment with Sho-saiko-to and its components. Jpn J Med Sci Biol 1995; 48: 79–87

43. Piras G, Makino M, Baba M. Sho-saiko-to, a traditional kampo medicine, enhances the anti-HIV-1 activity of Lamivudine (3TC) in vitro. Microbiol Immunol 1997; 41: 835–9

44. Xue YX, Liu CH, Zhang L, Yuan CS. Traditional Chinese medicine and AIDS. Am J Compreh Med 1999; 1: 542–4

45. Zhang L, Yue ST, Xue YX, et al. Effects of qian-kun-nin, a Chinese herbal medicine formulation, HIV positive subjects: a pilot study. Am J Chin Med 2002; 28: 305–12

46. www.chinadaily.com.cn/english/doc/2004-12/12/content_399505.htm

47. Wang J, Yu Z, Li G, et al. Clinical observation on the therapeutic effects of zhongyan-2 recipe in treating 29 HIV-infected and AIDS patients. J Tradit Chin Med 2002; 22: 93–8

48. Usha PR, Naidu MUR, Raju YSN. Evaluation of the anti-retroviral activity of a new polyherbal drug (Immu-25) in patients with HIV infection. Drugs R&D 2003; 4: 103–9

49. Hossain MS, Takimoto H, Hamano S, et al. Protective effects of hochu-ekki-to, a Chinese traditional herbal medicine against murine cytomegalovirus infection. Immunopharmacology 1999; 41: 169–81

50. Asiedu W, Asiedu F, Ennin M, et al. Compositions for treating AIDS and associated conditions from extracts of tropical herbs. US Patent 2004/0052868 A1

51. Kiem N, Kim RS. Khmer Angkor natural herb treatment for HIV infected and AIDS disease. US Patent 2003/0013082 A1

52. Wu TS. Herbal pharmaceutical composition for treatment of HIV/AIDS patients. US Patent 2003/0091658 A1

53. Chu CK, Cutler HG. Natural Products as Antiviral Agents. New York, NY: Plenum Press, 1992

54. Ng TB, Huang B, Fong WP, Yeung HW. Anti-human immunodeficiency virus (anti-HIV) natural products with special emphasis on HIV reverse transcriptase inhibitors. Life Sci 1997; 61: 933–49

55. Cragg GM, Boyd MR, Christini MA, et al. Screening of natural products of plant, microbial and marine origin: the NCI experience. Spec Publ R Soc Chem 1997; 200: 1–29

56. Vlietinck AJ, Bruyne TD, Apers S, Pieters LA. Plant-derived leading compounds for chemotherapy of human immunodeficiency virus (HIV) infection. Planta Med 1998; 64: 97–109

57. Lee KH. Antitumor agents.188. Highlights of research on plant-derived natural products and their analogs with antitumor, anti-HIV, and antifungal activity. In Cutler SJ, Cutler HG, eds. Biologically Active Natural Products: Agrochemicals and Pharmaceuticals. Symposium Series. Washington, DC: American Chemical Society, 2000: 73–94

58. Hanna L. Herbs for HIV. BETA Bull Exp Treatments AIDS 1998: 36–42

59. Sun IC, Kashiwada Y, Morris-Natschke SL, Lee KH. Plant-derived terpenoids and analogues as anti-HIV agents. Curr Topics Med Chem 2003; 3: 155–69

60. Wu JH, Morris-Natschke SL, Lee KH. Progress in the recent discovery and development of promising anticancer and anti-HIV agents from natural products in the United States. J Chin Chem Soc 2003; 50: 12–22

61. Lee KH. Modern research routes to new medicines from Chinese Materia Medica. Chin Pharmaceut J 2003; 55: 221–30

62. Wang JH, Zheng YT. Natural peptides and proteins with anti-HIV activity. Zhongguo Tianran Yaowu 2004; 2: 321–7

63. Lee KH. Current development in the discovery and design of new drug candidates from plant natural product leads. J Nat Prod 2004; 67: 273–83

64. Cos P, Maes L, Berghe DV, et al. Plant substance as anti-HIV agents selected according to their putative mechanism of action. J Nat Prod 2004; 67: 284–93

65. Wang HK, Xie Y, Yang ZY, et al. Recent advances in the development of flavonoids and their analogues as antitumor and anti-HIV agents. In Manthey JA, Buslig BS, eds. Flavonoids in the Living System. New York, NY: Plenum Press, 1998: 191–225

66. Mahmood N, Pizza C, Aquino R, et al. Inhibition of HIV by flavonoids. Antivir Res 1993; 22: 189–99

67. Lai GF, Chen JJ, Wang YF, et al. Advance in studies of flavonoids against HIV. Shangqui Shifan Xueyuan Xuebao 2002; 18: 83–7

68. Nishibe S, Ono K, Nakane H, et al. Studies on constituents of Plantaginis herba. 9. Inhibitory effects of flavonoids from Plantago species on HIV recverse transcriptase activity. Natural Med 1997; 51: 547–9

69. Kitamura K, Honda M, Yoshizaki H, et al. Baicalin, an inhibitor of HIV-1 production in vitro. Antivir Res 1998; 37: 131–40

70. Wu JA, Attele AS, Zhang L, Yuan CS. Anti-HIV activity of medicinal herbs: usage and potential development. Am J Chin Med 2001; 29: 69–81

71. Oho K, Nakane H, Fukushima M, et al. Inhibition of reverse transcriptase activity by a flavonoid compound, 5,6,7,-trihydroxyflavone. Biochem Biophy Res Commun 1989; 160: 982–7

72. Lee MJ, Kim M, Lee YS, Shin CG. Baicalein and baicalin as inhibitors of HIV-1 integrase. Yakhak Hoechi 2003; 47: 46–51

73. Zhang XQ, Tang XS, Chen HS. Inhibition of HIV replication by baicalin and S. baicalensis extract in H9 cell culture. Chin Med Sci J 1991; 6: 230–2

74. Cui L, Yuan J, Wang P. Pharmacological effect of baicalin. Zhongguo Yiyuan Yaoxue Zazhi 2000; 20: 685–6

75. Li BQ, Fu T, Yan YD, et al. Inhibition of HIV infection by baicalin – a flavonoid compound purified from Chinese herbal medicine. Cell Mol Biol Res 1993; 39: 119–24

76. Baylor NW, Fu T, Yan YD, Ruscetti FW. Inhibition of human T cell leukemia virus by the plant flavonoid baicalin (7-glucuronic acid, 5,6-dihydroxyflavone). J Infect Dis 1992; 165: 433–7

77. Zhao J, Zhang ZP, Chen HS, et al. Synthesis of baicalin derivatives and evaluation of their anti-human immunodeficiency virus (HIV-1) activity. Acta Pharmaceut Sin 1998; 33: 22–7

78. Raghavan K, Buolamwini JK, Fesen MR, et al. Three-dimensional quantitative structure–activity relationship (QSAR) of HIV integrase inhibitors: a comparative molecular field analysis (CoMFA). J Med Chem 1995; 38: 890–7

79. Wang Q, Wang YT, Pu SP, Zheng YT. Zinc coupling potentiates anti-HIV-1 activity of baicalin. Biochem Biophys Res Commun 2004; 324: 605–10

80. Muto R, Motozuka T, Nakano M, et al. The chemical structure of new substance as the metabolite of baicalin and time profiles for the plasma concentration after oral administration of Sho-saiko-to in human. Yakugaku Zasshi 1998; 118: 79–87

81. Ono K, Nakane H. Mechanisms of inhibition of various cellular DNA and RNA polymerases by several flavonoids. J Biochem 1990; 108: 609–13

82. Li BQ, Fu T, Dongyan Y, et al. Flavonoid baicalin inhibits HIV-1 infection at the level of viral entry. Biochem Biophys Res Commun 2000; 276: 534–8

83. Brinkworth RI, Stoermer MJ, Fairlie DP. Flavones are inhibitors of HIV-1 proteinase. Biochem Biophys Res Commun 1992; 188: 631–7

84. Shimizu I, Ma YR, Mizobuchi Y, et al. Effects of Sho-saiko-to, a Japanese herbal medicine, on hepatic fibrosis in rats. Hepatology (Phil) 1999; 29: 149–60

85. Geerts A, Rogiers V. Sho-saiko-to: the right blend of traditional oriental medicine and liver cell biology. Hepatology (Phil) 1999; 29: 282–4

86. Yoshino M, Ito M, Okajima H, et al. Role of baicalein compounds as antioxidant in the traditional herbal medicine. Biomed Res 1997; 18: 349–52

87. Tsutsumi M, Kitada H, Shiraiwa K, et al. Inhibitory effects of combined administration of antibiotics and anti-inflammatory drugs on lung tumor development initiated by N-nitrosobis(2-hydroxypropyl)amine in rats. Carcinogenesis 2000; 21: 251–6

88. Liu W, Kato M, Akhand AA, et al. The herbal medicine Sho-saiko-to inhibits the growth of malignant melanoma cells by upregulating Fas-mediated apoptosis and arresting cell cycle

through downregulation of cyclein-depedent kinases. Int J Oncol 1998; 12: 1321–6

89. Kato M, Liu W, Yi H, et al. The herbal medicine Sho-saiko-to inhibits growth and metastasis of malignant melanoma primarily developed in ret-transgenic mice. J Invest Dermatol 1998; 111: 640–4

90. Mizushima Y, Kashii T, Tokimitsu Y, Kobayashi M. Cytotoxic effect of herbal medicine Sho-saiko-to on human lung cancer cell lines in vitro. Oncol Rep 1995; 2: 91–4

91. Motoo Y, Sawabu N. Antitumor effects of saikosaponins, baicalin and baicalein on human hepatoma cell lines. Cancer Lett 1994; 86: 91–5

92. Inoue T, Jackson EK. Strong antiproliferative effects of baicalein in cultured rat hepatic stellate cells. Eur J Pharm 1999; 378: 129–35

93. Ono M, Miyamura M, Kyotani S, et al. Effects of Sho-saiko-to extract on liver fibrosis in relation to the changes in hydroxyproline and retinoid levels of the liver in rats. J Pharm Pharmacol 1999; 51: 1079–84

94. Yagura M, Murai S, Kojima H, et al. Changes of liver fibrosis in chronic hepatitis C patients with no response to interferon-α therapy: including quantitative assessment by a morphometric method. J Gastroenterol 2000; 35: 105–11

95. Shao ZH, Li CQ, Vanden Hock TL, et al. Extract from Scutellaria baicalensis Georgi attenuates oxidant stress in cadiomyocytes. J Mol Cardiol 1999; 31: 1885–95

96. Gao Z, Huang K, Yang, X, Xu H. Free radical scavenging and antioxidant activities of flavonoids extracted from the radix of Scutellaria baicalensis Georgi. BBA-Biomembranes 1999; 1472: 643–50

97. Minematsu S, Takei H, Sudo K, et al. A single oral dose toxicity study of TSUMURA Sho-saiko-to (TJ-9) in rats. Jpn Pharmacol Ther 1995; 23: 29–32

98. Inada Y, Watanabe K, Miyamoto K, et al. Regulatory activities of Sho-saiko-to in immune responses, eicosanoid pathway and HIV production. In Proceedings of the Tenth International Conference on AIDS Satellite Symposium. Yokohama, Japan, 1994

99. Maikeru R, Erena BK, Utopare M, et al. Anti-AIDS virus effect-enhancing agents containing Shosaikoto [Japanese patent]. Jpn Koka Tokkyo Koho 1996: 5

100. Fugh-Berman A. Herb–drug interactions. Lancet 2000; 355: 134–8

101. Halliwell B. Traditional Chinese Medicine: problems and drawbacks. Oxidat Stress Dis 2004; 14: 873–81

102. Williamson EM. Drug interactions between herbal and prescription medicines. Drug Safety 2003; 26: 1075–92

103. Power R, Gore-Felton C, Vosvick M, et al. HIV: effectiveness of complementary and alternative medicine. Prim Care 2002; 29: 361–78

104. Xie L, Takeuchi Y, Cosentino LM, Lee K-H. Anti-AIDS agents. 37. Synthesis and structure–activity relationships of (3′R,4′R)-(+)-cis-khellactone derivatives as novel potent anti-HIV agents. J Med Chem 1999; 42: 2662–72

105. Kashiwada Y. Studies on bioactive natural products: plant-derived natural products and analogues as anti-HIV agents. Nature Med 1999; 53: 153–8

106. Ovesna Z, Vachalkova A, Horvathova K, Tothova D. Pentacyclic triterpenoic acids: new chemoprotective compounds. Minireview. Neoplasma 2004; 51: 327–33

107. Yu D, Suzuki M, Xie L, et al. Recent progress in the development of coumarin derivatives as potent anti-HIV agents. Medicin Res Rev 2003; 23: 322–45

108. Wu JH, Morris-Natschke SL, Lee KH. Progress in the recent discovery and development of promising anticancer and anti-HIV agents from natural products in the United States. J Chin Chem Soc 2003; 50: 12–22

109. Zhang Q, Chen Y, Xia P, et al. Anti-AIDS agents. Part 62: Anti-HIV activity of 2′-substituted 4-methyl-3′, 4′-di-O-(-)-camphanoyl-(+)-cis-khellactone(4-methyl DCK) analogs. Bioorg Medicin Chem Lett 2004; 14: 5855–7

110. Huang L, Yuan X, Yu D, et al. Mechanism of action and resistant profile of anti-HIV-1 coumarin derivatives. Virology 2005; 332: 623–8

111. Yu D, Chen CH, Brossi A, Lee HK. Anti-AIDS agents. 60. Substituted 3′R, 4′R-DI-O-(-)-camphanoyal-2′, 2′-dimethyldihydropyrano[2,3-f] chromone (DCP) analogues as potent anti-HIV agents. J Med Chem 2004; 47: 4072–82

112. Oho K, Nakane H, Fukushima M, et al. Differential inhibitory effects of various flavonoids on the activities of reverse transcriptase and cellular DNA and RNA polymerases. Eur J Biochem 1990; 190: 469–76

113. Zhao J, Zhang ZP, Chen HS, et al. Preparation and anti-HIV activity study of baicalein and its benzylated derivates. Acta Pharmaceut Sin 1997; 32: 140–3

114. Hu CQ, Chen K, Shi Q, et al. Anti-AIDS agents 10. Acacetin-7-O-(-d-galactopyranoside, an anti-HIV principle from Chrysanthemum morifolium and a structure–activity correlation with some related flavonoids. J Nat Prod 1994; 57: 42–51

115. Cichewicz RH, Kouzi SA. Chemistry, biological activity, and chemotherapeutic potential of betulinic acid for the prevention and the treatment of cancer and HIV infection. Med Res Rev 2004; 24: 90–114

116. Huang L, Yuan X, Aiken C, Chen CH. Bifunctional anti-human immunodeficiency virus type 1 small molecules with two novel mechanisms of action. Antimicrob Agents Chemo 2004: 663–5

117. Sun IC, Chen CH, Kashiwada Y, et al. Anti-AIDS agents 49. Synthesis, anti-HIV and anti-fusion activities of IC95564 analogues based on betulinic acid. J Med Chem 2002; 45: 4271–5

118. Buckheit RW Jr, Russel JD, Xu ZQ, Flavin M. Anti-HIV-1 activity of calanolides used in combination with other mechanistically diverse inhibitors of HIV-1 replication. Antivir Chem Chemother 2000; 11: 321–7

119. Huerta-Reyes M, Basualdo MDC, Abe F, et al. HIV-1 inhibitory compounds from Calophyllum brasiliense leaves. Biol Pharm Bull 2004; 27: 1471–5

120. Xu ZQ, Barrow WW, Suling WJ, et al. Anti-HIV natural product (+)-calanolide A is active against both drug-susceptible and drug-resistant strains of Mycobacterium tuberculosis. Bioorg Medicin Chem 2004; 12: 1199–207

121. Lee JY, Yoon KJ, Lee YS. Catechol-substituted L-chicoric acid analogues as HIV integrase inhibitors. Bioorg Medicin Chem Lett 2003; 13: 4331–4

122. Lee DJ, Robinson WE Jr. Human immunodeficiency virus type 1 (HIV-1) integrase: resistance to diketo acid integrase inhibitors impairs HIV-1 replication and integration and confers cross-resistance to L-chicoric acid. J Virol 2004; 78: 5835–47

123. Reinke RA, Lee DJ, McDougall BR, et al. L-Chicoric acid inhibits human immunodeficiency virus type 1 integration in

vivo and is a noncompetitive but reversible inhibitor of HIV-1 integrase in vitro. Virology 2004; 326: 203–19

124. Johnson AA, Marchand C, Pommier Y. HIV-1 integrase inhibitors: a decade of research and two drugs in clinical trial. Curr Top Med Chem 2004; 4: 1059–77

125. Balzarini J, Hatse S, Vermeire K, et al. Mannose-specific plant lectins from the Amaryllidaceae family qualify as efficient microbicides for prevention of human immunodeficiency virus infection. Antimicrob Agents Chemo 2004: 3858–70

126. Miao B, Geng M, Li J, et al. Sulfated polymannuroguluronate, a novel anti-acquired immune deficiency syndrome(AIDS) drug candidate, targeting CD4 in lymphocytes. Biochem Pharmacol 2004; 68: 641–9

Index

Printed and bound by CPI Group (UK) Ltd, Croydon, CR0 4YY

23/10/2024

01777713-0001